Cognitive Behavioral Psychopharmacology

Cognitive Behavioral Psychopharmacology

The Clinical Practice of Evidence-Based Biopsychosocial Integration

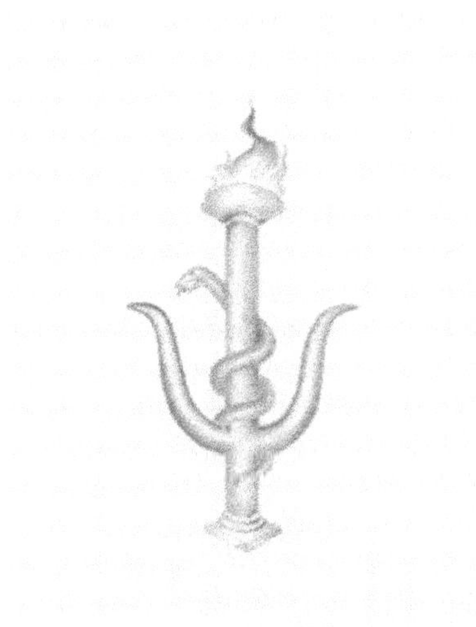

Edited by Mark Dana Muse

WILEY Blackwell

This edition first published 2018

Registered Office(s)
John Wiley & Sons, Inc., 111 River Street, Hoboken, NJ 07030, USA
John Wiley & Sons Ltd, The Atrium, Southern Gate, Chichester, West Sussex, PO19 8SQ, UK

Editorial Office
The Atrium, Southern Gate, Chichester, West Sussex, PO19 8SQ, UK

For details of our global editorial offices, customer services, and more information about Wiley products visit us at www.wiley.com.

Wiley also publishes its books in a variety of electronic formats and by print-on-demand. Some content that appears in standard print versions of this book may not be available in other formats.

Library of Congress Cataloging-in-Publication Data

9781119152569 [Hardback]
9781119152576 [ePDF]
9781119152583 [ePub]

Cover Design: Wiley
Cover Image: Cover illustration by Gloria Frigola: "The marriage of psychopharmacology and psychotherapy, under the light of evidence-based practice."

Set in 10/12, WarnockPro by SPi Global, Chennai, India.

10 9 8 7 6 5 4 3 2 1

Contents

Notes on Contributors

Donald Black, MD, is professor of psychiatry and director of the Psychiatry Residency Training Program at the University of Iowa Carver School of Medicine.

Taylor Bos, MA, was a junior fellow at the National Sleep Foundation before joining the Center for Sleep and Wake Disorders as clinical research coordinator.

James H. Bray, PhD, is former president of the American Psychological Association (APA), and former president of the American Society for the Advancement of Pharmacotherapy.

Christopher Brown, PsyD, ABPP, is a clinical psychologist who has published in the area of the integration of psychotherapy and psychiatric medication.

Ronald T. Brown, PhD, is professor of psychology and university president at the University of North Texas, Dallas. Dr. Brown chaired the APA work group on psychotropic medications for children and adolescents, and coauthored the work group's report in the publication *Psychopharmacological, Psychosocial, and Combined Interventions for Childhood Disorders: Evidence Base, Contextual Factors, and Future Directions* (2008, APA).

Kelly L. Cozza, MD, is an associate professor of psychiatry at Uniformed Services University, Bethesda, Maryland, and psychiatric consultant to the Department of Psychiatry, Walter Reed Army Medical Center. She is a senior author/editor of the *Handbook of AIDS Psychiatry* (2010, Oxford University Press) and the *Clinical Manual of Drug–Drug Interaction Principles for Medical Practice* (2009, American Psychiatric Publishing).

David F. Curtis, PhD, is an associate professor of psychology in the Department of Pediatrics at Baylor College of Medicine. He leads behavior therapy services for children with disruptive behaviors and he is the program director for Pediatric Primary Care Psychology at Texas Children's Hospital in Houston, Texas.

Catherine A. DeGood, DO, is the medical director of the Rhode Island-based Continuum Behavioral Health and faculty at the Warren Alpert Medical School of Brown University. She specializes in treating co-occurring chronic pain and substance use disorders.

Douglas E. DeGood, PhD, now a retired faculty, was previously director of psychology in the Pain Management Clinic at the University of Virginia Health Sciences Center. He has published extensively in the areas of biofeedback and pain assessment and treatment. He is author of *The Headache and Neck Pain Workbook* (1997, New Harbinger Publications) and senior co-author of *The Behavioral Medicine Treatment Planner* (1999, Wiley).

Samuel Dutton, PhD, MP, is a prescribing medical psychologist within the US Public Health Service at the United States Naval Academy, Annapolis, Maryland.

Helene A. Emsellem, MD, is medical director of the Center for Sleep and Wake Disorders and is clinical professor of neurology at George Washington University Medical Center.

Robert M. Julien, PhD, MD, is a retired research pharmacologist and anesthesiologist. His 13th edition of *Julien's Primer of Drug Action* (2014, Worth) is regarded as a definitive textbook of psychopharmacology.

George Kapalka, PhD, MP, is a pharmacologically trained medical psychologist who has written extensively on childhood disorders. His most recent books are *Collaboration between Pediatricians and Pharmacologically-trained Psychologists* (2010, Springer) and *Treating Disruptive Disorders: A Guide to Psychological, Pharmacological, and Combined Therapies (Clinical Topics in Psychology and Psychiatry* (2015, Routledge).

Mary Kelleher, MD, is clinical assistant professor, Department of Psychiatry at New York University. Her recent publications include *Dementia and Other Neurocognitive Disorders: An Overview* (2015, IGI Global), and *Psychosocial Studies of the Individual's Changing Perspectives in Alzheimer's Disease* (2015, IGI Global).

Mario Marquez, PhD, MP, is a prescribing child/adolescent medical psychologist in New Mexico. He is former president of the Society for the Advancement of Pharmacotherapy of the APA.

Robert E. McCue, MD,[1] was director of the Fellowship in Geriatric Psychiatry program and clinical associate professor of psychiatry at the New York University School of Medicine. He was also deputy chief of psychiatry/director of inpatient services, Woodhull Medical and Mental Health Center.

Kevin McGuinness, PhD, MP, is a retired captain with the United States Public Health Service. Dr Mc Guinness has practiced as a prescribing medical psychologist since 2006. He is a former president of the American Society for the Advancement of Pharmacotherapy.

Mikel Merritt, PhD, MP, is a prescribing medical psychologist with the United States Air Force.

1 Deceased.

Bret A. Moore, PsyD, MP, is a prescribing medical psychologist with the US Army. He co-edited *Pharmacotherapy for Psychologists: Prescribing and Collaborative Roles* (2010, APA), as well as the *Handbook of Clinical Psychopharmacology for Psychologists* (2012, Wiley).

Mark D. Muse, PhD, MP, is a prescribing medical psychologist and past president of the Maryland Academy of Medical Psychologists. He is author/editor of *Cognitive-Behavioral Therapy: Theoretical Foundations* (1996, MENSANA) as well as the *Handbook of Clinical Psychopharmacology for Psychologists* (2012, Wiley).

Joel Paris, MD, is professor in the Department of Psychiatry, McGill University, and author of *Treatment of Borderline Personality Disorder: A Guide to Evidence-Based Practice* (2010, Guilford Press).

Brenda J. B. Roman, MD, is professor of psychiatry at Wright State University School of Medicine. She is author of numerous book chapters and journal articles, including "Beyond Psychopharmacology for Bipolar Disorder: Psychotherapeutic Interventions for the Patient and Family" (2004).

Marla Sanzone, PhD, MP, is a former president of the Maryland Psychological Association and is a medical psychologist in private practice in Annapolis, Maryland. She has contributed to several books, including her recent chapter "Collaborative Treatment of Eating Disorders" in George Kapalka's (Ed.) *Pediatricians and Pharmacologically Trained Psychologists: Practitioner's Guide to Collaborative Treatment* (2011, Springer).

David Shearer, PhD, MP, is a civilian prescribing medical psychologist in the primary care clinic at Madigan Army Medical Center. He has researched and written on the topics of integrated psychotherapy and psychopharmacology in primary care settings.

Charles Schulz, MD, is professor of psychiatry at the University of Minnesota, where he has researched and taught on borderline personality disorder.

Peter Smith, PsyD, MP, is president of the Maryland Academy of Medical Psychologists, and chair of the workgroup on clinical psychopharmacology, Maryland Psychological Association.

Stephen M. Stahl, MD, PhD, is an internationally recognized clinician, researcher, and teacher in psychiatry, with subspecialty expertise in psychopharmacology. He has authored many books, including the seminal *Stahl's Essential Psychopharmacology* (4th ed., 2013, Cambridge University Press).

Randon Welton, MD, is director of the Residency Training Program, Boonshoft School of Medicine, Wright State University.

Tony C. Wu, PhD, ABPP, MP, is a pharmacologically trained medical psychologist and faculty member of clinical psychology, School of Social and Behavioral Sciences, Walden University.

Foreword

Science of Prescribing

The need for evidenced-based treatment guidelines is more important than ever, since mental illness affects one in five adults in the US each year, with nearly 10 million adults (4% of the US adult population) suffering with mental disorders serious enough to impact one or more areas of social and occupational functioning. There are nearly 4 million patients with depression followed by primary care in the US, with nearly four out of every five prescriptions for antidepressants being written by nonpsychiatrists. Clinicians and researchers must find a way to evaluate and disseminate the best treatments, individualized for each patient.

Treatments for behavioral and mental health disorders are an evolving area of science and practice that have substantial impact on the people who suffer from them. It is estimated that 47% of the US population will suffer from one or more mental health problem during their lifetime at a cost of over $57 billion (APA, 2016; Kessler et al., 2007). Research indicates that up to 25% of patients in primary care suffer from a mood disorder and this substantially impacts other health issues such as diabetes and hypertension (AHRQ, 2017). Prior to the 1990s the major treatments for behavioral health problems were psychotherapies, mainly based on psychodynamic theories, which had little evidence for their effectiveness. There were a few psychotropic medications available and many of them had significant and potentially severe side effects, and could be deadly with 1 month's prescription. The "Decade of the Brain" (Library of Congress/NIMH, 2000; Morris, 2000), and the focus on the neural and biological mechanisms of these disorders have radically changed treatment options since the 1990s. At the same time, research on evidence-based psychotherapies has increased, and proved that behavioral and other psychosocial therapies are also effective treatments for many mental health disorders.

Following the development of Prozac and the selective serotonin reuptake inhibitors (SSRIs), which provided a relatively safe treatment option, there has been a substantial increase in the use of psychotropic medications, especially by nonpsychiatric physicians in the United States (Wang et al., 2005, 2006). The National Institute of Mental Health's (NIMH) "Depression Awareness, Recognition, and Treatment (DART) Program" was a multiphase information and education program designed to educate health professionals and the general public that depressive disorders are prevalent and treatable (Regier et al., 1988). Part of the DART program targeted primary care physicians and coincided with the introduction of the SSRIs for treatment of depression. During the same period there was a dramatic decrease in the use of behavioral and other psychosocial therapies, despite evidence that they are effective (Wang et al., 2005). The increase in the use of psychotropic medications and decline in behavioral and psychotherapies is also linked to changes in reimbursement and the rise in managed mental healthcare by insurance companies (Phelps, Bray, & Kearney, 2017). The focus on either the exclusive use of psychotropic medications *or* the preferential use of behavioral therapies has not served the public well, and such a practice results in many people not getting the most effective treatments available. Hence the need for an integrated, evidenced-based approach.

An exciting recent study by Dunlop et al. (2017) provides enticing evidence that we are at a new and important watershed in our understanding of effective therapies for mental illness. This group has identified how to use imaging techniques like functional magnetic resonance imaging (MRI) to differentiate probable remission of depressive symptoms or failure of treatment with either cognitive-behavioral therapy (CBT) or medication before treatment by identifying "brain subtypes" in their research sample of patients with depression.

It is not very often that a book comes along that provides a new and innovative way to integrate two areas of science and practice, while providing a comprehensive and valuable review of the literature. Most books on psychopharmacology focus on the neurobiological aspects of medications and their use with specific disorders. There is relatively little about integration of how the psychosocial impact of taking a medication impacts its functioning and effectiveness, nor have psychopharmacology texts seriously looked at the *science of prescribing*; rather, they tend to focus on the chemical prescribed and its impact on symptoms. In this volume Muse and colleagues break away from the unidimensional, one-sided analysis of psychopharmacology as a stand-alone intervention. Indeed, they go even further by exploring the relative value of psychotherapy, and by integrating psychosocial interventions with pharmacotherapy according to the evidence at hand. There are chapters on each of the major categories of mental and behavioral health problems that review the existing literature and provide recommendations for the appropriate use of psychotropic medications and behavioral therapies for these disorders. What is refreshing is the perspective on the integration of the two approaches, while relying on the existing evidence for making recommendations.

The first chapter by Mark Muse provides an overview and summary of each of the chapters in the book. He provides a conceptual framework to understand the chapters and outlines the criteria for the evidence-based reviews that rely on the recommendations of Sackett, Rosenberg, Gray, Haynes, and Richardson (1996). He then summarizes the major, first-line recommendations for each of the disorders. This chapter alone is worth the price of the book and is an excellent reference chapter. The remaining chapters provide in-depth coverage of all recommended treatments, first-line, as well as secondary and tertiary treatments, for all major mental conditions that are seen in behavioral health and general medical settings. The last chapter by Dr. Muse provides an innovative perspective on integrating behavioral perspectives and the science of prescribing with psychopharmacology. This book will serve as an important reference for a variety of healthcare providers. All of the many authors who collaborated on this project are to be congratulated for developing a framework on integrating behavioral therapies with psychopharmacology. This integration fits well with the move toward an integrated healthcare system in the United States.

Cognitive Behavioral Psychopharmacology: The Clinical Practice of Evidence-Based Biopsychosocial Integration is an important collaborative step in the push toward a clearer understanding of the interplay between psychopharmacology and psychotherapy, with an ever-diligent eye toward evidence-based decision-making. The chapters follow the format of reviewing the literature concerning effective psychotherapies, psychopharmacological interventions, and combinations of both for each diagnostic category, managing to include the relevant meta-analyses and randomized clinical trials down to case reports, rounded out by discussions of available published clinical guidelines. Outstanding chapters, able to stand alone as definitive reviews for all providers, are those addressing insomnia, attention deficit hyperactivity disorder (ADHD) and disruptive disorders in childhood and adolescence, chronic nonmalignant pain, and depression and dementia-related disorders in the elderly. This book is an important milestone in the quest to better predict and achieve therapeutic outcomes in the management of mental illness with well-studied medication and behavioral interventions. It will be exciting to see where the second edition of this important first round will lead us.

James H. Bray, PhD
Former President of the American Psychological Association
and American Society for Advancement of Pharmacotherapy.

Kelly L. Cozza, MD, DFAPA, FAPM[1]
Associate Professor, Department of Psychiatry
Director, Psychiatry Clinical Clerkship
Scientist, Center for the Study of Traumatic Stress
Uniformed Services University of the Health Sciences
Bethesda, Maryland

References

Agency for Healthcare Research and Quality (AHRQ) (2017). *Behavioral and mental health*. Retrieved from http://www.ahrq.gov/professionals/prevention-chronic-care/improve/mental/index.html

American Psychological Association (APA) (2016). *Data on behavioral health in the United States*. Retrieved from http://www.apa.org/helpcenter/data-behavioral-health.aspx

Dunlop, B. W., Rajendra, J. K., Craighead, W. E., Kelley, M. E., McGrath, C. L., . . . & Mayberg, H. S. (2017). Functional connectivity of the subcallosal cingulate cortex and differential outcomes to treatment with cognitive-behavioral therapy or antidepressant medication for major depressive disorder. *AJP in Advance*, 1–13. doi:10.1176/appi.ajp.2016.16050518

1 The opinions or assertions contained herein are the private views of the author and are not to be construed as official or as reflecting the views of The Uniformed Services University of the Health Sciences, the Department of the Navy or the Department of Defense. The author has no conflicts to disclose, and has not received payment nor honorarium for this foreword.

Kessler, R. C., Angermeyer, M., Anthony, J. C., De Graff, R., Demyttenaere, K., Gasquet, I., . . . & WHO World Mental Health Survey Consortium (2007). Lifetime prevalence and age of onset distributions of mental disorders in the World Health Organization's World Mental health Survey Initiative. *Word Psychiatry, 6*, 168–176.

Library of Congress (2000). *Project on the decade of the brain.* Retrieved from http://www.loc.gov/loc/brain/

Morris, K. (2000). Advances in "brain decade" bring new challenges. *Lancet, 355*, 45. doi:10.1016/S0140-6736(99)90222-2

Phelps, R., Bray, J. H., & Kearney, L. K. (in press, *2017). A* quarter century of psychological practice. *American Psychologist.*

Regier, D. A., Hirschfeld, R. M., Goodwin, F. K., Burke, J. D., Lazar, J. B., & Judd, L. L. (1988). The NIMH depression awareness, recognition, and treatment program: Structure, aims, and scientific basis. *American Journal of Psychiatry, 145*, 135101357. doi:10.1176/ajp.145.11.1351

Sackett, D., Rosenberg, W., Gray, J., Haynes, R. B., & Richardson, W. S. (1996). Evidence based medicine: What it is and what it isn't. *British Journal of Medicine, 312*, 71.

Wang, P. S., Lane, M., Olfson, M., Pincus, H. A., Wells, K. B., & Kessler, R. C. (2005). Twelve-month use of mental health services in the United States: Results from the National Comorbidity Survey Replication. *Archives of General Psychiatry, 62*, 629–640. doi:10.1001/archpsyc.62.6.629

Wang, P. S., Demler, O., Olfson, M., Pincus, H. A., Wells, K. B., & Kessler, R. C. (2006). Changing profiles of service sectors used for mental health care in the United States. *American Journal of Psychiatry, 163*, 1187–1198. doi:10.1176/appi.ajp.163.7.1187

Preface

The present volume has had to wait until now to be written because a truly unbiased, evidence-based look at the weighted value of treatments and combinations of treatments within behavioral health has required time to mature while evidence slowly amassed and practitioners' acceptance of the integrated biopsychosocial paradigm increased. We now know, more than ever, that the biopsychosocial model is strongly supported by the data. Indeed, it would be remiss at this stage of our understanding to exclude *a priori* either medications or psychotherapies when evaluating the effectiveness of the entire array of treatment approaches available for any given condition or patient.

This book brings together experts of renown who have made exhaustive searches of evidence-based studies within their respective specialties, and weighed their findings according to the quality of each study to be able to present to you summaries of their investigations as well as practice recommendations based upon the evidence. In analyzing the data, authors were encouraged to use a system of classification in which each article reviewed was rated according to its strength of design and clarity of findings.

Chapter 1 summarizes all major findings of the individual chapters that comprise this volume, and it culminates in a single table that specifies first-line, integrated approaches for each major diagnosis. Each of the following chapters, authored in large part by teams made up of both prescriber and therapist, targets a specific diagnostic area, and also generates a concise table of detailed findings for its respective domain; within each chapter the reader will find a summary table with not only the first-line treatments for the condition under study, but also alternative treatments that may be indicated for particular nuances of the presenting problem, or because the condition has proved resistant to first-line approaches for a given patient.

The final chapter, Chapter 13, presents a new conceptualization for the integration of pharmacotherapy and psychosocial therapies through behaviorally managed medications. The final chapter departures from the rigorous substantiation of recommendations based on randomized clinical trials and metanalyses found in the previous chapters, as there simply is not, at this juncture, a body of controlled clinical studies investigating the systematic application of behavioral principals of learning in the integration of pharmacotherapy with psychotherapy. Notwithstanding this limitation, the chapter, while falling short of authoritative best-practice recommendations, presents numerous possibilities for innovative prescribing within the cognitive behavioral approach, and presents nine case studies to illustrate the potential of prescribing medications from the cognitive-behavioral paradigm.

The idea of behaviorally prescribed medication as an interface that overarches the integration of pharmacotherapy with psychotherapy provides a new direction of inquiry from which clinical trials might eventually substantiate the basic tenant that learning is the basis of therapeutic change, and that learning can be enhanced by employing conditioning contingencies, based on cognitive-behavioral methods, when prescribing medications.

I am grateful to each and every contributor to this volume. It has been a rare privilege to work with some of the world's sharpest minds, and to learn how they view the practice of integrated biopsychosocial diagnosis and treatment within their specialties. I have received a great deal of support in preparing this book, and my gratitude extends especially to Wiley-Blackwell for believing in the value and uniqueness of the project, and to my colleagues at the Maryland Academy of Medical Psychologists, who provided moral as well as intellectual support.

Special thanks is due Professor Robert McGrath, past president of the American Society for the Advancement of Pharmacotherapy, for reviewing and encouraging Chapter 13.

Mark Dana Muse

Cognitive Behavioral Psychopharmacology

1

Evidence-Based Biopsychosocial Treatment through the Integration of Pharmacotherapy and Psychosocial Therapy

Mark D. Muse

The integration of psychotropics into a broader psychosocial therapeutic plan would seem more than justified by previous reviews of the benefits associated with such a multimodal approach to coordinated behavioral health treatment (Reis de Olivera, Schwartz, & Stahl, 2014). It is no longer enough to think along traditional lines of which is the best medication for a particular diagnosis, nor is it sufficient to adhere to one school of psychotherapy and apply it without much regard to diagnosis. Thus, CBT (cognitive-behavioral therapy) for CBT's sake, just as pharmacotherapy as a standalone, would appear to be paradigms with diminished futures. Evidence-based therapeutic strategies argue that treatments, or a combination of treatments, might best be selected according to their relative impact on a certain constellation of symptoms, together with accompanying psychosocial variables, not the least among these being subject variables. Such an approach advocates integrating different biopsychosocial approaches to optimize therapeutic result. In some instances it is a question of selecting one treatment over another, while in the majority of cases it is more a question of combining treatments, and often this means coordinating multimodal therapeutic interventions (Lazarus, 1981).

"Evidence-based" is a lure that does not always provide us with clear-cut distinctions among multiple intervention strategies because, quite often, the evidence is not there. The evidence that is available, and it is substantial, is limited by its designs, which are driven by the interests of the investigators. Medications are largely tested against placebo, while CBT has rarely been pitted head-to-head against other psychosocial therapies, and where this has been done by resurrecting past studies in meta-analyses, the results are confoundingly ambiguous (Tolin, 2010), which is not a state to be cherished in science. Meta-analyses incorporate all of the shortcomings of the original randomized controlled trials (RCTs) that they attempt to digest (Kennedy-Martin, Curtis, Faries, Robinson, & Johnston, 2005; Walker, Hernandez, & Kattan, 2008). Oftentimes, meta-analyses find no difference between medication and psychotherapy, and no discernable advantage among various medications or among different psychotherapies. And, just as obfuscating is the fact that many studies are kept from public knowledge through selective publication, leading to a skewing of data toward a spurious impression of greater effectiveness than might otherwise be the case if all data were reported (Turner, Matthews, Linardatos, Tell, & Rosenthal, 2008). Still, one often finds that CBT

Cognitive Behavioral Psychopharmacology: The Clinical Practice of Evidence-Based Biopsychosocial Integration, First Edition. Edited by Mark Dana Muse.

is presented as having accumulated substantial data to support it as an efficacious therapy for the majority of psychiatric disorders (Butler, Chapman, Forman, & Beck, 2006), and this is certainly true because the number of studies completed with CBT as the independent variable far outweigh studies conducted on other psychotherapies. However, it is a stretch to say, based on the present data, that CBT is *more* efficacious than other psychotherapies. Hofmann, Asnaani, Imke, Sawyer, & Fang (2012), in a review of 269 meta-analyses concluded that CBT generally showed higher response rates than other psychosocial therapies, but the nature of the other therapies examined was often vague, and in several cases no superiority of CBT over the other psychosocial approaches was demonstrated, while in at least one case psychodynamic therapy was shown to be superior to CBT; indeed, when psychoanalysis is studied for effectiveness, it compares well with other therapies (de Maat et al., 2013), although the rigor of such studies leaves much to be desired.

What is the researcher, not to mention the clinician hoping to hang his shingle on tangible data, to derive from such a state of affairs? I submit that we have many wonderful meta-analyses that have given us a glimpse of where the truth lies, but we need to go back and design hard-hitting RCTs to fill in the blanks. Perhaps we have mined the data sufficiently at this point, and need more data. Well-designed RCTs that compare head-to-head the different psychosocial therapies are needed, just as are RCTs that pit different medications against psychosocial therapies, and not just placebo-controlled groups. And, the reciprocal influence among various therapies—such as pharmacological agents with other psychotropics (so-called polypharmacy) as well as such agents with a multitude of psychosocial therapies (what analysis of variance calls "interactions")—is where the hope for integration lies. Having said this, one is often struck by the commonalities of the various therapeutic approaches (Frank & Frank, 1991), be they pharmacologic or psychotherapeutic; and, until we are able to determine more precisely what components of a given approach endow it with an advantage over its brother, we are likely to run a lot of RCTs with equivocal results, since, in the end, the common response to therapeutic intervention, placebo included, is a global one in which patients tend to get better.

For years the movement toward integrating psychopharmacology with psychotherapy has moved forward on sound judgment alone: even with a paucity of substantiating research, a multimodal approach where pharmacotherapy is coordinated with psychological treatments has appeared to make sense at face value. Only recently has sufficient data accumulated to allow evidence-based pronouncements on the value of combining these two approaches, and the data available at this time have vindicated the theory to a large extent, while certain exceptions have also been found. The efficacy of combining pharmacotherapy and psychotherapy as a practice is borne out to a large extent by research; yet, as we shall see in the coming chapters, medication is sometimes contraindicated as an add-on to psychotherapy, and therapy is not always a benefit when added to medication management. As more investigations are completed in the area of biopsychosocial integration, it will become increasingly apparent that a multitude of variables are implicated in outcome, the patient population under consideration being one of the most important (Arnold, 1993).

We have elucidated here, as far as the evidence takes us to date, which combination of treatments is recommendable for each of the major psychiatric diagnoses. Never before has a single volume embarked upon coordinating psychopharmacological and psychotherapeutic treatments for the major psychiatric diagnoses from the evidence-based cognitive-behavioral perspective. Yet, diagnostic categorizations only take us so far, for it is, ultimately, the person whom we are treating, and the appreciation of the importance of patient variables is what distinguishes the astute practitioner from the mere technician.

There is a burgeoning movement in mental health to acknowledge the entire person's functioning across physical, psychological, and social spheres, and to integrate medical as well as psychological and social interventions in order to address the entire spectrum of the patient's life (McHugh & Slavney, 1998; McHugh, 2012a; McHugh, 2012b) presenting problems being, perhaps, the more important aspect of that life to the clinician. This book approaches the movement toward biopsychosocial integrative care from an evidence-based perspective, and goes beyond to offer a new way of conceiving of the interface between pharmacotherapy and psychotherapy by spelling out proven coordinated approaches for all of the major psychiatric diagnoses.

Methodology

The present volume has attempted to reduce bias by avoiding all pre-established search filters when sifting through the evidence as it exists today, but instead relied heavily on unfettered RCTs and meta-analyses to complete an exhaustive nonquantitative systematic review of the literature (Siwek, Gourlay, & Slawson, 2002). Cognizant of the variability in the quality inherent in clinical trials (Juni, Altman, & Egger, 2001), we endeavored to be all inclusive (Edinger & Cohen, 2013) while, ultimately, distilling our findings in a way that leads to basic best-practice recommendations, based upon evidence and upon the expert opinion of each chapter's authors. While some of the indications in this book arrive at the level of research-validated best practices, others are meant only as a starting place for the clinician to build his or her own therapeutic prescription for a given patient. In any case, we hold to the definition of evidence-based clinical practice as more than the mere application of treatments according to their proven effectiveness in controlled trials, rather, we accept evidence-based practice as "the conscientious, explicit, and judicious use of current best evidence in making decisions about the care of individual patients, while integrating individual clinical expertise with the best available external clinical evidence from systematic research" (Sackett et al., 1996).

The chapter authors each collected current research in their respective domain, and categorized the quality of the research according to the following hierarchy:

Level 1a: Evidence derived from a high-quality meta-analysis of RCTs.
Level 1b: Evidence derived from at least one well-controlled RCT.
Level 2a: Evidence derived from at least one randomized study without double-blind controls.
Level 2b: Evidence derived from at least one controlled, non-randomized quasi-experimental study.
Level 3: Evidence based on a case study or correlation study.
Level 4: Evidence based on a committee report or panel of experts.

After weighting and weighing the evidence, best-practice recommendations were arrived at by using the criteria outlined in Table 1.1.

Table 1.1 Best-practice recommendation criteria.

Level of value	Best-practice status	Criteria
Level A	Recommended	Assessment supported by a substantial amount of high-quality evidence (Level 1 or 2) and based upon a consensus of the clinical judgment of the chapter authors
Level B	Suggested	Assessment supported by sparse, but high-grade data (Level 1 or 2), or a substantial amount of low-grade data (Level 3 or 4) and the clinical consensus of the chapter authors
Level C	May be considered	Assessment supported by low-grade data (Level 3 or 4), or the clinical consensus of the chapter authors

Results

The results of each chapter's survey of the evidence, as intriguing and valuable in guiding clinical interventions as they may be, generated varying degrees of confidence. It is a given that no result presented itself with unequivocal certainty, and a great deal is left up to interpretation. The evidence, as might be predicted, was more substantial for the major psychiatric diagnoses (psychosis, mood disorder, anxiety) than for those diagnoses treated within subspecialties (pain, eating disorders, sleep disorders).

We summarize in Table 1.2,[1] at the cost of oversimplification, the major findings of the various chapters that comprise this book, keeping in mind that only those practice recommendations that are considered first-line are presented here. Apart from Table 1.2, each chapter presents a more detailed table of its respective findings and practice recommendations; in the summary tables of the individual chapters the reader will find not only first-line treatments for the condition under study, but also alternative treatments that may be suggested for an array of reasons. In developing our recommendations and suggestions, we have remained cognizant of the principle that "first-line" treatments are only a starting point, and that there are numerous circumstances in which an alternative treatment should be considered preferable to the standard first-line approach.

There is, without a doubt, much left to be discovered in the effectiveness of various approaches for the treatment of mental health diagnoses, conditions, symptoms, and issues, and a recurrent call for greater investigation permeates each and every chapter of this volume. Consequently, what our survey has revealed is that we have a way to go before we identify condition-specific effective and efficacious treatments. Until then, it is reassuring that all treatments, regardless of the condition, tend to be effective to a degree. Globally, medication is about on par with psychotherapy, which is on par with social/family approaches, and many drugs and psychotherapies are equivalent among themselves (Cuijpers, 2016). That is not to say that there are no differences; rather, the differences are less impressive than the similarities. It would seem that any treatment is better than none (Kelly, 1955), including placebo. And let us be clear, placebo is not the absence of treatment, but treatment without any particular intervention.

What we don't know is humbling, but what we do know from previous studies (MacKenzie, 1998; Sinyor, Schaffer, & Levitt, 2010; Soderberg, & Tungstrom, 2007) is that about one-third of patients treated will initially get better, while one-third of those

Table 1.2 Evidence-based findings and derived first-line clinical practice recommendations for the integration of pharmacotherapy and psychosocial therapy in the biopsychosocial treatment of major psychiatric diagnoses.

Psychosis

- Treatment of psychotic disorders should not be delayed, but begin early in the patient's life, and should involve both medications and psychosocial components that are tailored to each patient's specific needs and circumstances
- Antipsychotic medication use is nearly universally indicated in the management of psychoses
- CBT is more effective in reducing positive symptoms than in reducing negative symptoms, and is particularly indicated as adjunctive therapy where medication has not improved positive symptoms
- There is some evidence that preceding CBT with cognitive remediation (CR) may shorten therapy duration and reduce costs
- Relapse after successful initial treatment is prevalent with psychosis, and there is some evidence that cognitive-based and family therapies that specifically target relapse may improve longer outcomes

Major depressive disorders

- MILD: Talk therapy should be the primary intervention. CBT, cognitive therapy (CT), and interpersonal therapy (IPT) have been well researched
- MODERATE: Combined medication and talk therapy is preferred starting point. If a combined approach is not available, talk therapy and pharmacotherapy are both first-line.
- SEVERE WITHOUT PSYCHOTIC FEATURES: First-line interventions include CBT, CT, IPT, selective serotonic reuptake inhibitors (SSRIs), serotonin–norepinephrine reuptake inhibitors (SNRIs), and bupropion
- SEVERE WITH PSYCHOTIC FEATURES: SSRI/SNRI augmented with aripiprazole

Bipolar disorder

- MANIA: Patients diagnosed with mania should be started on medications with proven efficacy: specifically, carbamazepine, lithium, valproate, and second-generation antipsychotic medications, including aripiprazole, olanzapine, quetiapine, risperidone, and ziprasidone. For severe mania, combinations of mood stabilizers and second-generation antipsychotic medications should be considered, while providing psychoeducation over an extended period. Psychotherapy is not effective in controlling acute mania
- DEPRESSION: Electroconvulsive therapy should be considered for severely depressed patients, and for patients with severe mania accompanied by psychotic symptoms, significant suicidality, life-threatening malnutrition, or catatonia, and in those patients who fail to respond to medications. Traditional antidepressants should be avoided since they increase risk of switching to a manic or hypomanic mood

Dysthymia and adjustment disorder

- DYSTHYMIA: Combination therapy, consisting of CBT and pharmacotherapy, is first-line treatment for dysthymia
- ADJUSTMENT DISORDER with DEPRESSION: The first-line treatment for adjustment disorders is psychotherapy, especially problem-solving therapy (PST). Medications are overused in the primary care setting for treating adjustment disorders

(*Continued*)

Table 1.2 (Continued)

Anxiety disorders

- GENERALIZED ANIXETY DISORDER: First-line treatment should be psychotherapeutic, and CBT is a reasonable first choice
- SPECIFIC PHOBIAS: First-line treatment for simple phobias should be CBT, with exposure techniques emphasized. No psychotropic medication is recommended on a continuous basis for the treatment of phobias
- SOCIAL ANXIETY DISORDER: Social anxiety disorder is more resistant to treatment than other anxiety disorders, and it responds about equally well to pharmacological and psychosocial treatment. SSRIs are considered first-line pharmacological treatment for social anxiety disorder, whereas benzodiazepines or beta blockers may provide effective p.r.n. coverage for performance anxiety. CBT is recommended as a first-line psychosocial treatment, with a group therapy approach particularly indicated
- PANIC DISORDER: CBT is the treatment of choice for panic disorder. Psychodynamic therapy should be considered for those patients unable to tolerate CBT for panic disorder
- POSTTRAUMATIC STRESS DISORDER (PTSD): Monotherapy with medication is not indicated with PTSD since there is no drug treatment at this time for this disorder. Psychotherapy is first-line, with CBT and trauma-focused being equally as effective. Medications play only an adjunctive role in the management of PTSD
- OBSESSIVE COMPULSIVE DISORDER: CBT is the treatment of choice, and should be prescribed as monotherapy since combining it with pharmacotherapy provides no real advantage

Borderline personality disorder (BPD)

- Psychotherapy is the first-line treatment. No given psychosocial approach, however, has proved more effective than other approaches. While dialectical behavioral therapy (DBT) and mentalization-based therapy (MBT) have proved effective interventions with BPD, systems training for emotional predictability and problem solving (STEPPS) is a much shorter intervention with similar effectiveness
- No medication is indicated for the treatment of BPD, *per se*, and benzodiazapines in particular should be avoided with this patient population.

Sleep disorders

- For the treatment of insomnia, CBT for insomnia (CBT-i) techniques should be considered first-line treatment due to the durability of treatment gains and lack of adverse effects associated with such treatment
- Of the medications for insomnia, benzodiazepines, Z-drugs, and orexin/hypocretin antagonists appear to have the greatest efficacy, but all of these drugs may cause significant side effects and interact with other medications

Chronic pain disorders

- Integration of multidisciplinary approaches is essential to chronic pain management; this entails coordinating combination therapies of CBT with pharmacological approaches, physical therapy, exercise, and nutrition
- CBT is first-line intervention for chronic pain, with pharmacological forming an essential, but adjunctive, role for many patients
- Antidepressant medication, especially tricyclic medication and mood stabilizers, are considered first-line among pharmacological treatments of chronic pain
- Combined therapy is generally indicated over monotherapy for the management of chronic, benign pain

Table 1.2 (Continued)

Eating disorders

- ANOREXIA NERVOSA: CBT is demonstrated to be the most efficacious first-line treatment for adults. Family psychotherapy is indicated as first-line for children under 16 with the inclusion of CBT and other psychotherapy approaches when the young patient is cognitively and developmentally capable of using these methods. Nutritional education and behavioral intervention are recommended when patients are insufficiently nourished/significantly malnourished such that they are cognitively compromised and unable to make use of psychotherapy. Adding insight-oriented forms of psychosocial intervention to CBT is appropriate when a patient of any age exhibits co-morbidities or life concerns necessitating the integration of interpersonal and dynamic change processes
- BULIMIA NERVOSA: First-line treatment should be CBT and interpersonal psychotherapy or, alternatively, DBT when presenting with BPD. Fluoxetine or another SSRI, in combination with psychotherapy, should be considered when co-morbid with depressive and/or anxiety disorders. Family psychotherapy is indicated as first-line for children under 16
- BINGE EATING DISORDER: Combination therapy, with CBT plus SSRI, is first-line treatment. If response to CBT and SSRI is insufficient, shift SSRI to SNRI or augment with dopamine norepinephrine reuptake inhibitor (DNRI), provided no self-induced vomiting. Psychostimulants to improve appetite management may be indicated in combination with antidepressant and CBT or other psychosocial therapy

Childhood Disorders: ADHD and behavioral disorders

- ATTENTION DEFICIT/HYPERACTIVITY DISORDER (ADHD): There is compelling evidence that combined treatment, consisting of stimulant medication and behavioral management methods, are especially efficacious in the management of ADHD
- OPPOSITIONAL DEFIANT DISORDER (ODD): Psychosocial interventions should be first-line treatments for ODD. Behavioral Parent Training (BPT) has demonstrated the greatest benefits and is recommended across all age groups. Problem-solving skills training (PSST) and anger control skills training (ACST) are also well-established interventions, but they typically complement BPT for ages 7 and up. Pharmacological treatments are not recommended as solitary or even combined treatments for ODD due to an inability to reduce core symptoms and risk of negative side effects
- CONDUCT DISORDER (CD): The first-line treatment for CD should be psychosocial; CBT is particularly indicated when it incorporates a systemic component that targets patient, parent, and family dynamics

Disorders of elder population: Depression, dementias and cognitive disorders

- LATE-LIFE DEPRESSION: Antidepressant for major depressive disorder if ≤ 75 years and no executive dysfunction. May be augmented with aripiprazole. Psychotherapy is indicated, especially CBT, PST, or brief psychodynamic therapy
- COGNITIVE DEFICITS OF DEMENTIA: Acetylcholinesterase inhibitors (AChEIs) for Alzheimer's disease, up to 2 years. Memantine + AChEI for moderate–severe Alzheimer's disease. Reality-oriented psychotherapy
- DEPRESSION CONCOMITANT WITH DEMENTIA: Antidepressants if major depressive disorder criteria met. Behavioral therapy groups, and effort to enhancing social engagement of patients. Teaching behavioral approaches to residential staff
- PSYCHOTIC SYMPTOMS CONCOMITANT WITH DEMENTIA: No interventions meet level A of evidence
- BEHAVIORAL SYMPTOMS CONCOMITANT WITH DEMENTIA: Caregiver training and psychoeducational counseling

who do not respond to the initial treatment will, in turn, respond to a second treatment, and so on, regardless of the treatment employed. While such results are based on group studies and cannot be translated directly to any given patient or condition, the overall positive outcome, although less than perfect, is of great solace to those trying to help others in need. It is also reason to pause and reflect before championing any given therapeutic school, method, or substance.

That being said, Table 1.2 generally finds that psychotherapy is as effective, while posing less risk of pernicious iatrogenic outcomes, as pharmacotherapy, and, therefore, psychosocial interventions are indicated as first-line treatment over pharmacotherapy in the majority of psychological problems. The exception, in which pharmacotherapy might be considered to trump psychotherapeutic approaches as first-line interventions, consist largely of the treatments of major mood and thought disorders. Combination treatments, on the other hand, are generally indicated for the majority of conditions, with anxiety disorders, adjustment disorders, and personality disorders being the exception. Yet, each condition has its own indications and contraindications, and all are full of caveats.

For example, antipsychotic medication use is generally indicated in the management of psychoses, while combined treatments that involve both medications and psychosocial components are best tailored to each patient's specific need and circumstance. Relapse is particularly prevalent with schizophrenia, and the use of cognitive and family therapies that specifically target relapse should form an integral part of treatment with this patient population. In the treatment of major depression, combined treatments can provide greater benefit when patient expectations are addressed to ensure that there is a realistic understanding of the degree and pacing of improvement; the combined use of selective serotonin reuptake inhibitors (SSRIs) together with CBT should be considered first-line. Bipolar disorder, by and large, requires the use of mood-stabilizing medication during manic episodes, and antidepressant agents (excepting SSRIs and serotonin–norepinephrine reuptake inhibitors (SNRIs)) during the depression phase of the disorder, while psychotherapy is essential as an adjunct for educating the patient on compliance with psychopharmacology and for facilitating a eurhythmic lifestyle. Dysthymia responds best to combination therapy of psychopharmacology and CBT, while adjustment disorder with depressed mood responds well to psychotherapy (especially problem-solving therapy and CBT). Pharmacotherapy should generally be avoided in chronic depression that manifests with a large psychosocial adjustment component, such as in the case of adjustment disorder with depression, as well as in some forms of depression not-otherwise-specified (NOS).

Personality disorders, and more particularly borderline personality disorder (BPD), are best treated with psychosocial approaches, while medication, at best, might be used for co-existing symptoms outside the classic borderline constellation of symptoms; nonetheless, no one psychotherapy has proved more effective than the others used in the treatment of BPD. Chronic benign pain is optimally treated with an integrative, multidisciplinary approach, and CBT is the first-line psychotherapeutic intervention among such a multimodal treatment regimen, with pharmacological interventions forming an essential, but adjunctive, role for many patients. Opioids are of limited utility in the treatment for chronic pain, but should be reserved as a tertiary approach.

For the optimal treatment of insomnia, integrated cognitive-behavioral therapy for insomnia (CBT-i) with pharmacotherapy, in proper sequencing, appears to provide the most effective response. Pharmacotherapy may initially lead to faster alleviation of symptoms of insomnia but it is typically associated with adverse effects and the return of symptoms upon discontinuation of medications. Supplementing CBT-i with medication, however, can lead to better treatment compliance in the early stages of therapy. Eating disorders respond well to CBT when personality disturbance is not severe. Notwithstanding psychosocial approaches as first-line, combined pharmacotherapy and psychosocial therapies are indicated in most clinical presentations of eating disorders, including bulimia and anorexia. On the other hand, monotherapy with medication alone has not been shown to be effective in long-term treatment in any of the eating disorders, while group therapy is a useful adjunct to individual psychotherapy for all eating disorders, but is not sufficient as monotherapy.

A common factor found across ADHD, oppositional defiant disorder (ODD), and conduct disorder (CD) is that effective interventions rely upon the support of adult caregivers, with the most robust, long-lasting treatment effects achieved when parents and teachers are involved in intervention efforts. Psychostimulants are the gold standard for the pharmacological treatment of ADHD, yet first-line pharmacological intervention is recommended for ADHD only, and is not recommended as monotherapy for either ODD or CD. Psychosocial therapies are considered first-line interventions for ODD and CD, achieving significant positive outcomes with lasting intervention effects. In the treatment of the elderly, with or without dementias or cognitive disorders, evidence shows that antidepressants and psychotherapy are equally efficacious in addressing late-life depression. With demented patients, antidepressants are effective for the treatment of major depressive disorder, particularly with those diagnosed with Alzheimer-related dementia. When treating psychosis associated with cognitive disorders, however, psychosocial/nonpharmacological methods are preferred due to their low side effect profile with this medically vulnerable population. When behavioral disturbances occur concomitant with dementia, nonpharmacological interventions may be the first treatment tried.

The State of the Art of Clinical Research and its Derived Evidence-Based Practice Guidelines

In summary, the preceding indications are not meant to be taken as a cookbook. There are, in fact, few specific recommendations, other than pointing out what might be best practices, and other practices that are best avoided. The indications are largely for first-line treatments, with further recommendations when patients are initial nonresponders. However, "difficult" patients, which may make up a sizable part of some challenging practices, require creative thinking, and may justify, indeed, compel the use of minority therapeutic approaches that are not ordinarily recommended, or the occasional implementation of polypharmacy when such practices are best not adopted by default. The individual chapters, dedicated to their respective major disorder or patient population, provide practice guidelines for second- and third-line interventions for just such complex or resistant cases.

Practice guidelines in general vary considerably in quality, and have been noted to reflect in many cases the bias of professional and governmental organizations that devise them (Stricker, Abrahamson, & Bologna, 1999). In this regard, we have given free rein to the experts who author each chapter in this book, knowing full well that bias will exist to a certain degree, but, in avoiding institutional input, we have confided in the individual professionals' assessment of the evidence as they found it in their respective inquiries. If there is an overriding bias to the present volume, it is in insisting on evidence in formulating treatment guidelines rather than on theoretical considerations.

Practice guidelines might best be developed in accordance with American Psychological Association standards (APA, 1999, 2002), which place emphasis on demonstrating that recommended specific treatments offer benefit beyond the patient simply being "in treatment", because, as we have seen, most patients get better when in treatment, regardless of the type of treatment. Until then, evidence-based practice (APA Presidential Task Force on Evidence-Based Practice, 2006) is an ideal that is slowly becoming reality as research strives to provide more discerning results. In its current state, moreover, it requires that the practitioner be aware of the kind of research data that may be relevant to decisions made in the office, and it also cries out for further institutional investment in research if evidence is to continue to refine our decision-making.

The Cochrane Library (Higgins & Green, 2011) has, as of 2008, over a half million registered controlled trials, and yet we have seen that there is a need for much more research to fill in the gaps in our knowledge. With the evidence that we have to date, certain indications, recommendations, and directions suggest themselves. Guidelines have been offered in the past for integrating pharmacotherapy with CBT (Veale & Stout, 2010), with caution being recommended when combining treatment for integrative care of depression, obsessive compulsive disorder, posttraumatic stress disorder, generalized anxiety disorder, panic, body dysmorphia, eating disorders, and personality disorders. Based largely on National Institute of Clinical Excellence recommendations (NICE, 2004, 2005, 2007), Veale and Stout (2010) suggest medication might be integrated with psychosocial therapies when one or the other has proved insufficient. Busch and Malin (1998) point out, however, that even when a given treatment or combination of treatments increases effective management of presenting symptoms, an initial improvement in symptoms may obviate further therapeutic follow up, and interfere with the patient's motivation to address more long-term issues.

A different challenge is how to operationalize evidence and its derived recommendations, and transfer guidelines into established practices. A growing body of evidence suggests that psychiatric medication outcomes are shaped significantly by psychological and social factors surrounding the prescribing process; however, there have also been consistent findings demonstrating a gap between evidence-based emphasis on the importance of the prescribing environment and actual prescribing practices among professionals who work in environments that tend to limit personal engagement of patient with professional (Grol & Grimshaw, 2002). While psychiatric training program directors purport to value highly the importance of psychosocial factors in the prescribing process (Mallo, Mintz, & Lewis, 2014), there is limited emphasis of these factors being incorporated into psychopharmacology training (McGrath & Muse, 2010; Muse & McGrath, 2010). Until a more comprehensive training model emerges in schools of medicine and/or psychology, it is our impression that most professional development in the area of integrated practices will occur postspecialization, largely through the continuing education pursuits of the most motivated practitioners. This leaves us with the feeling that a lot of lip service is given to evidence-based practice, while it is, perhaps, the unusual practitioner who actually does the homework necessary to be able to apply research findings to his or her trade.

Finally, we offer a field-wide look at the state of research in mental health treatment through our survey of the various psychiatric groupings. Table 1.3 summarizes the

Table 1.3 The state of research in evidence-based behavioral health treatments of major psychiatric diagnoses.

General observations across all diagnoses

- Research results are difficult to transfer directly to clinical practice due to the limitations found in many research studies. Specifically, research conditions are quite different from practice conditions, which begs the question of whether research results, due to their restrictive protocols, underestimate the effectiveness of treatment in a flexible, accommodating clinical setting
- The selection of patients in randomized controlled trials (RCTs) is exclusionary, and does not necessarily represent the patient population served in clinical practice
- Patients' preference for a given treatment method is ignored in research employing randomized assignment. Patient preference, however, plays a large role in treatment outcomes, and may account for clinical improvements due to goodness of fit that is absent in research designs
- Outcome data in research, such as rating scales, may miss the quality-of-life issues that motivate people to seek treatment
- Many studies of medication impact utilize only one medication, and some do not allow for dose titration. In a few studies there is flexible dosing, and an occasional "second step" medication when a first medicine does not bring about symptom resolution, but the treatment options are still limited
- There is a large variety of treatment approaches that in the research are often treated as equivalent. Many of these have not truly undergone head-to-head trials
- CBT is a broad term that is used to describe therapies that may have little in common, but are often aggregated into meta-analyses without verification that the protocols are comparable
- In both therapy and medication the majority of studies compare to a placebo. In the few studies that do compare medicines in a head-to-head trial, such comparisons are often limited to pairing a new drug with an older one. Research would ideally compare multiple psychosocial and pharmacologic treatments with other comparable therapies, rather than simply showing superiority over placebo
- Research has lagged behind practice, where patients often choose their mode of therapy or elect for combined therapy. Much more research needs to be done involving combined therapy
- Many studies that result in inconclusive or negative findings are not made public, creating an inflated sense of the effectiveness of treatments based only on positive, confirmatory studies

Diagnosis-specific observations

- *Psychoses*: There is significant demographic variation based on the particular diagnostic criteria and research sampling methodology utilized in identifying schizophrenia. Findings are limited by the small size of the compared groups. Well-controlled investigations of the combination of psychotropic medication plus nonmedicine treatments versus medication or psychotherapy alone are limited because the use of add-on nonmedicine treatment has become the standard practice for most patients suffering from psychosis; therefore, there are many confounds that obscure the true effectiveness of each treatment, *per se*. Research contains several specific models for integrated clinic operations, but it has not advanced to the stage of reliably unpacking individual psychosocial components within those models
- *Major depressive disorder*: Antidepressant medications in research are grouped based on category (i.e., selective serotonin reuptake inhibitor (SSRI), tricyclic, serotonin norepinephrine reuptake inhibitor (SNRI), etc.). These medicines also often get aggregated in meta-analyses, ignoring potential differences. CBT studies limit therapy to a number of sessions far below the number generally employed in other therapies such as psychoanalysis, making head-to-head comparisons difficult

(*Continued*)

Table 1.3 (Continued)

- *Bipolar disorder*: Traditionally, research into bipolar disorders focused mostly on controlling acute mood symptoms using physical interventions such as medication or electroconvulsive treatments, and only recently have psychosocial components come under investigation. The research into psychosocial interventions for bipolar depression, however, has mainly focused on its use as adjunctive treatment. Research has focused on medication adherence and very little emphasis has been directed toward behavioral adherence
- *Dysthymia and adjustment disorders*: There is little research on dysthymia, and even less on adjustment disorder with depressed mood. What little research is available has largely been done through drug studies, leaving little evidence as to the effectiveness of psychosocial treatment of chronic depression
- *Anxiety disorders*: More research on psychosocial approaches other than CBT is needed. Such research would ideally compare different psychosocial therapies, rather than simply show superiority over placebo. Much more research is needed with the child and adolescent population to show benefits and adverse reactions to pharmacotherapy in anxiety disorders
- *Personality disorder*: Structured interviews and self-report assessments are helpful in properly diagnosing borderline personality disorder (BPD), but they are rarely used outside of research settings. Although there is no Food and Drug Administration (FDA) approved medication for BPD, many patients seen in clinical trials for psychosocial interventions are on psychotropics, confounding the results obtained. Future research should begin to test models that integrate what are considered the best ideas from different programs, thereby drawing on some of the most fertile areas as we continue exploring better treatments
- *Insomnia*: More research is needed to make specific comparisons between different pharmacological interventions, comparing pharmacological interventions to CBT, and examining the efficacy of different sequences of treatment combinations. As benzodiazepines are used in the treatment of insomnia, more research is needed to evaluate the potential relationship between this class of medication use and dementia. More research on polypharmacy for insomnia and depression is needed in order to development specific guidelines regarding safe and effective combinations
- *Chronic pain*: Research to date has not entirely clarified the benefit/risk ratio of the intrathecal opioid drug pump. Medications for pain can be particularly risky for older adults, yet there is little research on alternatives. Future research should be directed at the identification of which components of CBT work for what type of patient and why. Furthermore, future research should include more direct comparisons of adverse outcomes associated with mainstream treatments vs. the relative safety of alternative medicine treatments
- *Eating disorders*: The preponderance of research is on anorexia nervosa, while bulimia has been relatively neglected
- *Child and adolescent population*: Much more research is needed with the child and adolescent population to show benefits and adverse reactions to pharmacotherapy. Few studies have examined the efficacy of pharmacotherapies on children with comorbidity of attention deficit hyperactivity disorder (ADHD) and aggression. Pharmacological research dedicated exclusively to the treatment of oppositional defiant disorder (ODD) is very limited
- *Geriatric population*: Very few studies have examined the efficacy of psychotherapy as a treatment for a formally diagnosed depressive syndrome in people with dementia. The FDA has not approved any medication to treat psychotic symptoms concomitant with dementia, making all medication use off-label

quality of research discovered by the different teams that authored the individual chapters. While there are many limitations in the design and findings of past and present studies, the recent interest in research-based evidence in the selection of treatment modalities is, itself, an indication of practitioners' desire to be guided by rational decision-making in providing recommendations to their patients. It is our hope that the behavioral sciences will continue to improve the research effort to reduce ambiguities among evidence, and to further clarify effective and efficacious treatment options.

Evidence-based practice of behavioral health intervention is wrought with caveats of inadequate research and insufficient guidelines for translating what evidence exists into clinical practice recommendations. Still, given that the emphasis on linking practice to research is essentially nascent at this time, the future is left to imagine. One of the inspiring trends is the blurring of traditional professional difference between "prescribers" and "therapists." It is not difficult to imagine a future in which clinicians in the behavioral health field are educated in the biological foundations as well as the psychological and sociological foundations of mental illness and health. Such a generation of practitioners, integrated into the entire extant body of knowledge and eager to expand its limits, may better ask the right questions and find the correct answers on how to best bring science to bear on matters of mental/emotional suffering and wellbeing.

Note

1 Table 1.2 reviews the first-line practice recommendations for each major diagnosis and/or patient population. The individual chapters delve further into the details of each condition, and present in their respective summary tables not only first-line treatments, but suggested alternative treatments of merit to be considered when matching approach with the individual patient.

References

American Psychological Association (APA). (1995). *Template for developing guidelines: Interventions for mental disorders and psychosocial aspects of physical disorders.* Washington, DC: APA.

American Psychological Association (APA). (2002). Criteria for evaluating treatment guidelines. *American Psychologist, 57,* 1052–1059.

APA Presidential Task Force on Evidence-Based Practice (2006). Evidence-based practice in psychology. *American Psychologist, 61,* 271–285.

Arnold, L. (1993). A comparative overview of treatment research methodology: Adult vs. child and adolescent, psychopharmacological vs. psychosocial treatments. *Psychopharmacology Bulletin, 29,* 5–17.

Busch, F., & Malin, B. (1998). Combining psychopharmacology, psychotherapy and psychoanalysis. *Psychiatric Times,* May 1.

Butler, A., Chapman, J., Forman, E., & Beck, A. T. (2006). The empirical status of cognitive-behavioral therapy: A review of meta-analyses. *Clinical Psychology Review, 26,* 17–31.

Cuijpers, P. (2016). Are all psychotherapies equally effective in the treatment of adult depression? The lack of statistical power of comparative outcome studies. *Evidence-Based Mental Health Online First, 19*, 39–42.

de Maat, S., de Jonghe, F., de Kraker, R., Leichsenring, F., Abbass, A., Luyten, P., . . . & Dekker, J. (2013). The current state of the empirical evidence for psychoanalysis: A meta-analytic approach. *Harvard Review of Psychiatry, 21*, 107–137.

Edinger, T. & Cohen, A. (2013). A large-scale analysis of the reasons given for excluding articles that are retrieved by literature search during systematic review. *AMIA Annual Symposium Proceedings*, 379–387.

Frank, J. D., & Frank, J. B. (1991). *Persuasion and healing: A comparative study of psychotherapy*. Baltimore, MA: Johns Hopkins University Press.

Grol, R., & Grimshaw, J. (2002). From best evidence to best practice: Effective implementation of change in patients' care. *The Lancet, 362*, 1225–1230.

Higgins, J., & Green, S. (2011). *Cochrane handbook for systematic reviews of interventions*. Retrieved from www.cochrane-handbook.org

Hofmann, S., Asnaani, A., Imke, J., Sawyer, A. T., & Fang, A. (2012). The efficacy of cognitive behavioral therapy: A review of meta-analyses. *Cognitive Therapy and Research, 36*, 427–440.

Juni, P., Altman, D., & Egger, M. (2001). Systematic reviews in health care: Assessing the quality of controlled clinical trials. *British Medical Journal, 323*, 42–46.

Kelly, G. (1955). *The psychology of personal constructs*. London; New York: Routledge in association with the Centre for Personal Construct Psychology.

Kennedy-Martin, T., Curtis, S., Faries, D., Robinson, S., & Johnston, J. (2005). Literature review on the representativeness of randomized controlled trial samples and implications for the external validity of trial results. *Trials,16*, 495.

Lazarus, A. (1981). *The practice of multimodal therapy*. New York: McGraw-Hill.

MacKenzie, K. R. (1998). Treatment outcomes in psychotherapy and psychiatric interventions. *Journal of Psychotherapy Practice and research, 7*, 87–89.

Mallo, C., Mintz, D., & Lewis, K. (2014). Integrating psychosocial concepts into psychopharmacology training: A survey study of program directors and chief residents. *Psychodynamic Psychiatry, 42*, 243–254.

McGrath, R., & Muse, M. (2010). Room for a new standard: Response to comments by Heiby. *Journal of Clinical Psychology, 66*, 112–115.

McHugh P. R., & Slavney, P. R. (1998). *The Perspectives of Psychiatry* (2nd ed.). Baltimore: Johns Hopkins Press.

McHugh, P. R. (2012a). Rendering mental disorders intelligible: Addressing psychiatry's urgent challenge. *In Philosophical Issues in Psychiatry II: Nosology*. Oxford University Press. DOI: 10.1093/med/9780199642205.003.0038

McHugh, P. R. (2012b). The Perspectives of Psychiatry: The Public Health Approach. *In Public Mental Health*. Oxford University Press. DOI: 10.1093/acprof:oso/9780195390445.003.0002

Muse, M., & McGrath, R. (2010). Training comparison among three professions prescribing psychoactive medications: Psychiatric nurse practitioners, physicians, and pharmacologically-trained psychologists. *Journal of Clinical Psychology, 66*, 1–8.

National Institute for Health and Clinical Excellence (NICE) (2004). *Anxiety: Management of anxiety (panic disorder, with or without agoraphobia, and generalised anxiety disorder) in adults in primary, secondary and community care*. Retrieved from http://www.nice.org.uk/CG22. London: National Institute for Health and Clinical Excellence.

National Institute for Health and Clinical Excellence (NICE) (2005). *Obsessive-compulsive disorder: Core interventions in the treatment of obsessive compulsive disorder and body dysmorphic disorder*. Retrieved from http://www.nice.org.uk/CG031). London: National Institute for Health and Clinical Excellence.
National Institute for Health and Clinical Excellence (NICE) (2007). *Depression: Management of depression in primary and secondary care*. Retrieved from http://www.nice.org.uk/CG023. London: National Institute for Health and Clinical Excellence.
Noyes, R., & Perry, P. (1990). Maintenance treatment with antidepressants in panic disorder. *Journal of Clinical Psychiatry, 51*, 24–30.
Reis de Olivera, I., Schwartz, T., & Stahl, S. (2014). *Integrating psychotherapy and psychopharmacology: A handbook for clinicians*. Abingdon: Routledge.
Sackett, D., Rosenberg, W., Gray, J., Haynes, R. B., & Richardson, W. S. (1996). Evidence based medicine: What it is and what it isn't. *British Journal of Medicine, 312*, 71.
Siwek, J., Gourlay, M., & Slawson, D. (2002). How to write an evidence-based clinical review article. *American Family Physician, 65*, 251–258.
Stricker, G., Abrahamson, D., & Bologna, N. (1999). Treatment guidelines: The good, the bad, and the ugly. *Psychotherapy, 36*, 69–79.
Sinyor, M., Schaffer, A., &Levitt, A. (2010). The Sequenced Treatment Alternative to Relieve Depression (STAR*D) trial: A review. *The Canadian Journal of Psychiatry, 55*, 126–135.
Soderberg, P., & Tungstrom, S. (2007). *Outcome in psychiatric outpatient services*. Umea, Sweden: Umea University.
Tolin, D. (2010). Is cognitive-behavioral therapy more effective than other therapies? A meta-analytic review. *Clinical Psychology Review, 30*, 710–720.
Turner, E., Matthews, A., Linardatos, E., Tell, R. A., & Rosenthal, R. (2008). Selective publication of antidepressant trials and its influence on apparent efficacy. *New England Journal of Medicine, 358*, 252–260.
Veale, D., & Stout, A. (2010). Cognitive behaviour therapy meets psychopharmacotherapy. *The Cognitive Behavioral Therapist, 3*, 1–15.
Walker, E., Hernandez, A, & Kattan, M. (2008). Meta-analysis: Its strengths and limitations. *Cleveland Clinic Journal of Medicine, 75*, 431–439.

2

Psychoses: Evidence-Based Integrated Biopsychosocial Treatment

David Shearer, Bret A. Moore, and Christopher Brown

The changes in diagnostic criteria for psychotic disorders in the transition from the Diagnostic and Statistical Manual of Mental Disorders, fourth edition (DSM-IV-TR) to the fifth edition (DSM-5) were relatively piecemeal when compared to major shifts in other diagnostic categories (American Psychiatric Association, 2000, 2013). Schizophrenia subtype categories (paranoid, disorganized, catatonic, undifferentiated, and residual) were eliminated due to poor empirical support, and replaced with a dimensional rating system to describe symptom severity. A requirement was added that at least one of the core positive symptoms of schizophrenia be present, and the diagnostic requirements of differentiating bizarre from nonbizarre delusions and "Schneiderian" auditory hallucinations (e.g., two or more voices conversing) were eliminated. The requirement was added for the diagnosis of schizoaffective disorder that a relevant mood episode be present for a majority of the disorder's total duration. The criteria for delusional disorder eliminated the requirement that delusions be nonbizarre, and instead added a specifier for bizarre delusions. There is no longer a distinction between shared and nonshared delusional disorder, and, finally, the criteria for catatonia were simplified to eliminate different symptom requirements for different contexts (e.g., psychotic, bipolar, depressive, other medical, or undifferentiated medical conditions). Unless otherwise specified above, the International Statistical Classification of Diseases and Related Health Problems, 10th revision (ICD-10; WHO, 1992) and DSM-5 criteria for the disorders discussed in this section are equivalent.

The classification of psychotic disorders is based upon core symptoms that include delusions, hallucinations, disorganized thinking and/or speech, grossly disorganized or abnormal motor behavior (including catatonia), and negative symptoms (American Psychiatric Association, 2013). Delusions are defined as "fixed beliefs that are not amenable to change in light of conflicting evidence," and hallucinations as "perception-like experiences that occur without an external stimulus." The degree of thought disorganization is often inferred from speech. Relevant motor behaviors can include "silliness," agitation, difficulties learning motor behaviors or directing them toward goals, and catatonic decrease in environmental reactivity. Negative symptoms can include diminished emotional expression, decreased self-initiated purposeful activities (avolition), diminished speech (alogia), decreased pleasure from positive stimuli or recollections (anhedonia), and decreased interest in social interactions (asociality).

Cognitive Behavioral Psychopharmacology: The Clinical Practice of Evidence-Based Biopsychosocial Integration, First Edition. Edited by Mark Dana Muse.

Schizotypal (personality) disorder is referenced in the DSM-5 section for schizophrenia spectrum and other psychotic disorders, because it is considered a part of the schizophrenia spectrum despite being formally classified among the personality disorders. Its estimated prevalence is up to 1.9% in clinical populations and 3.9% in the general population. This disorder is marked by a combination of difficulty maintaining close relationships, cognitive and perceptual distortions, and eccentricities of behavior. These symptoms must not occur exclusively during a psychotic disorder, mood disorder with psychotic features, or autism spectrum disorder.

Delusional disorder includes the following subtypes: erotomanic, grandiose, jealous, persecutory, somatic, mixed, and unspecified. This disorder has an estimated prevalence rate of around 0.2% (most commonly the persecutory subtype), and although the DSM-5 authors speculate that the jealous subtype may be more common in males, overall no significant gender differences are noted. This disorder is characterized by one or more prominent delusions in the absence of significant hallucinations, and by any functional impairment and mood disturbance closely linked to the delusion(s). Unlike the DSM-5, the ICD-10 still distinguishes between shared (induced delusional disorder) and nonshared variants of this diagnosis.

Brief psychotic disorder involves one or more core positive symptoms of psychosis (delusions, hallucinations, disorganized speech, and/or grossly disorganized or catatonic behavior) lasting for more than a day but less than a month and leading to full return to premorbid functional level. The disorder has about twice as high an incidence rate among females as males. Relevant specifiers include "with/without marked stressor(s)," "with postpartum onset," and "with catatonia." The ICD-10 has a greater variety of diagnostic labels than the DSM-5, and includes acute polymorphic psychotic disorder without symptoms of schizophrenia; acute polymorphic psychotic disorder with symptoms of schizophrenia; acute schizophrenia-like psychotic disorder; other acute predominantly delusional psychotic disorders; other acute and transient psychotic disorders; and acute and transient psychotic disorder, unspecified.

Schizophreniform disorder involves two or more core positive or negative symptoms of psychosis (delusions, hallucinations, disorganized speech, grossly disorganized or catatonic behavior, and/or negative symptoms) lasting between 1 and 6 months, and not meeting criteria for a more severe psychotic disorder. The estimated prevalence rate globally is similar to schizophrenia (0.3–0.7%), but in the US is approximately five times less prevalent than schizophrenia. In the ICD-10, this diagnosis is classified under "other schizophrenia."

Schizophrenia is the most widely researched and publicly recognized psychotic diagnosis, and its history includes significant shifts in theoretical conceptualization, neurobiological understanding, and diagnostic criteria. DSM-5 criteria for diagnosing schizophrenia involve the occurrence of two or more of the symptoms of schizophreniform disorder that last for at least 6 months, with at least 1 month of active-phase symptoms. The lifetime incidence rate of schizophrenia, according to the DSM-5, is estimated at 0.3–0.7%, with significant demographic variation based upon the particular diagnostic criteria and research sampling methodology utilized. The most inclusive diagnostic criteria appear to show equivalent risk between females and males. In contrast to the DSM-5, the ICD-10 still includes schizophrenic subtypes (paranoid, hebephrenic (disorganized), catatonic, undifferentiated, residual, simple, other, and unspecified), as well as a diagnosis of postschizophrenic depression.

Schizoaffective disorder is the most severe psychotic disorder, involving concurrent major mood episodes (major depressive or manic) and active-phase schizophrenia. Its incidence rate is estimated to be a third of that of schizophrenia, with higher incidence among females because of the higher incidence of major depressive episodes among females.

Substance/medication-induced psychotic disorder involves delusions and/or hallucinations developing during or soon after relevant substance exposure, intoxication, or withdrawal. A concurrent substance-related diagnosis is customarily made. Although the DSM-5 states that prevalence in the general population is unknown, between 7 and 25% of individuals presenting with first-episode psychosis may meet criteria for this diagnosis.

Psychotic disorder due to another medical condition includes prominent hallucinations or delusions that are the direct pathophysiological consequence of another medical condition such as transient infection or chronic cephalopathy, and that do not occur exclusively during the course of a delirium. Lifetime prevalence estimates are 0.21–0.54%, with the highest incidence among people over 65 years of age, and with significant variability between underlying medical etiologies.

Catatonia can occur with a variety of psychiatric disorders and medical conditions, and includes symptoms of stupor, catalepsy, waxy flexibility, mutism, negativism, posturing, mannerism, stereotypy, agitation, grimacing, echolalia, and echopraxia. The incidence rate of catatonia among schizophrenic patients is estimated as being about 35%, with a majority of catatonic cases occurring as part of depressive and bipolar disorders rather than psychotic disorders. Three catatonic diagnoses are recognized among the psychotic disorders in the DSM-5: catatonia associated with another mental disorder; catatonic disorder due to another medical condition; and unspecified catatonia.

A diagnosis of "other specified schizophrenia spectrum" and "other psychotic disorder" may be made when full criteria are not met for any other psychotic disorder, and when a clinician wishes to communicate a specific reason for this. Examples of such circumstances provided in the DSM-5 include persistent auditory hallucinations in the absence of other symptoms, delusions with significant overlapping mood episodes, attenuated psychosis syndrome, and delusional symptoms in the partner of a person with delusional disorder. A diagnosis of "unspecified schizophrenia spectrum" and "other psychotic disorder" may be made when full criteria are not met for any other psychotic disorder, and when a clinician wishes not to communicate the specific reason for this.

Historical Perspective

The modern scientific conceptualization of psychosis is often referenced as beginning with the work of Emil Kraepelin in the late 19th century and Eugen Bleuler in the early 20th century (Kyziridis, 2005). Kraepelin coined the term "dementia praecox" ("early dementia") to characterize a syndrome of emotional, social, cognitive, and neurological symptoms that are now understood as psychotic in nature. Bleuler, a critic of the conceptualization of dementia praecox, coined the term "schizophrenia" and described positive and negative symptoms, including four "As" (blunted **A**ffect, loose **A**ssociations, **A**mbivalence, and **A**utism). Although modern understanding of psychotic disorders has evolved beyond the work of Kraepelin and Bleuler, these early pioneers are understood to have brought a greater level of science to the study of such disorders.

The rise of psychoanalysis included a focus on early childhood experiences as possible progenitors of psychosis (Kyziridis, 2005). Parenting dynamics such as the "schizophrenogenic mother" and the "double bind" scenario featured prominently in psychoanalytic understanding of unconscious patterns underlying psychotic, cognitive, and emotional patterns. The discovery of first-generation antipsychotic medications during the 1950s spurred a more biologically based investigation of psychosis, a movement that grew considerably in the 1970s with the rise of cranial imaging technology such as computed tomography (CT). Findings of increased ventricular size and responsiveness to dopamine-modulating agents provided compelling evidence of the biological basis of psychotic disorders. Even more recently, genetic studies of psychosis have increased scientific knowledge of heritability and distinction between subtypes (Insel, 2010).

Social and political developments have played as much of a role as scientific advances in the landscape of psychosis in the US. For the first half of the 20th century, institutional treatment of serious mental illness was far more widespread, culminating in a population maximum of 559,000 psychiatrically institutionally individuals in 1955 (Lamb & Bachrach, 2001). Institutional environments were able to support intensive interventions, such as neurosurgery, electroconvulsive therapy, and management of the serious side effects of first-generation antipsychotics.

Despite the prominence of long-term inpatient institutions in American mental health care, ethical controversies with this approach led to a movement of widespread deinstitutionalization in the second half of the 20th century (Lamb & Bachrach, 2001). Notwithstanding intentions of increased patient autonomy and social integration, deinstitutionalization has itself been controversial. This is both because the population of chronically psychotic individuals has been met with high rates of incarceration and homelessness, and because a nationwide system of outpatient community mental health centers has never materialized as fully as had been envisioned. The interventions discussed in this chapter can only be understood within a healthcare system still struggling with the tension of how to best provide care for chronically mentally ill patients who often cycle between brief inpatient stays, tenuous housing situations, and interaction with law enforcement.

Present-day evidence-based psychosis treatment continues to require antipsychotic pharmacotherapy as the standard of care (Patterson & Leeuwenkamp, 2008), but also uniformly acknowledges the need for psychosocial as well as biochemical intervention (American Psychiatric Association, 2004; Canadian Psychiatric Association, 2005). Assertive community treatment, supported employment, cognitive-behavioral therapy (CBT), family-based services, token economy behavioral modification, skills training, psychoeducation, cognitive remediation, and treatment of co-occurring addiction and weight management conditions all show varying degrees of promise in conjunction with antipsychotic medication, as does close case management to ensure adherence and consistency.

Evidence-Based Findings

Many of the more recent randomized controlled trials (RCTs) have evaluated the efficacy of treatment early in the disease process of psychosis. The trend has been toward evaluating treatment of first-episode psychosis to determine if earlier intervention might improve long-term outcomes. Well controlled investigations of the combination of psychotropic medication plus nonmedicine treatments versus medication alone are limited (e.g., Guo et al., 2010) because the use of nonmedicine treatment (e.g., CBT, psychoeducation, family-based services) has become the standard practice for most patients suffering from psychosis. Therefore, the majority of recent RCTs compare medication plus a nonmedicine treatment of interest vs. treatment as usual (TAU); and TAU most often includes both medication (most often an atypical antipsychotic) and some form of psychosocial intervention. For instance, patients with psychosis who are treated with antipsychotics in the US and other western countries are typically offered some form of community treatment in addition to the medication, such as case management.

Pertinent to our discussion here are the findings of Jääskeläinen et al. (2013) in a review and meta-analysis of recovery in schizophrenia. These authors found that in their review of 50 studies, only one in seven patients with schizophrenia met their criteria for recovery. They concluded that "Despite major changes in treatment options in recent decades, the proportion of recovered cases has not increased" (p. 1296). Ventura et al. (2011) evaluated remission and recovery rates for medication treatment of early schizophrenia. The 77 patients in this study were followed for 1 year after hospital discharge with continuous antipsychotic treatment. The results were discouraging, with only 36% maintaining full remission at 6 months of which 10% achieved full recovery. At 1 year 22% had maintained full symptom remission and only 1% had a full recovery. This emphasizes the importance of investigating and increasing the efficacy of treatments for psychosis, particularly the combination of antipsychotic medication plus psychological/psychosocial interventions. The question is less about whether we should combine medication and psychosocial intervention and more about which combination has the best results.

Level 1 Evidence: RCTs and Meta-analyses

Randomized Controlled Trials

One approach to treatment can be termed "integrated treatment" (IT). The rational for IT is based on an assumption that a combination of diverse treatment approaches may be more effective than a single intervention alone. Such IT programs of intervention may include case management, family intervention, individual therapy, and antipsychotic medication. These studies ask the question "which combination of psychosocial interventions results in the best outcomes when used as an adjunct to antipsychotic medication?"

Srihari et al. (2015) investigated the efficacy of an IT approach (clinic for specialized treatment early in psychosis (STEP) program) plus antipsychotic medication versus TAU in an RCT. There were 120 participants receiving first-episode treatment for psychosis. The STEP program integrated psychotropic medication, family education, CBT, and case management, whereas TAU involved psychotropic medication plus the typical services provided in the community or clinic. No guidelines were provided for the TAU group and providers were free to utilize their standard approach. At a 1-year follow up they found that participants randomly assigned to the STEP program, as compared to those in the TAU group, showed reductions in total hospitalizations, hospital days, bed days, likelihood of hospitalization, and improvement in vocational outcomes.

Mueller, Schmidt, and Roder (2015) evaluated a specific cognitive remediation therapy called integrated neurocognitive therapy (INT) versus "standard care" (TAU), which could include medication as well as a variety of psychosocial programs and case management. However, the standard care group could not include treatments that might be considered a version of cognitive remediation, such as CBT or social skills training. The participants were 156 outpatient schizophrenic patients, across eight sites, randomly assigned to INT and TAU. INT was provided in 30 bi-weekly therapy sessions lasting 90 min that is described as targeting "multiple neuro and social cognitive domains with a special focus on generalization of therapy effects to functional outcome" (p. 604). The results revealed that at the 9-month follow up assessment participants in the INT group vs. the TAU group evidenced significant improvement in some of the neuro and social cognitive domains, and in some measures of negative symptoms and functional outcome. When INT was utilized, the number needed to treat (NNT) was 5 to improve functional outcome by 10–50% as measured by global assessment of functioning (GAF) scores. Initial improvement in positive symptoms at the conclusion of treatment found for the INT group was not maintained at a significant level at the 9-month follow up.

The National Institute of Mental Health (NIMH) funds the Recovery After an Initial Schizophrenia Episode (RAISE) Early Treatment Program in which Kane and colleagues (2015) investigated the use of a specialty care treatment program called NAVIGATE. Four hundred and four first-episode psychosis patients participated in the study of 223 clinics using the NAVIGATE program versus 181 clinics engaging in "typical care" (TAU). The NAVIGATE program is a team-based, coordinated specialty care program that personalizes a treatment plan for each patient by integrating components of psychotherapy, low-dose antipsychotic medications, case management, and work or educational support. The patient is actively involved in the selection of their personalized treatment plan (Mueser et al., 2015). Kane et al. (2015) found that the duration of untreated psychosis (DUP) moderated outcome. Participants with less than 74 weeks DUP in the NAVIGATE program showed more improvement in overall symptoms and quality of life measures as compared to those in the TAU group or those with longer than 74 weeks DUP. This suggests that identifying and commencing treatment rapidly for first-episode psychosis may be a key variable in achieving more positive outcomes.

The Guo et al. (2010) study is particularly important because it compares a medication-only treatment group with a medication plus psychosocial intervention treatment group for early-stage schizophrenia. In this study, conducted in China, there were 1,268 participants randomly assigned to one of the two treatments. The well-defined, manualized psychosocial intervention included CBT, skills training, psychoeducation, and family intervention. TAU was antipsychotic medication-only. After 1 year of 48 psychosocial group sessions for the experimental group, outcomes for the two groups were assessed. At 1 year of treatment the combined group, as compared to the medication-only group, had a lower risk of relapse, less discontinuation of treatment, and improved quality of life, social functioning and insight.

The OPUS Trial is a Danish RCT study comparing an IT to "standard treatment" of 547 patients with first-episode psychosis (Petersen et al., 2005; Thorup et al., 2005). The "standard treatment" group received medication management plus a community mental health nurse and possibly social work support. The IT group involved medication management plus "assertive community treatment," which included family education and involvement, as well as social skills training. Follow up assessments at 1 and 2 years showed that those in the IT group improved on psychotic and negative symptoms, as compared to the standard treatment group. Additionally, patients in the IT vs. standard treatment had less substance misuse, were more satisfied with treatment, and showed better adherence to treatment. However, at a 5-year follow up the advantages seen for the IT group vs. the standard treatment group were not maintained (Bertelsen et al., 2008). This could bring into question the long-term effects of combined treatment strategies, at least after a significant time period has elapsed after the initial treatment intervention.

The Lambreth Early Onset (LEO) Team similarly conducted a randomized, controlled clinical trial for early psychosis comparing specialized care vs. standard care (Craig et al., 2004). In this trial 144 early psychosis patients were randomly assigned to groups and followed up at 18 months. The specialized care group received evidence-based biopsychosocial interventions that included low-dose antipsychotics, manualized CBT, family counseling, and vocational support. Participants in the standard care group received treatment from community mental health teams. At 18 months there was some evidence that the specialized care group had an advantage over the standard care group for reducing hospital readmissions and treatment dropout. There was no difference in rate of relapse. In a 5-year follow up of the LEO trial participants, Gafoor and colleagues (2010) found no differences between groups in number of hospital bed days or readmissions. These findings are consistent with the OPUS trial data suggesting that shorter term gains were not maintained at 5-year follow ups.

Kuipers, Holloway, Rabe-Hesketh, & Tennakoon (2004) compared the locally available community mental health services (TAU) versus an early intervention program delivered by the COAST team (Croydon Outreach and Assertive Support Team) for 59 patients randomly assigned to one of the conditions. The COAST team offered a range of treatment options including medication management, CBT, family interventions, vocational and welfare assistance. Both groups improved over time (baseline, 6 and 9 months) with no significant differences between groups on all measures used.

In an RCT of 50 recent onset schizophrenic patients, Grawe, Falloon, Widen, & Skogvoll (2006) compared an IT to standard treatment (ST). ST included medication management and case management. IT included medication management and case management plus cognitive-behavioral family treatment with skills training, cognitive-behavioral treatment formulated for psychosis (CBTp), and home-based crisis management. Over a 2-year follow up period, the authors found advantages for IT over ST in reducing negative symptoms, minor psychotic episodes, and managing positive symptoms. However, there was no advantage to IT over ST in reducing the occurrence of major psychotic events or number of hospital admissions. Finally, IT was superior to ST in a composite index of general functioning that included measures of suicidal behavior, psychopathology, and general functioning.

Patients with co-morbid substance use disorders and schizophrenia were investigated by Barrowclough et al. (2001) in a small RCT involving 36 participants. The authors compared routine care (RC) vs. RC plus integrated care (IC) and 12 months posttreatment. RC included medication management, case management, monitoring, and access to community rehabilitation activities. The IC group included all the elements of RC, but added motivational interviewing, CBT, and family intervention. The IC group showed greater improvement in general functioning, reduced positive symptoms, reduced symptom exacerbation, and an increase in drug or alcohol abstinence. The findings are limited by the small size of the compared groups, and more research is needed to tease out the relative contribution of the different interventions included in the IC group.

Lecomte and colleagues (2009) conducted an RCT with 129 patients with recent onset psychosis. Individuals were randomly assigned to one of three groups: CBT group, social skills group, or a wait list control group. All participants were receiving antipsychotic treatment at the onset of the study. The research team evaluated outcomes at baseline, 3 and 9 months posttreatment. Outcomes measures included positive and negative symptoms, self-esteem, overall symptoms, active coping skills, and dropout rate. The CBT group showed an advantage over the social skills group for overall symptoms, self-esteem, and active coping skills. Both treatment groups were superior to the wait list group on measures of positive and negative symptoms. Finally, there was a lower drop-out rate for the CBT vs. social skills group. In this sample, when medication management was provided, the addition of CBT resulted in a superior outcome as compared to adding social skills.

Lewis et al. (2002) found no lasting differences between a control group and experimental CBT group in acute phase responses in an RCT of 315 patients after their first or second admission for schizophrenia. In the experimental group, a 5-week CBT program was added to RC and compared to RC plus supportive counseling. Medication management was provided to both groups. Benefits, as measured by reduction in positive and negative symptoms, showed some advantages for the CBT group over the RC group at 4 weeks. However, the advantage was not maintained at the 6-week follow up. There was a nonsignificant trend suggesting that the CBT group may have improved faster than the routine group.

The study by Leavey et al. (2004) had the primary aim of evaluating the impact of a brief family intervention on caregiver's satisfaction. However, the number of patient days in the hospital was also tracked. This was compared to TAU (normal care provided by community psychiatric services) for 106 first-episode patients with psychosis in an RCT. Seven 1-h sessions of education and advice were provided to patient givers in addition to TAU in the experimental group. The results showed no difference between groups on caregiver satisfaction and no difference between groups on number of hospital bed days.

In another evaluation of adding a family intervention group to medication management, Zhang, Wang, Li, and Phillips (1994) conducted a RCT for 78 first-episode, male schizophrenia patients in China discharged from their first hospital stay. Both the experimental and control groups received TAU with medication management, but the experimental group also received family individual and group sessions with the primary focus being on the family members. Patients were not invited to the first session, but were invited for the ongoing family group sessions, with sessions occurring at least once every 3 months for 18 months. The experimental group was superior to the control on measures of hospital readmission, and on the number of hospital-free days for those readmitted. For patients in both groups who were not readmitted to the hospital in the 18-month follow up period, the level of overall functioning was estimated to be better in the experimental versus the control group.

Reeder et al. (2014) examined the impact on cost of care for schizophrenia patients randomly assigned to a cognitive remediation (CR) treatment plus medication vs. TAU for 85 participants. TAU included medication management. Two of the four models showed a cost advantage for the CR group associated with cognitive improvement.

The authors conclude that change in executive functioning of schizophrenic patients may reduce disability as well as cost of care.

Drake and colleagues (2014) investigated the use of CR preceding CBT for psychosis (CBTp) for first episodes of nonaffective psychosis. This was compared to social contact (SC) preceding CBTp in 61 patients randomly assigned to these conditions. Presumably, patients in both groups were receiving antipsychotic medication as they were on a clinic wait list for CBTp. Outcome measures at baseline, after CR at 12 weeks, and after completion of CBTp (42 weeks) included psychotic symptoms, CBTp progress, insight, cognition, and self-esteem. There was no difference between groups on psychotic symptoms, but when CR preceded CBTp, the CBTp courses were significantly shorter than when preceded by SC. The authors conclude that CR preceding CBTp may enhance CBTp as well as reduce overall treatment costs.

An interesting study by Hogarty and colleagues (2004) involved two concurrent trials. The study compared schizophrenic patients randomly assigned to personal therapy (PT) vs. one of the contrasting control therapies, either family or supportive therapy (FT, ST). All patients received adequate antipsychotic medication management. One trial followed 97 patients randomly assigned to PT or control therapy who were living with family. The other trial followed 54 patients also randomly assigned to PT or control therapy living independent of family. The patients were followed for 3 years on measures of relapse and treatment noncompliance. The results for the group living with family revealed that PT was more effective than the control therapies in preventing psychotic relapse and noncompliance. However, for the group living independently of family, PT was less effective than ST. In addition, the rate of psychotic relapse was actually higher in the PT group for this sample living independently of family. This suggests that living with family may be a protective factor and the authors conclude that PT is probably best applied for patients with stable symptoms and stable residential status.

In summary, IT approaches make rational sense in the treatment of schizophrenia. Evidence from RCTs shows mixed results with some combinations of psychosocial intervention plus medication outperforming TAU. However, it appears there may be a trend toward diminishing results when outcomes for these comparisons are evaluated in the long run (e.g., 5 years). The results of the study by Kane et al. (2015) suggest that reducing the DUP for first psychosis may be a major moderating factor in treatment outcome. Evidence supporting CBT was mixed, but there appears to be some advantage of CBT over TAU (Lecomte et al., 2009; Lewis et al., 2002). Interestingly, there is some evidence that preceding CBT with CR may shorten therapy duration and reduce costs and disability (Drake et al., 2014; Reeder et al., 2014). The addition of PT to antipsychotic medication may be best reserved for medically stable patients living in stable residential status.

Meta-Analyses

In a recent meta-analysis and meta regression of 30 studies ($n = 2312$) evaluating the utility of CBT adapted for treatment of negative symptoms in schizophrenia, Velthorst et al. (2015) found no significant effect of CBT on negative symptoms. They note that earlier studies had shown some benefit for CBT for negative symptoms, but more recent studies are consistent with no significant effect.

In a meta-analysis and review of CBT for schizophrenia, Jauhar and colleagues (2014) found only minimal therapeutic effect. Fifty-two studies met the criteria for meta-analysis in this review that evaluated negative, positive, and overall symptom outcomes. The therapeutic effect of CBT was even smaller when sources of bias were considered in the analysis.

Burns, Erickson, and Brenner (2014) evaluated the effect of CBT on patients with medication-resistant psychosis. In a meta-analysis of 12 RCTs (n = 552), the authors found that "For patients who exhibit symptoms of psychosis despite adequate trials of medication, CBT for psychosis can confer beneficial effects above and beyond the effects of medication" (p. 874), especially for positive and general symptoms of psychosis.

Zimmerman, Favrod, Trieu, & Pomini (2005), in a meta-analysis of CBT for the treatment of positive symptoms of schizophrenia spectrum disorders, found that CBT, when added to antipsychotic medication, can result in a significant improvement in positive symptoms as compared to other "adjunctive measures." Other "adjunctive measures" included supportive therapy, wait-listing, and manual-based therapies. They included 14 RCTs (n = 1,484) and emphasized that the improvement in positive symptoms was more relevant for acute vs. chronic psychosis.

Pilling and colleagues (2002) conducted a meta-analysis of RCTs investigating either family intervention or CBT for schizophrenia as compared to ST. Both the experimental and control groups included medication management. There were 18 family intervention studies (n = 1,467) included in the meta-analysis and 8 CBT studies (n = 528). The results showed that as compared to the control groups family intervention groups showed an advantage for increasing medication compliance and reducing relapse and readmission rates. The CBT groups benefited from lower dropout rates and improvements in "mental state" as measured by commonly used scales as compared to the control groups.

Bird and colleagues (2010) conducted a meta-analysis and review of early intervention (EI) services, CBT, and family intervention for early psychosis, as compared to standard care that included medication management. Four studies met their inclusion criteria for EI (n = 800), three studies for family interventions (n = 288), and four studies for CBT (n = 620). Patients in the experimental groups received antipsychotic medication management as part of their treatment regimen. Elements of EI included case management, psychosocial intervention that might include CBT, social skills training, family interventions, and vocational strategies. Family interventions varied across studies but all included some element of psychoeducation and problem solving in an individual and/or group format. CBT approaches were also mixed with some studies targeting positive symptoms and insight, while other studies comprising the meta-analysis of CBT were adapted specifically for treatment of early psychosis. As compared to standard care, EI resulted in reductions in symptom severity, hospital admissions, and relapse. Family intervention also reduced hospital admissions and relapse, whereas CBT reduced symptom severity with no significant reduction in hospital admission or relapse.

The study by Alvarez-Jiménez, Parker, Hetrick, McGorry, and Gleeson (2011) is a somewhat complex meta-analysis of different psychosocial and medication RCTs for first-episode psychosis. Nine of 18 RCTs included in the meta-analysis were specific to psychosocial interventions that included specialized first-episode psychosis (FEP) interventions, CBT, individual and family cognitive-based relapse prevention therapy, family therapy, and TAU. Specialist FEP treatments may include elements such as a multidisciplinary team, community outreach, evidence-based treatment, low-dose atypical antipsychotics, manualized CBT, crisis plans, family counseling, and psychoeducation. The authors conclude that specialist FEP treatments prevent relapse better than TAU; CBT did not show advantages over specialist FEP treatments, but did not specifically target relapse in these studies. They further conjecture that "Cognitive-based individual and family interventions may need to specifically target relapse to obtain relapse prevention benefits that extend beyond those provided by specialist FEP programs" (p. 619).

Pitschel-Walz, Leucht, Bäuml, Kissling, and Engel (2001) investigated the effect of family interventions on relapse and rehospitalization for schizophrenic patients in a meta-analysis of 25 studies with participants ranging in number from 23 to 418. Family interventions plus medication were compared with medication-only, and the authors found reductions in relapse of up to 20% when patients' relatives were included in the treatment of schizophrenic patients.

A less recent meta-analysis included 106 studies of psychosocial treatment plus medication vs. medication-only in the management of schizophrenia. The authors found adding psychosocial treatment to medication alone resulted in greater improvement in symptoms that were maintained over time; lower relapse frequencies were also found (Mojtabai, Nicholson, & Carpenter, 1998). The psychosocial treatment included modalities such as traditional psychotherapy, family psychoeducation, cognitive training, and community treatment.

In a separate meta-analysis of 40 RCTs (n = 2104), CR for schizophrenia was found to have a "small to moderate" effect on cognitive outcomes at both posttreatment and follow up assessments (Wykes, Huddy, Cellard, McGurk, & Czobor, 2011).

In summary, there appears to be some historical support for CBT combined with medication for psychosis, perhaps especially for improvement in positive symptoms of schizophrenia (Alvarez-Jiménez et al., 2011; Bird et al., 2010; Burns et al., 2004; Pilling et al., 2002; Zimmerman et al., 2005). However, more recent meta-analyses have been less supportive, showing minimal effect for CBT for psychoses, especially negative vs. positive symptoms (Jauhar et al., 2014; Velthorst et al., 2015). In sum, we may cautiously conclude that CBT for psychosis may have an advantage for treating positive vs. negative symptoms, perhaps be preferred when encountering treatment-resistant schizophrenia, may be better for acute vs. chronic psychosis, and may have better efficacy when CBT is specifically designed to address an identified outcome (e.g., relapse rates).

In addition, there appears to be solid evidence that family interventions are helpful as an adjunct to antipsychotic medication for schizophrenia (Bird et al., 2010; Mojtabai et al., 1998; Pilling et al., 2002; Pitschel-Walz et al., 2001). Family interventions vary across studies but often include at least a psychoeducational component and potentially individual family therapy, group family therapy, crisis planning, or other support. Family interventions appear to reduce relapse rates, likely increase medication compliance, and reduce hospital readmission rates. Bird and colleagues (2010) provide good evidence that early intervention may improve outcomes as well. CR has small to moderate effects on cognitive outcomes for schizophrenic patients (Wykes et al., 2011).

Level 2 Evidence: Less Well Controlled Trials or High Quality Cohort Studies

In a nonrandomized study Cullberg, Levander, Holmqvist, Mattsson, & Wieselgren (2002) compared a treatment system for FEP patients (n = 175, Swedish Parachute Project) to a historical cohort group (n = 71) and a prospective cohort group (n = 64). The main tenets of the Parachute Project system for FEP were to minimize use of high-dose neuroleptics, increase continuity of care, minimize reliance on hospital care, and not to mix chronic with FEP patients in treatment. An emphasis was placed on rapid engagement in treatment with psychosocial and support elements that included crisis planning and care, psychotherapy, and family involvement including psychological support, treatment, and psychoeducation. The authors found that GAF scores in the first year of treatment were significantly higher for the historical group and similar to those found for the prospective group. After treatment, inpatient care and neuroleptic use were lower for the Parachute group, and the authors conclude that these results can be obtained by providing intensive psychosocial treatment and support.

Dixon and colleagues (2015) describe the RAISE Connection Program for 65 patients in Baltimore and New York. Treatment elements included a range of options including vocational support, family support, family education, psychoeducation, skills training, CBT-based support, substance abuse treatment, and suicide prevention. These patients with early psychosis were followed for 2 years and results showed that, as compared to initial base rates, occupational functioning, social functioning, and remission rates improved significantly over time, whereas symptoms declined.

Uzenoff et al. (2012) describe results at 1 year of a multielement treatment center for early psychosis. One hundred and sixty-three patients were treated at the Outreach and Support Intervention Services (OASIS) clinic in North Carolina. The treatment program includes assessment, case management, and medication management, with a focus on developing autonomy and stability. Based on individual needs, a wide variety of additional services are offered and provided in the clinic, community, and home. These can include supportive or CBT, connection to community resources (e.g., vocational rehabilitation), group therapy, family and/or multifamily therapy, and substance use treatment. The authors found significant improvements in measures of symptoms (positive and negative), role functioning, and global functioning. In addition there were advantages in symptom remission, functioning, and increased school attendance.

In an investigation of early intervention for FEP patients, Linszen, Dingemans, & Lenior (2001) found that a 15-month intervention program for 71 patients kept the relapse rate to a low 15%. The same patients were then referred to other community agencies and followed for 5 years, and it was subsequently found that the low relapse rate was not maintained. The authors conclude that it may the continuity of outpatient care and caregivers that is most important, rather than the early identification and intervention when considering longer-term outcomes with schizophrenia.

Level 3 Evidence: Case Controlled Studies and Reviews

Jones, Hacker, Cormac, Meaden, and Irving (2014) reviewed RCTs comparing CBT to other psychosocial interventions for schizophrenia and concluded that there is no clear advantage for CBT over these other forms of therapy. A separate review by Turkington,

Kingdon, and Weiden (2006) suggests that research, particularly in the UK, has shown some promise for CBT in schizophrenia, but more investigation is needed.

In a review of the literature assessing adjunctive psychosocial therapies for schizophrenia, Patterson and Leeuwenkamp (2008) concluded that the addition of psychosocial therapy to pharmacotherapy improves medication adherence, reduces relapse, and significantly improves quality of life and social functioning.

Patterson and Leeuwenkamp (2008) reviewed the evidence for adding psychosocial interventions to antipsychotic medication and found significant advantage across important outcomes. In a different review, Jones et al. (2014) found CBT to be no better than other forms of psychosocial intervention in the treatment of schizophrenia.

Level 4 Evidence: Case Series, Case Reports, Panel of Experts, Institutional Guidelines

The American Psychiatric Association (2004, Dixon, Perkin, & Calmes, 2009) has provided guidelines and recommendations for the treatment of patients with schizophrenia. The American Psychiatric Association identifies the primary targets of treatment as reducing or eliminating symptoms, maximizing quality of life and adaptive functioning, and to promote and maintain recovery to the greatest level possible. There is clear recognition in the guidelines that adding psychosocial treatment to psychotropic management enables recovery and reduces relapse. Nonetheless, according to this guideline, psychosocial treatments should be selected based on individual patient needs and the social context in which they live. These interventions are best applied during the stable phase of treatment. The American Psychiatric Association recommends the following psychosocial treatments: family interventions, supported employment, assertive community treatment, social skills training, and CBT-oriented psychotherapy. The authors note that at the time of publication CR, peer support, and peer-delivered services required additional investigation.

The Canadian Psychiatric Association (2005) recommends that optimal treatment of schizophrenia requires the addition of psychosocial treatment to pharmacologic treatment. The Canadian Psychiatric Association (CPA) indicates that this combined approach can result in improvements in medication adherence, reduce relapse and readmission, reduce distress, improve functioning, and provide support for patient, families, and caregivers. Similar to the American Psychiatric Association (2009) recommendations, the CPA suggests that psychosocial interventions be applied after the acute symptoms are stabilized on medication. It further highlights the importance of having service providers demonstrate proficiency and familiarity with this population and the treatments applied. Recommended psychosocial treatments to use in combination with pharmacotherapy include psychoeducation, vocational interventions, skills training, CBT, family interventions, and treatment of co-morbid symptoms. Peer support strategies lacked adequate support at the time of publication.

The Royal Australian and New Zealand College of Psychiatrists (2005) also provides guidelines for the treatment of schizophrenia. The College states that while antipsychotic medication management is the cornerstone of treatment, all patients treated for schizophrenia and their families should also be offered comprehensive psychosocial interventions. The need for competent and well-trained providers is emphasized as well as the importance of tailoring treatment to patient goals, stage of illness, and patient preferences. Recommended psychosocial treatments include family interventions, CBT, vocational rehabilitation, and treatment of co-morbid conditions (e.g., substance abuse).

The 2009 Schizophrenia Patient Outcomes Research Team (PORT) represents the third set of PORT recommendations based on a comprehensive summary of evidence-based psychosocial and pharmacological treatment for persons with schizophrenia (Buchanan et al., 2009; Dixon et al., 2009). These summaries make specific recommendations for pharmacologic treatment as the cornerstone of intervention for schizophrenia, with eight adjunctive treatment recommendations for psychosocial interventions. The recommended psychosocial interventions include assertive community treatment, supported employment, CBT, family-based services, token economy, skills training, psychosocial interventions for alcohol and substance use disorders, and psychosocial interventions for weight management. Treatment options that did not have enough evidence for recommendation at the time of publication included interventions with a focus on medication adherence, CR, psychosocial treatments for recent onset schizophrenia, and peer support and peer-delivered services (Dixon et al., 2009).

The British National Institute for Health and Care Excellence (NICE) guidelines for the management of psychosis and schizophrenia in adults were updated in 2014 (Kuipers, Yesufu-Udechuku, Taylor & Kendall, 2014; NICE, 2014). These recommendations are based on review of available evidence and expert consensus. The recommendations include a focus on physical health, support for careers, preventing psychosis, management of first-episode and chronic psychosis, antipsychotic medication management considerations, and promotion of recovery and overcoming barriers to treatment. NICE guidelines recommend the use of family intervention and individual CBT for first-episode and acute episodes of psychosis in conjunction with antipsychotic medication.

In summary, all expert panels and institutional guidelines reviewed in this chapter recommend that schizophrenia be treated with a combination of medication and some form or forms of psychosocial/psychological intervention (American Psychiatric Association, 2009; Canadian Psychiatric Association, 2005; PORT 2009; Royal Australian and New Zealand College of Psychiatrists, 2005; NICE, 2014). Types of psychosocial/psychological interventions recommended include family intervention, CBT, vocations support, social or other skills training, treatment of co-morbid disorders, assertive community treatment, and psychoeducation.

Practice Guidelines

The available evidence suggests that combining psychosocial interventions with antipsychotic medication is the treatment of choice for psychosis. Treatment protocols that integrate a range of psychosocial interventions with appropriate medication management appear to show great promise. However, there are some excellent studies that suggest that initial positive results using this combined approach may not yield significant longer-term benefits (e.g., Bertelsen et al., 2008; Gafoor et al., 2010). Kane et al. (2015) emphasized the importance of commencing treatment rapidly for FEP as a potential key variable in achieving more positive outcomes. These authors suggest that reducing the DUP may magnify the impact of effective treatment, perhaps leading to better long-term outcomes. The preponderance of high quality evidence, which is limited, suggests that in addition to appropriate medication management, psychosocial interventions should be implemented based on the individual needs of the patient. Such psychosocial treatments could include one or more of the following interventions: family involvement in treatment, supportive and/or skills-based therapy such as CBT, psychoeducation, case management, proactive crisis management, skills training, and vocational support or training.

Expert panels, consensus statements, and practice guidelines all suggest that schizophrenia be treated with a combination of medication and some form or forms of psychosocial/psychological intervention. In addition there is emerging evidence that, in addition to the "best practices" psychosocial interventions identified above, the following interventions should be considered as well: co-morbid substance abuse treatment, connections to community resources, suicide prevention, CR, and emphasizing continuity of caregivers over time.

Table 2.1 summarizes practice guidelines for evidence-based treatment of psychosis.

Table 2.1 Integrative biopsychosocial intervention with psychosis: Summary of best practice recommendations by level of confidence derived from strength of evidence.

Practice guidelines for psychosis		
Level A	Recommended	• Treatment of psychotic disorders should not be delayed, but begin early in the patient's life, and should involve both medications and psychosocial components that are tailored to each patient's specific needs and circumstances • Antipsychotic medication use is nearly universally indicated in the management of psychoses • CBT is more effective in reducing positive symptoms than in reducing negative symptoms, and is particularly indicated as adjunctive therapy where medication has not improved positive symptoms • There is some evidence that preceding cognitive-behavioral therapy (CBT) with cognitive remediation (CR) may shorten therapy duration and reduce costs • Relapse after successful initial treatment is prevalent with psychosis, and there is some evidence that cognitive-based and family therapies that specifically target relapse may improve longer outcomes
Level B	Suggested	• Rapid treatment response to first-episode psychosis may yield long-lasting benefits • Reduction of the duration of untreated psychosis may improve outcomes • Consider implementation of co-morbid substance abuse treatment • To the degree possible, involve family members and/or caregivers in treatment
Level C	May be considered	• Psychosocial interventions form an integral part of therapy, but are best instituted after stabilization with pharmacotherapy • Emphasize continuity of caregivers over time to reduce relapse

Illustrative Case Studies

Rob is a 27-year-old, Caucasian male who was recently diagnosed with schizophrenia during a 1.5-year prison term for drug distribution. He has a history of polysubstance abuse and several shorter jail sentences. His prison sentence was the longest period of his life in which he has had consistent healthcare, including his first trial of antipsychotic medication. He responded favorably to this treatment, but continued to abuse substances that resulted in psychotic symptoms. Rob now lives with a girlfriend, and child protective services (CPS) has custody of their 2-year-old child. He shows little insight into his symptoms, primarily because he confuses them with the effects of recreational substances. Medically, he is Hepatitis C positive and shows signs of liver damage. He is being monitored on a weekly basis by a parole officer.

Rob's treatment must involve substance abuse treatment and monitoring, as well as continued use of antipsychotic medication. His parole officer and/or CPS caseworker could assist him in securing Medicaid coverage and enrollment in a community mental health program, both for medications and counseling. At that point, consistent contact with a nurse case manager (who could coordinate substance abuse screening with his parole officer) will be critical to his successful treatment. It would be helpful for Rob's girlfriend to attend his health care appointments when possible so that she feels involved and invested in his health.

Susan is a 43-year-old, Alaskan Native woman who has been diagnosed with schizoaffective disorder since she was a teenager in residential treatment. She has a history of being abused in domestic relationships and of periods of homelessness. She has no history of substance abuse, and her insight into her psychiatric condition has improved during the past decade. She pursues medical care during periods of coverage by her state Medicaid program, but has experienced great difficulty finding an outpatient psychiatrist who will accept her case. Her medical conditions include obesity, diabetes with variable control, and chronic orthopedic pain from past injuries. She has regular visits with a daughter, who is a supportive and stable influence in her life.

Susan's difficulty in finding specialty psychiatric care means that her antipsychotic medication will likely be prescribed by a primary care provider (PCP). Her daughter could assist in her care by attending appointments with her when she is able to do so, and by working with a mental illness advocacy organization to assist the PCP in staying current with new medication options. Susan and her daughter would also benefit from psychosocial support groups, whether through healthcare organizations, advocacy groups, or cultural organizations.

Cynthia is a 35-year-old, African-American woman who has a history of psychotic symptoms, but not of conclusive diagnosis. She utilizes emergency medical care when in crisis (suicide attempts and/or florid psychotic symptoms), but has never had sustained engagement with outpatient treatment. Her sister's family is raising her two children, and her sister determines when Cynthia is psychiatrically stable enough to visit them. Her large extended family lives in the area and often acts as a stabilizing influence, as well as providing her with material support. She is religiously devout and at times views her symptoms as spiritual experience. Her physical health is fairly good at present, but her family is very concerned about her ability to deal with any future injuries or illnesses safely.

Cynthia would benefit from a thorough, outpatient evaluation of her condition during a period of relative stability, both to inform healthcare decisions and to assist in securing disability benefits and services. Enrollment in a community mental health program would allow for case management that she has not had previously, as well as for consideration of newer antipsychotic medications that may not be commonly prescribed in emergency departments. She is fortunate to have many family members who could attend appointments with her, perhaps on a rotating basis to ease the stress of caregiving, and who could communicate with each other about any changes in her condition or treatment plan.

Final Observations

The disease of schizophrenia and related psychotic disorders can be life-shattering for patients and their families. Advances in antipsychotic medication treatment with lower side effect profiles and, therefore, greater tolerability have made treatment of psychosis more effective and acceptable to patients. In addition, research and clinical practice have shown that adding psychosocial interventions and support for patients, their families, and caregivers can have a substantial impact on recovery and functioning. However, the potential for lifelong disability and high rates of relapse (e.g., Harvey et al., 2012; Weiden & Olfson, 1995) remain substantial barriers to successful treatment. While there is essentially universal agreement that antipsychotic medication should be combined with psychosocial intervention, there is no clear evidence that any one psychosocial intervention is best. Rather, the trend toward combining psychosocial interventions rationally, based on individual patient needs and preferences, seems to be the most promising avenue. However, when these psychosocial interventions are combined it is more difficult to tease apart which components of these "integrated" treatment protocols are most effective. More research will be needed to clarify the most important aspects of treatment. There is a growing acceptance that aggressive and rapid treatment of FEP may be a vital step in both the short- and long-term treatment of psychosis. This emphasizes the need for readily available community resources including rapid access to medication management and specialized treatment teams to work with this population. Reducing barriers and DUP may become one of the primary components of effective treatment in the long run. In the meantime, the capability to individualize treatment plans based on individual patient needs, circumstances, and preferences will be an essential first step in effective interventions that include medication and psychosocial treatment.

References

Alvarez-Jiménez, M., Parker, A. G., Hetrick, S. E., McGorry, P. D., & Gleeson, J. F. (2011). Preventing the second episode: A systematic review and meta-analysis of psychosocial and pharmacological trials in first-episode psychosis. *Schizophrenia Bulletin, 37*, 619–630.

American Psychiatric Association. (2000). *Diagnostic and Statistical Manual of Mental Disorders* (4th ed., text rev.). Washington, DC: American Psychiatric Association.

American Psychiatric Association (2004). Practice guidelines for the treatment of patients with schizophrenia, second edition. *American Journal of Psychiatry, 161*, 1–56.

American Psychiatric Association. (2013). *Diagnostic and statistical manual of mental disorders* (5th ed.). Washington, DC: American Psychiatric Association.

Barrowclough, C., Haddock, G., Tarrier, N., Lewis, S. W., Moring, J., O'Brien, R., . . . & McGovern, J. (2001). Randomized controlled trial of motivational interviewing, cognitive behavioral therapy, and family intervention for patients with comorbid schizophrenia and substance use disorders. *American Journal of Psychiatry, 158*, 1706–1713.

Bertelsen, M., Jeppesen, P., Petersen, L., Thorup, A., Øhlenschlaeger, J., le Quach, P., . . . & Nordentoft, M. (2008). Five-year follow-up of a randomized multicenter trial of intensive early intervention vs standard treatment for patients with a first episode of psychotic illness: The OPUS trial. *Archives of General Psychiatry, 65*, 762–771.

Bird, V., Premkumar, P., Kendall, T., Whittington, C., Mitchell, J., & Kuipers, E. (2010). Early intervention services, cognitive-behavioural therapy and family intervention in early psychosis: Systematic review. *British Journal of Psychiatry, 197*, 350–356.

Buchanan, R. W., Kreyenbuhl, J., Kelly, D. L., Noel, J. M., Boggs, D. L., Fischer, B. A., . . . & Keller, W. (2010). The 2009 schizophrenia PORT psychopharmacological treatment recommendations and summary statements. *Schizophrenia Bulletin, 36*, 71–93.

Burns, A. M. N., Erickson, D. H., & Brenner, C. A. (2014). Cognitive-behavioral therapy for medication-resistant psychosis: A meta-analytic review. *Psychiatric Services, 65*, 874–880.

Drake, R. J., Day, C. J., Picucci, R., Warburton, J., Larkin, W., Husain, N., . . . & Marshall, M. (2014). A naturalistic, randomized, controlled trial combining cognitive remediation with cognitive-behavioural therapy after first-episode non-affective psychosis. *Psychological Medicine, 44*, 1889–1899.

Canadian Psychiatric Association (2005). Clinical practice guidelines: Treatment of schizophrenia. *Canadian Journal of Psychiatry, 50* (Supp 1), 1S–59S.

Craig, T. K. J., Garety, P., Power, P., Rahaman, N., Colbert, S., Fornells-Ambrojo, M., & Dunn, G. (2004). The Lambreth Early Onset (LEO) Team: Randomized controlled trial of the effectiveness of specialized care for early psychosis. *British Medical Journal, 329*, 1067–1073.

Cullberg, J., Levander, S., Holmqvist, R., Mattsson, M., & Wieselgren, I. M. (2002). One-year outcome in first episode psychosis patients in the Swedish Parachute project. *Acta Psychiatrica Scandinavica, 106*, 276–285.

Dixon, L. B., Dickerson, F., Bellack, A. S., Bennett, M., Dickinson, D., Goldberg, R. W., . . . & Kreyenbuhl, J. (2009). The 2009 schizophrenia PORT psychosocial treatment recommendations and summary statements. *Schizophrenia Bulletin, 36*, 48–70.

Dixon, L. B., Goldman, H. H., Bennett, M. E., Wang, Y., McNamara, K. A., Mendon, S. J., . . . & Essock, S. M. (2015). Implementing coordinated specialty care for early psychosis: The RAISE Connection Program. *Psychiatric Services, 66*, 691–698.

Dixon, L., Perkins, D., & Calmes, C. (2009). Guideline Watch: Practice guideline for the treatment of patients with schizophrenia. *American Psychiatry Association*. Retrieved from psychiatryonline.org

Gafoor, R., Nitsch, D., McCrone, P., Craig, T. K., Garety, P. A., Power, P., & McGuire, P. (2010). Effect of early intervention on 5-year outcome in non-affective psychosis. *British Journal of Psychiatry, 196*, 372–376.

Grawe, R. W., Falloon, I. R., Widen, J. H., & Skogvoll, E. (2006).Two years of continued early treatment for recent-onset schizophrenia: A randomised controlled study. *Acta Psychiatrica Scandinavica, 114*, 328–336.

Guo, X., Zhai, J., Liu, Z. Fang, M., Wang, B., Hu, B., . . . & Zhai, J. (2010). Effect of antipsychotic medication alone vs combined with psychosocial intervention on outcomes of early-stage schizophrenia: A randomized, 1 year study. *Archives of General Psychiatry, 67*, 895–904. D]doi:10.1001/archgenpsychiatry.2010.105.

Harvey, P. D., Heaton R. K., Carpenter, W. T. Jr., Green, M. F., Gold, J. M., & Schoenbaum, M. (2012). Functional impairment in people with schizophrenia: Focus on employability and eligibility for disability compensation. *Schizophrenia Research, 140* (1–3), 1–8. doi:10.1016/j.schres.2012.03.025

Hogarty, G. E., Kornblith, S. J., Greenwald, D., DiBarry, A. L., Cooley, S., Ulrich, R. F., . . . & Flesher, S. (2004). Three-year trials of personal therapy among schizophrenic patients living with or independent of family, I: Description of study and effects on relapse rates. Focus: *The Journal of Lifelong Learning in Psychiatry, 2*, 146–157.

Insel, T. R. (2010). Rethinking schizophrenia. *Nature, 468*(7321), 187–193.

Jääskeläinen, E., Juola, P., Hirvonen, N., McGrath, J. J., Saha, S., Isohanni, M., . . .& Miettunen, J. (2013). A systematic review and meta-analysis of recovery in schizophrenia. *Schizophrenia Bulletin, 39*, 1296–1306.

Jauhar, S., McKenna, P. J., Radua, J., Fung, E., Salvador, R., & Laws, K. R. (2014). Cognitive-behavioural therapy for the symptoms of schizophrenia: Systematic review and meta-analysis with examination of potential bias. *British Journal of Psychiatry, 204*, 20–29.

Jones, C. Hacker, D. Cormac, I., Meaden, & Irving, C.B. (2014). Cognitive behavioural therapy versus other psychosocial treatments for schizophrenia, *Cochrane Database Systems Review, 4*, 1–155.

Kane, J. M., Robinson D. G., Schooler, N. R., Mueser, K. T., Penn, D. L., Rosenheck, R. A., . . . & Heinssen, R. K.(2015). Comprehensive versus usual community care for first-episode psychosis: 2-year outcomes from the NIMH RAISE early treatment program. *American Journal of Psychiatry, 173*(4), 362–372.

Kuipers, E., Holloway, F., Rabe-Hesketh, S., & Tennakoon, L. (2004). Croydon Outreach and Assertive Support Team (COAST): An RCT of early intervention in psychosis. *Social Psychiatry and Psychiatric Epidemiology, 39*, 358–363.

Kuipers, E., Yesufu-Udechuku, A., Taylor, C., & Kendall, T. (2014). Management of psychosis and schizophrenia in adults: Summary of updated NICE guidance. *British Medical Journal, 348*, 1173.

Kyziridis, T. C. (2005). Notes on the history of schizophrenia. *German Journal of Psychiatry, 8*, 42–48.

Lamb, H. R., & Bachrach, L. L. (2001). Some perspectives on deinstitutionalization. *Psychiatric Services, 52*, 1039–1045.

Leavey, G., Gulamhussein, S., Papadopoulous, C. Johnson-Sabine, E., Blizard, B., & King, M. (2004). A randomized controlled trial of a brief intervention for families of patients with a first episode of psychosis. *Psychological Medicine, 34*, 423–431.

Lecomte, T., Leclerc, C., Corbiere, M., Mykes, T., Wallace, C. J., & Spidel, A. (2009). Group cognitive behavioral therapy or social skills training for individuals with a recent onset of psychosis? Results of a randomized controlled trial. *Journal of Nervous and Mental Disorders, 196*, 866–75.

Lewis, S., Tarrier N., Haddock, G., Bentall, R., Kinderman, P., Kingdon, D., . . . & Dunn, G. (2002). Randomised controlled trial of cognitive behavioral therapy in early schizophrenia: Acute phase outcomes. *British Journal of Psychiatry, 181*(suppl 43), s91–97.

Linszen, D., Dingemans, P., & Lenior, M. (2001). Early intervention and a five year follow up in young adults with a short duration of untreated psychosis: Ethical implications. *Schizophrenia Research, 51*, 55–61.

Mojtabai, R., Nicholson, R. A., & Carpenter, B. N. (1998). Role of psychosocial treatments in management of schizophrenia: A meta-analytic review of controlled outcome studies. *Schizophrenia Bulletin, 24*, 569–587.

Mueller, D. R., Schmidt, S. J., & Roder, V. (2015). One-year randomized controlled trial and follow-up of integrated neurocognitive therapy for schizophrenia outpatients. *Schizophrenia Bulletin, 41,* 604–616.

Mueser, K. T., Penn, D.L., Addington, J., Brunette, M. F., Gingerich, S., Glynn, S. M., . . . & Kane, J. M. (2015). The NAVIGATE program for first-episode psychosis: Rationale, overview, and description of psychosocial components. *Psychiatric Services, 66,* 680–690.

Patterson, T. L., & Leeuwenkamp, O. R. (2008). Adjunctive psychosocial therapies for the treatment of schizophrenia. *Schizophrenia Research, 100,* 108–119. doi:10.1016/j.schres.2007.12.468

Petersen, L., Jeppesen, P., Thorup, A., Abel, M. B., Øhlenschlaeger, J., Christensen, T. Ø., . . .& Nordentoft, M. (2005). A randomised multicentre trial of integrated versus standard treatment for patients with a first episode of psychotic illness. *British Medical Journal, 331,* 602.

Pilling, L., Bebbington, P., Kuipers, E., Garety, P., Geddes, J., Orbach, G., & Morgan, C. (2002). Psychological treatments in schizophrenia: I. Meta-analysis of family intervention and cognitive behavior therapy. *Psychological Medicine, 32,* 763–782.

Pitschel-Walz, G., Leucht, S., Bäuml, J., Kissling, W., & Engel, R. R. (2001). The effect of family interventions on relapse and rehospitalization in schizophrenia: A meta-analysis. *Schizophrenia Bulletin, 27,* 73–92.

Reeder, C., Harris, V., Pickles, A., Patel, A., Cella, M., & Wykes, T. (2014). Does change in cognitive function predict change in costs of care for people with a schizophrenia diagnosis following cognitive remediation therapy? *Schizophrenia Bulletin, 40,* 1472–1481.

Royal Australian and New Zealand College of Psychiatrists (2005). Clinical practice guidelines for the treatment of schizophrenia and related disorders. *Australian and New Zealand Journal of Psychiatry, 39*(1–2), 1–30. doi: 10.1090/j.1440-1614.2005.011516.x

Srihari, V. H., Tek, C., Kucukgoncu, S., Phutane, V. H., Breitborde, N. J., Pollard, J., . . . & Woods, S.W.. (2015). First-episode service for psychotic disorders in the U.S. public sector: A pragmatic, randomized control trial. *Psychiatric Services, 66,* 705–712.

Thorup, A., Petersen, L., Jeppesen, P., Øhlenschlaeger, J., Christensen, T., Krarup, G., . . . & Nordentoft, M. (2005). Integrated treatment ameliorates negative symptoms in first episode psychosis: Results from the Danish OPUS trial. *Schizophrenia Research, 79,* 95–105.

Turkington, D., Kingdon, D., & Weiden, P.J. (2006). Cognitive behavior therapy for schizophrenia. *American Journal of Psychiatry, 163,* 365–373.

Uzenoff, S. R., Penn, D. L., Graham, K. A., Saade, S., Smith, B. B., & Perkins, D. O. (2012). Evaluation of a multi-element treatment center for early psychosis in the United States. *Social Psychiatry and Psychiatric Epidemiology, 47,* 1607–1615.

Velthorst, E., Koeter, M., van der Gaag, M., Nieman, D. H., Fett, A. K. J., Smit, F., . . . & de Haan, L. (2015). Adapted cognitive-behavioural therapy required for targeting negative symptoms in schizophrenia: Meta-analysis and meta-regression. *Psychological Medicine, 45,* 453–465.

Ventura, J., Subotnik, K. L., Guzik, L. H., Hellemann, G. S., Gitlin, M. J., Wood, R. C., & Nuechterlein, K. H. (2011). Remission and recovery during the first outpatient year of the early course of schizophrenia. *Schizophrenia Research, 132,* 18–23.

Weiden, P.J. &, Olfson, M. (1995). Cost of relapse in schizophrenia. *Schizophrenia Bulletin, 21*, 419–429.

World Health Organization (1992). *International Statistical Classification of Diseases and Related Health Problems, 10th Revision (ICD-10)*. Geneva: WHO.

Wykes, T., Huddy, V., Cellard, C., McGurk, S. R., & Czobor, P. (2011). A meta-analysis of cognitive remediation for schizophrenia: Methodology and effect sizes. *American Journal of Psychiatry, 168*, 472–485.

Zhang, M., Wang, M., Li, J., & Phillips, M. R. (1994). Randomised control trial of family intervention for 78 first episode male schizophrenic patients. An 18 month study in Suzhou, *Jiangsu. British Journal of Psychiatry, 165*(Suppl), 96–102.

Zimmermann, G., Favrod, J., Trieu, V. H., & Pomini, V. (2005). The effect of cognitive behavioral treatment on the positive symptoms of schizophrenia spectrum disorders: A meta-analysis. *Schizophrenia Research, 77*, 1–9.

3

Mood Disorders: Evidence-Based Integrated Biopsychosocial Treatment of Major Depressive Disorder

Mikel Merritt

"Evidence-based" is an attractive and alluring term that, at its best, assures the practitioner that the treatments available have been duly evaluated, and that their relative merit has been proved through a nonbiased, empirical methodology. The research cited throughout this chapter and, indeed, throughout this book is sound research, and research that is vital to improving the base of knowledge for the field of mental health and, ultimately, for the treatment of mental health conditions; in our case at hand, we wish to allow research to guide our clinical practice in the treatment of major depression. Still, as we evaluate the studies and treatment methodologies, it is incumbent upon us to keep a few important matters in mind about the research that we are relying on to draw our best-practice conclusions.

First, the "Gold Standard" in treatment research involves randomized controlled trials (RCTs). Participants who are deemed appropriate for a study are randomly assigned to a treatment group, and in many of these studies that means that they are assigned to a medication treatment group, a psychotherapy treatment group, or a combination treatment group. While this practice has significant benefit in helping to ensure that each treatment arm has a similar make up, and it certainly represents quality methods for limiting the influence of confounding variables, this is not how clinical practice works. In actual treatment, patients do in fact self-select for medication by speaking first with their primary care provider, or they may initially seek therapy from a psychologist, social worker, or other licensed psychotherapist. An increasing number of patients in therapy are also taking psychotropic medication adjunctively (Barnett & Neel, 2000), and such patients are making these decisions based on what they believe will be most helpful, least intimidating, or perhaps what is most accessible to him/her. The value of self-selection to a particular mode of treatment is mentioned here not to dissuade the reader from reading the research, but rather to highlight the importance of considering how expectations may impact results. Research (Carlino, Pollo, & Benedeti, 2012) has demonstrated that a patient's expectations may impact the utility or effectiveness of treatment. Thus, in an RCT, if a patient is assigned to a treatment method that he or she perceives will be ineffective, the results are likely to reflect those attitudes. This is just as true for medications (Colloca & Miller, 2011) as it is for psychotherapy. The result may be that in clinical practice we see therapies, both talk therapy and

Cognitive Behavioral Psychopharmacology: The Clinical Practice of Evidence-Based Biopsychosocial Integration, First Edition. Edited by Mark Dana Muse.

pharmaceutical interventions, outperforming the research data. The benefit of the RCT, however, is that we would expect this same factor to influence all treatment arms equally, but without research to determine current attitudes toward the various treatments offered, it is difficult to tell if any one form of therapy would be more likely that another to suffer bias in pre-assigning it.

Second, a majority of treatment studies that involve medication, in either a head-to-head comparison with psychotherapy or as a part of a combined treatment arm, evaluate only one psychotropic, or, in the case of major depression, antidepressant. Using only one medication is problematic, as some estimates (Bauer, Whybrow, Angst et al., 2002) demonstrate that approximately 40% of patients do not respond to the initial treatment with psychotropic medication, and of the nonresponders approximately half of those do not have symptom remission with a second agent. A study comparing a therapeutic algorithm with "treatment as usual" (TAU) (Bauer et al., 2009) found that under TAU patients were administered an average of three different medications. While we don't yet have a full understanding of why a patient might respond to one medication better than another, it is common in clinical practice to change medications if there is no symptom remission on the initial pharmaceutical tried. Again, the difference between clinical practice and research may lead to improved outcomes in the clinic over what is seen in research findings, and it is important for clinicians to note this difference in thinking about the treatment of their patients.

Third, remember that research studies require outcome data; with depression many researchers use the Hamilton Rating Scale for Depression (or HAM-D), or the Beck Depression Inventory (BDI). While these are valuable sources of information, with great clinical utility, we should keep in mind that no patient comes to the clinic requesting treatment to lower their BDI! Clinicians might wish to remain mindful of the quality of life of their patients (IsHak et al., 2011) and not focus solely on depression ratings. When evaluating research, it is good to examine if the research reports score reduction to below a predetermined cutoff score or if the study is examining overall reduction in scores. Of course, these scores combined with quality-of-life improvements are even better. A severely depressed patient who goes from a high HAM-D score to a moderate score may still be scoring in the "depressed" range, but the impact of treatment on quality of life could be rather large. Similarly in "mildly depressed" patients a score that drops from one point over to one point under the predetermined cutoff may have little impact on quality of life.

Finally, as is always the caveat in reviewing research, the exclusion criteria can result in studies on individuals who don't look like the patients that we may serve clinically. Often patients in research studies have a cleaner diagnostic picture, may be receiving services at no cost or a reduced cost, and efforts are made to control dropout that may not be feasible in clinical practice. At times it feels to us like the patients walking through our door bear little resemblance to those with whom a treatment was validated or assessed.

Such concerns notwithstanding, it is vital that the field of mental health continues to engage research questions and evaluate the growing body of evidence to ensure that we are providing the best care available to our treatment population.

Review of Depression Prevalence, Typical Course of Illness

According to the World Health Organization (WHO, 2016) an estimated 350 million people globally are affected by depression, with over 800,000 people dying from suicide. Less than half of those affected by depression receive formal treatment. In the US, major depressive disorder has a lifetime prevalence rate from 14.4% (Kessler, Petukhova, Sampson, Zaslavsky & Wittchen, 2012) to 17% (Kessler, Chiu, Demler, & Walters, 2005), indicating that approximately 15% of people will meet diagnostic criteria for major depressive disorder at some point in their lifetime.

Based on the Diagnostic and Statistical Manual of Mental Disorders, fifth edition (DSM-5) (American Psychiatric Association, 2013) the current diagnostic criteria for major depressive disorders are:

A) Five (or more) of the following symptoms have been present during the same 2-week period and represent a change from previous functioning; at least one of the symptoms is either a depressed mood or a loss of interest or loss of pleasure. Symptoms that are clearly attributable to another medical condition should not be included for the purpose of making a major depressive disorder diagnosis.
   1) Depressed mood most of the day, nearly every day, as indicated by either subjective report (e.g., feels sad, empty or hopeless) or observation made by others (e.g., appear tearful).
   2) Markedly diminished interest or pleasure in all, or almost all, activities most of the day, nearly every day (as indicated by either subjective account or observation).
   3) Significant weight loss when not dieting, or weight gain (e.g., a change of more than 5% of body weight in a month), or decrease or increase in appetite nearly every day.
   4) Insomnia or hypersomnia nearly every day.
   5) Psychomotor agitation or retardation nearly every day (observable by others, not merely subjective feelings of restlessness or being slowed down).
   6) Fatigue or loss of energy nearly every day.
   7) Feelings of worthlessness, or excessive/inappropriate guilt (which may be delusional) nearly every day (not merely self-reproach or guilt about being sick).
   8) Diminished ability to think or concentrate, or indecisiveness nearly every day (either by subjective account or as observed by others).
   9) Recurrent thoughts of death (not just fear of dying), recurrent suicidal ideation without a specific plan, or a suicide attempt or a specific plan for committing suicide.

B) The symptoms cause clinically significant distress or impairment in social, occupational, or other important areas of functioning.

C) The episode is not attributable to the physiological effects of a substance or to another medical condition.

D) The occurrence of the major depressive episode is not better explained by schizoaffective disorder, schizophrenia, schizophreniform disorder, delusional disorder, or other specified and unspecified schizophrenia spectrum disorders, or by other psychotic disorders.

E) There has never been a manic or hypomanic episode.

These diagnostic criteria essentially hold true for the International Classification of Diseases, 10th edition (ICD-10), which describes this diagnosis in the following way on its web-based reference resource designed to give current diagnostic ICD-10 criteria (www.icd10data.com):

- A disorder characterized by melancholic feelings of grief or unhappiness.
- A melancholy feeling of sadness and despair.

- A mental condition marked by ongoing feelings of sadness, despair, loss of energy, and difficulty dealing with normal daily life. Other symptoms of depression include feelings of worthlessness and hopelessness, loss of pleasure in activities, changes in eating or sleeping habits, and thoughts of death or suicide.
- Affective disorder marked by dysphoric mood, inactivity, lack of interest, insomnia, feelings of worthlessness, diminished ability to think, and thoughts of suicide.
- An affective disorder manifested by either a dysphoric mood or loss of interest or pleasure in usual activities. The mood disturbance is prominent and relatively persistent.
- Symptoms can include: sadness, loss of interest or pleasure in activities one used to enjoy, change in weight, difficulty sleeping or oversleeping, energy loss, feelings of worthlessness, thoughts of death or suicide.

Pharmacotherapy of Major Depressive Disorders

Historical Perspective

In the 1950s it was posited that the neurotransmitters known as monoamines were responsible for depression. This arose from the finding that patients treated with reserpine for hypertensive vascular disease developed depressive symptoms (Muller, Pryor, Gibbons, & Orgain, 1955). Once it was discovered that reserpine had an inhibitory effect of vesicular monoamine transporters, researchers began to wonder if depression could be ameliorated using medicines to boost monoamine availability. The first medications that were used to treat major depression were monoamine oxidase inhibitors (MAO-Is). This class of medication serves to inhibit the action of the enzyme that breaks down the monoamines serotonin, norepinephrine, and dopamine. The success of MAO-Is led to increased research and the development of tricyclic antidepressants (TCAs, so named due to the three benzene rings at their molecular core). Eventually, serotonin was identified as playing a significant role in depression, in part through postmortem studies that revealed decreased concentrations of serotonin in depression-related suicides (Shaw, Camps, & Eccleston, 1967). Research subsequently focused on the development of selective serotonin reuptake inhibitors (SSRIs), which are the most common antidepressant used today. The first SSRI, fluoxetine or Prozac, was approved by the Food and Drug Administration (FDA) for treatment of major depression in 1987.

The next class of medication discovered was the “atypical antidepressants” so named because they do not act directly on serotonin. The most prevalent of these is bupropion or Wellbutrin, which has its primary action on the dopamine reuptake, but also inhibits the reuptake of norepinephrine. Bupropion was initially approved by the FDA for the treatment of depression in 1989; other sustained release and extended release formulations have since been approved in 1996 and 2003, respectively.

A separate class of antidepressant medications is found in serotonin–norepinephrine reuptake inhibitors (SNRIs). Venlafaxine was the first of these approved by the FDA in 1993 for use in major depression. These medicines act to block the reuptake of both serotonin and norepinephrine. Some studies have indicated superior performance, however, the gains are modest (Papakostas, Thase, Fava, Neslon & Shelton, 2007; Stahl, Grady, Moret & Bradley, 2005) (see Chapter 5 for a comparison of the effectiveness of multiple antidepressant medications). For a more thorough review of the history of antidepressant medications, Hillhouse & Porter (2015) have an excellent article.

TCAs are still used periodically. They have, nonetheless, fallen out of favor due to the newer SSRIs' reduced side effect profile (Weihs & Wert, 2011). In addition, large doses of tricyclic antidepressants can be more lethal than the SSRIs; with TCAs there is an increased risk of overdose. On the other hand, MAO-Is can be very beneficial in the treatment of major depression, although their one rather large caveat is that they bond with the enzyme that breaks down other substances, and thus can lead to heightened levels of potentially toxic substances. Most significant among these is tyramine. The use of MAO-Is requires strict diet adherence, as potentially fatal levels of tyramine can occur if the patient consumes high levels of dairy or soy.

As mentioned above, SSRIs have enjoyed increased favor among prescribers and among insurance companies. This is largely due to their improved side effect profile, reduced risk of toxicity, and as patents expire, increased affordability. Most also only require once-daily dosing. Nevertheless, SNRIs have grown in use when SSRIs have produced suboptimal results in a given patient. Their dual system of action may make them more potent in the resolution of depressive symptoms, although the data are not entirely conclusive in this area.

Of the atypical antidepressants, bupropion is the most popular, likely due to having been on the market longer and also being used for a variety of concerns. Bupropion has been marketed for smoking cessation, under the brand name Zyban, and is also a potential first-line treatment for attention deficit hyperactivity disorder (ADHD). Vilazodone, one of the newer atypical antidepressant medications, works by not only selectively inhibiting serotonin reuptake, but also by acting as an agonist at the 5-HT1A receptor.

Pharmacotherapy carries an inherent risk of side effects. Most prominently, many of these medications currently carry a black box warning from the FDA stating that there is a risk of suicidality, particularly for males under 25 years of age. Many of these medications also have a high risk of sexual dysfunction, ranging from decrease in arousal to delayed orgasm.

Other potentially problematic risks include that of serotonin syndrome (especially with SSRIs) and prolonging the Q-T interval (especially with TCAs). Either of these two side effects is potentially life threatening. Reduced seizure threshold is a concern with bupropion, and should be avoided in patients with a history of seizure disorder or epilepsy. There is also a risk of developing Stevens–Johnson syndrome with many of the antidepressants.

The potential for adverse reactions with antidepressant medications may contribute to relatively high rates of dropout from pharmacotherapy. The dropout rates for pharmacotherapy are typically higher than for traditional psychotherapy (Gartlehner et al., 2016). Another drawback to pharmacotherapy is the number of medications that may be required to achieve symptom remission. In TAU conditions, patients are tried on three different medications on average before symptoms improve. This delay can be disheartening, and may lead to patient dropout. To date there are no good assessments to indicate which medicines will work best for different patients. There are treatment algorithms that indicate which types of antidepressant may be best for certain symptom constellations, but no test for response to a specific agent has been developed. That being said, there are guidelines (*VA/DoD Clinical Practice Guideline for the Management of Major Depressive Disorder*, Management of Major Depressive Disorder Working Group, 2016) which suggest that if a first-degree family member has a similar diagnosis and has responded well to a medication, there is an increased likelihood of response to the same agent in the new patient.

Comparisons Among Psychopharmacological Agents

When a new medication to treat depression is developed, and particularly a new drug that operates within a defined class of medications, there are a number of trials that the medicine undergoes. Willetts, Lippa, and Beer (1999) present a discussion of the development of one such medication, citalopram, and the various studies that went into proving the efficacy of the medication. The authors briefly discuss uncontrolled trials in which citalopram was shown to reduce scores on depression screeners for both short- and long-term use. They then turned to examining placebo-controlled trials, one of the more common types of trials, where patients are assigned to receive either an active medication or a placebo. In these trials, patients taking citalopram had significantly lower Hamilton Rating Scale for Depression (HAM-D) scores than did patients receiving the placebo. The differences were evident within the first week of treatment. The authors next reviewed a series of controlled trials in which citalopram is compared with other SSRIs that have a proven record of treating depression. Comparison with fluoxetine is provided as a demonstration of the results of such studies, which demonstrate that citalopram is "at least as effective as other SSRIs."

In a meta-analysis done by Montgomery (2001), a comparison was made between outcomes achieved with the SSRI paroxetine to those achieved with TCAs. The author found that across 39 studies paroxetine performed equally as well as did all TCAs in regards to depression reduction as measured on the HAM-D. Paroxetine did have a slight advantage over TCAs (excluding clomipramine) in reduction of the HAM-D anxiety factor score, but this was the only statistically significant difference among the medications as assessed by symptom improvement. The real benefit of paroxetine as compared to the TCAs came in the investigation of adverse reactions: the SSRI paroxetine had significantly lower instances of adverse effects than the TCAs. Additionally, the dropout rates due to adverse effects were higher among the TCAs than with paroxetine. It should be noted, however, that this difference was not statistically significant.

Another meta-analysis evaluated the speed of symptom remission in patients with depression and found that the atypical antidepressant mirtazapine had more rapid effects than SSRIs. Thase et al. (2010) examined 15 studies that compared mirtazapine to different SSRIs. The authors defined medication effect as any change on the assessment measures (the HAM-D-17 and the Montgomery–Asberg Depression Scale, MADRS). Depression remission was defined as HAM-D-17 (this version of the HAM-D only scores the first 17 items of the list of 21 items) score equal or below 7, or a MADRS score equal or below 12. Scores were evaluated at weeks 1, 2, 4, and 6 to assess the speed of change and or remission. The results of the meta-analysis revealed that patients in the mirtazapine groups showed faster response rates, and faster remission rates over the course of 6 weeks of treatment, when compared with SSRIs. The authors highlighted the fact that using mirtazapine gave patients a 74% higher probability of remission within 2 weeks. These authors did not specifically look at side effects or adverse events. Nevertheless, they found a higher dropout rate for patients in the mirtazapine conditions than the SSRI conditions with $p < .05$.

There are relatively few studies that provide head-to-head comparisons of medications. In one such study, Aberg-Wistedt, Agren, & Ekselius, Bengston, and Akerblad (2000) compared the two SSRIs, sertraline and paroxetine, over the course of 6 months of continuous treatment. This study randomly assigned 353 patients to either receive sertraline or paroxetine for the duration of 6 months. Of note in this study is the fact that the dosing was flexible (meaning that the treating provider could increase the dose of the medicine for initial nonresponders). The results of their study showed the best predictor of remission was an early response to the medication, regardless of which medication the patients were taking. They did find a slightly higher incidence of adverse events among patients in the paroxetine condition, but the overall results indicated that both medications were equally effective in the short term, and for long-term maintenance therapy.

Initial treatments, however, are frequently unsuccessful. Rush et al. (2004) found that 70% of patients did not achieve remission, and Trivedi et al. (2006) found that 50% of patients did not experience a treatment response, in both cases after an adequate trial of an SSRI. Faced with this data, Lenox-Smith and Jiang (2007) sought to compare the SNRI venlafaxine, extended release, with the SSRI citalopram as second-step agents in an RCT. A total of 406 patients who had failed a previous trial of an SSRI (not citalopram) were randomly assigned to receive either venlafaxine extended release (ER) or citalopram. The researchers initially found that the two medications were equivalent in their impact as a second-step treatment for major depression. There were no significant differences in the dropout rates due to adverse events. Upon secondary analysis, however, the researchers found that for patients with a higher HAM-D scores (over 31) venlafaxine was more effective than citalopram at 12 weeks. Scores on the HAM-D were statistically significantly lower in the venlafaxine condition.

In a pooled analysis of three studies involving a comparison of escitalopram with either venlafaxine or duloxetine (both SNRIs), Lam, Lohn, and Despiégel (2010) found that escitalopram had improved efficacy as a second-step agent after patients had failed a trial of an SSRI. These researchers also found that venlafaxine had a significantly higher dropout rate due to adverse events than did escitalopram. These results would seem to indicate that, taking dropout rate into account along with efficacy of treatment, escitalopram may be more beneficial than switching to an SNRI, when used as a second trial treatment.

Research studies have yet to yield unequivocal results, and it remains difficult to determine which medicines would be most effective as a first- or even second-line treatment. Some research has suggested that all of the SSRIs are equally effective (Kroenke, West, & Swindle, 2001), while others have found that there may be some differences (Montgomery et al., 2007). In a review of antidepressant literature, Montgomery et al. (2007) evaluated the available evidence of medication superiority. These reviewers enumerated the three classes of evidence they categorized studies into: Class A evidence included studies from an RCT that showed, under fair comparison conditions, a significant advantage for one medication over another, noting that the evidence is more persuasive if the size of the study is comparable to studies needed to find a difference from placebo. Drugs that had two positive RCTs were considered to have demonstrated "definite superiority." Class B evidence demonstrated superiority of a medication over another in a meta-analysis that includes head-to-head RCTs. If there was consistent evidence from more than one meta-analysis, this was deemed evidence of "probable superiority." If there were one positive class A study paired with one positive class B study the authors deemed this evidence of "definite superiority." Class C evidence was evidence from uncontrolled trials, or RCTs that did not meet the class A criteria. These studies were considered hypothesis-generating studies, and were deemed evidence of "possible superiority." Based on these criteria the authors identified several medications that were deemed "definitely superior" for the treatment of depression. These medications were: clomipramine, venlafaxine, and escitalopram. Escitalopram was also the only medication that the authors found to have evidence of "definite superiority" for the treatment of severe depression, with venlafaxine having "probable superiority" in treating severe depression.

Psychosocial Treatments of Major Depressive Disorder

Behavioral therapy involves the therapist and patient focusing on the behaviors that the patient is engaging in. In this type of therapy the provider develops behavioral homework and activation exercises for the patient to engage in. There is little to no focus on the thought processes that underlie the behavior.

Psychodynamic systems of therapy focus on internal psychic conflicts. The theory behind psychodynamic therapy is derived from the work of Freud and postulates that when there are competing intra-psychic drives that are incompatible with one another the result is the outward presentation of psychological symptoms. The therapy focuses on resolving these intra-psychic conflicts, which is believed to then resolve the external expression of the conflict.

Cognitive-behavioral therapy (CBT) is perhaps one of the most researched forms of therapy. This particular practice grew out of the work of Aaron Beck. Beck focused on the cognitions that a patient may have that led to emotional responses. He postulated that individuals had basic core beliefs about themselves, which in the case of depression are negative, enduring beliefs. This leads to intermediate beliefs that impact attitudes, rules, and assumptions. The most surface level of these beliefs are automatic thoughts, which are brief transient images or thoughts that often go unrecognized, but which have consequences for the feelings and behavior of the individual. In this system of therapy the provider combines an analysis of the patient's thoughts and beliefs with behaviors designed to engage and alter those thoughts and behaviors.

While CBT is highly researched, it can also be difficult to assess what form it is taking in various research articles. Several systems of therapy have adopted the overarching umbrella of CBT. It is incumbent on the practitioner to evaluate the research critically to determine if research addresses CBT as theory, or is examining a specific form or modality of CBT, which may or may not be generalizable to the field at large.

Interpersonal therapy (IPT) is a system of therapy that focuses on how life events and interpersonal roles impact mood. The therapeutic technique encourages the patient to alter problematic relationships and roles that the patient has adopted in order to alleviate depressive symptoms.

Psychotherapy, in general has a lower incidence of side effects or iatrogenic impact than do pharmacological interventions (Gartlehner et al., 2016). That is not to say that there is no incidence of negative outcomes from psychotherapy. There have been instances of iatrogenic impact from some forms of therapy, most notably, "rebirthing" therapy for attachment disorders has been tied to significant psychological harm (Lilienfeld, 2007; O'Donohue & Engle, 2013).

While psychotherapy does have a lower incidence of dropout rates when compared to psychotropic treatment in research studies (a meta-analysis by Gartlehner et al., 2016, found that for second-generation antidepressants discontinuation was nearly twice as likely due to adverse events as compared to any psychological treatment), there is still patient dropout in studies of psychotherapy.

Comparisons Among Various Psychotherapeutic Approaches

While there is a variety of therapeutic approaches, knowing how these various techniques compare can be highly beneficial in determining which approaches have the best outcomes for patients. Even among the overarching categories presented earlier there exist variations that fall within each category, which can involve specific technical applications, or even the mode of delivery (i.e., telephonic therapy vs. individual therapy vs. group therapy).

Hans and Hiller (2013) took an interesting approach to this question by conducting a meta-analysis to evaluate the effectiveness of CBT delivered in both group and individual settings, and then benchmarking their effectiveness against RCTs of other types of intervention, again in both group and individual delivery systems. The authors based their evaluation on efficacy evaluations using Seligman's (1995) differentiation as a road map. Seligman had posited the operational definition that "efficacy studies" were well-controlled RCTs with strict exclusion criteria, high therapist fidelity to a treatment protocol, therapists trained for the purpose of delivering the treatment in the study, and a well-defined number of sessions. Conversely, effectiveness studies involved more "real-world" conditions with flexible use of a protocol, no set number of sessions, no assessment of therapist adherence, and no specific therapist training for the study. The results indicated that both for group and individual CBT there were statistically significant effect sizes indicating that both types of therapy reduced depression severity. When Hans and Hiller benchmarked these results against efficacy studies, however, the efficacy studies had much larger effect sizes. For example, in an effectiveness meta-analysis, CBT delivered individually had an overall effect size of $d = 1.12$, while an efficacy study where cognitive therapy and behavioral activation were used the effect size $d = 2.22$. Similar results were found for the group therapy format. In addition Hans and Hiller found higher dropout rates from effectiveness studies than from efficacy studies. One benefit of this meta-analysis is the finding that CBT can be transported to clinical practice with positive outcomes. The attempt to benchmark against other therapies, however, falls short as there are many potential confounds in this comparison, which the authors freely admit. In this sense, the study is not as beneficial as a true "head-to-head study" where therapies are compared within one study, and subject to identical constraints.

In a different study that attempted to compare treatment types using RCT procedures, Kramer, Roten, Perry, and Despland (2013) sought to compare psychoanalysis, psychodynamic psychotherapy, cognitive therapy, and clinical management, on their respective ability to mitigate depressive symptoms. Their study was only a pilot intended to prove the ability to conduct a larger study at a later point, and so the sample size was very small (eight total patients) and the duration of therapy was quite extensive, 2 years of treatment for all conditions. The results indicated that for each type of therapy one patient had significant gains while the other did not (there were two patients in each condition). One notable aspect was that the measures of coping and defensive functioning (typically constructs more related to psychodynamic treatments than CBT) showed improvement along the same pattern as the depression ratings from the HAM-D. Also notable in this comparison was the dosing of treatment. Psychoanalysis was delivered three times a week for 2 years, the psychodynamic psychotherapy was delivered twice per week for 2 years, while CBT was delivered once per week over 2 years. While this particular study does not produce results that will help to differentiate between how effective each therapy was in treating depression, it does help to elucidate the difficulties in comparing therapies within the same study. Many CBT studies limit therapy to a number of sessions far below the 2 years provided, while for psychoanalysis this time frame is not uncommon. This difference alone can make head-to-head comparisons difficult.

An attempt at comparing CBT head-to-head with other forms of therapy is found in the meta-analysis conducted by Cuijpers, van Straten, Andersson, & van Oppen (2008), who noted that despite several other meta-analyses finding CBT to be a superior treatment for depression (e.g., Gloaguen, Cottraux, Cucherat, & Blackburn, 1998) further scrutiny revealed that therapeutic benefits were reduced when compared with high-quality treatments that had not been explicitly designed as a control condition (Wampold, Minami, Baskin, & Callen Tierney, 2002). Cuijpers et al. (2008) examined seven different types of therapy, which included CBT, nondirective supportive therapy, behavioral activation therapy, psychodynamic therapy, problem-solving therapy, interpersonal psychotherapy, and social skills training through a meta-analysis of 53 studies. When comparing these studies the authors found that a majority of the treatments did not have statistically different effect sizes. The notable exceptions to this were nondirective supportive therapy, which had a significantly ($p < .05$) smaller effect size, and interpersonal therapy, which was showed to be significantly more efficacious. Meta-analysis at follow up, however, did not indicate a significant difference between any of the treatments. The only other difference between the seven types of therapies was a higher dropout rate for CBT than for the other types of therapy.

Examination of the studies included in the meta-analysis shows some interesting considerations. First, and most notably, some of the studies focused on narrow groups; for example "Behavioral treatment of depression in dementia patients" (Teri, Logsdon, Uomoto, & McCurry, 1997). And, several studies included only HIV positive patients, or only patients with low socio-economic status, etc. It could certainly be argued that narrowly focused studies, even when combined with studies that are more representative of the general population, could have an unknown impact on the overall outcome. Conversely, taking samples that include only subgroups that would often be excluded from "general population" samples serves to round out the representation of patients that may actually present in the clinical setting, which, after all, is what the practicing clinician will find relevant.

In an RCT examining the impact of cognitive therapy, behavioral activation, and antidepressant medication on relapse rates, Dobson et al. (2008) found that cognitive therapy and behavioral activation had a positive impact on reducing relapse, or future instances of depression, while antidepressants only had that effect when they were continued. The authors noted that at 1-year follow up the cost of continued medication management was higher than the overall cost of either type of therapy. They did not, however, find any statistically significant differences between the two types of therapy.

Wampold et al. (1997) compared only "bona fide" psychotherapies, and included only studies that involved direct comparisons of two or more therapies. The authors posit that often therapies are compared against other "treatments" that do not actually contain an active therapy component and are, in effect, placebo control groups. Their meta-analysis found that the actual effect size difference between "bona fide" therapies is zero. They note that when their data are compared with data from meta-analyses that do include these other "non-therapies" the effect sizes of other studies are about double what Wampold et al. found. Wampold and colleagues do not suggest that therapeutic approaches are ineffective, but rather that bona fide therapies do not significantly differ from one another. Thus the conclusion is that therapy works, but which kind of therapy is nearly irrelevant.

Building on this idea, Laska, Gurman, and Wampold (2014) present data on a "common factors approach" to therapy. The authors believe that common factors have become viewed as nonscientific and have not been adequately studied. They identify five factors that make up the common factors approach: (1) an emotionally charged bond between therapist and patient, (2) a confiding healing setting in which therapy takes place, (3) a therapist who provides a psychologically derived and culturally embedded explanation for emotional distress, (4) an explanation that is adaptive (provides believable options for overcoming the difficulties) and is accepted by the patient, and (5) a set of procedures engaged in by the patient and therapist that lead the patient to enact something that is positive, helpful, or adaptive (Frank & Frank, 1993; Wampold, 2001). Throughout their article the authors suggest that no single therapy is more effective than another, and that many of the studies that indicate this have flaws. Their analysis, built on the previous findings of Wampold et al. (1997), suggests that there is much more to therapy than learning an approach or following a protocol. The authors do not discuss the implications for medication, but given evidence on placebo (Carlino et al., 2012), and nocebo effect (Colloca & Miller, 2011), it is likely that common factors may play a role in pharmacological interventions as well.

Combined Treatment of Major Depressive Disorder

Happily, there is a large volume of research focused on various methods for combining psychotherapy and pharmacological intervention in the treatment of major depression.

Based on a review, Huhn et al. (2014) found that in general the literature favored pharmacotherapy slightly in the acute phase of a major depressive disorder, but that psychotherapy had a larger advantage when assessing for relapse. These findings may also help to explain that when combined therapy was examined (again looking at meta-analyses of treatment for depression), the studies reviewed evidenced favor for combined therapy over monotherapy. This was true whether combined treatment was pharmacotherapy added to a regimen of psychotherapy, or psychotherapy added to a regimen of pharmacotherapy. In either condition, effects were similarly in magnitude. The greatest weakness of this article is that the authors do not differentiate between types of pharmacotherapy or psychotherapy. So while the evidence is helpful in arguing the merits of combined treatments, there certainly isn't evidence of which type of each was used.

Several meta-analyses have been done to examine the impact of combined treatment (Cuijpers, Dekker, Hollon, & Andersson, 2009 Cuijpers, van Straten, Hollon, & Andersson, 2010) on major depressive disorder. These meta-analyses have looked at the question of combined therapy in several different ways. In one review (Cuijpers et al., 2009), which involved a total of 25 studies that utilized RCTs, the authors examined effect sizes of differences seen between pharmacotherapy as a monotherapy and combined pharmacotherapy and psychotherapy. The 25 studies included involved a total of 2,036 patients, and the synthesized data resulted in a mean effect size of d = 0.31, in favor of combined therapy. The authors note that this difference represented a small favoring of combined treatments over pharmacotherapy alone. They also noted that when looking at treatments for patients with dysthymia the effect sizes were much lower than for those targeting only major depressive disorder.

Cuijpers et al. (2009) also examined studies that compared psychotherapy alone to combined psychotherapy and pharmacotherapy. This meta-analysis examined a total of 18 studies comprising 1,838 participants. This meta-analysis again found a small to moderate overall effect size of d = 0.35. The authors then sought to determine if this impact was clinically relevant by examining the binomial effect size, and they found that success rates increased from .41 to .59, indicating that there may be an added benefit of combined therapy over psychotherapy. There were some significant limitations and drawbacks to this meta-analysis. The most salient was the authors' decision to include studies of highly specific subpopulations (e.g., two studies involved adults who were HIV positive, one included only patients with multiple sclerosis, one was only patients with generic "chronic" depression, and one study only included older adults).

Another meta-analysis of combined therapy examined the difference between psychotherapy combined with placebo, and psychotherapy combined with an active agent. This meta-analysis (Cuijpers et al., 2010) highlights an important element missing in previous meta-analyses in that when comparing psychotherapy or pharmacotherapy with combined treatments it is impossible to maintain even a single blind condition as the participants know when they are receiving psychotherapy and when combined treatments. The addition of a placebo allows at a minimum the potential for a single blind where participants do not know if they are receiving only psychotherapy or psychotherapy plus medication. This meta-analysis combined the results of 16 studies involving a total of 852 patients. The results of the study indicated that overall treatment was beneficial for both conditions with an effect size of d = 1.73, but the overall effect of an active agent versus placebo was only d = 0.25. While the use of a placebo would allow for at least a single blind, only 14 studies reported explicitly that participants were blind, 12 reported that assessors did not know what condition the participants were in, and a mere five reported that assignment to conditions was completed by an independent party. This meta-analysis again included several studies that were aimed at specific subpopulations. Specifically, of the 16, only six were aimed at adults in general, four focused on adults with a general medical condition (e.g. HIV, multiple sclerosis, and coronary disease), four involved patients who were dual diagnosed with a co-morbid substance use disorder, and the last two studies focused on older adults who had lost their spouse, and women with postpartum depression. The results favored, although only slightly, the combination of an active pharmacological agent and psychotherapy over placebo paired with psychotherapy.

In a separate study (IsHak et al., 2011) an attempt was made to examine not just treatment outcomes, but quality-of-life measures between psychotherapy, pharmacotherapy, and combined treatment. While the authors did not actually perform a meta-analysis, they conducted a review of multiple studies that assessed quality of life and found that the remission of depressive symptoms, through medication, psychotherapy, and combined treatments, all led to improvements in quality of life. The authors reviewed six studies of psychotherapy as a monotherapy, 23 studies of medication as monotherapy, and eight studies of combined treatment. While the review presents helpful information in regard to assessing quality of life and ensuring that improvements on depression rating scales are actually meaningful in the patient's life, only three of the studies actually performed any type of "head-to-head" comparisons. All three demonstrated that combined therapy was associated with a statistically significant higher quality of life than in pharmacotherapy alone. Again the review demonstrates a need for more research on combined therapies to ascertain the degree of improvement that may or may not be gained from combined therapies; still, the initial results continue to be positive in favor of combining psychotherapy with pharmacotherapy.

In a 2007 study, Ludman, Simon, Tutty, and Von Korff examined whether adding a CBT tele-therapy protocol to TAU for patients receiving psychotropic therapy for depression from their primary care clinic would improve outcomes (Ludman et al., 2007). They found that participants who had been assigned to the phone therapy group had significantly lower scores on the Hopkins Symptom Checklist (HSCL) over the course of treatment, and were able to maintain lower scores at an 18-month follow up. While the differences at follow up were not statistically significant, the researchers found that participants in the combined treatment conditions were statistically significantly more likely to describe themselves as "much improved" or "very much improved" over the medication-only patients. The results of this study indicate that the addition of even a tele-mental health protocol as a form of combined therapy can have a significant impact on the improvement of patients and, perhaps more strikingly, on their perception of how improved they are. As it has increasingly become the case that patients with major depressive disorder seek treatment from their primary care providers, it is helpful to look at how therapies that are specifically adjunct to this context can be beneficial beyond care as usual.

The timing of adding psychotherapy, and specifically a CBT protocol, to a medication regimen was studied by Rizvi and colleagues (Rizvi, Zaretsky, Schaffer & Levitt, 2015). Approximately 90% of patients were already receiving pharmacotherapy, and those who were not were initiated on pharmacotherapy (the various agents used were either SSRIs, SNRIs, or bupropion). Participants were then randomly assigned to either receive CBT immediately, or were placed on a wait list for 6 months and then received CBT. At the conclusion of treatment, CBT patients were followed for 12 months. The researchers found that during the active treatment phase both groups experienced reductions in BDI scores that were not significantly different from each other (the immediate group scores during CBT and the delayed group scores from 6 months later who were in the active treatment phase). The authors noted that the immediate group had lower scores during follow up, but this difference was only statistically significant during the 10th month of follow up. When the researchers compared the immediate group to only those in the delayed group who were still experiencing a depressive episode, the magnitude of change was significantly better for the immediate group. These results may suggest that patients with a more enduring depression benefit from earlier intervention, or it may be an indication that enduring depression is more resistant to treatment. Noteworthy is the fact that the authors found that overall the BDI scores of the immediate treatment were lower than for the delayed treatment group, which lends support to the notion that greater levels of improvement are attained when treatment is immediately available.

Manber et al. (2008) found that remission from depressive symptoms occurred significantly more rapidly with a combined therapy than in either psychotherapy or pharmacotherapy administered as a monotherapy. The authors did not find a significant difference between the two monotherapies. In addition they found that the combined therapy condition had a significantly larger proportion of patients experiencing symptom remission. The authors used archival data to examine the Keller et al. (2000) study in which patients were randomly assigned to receive either nefazodone, a course of psychotherapy (cognitive behavioral analysis system of psychotherapy or CBASP), or a combined condition involving both. They found that in the medication-only condition 14.2% of patients attained symptom remission, while in the CBASP-only condition 13.9% of patients achieved remission, and in the combined-medication–CBASP condition 28.9% of patients achieved remission. The differences proved to be statistically significant. They also found that time to remission was less for patients in the combined condition, while the two monotherapy groups were not significantly different in time to remission. Finally, the authors conducted a secondary or exploratory analysis to determine if there were characteristics of patients that led to improved outcomes in any of the three treatment conditions. What they found was that for patients in combination therapy there were significantly improved outcomes for those who had low levels of depression, and for those who had high levels of depression with low levels of anxiety; patients who had high levels of depression *and* high levels of anxiety showed less favorable results. In both of the monotherapies there were no significant differences between any of the identified subgroups.

In another analysis of the same data set (data from Keller et al. 2000), Stulz, Thase, Klein, Manber, and Christoph (2010) examined in greater depth the notion of subgroups within the study. While the treatment conditions were similar with regard to the level of depressive symptoms, participants in each treatment condition were separated into "low," "moderate," and "severe" with regard to the level of depression symptoms. The authors plotted scores for each of the three groups within the three treatment conditions (CBASP, nefazodone, and combined treatment) across the 12 weeks of the study. The authors then used a slope regression analysis to compare the results. They found that there was a significantly steeper negative slope (ratings of depression symptoms reduced faster) in the combined therapy condition than in either of the monotherapy conditions (which did not differ from each other significantly) in both the low and moderate depressive symptom subgroups. For patients with severe levels of depression symptoms there was no significant difference between any of the treatment conditions.

One of the largest studies undertaken in recent years to evaluate treatments for depression was the Sequenced Treatment Alternatives to Relieve Depression (STAR*D) Study. The STAR*D was a 7-year study that evaluated various treatment modalities over a course of time progressing through four levels of treatment. At each level of treatment if patients became asymptomatic they were placed into a 12-month follow up program to assess duration of improvement. Level 1 of the study involved placing patients on citalopram (Celexa) for 12–14 weeks. The study began with 4,041 participants, but after exclusion criteria were applied 2,876 participants entered level 1. Of those individuals 1,439 did not become symptom free and were moved into the level 2 portion of the study. In level 2, patients were given the option to switch from citalopram to another treatment, either a different medication or cognitive therapy (CT), or to augment the citalopram with either another medication or CT. Of the sample, 147 elected to either switch to CT or augment citalopram with CT. Of those patients, 25% who switched to CT alone became symptom free, and 23% of those who augmented became symptom free. These results were not significantly different from patients who were in medication-only paths in level 2 (i.e., patients who either switched to another medication or augmented citalopram with another medication). Of note, researchers found that those in the CT augmentation group took longer (55 days) for symptom remission than those who chose medication augmentation (26 days). The CT-only group was not significantly different from those who switched to a new medication in time to remission, but the authors note that they were spared the side effects experienced by those who switched to another medication. Some of the limitations of the STAR*D, when used to compare psychotherapy with medication or combination treatments, include: (1) patients had no option regarding the initial treatment tried: all were given an SSRI. (2) The evaluation between and among different types of therapy was only for patients who had already "failed" a trial of medication and were deemed "non-responders." These limitations make it difficult to assess the role of therapy and combined treatments on the general population. Adding to this, the number of patients electing to undergo psychotherapy was relatively small when compared with the total number of participants in the study.

Conclusions

The literature presented and reviewed in this chapter indicates a strong rationale for combined treatments. In addition, many of the findings point to the merits of combined treatment early, as this may lead to faster and more complete remission; in this vein, a case can be made for the cost effectiveness of combined treatments. Given the weight of the evidence, a reasonable recommendation would be to initiate both pharmacotherapy and psychotherapy as soon after a diagnosis is made as possible.

Of course the therapist must also take into account the patient's desires and beliefs in what will be beneficial for treating his or her depression. This is one of the most striking absences in the literature. Even with scores of studies comparing psychotherapy, medication, and combined therapies, few studies have evaluated patient preference and how that might impact outcomes. When patients are randomly assigned to a condition that they do not believe will be beneficial, what is the impact on outcomes? Patient choice is a vital part of what practitioners in the field must navigate in electing and implementing treatments and, yet, in the literature it is treated as though randomization will cancel out the effects. While this may be true in large, high powered studies, for the patient sitting in front of us, his/her preference is not an artifact but a matter of autonomy and an essential ingredient that promotes involvement in a collaborative relationship.

Table 3.1 summarizes our findings and conclusions.

Final Observations

Many prescriptions for antidepressant medications are written by primary care physicians. It is common for the patients receiving these therapies to not be involved in any type of psychotherapy despite evidence in the literature suggesting that combining efforts may lead to faster and greater improvements over time. When patients are provided with CBT at the time they are diagnosed and started on medication the outcomes are better. If CBT is used as an adjunct only after medicine has failed to bring about full symptom resolution the outcomes are still present, but less impressive.

Providers, especially those who have the first contact with a patient regarding complaints of major depression, need to be mindful of the expectations of their patients.

Table 3.1 Integrative biopsychosocial intervention with major depressive disorders: Summary of best-practice recommendations by level of confidence derived from strength of evidence.

Major depressive disorder—mild		
Level A	Recommended	• Talk therapy should be the primary intervention • Cognitive behavioral therapy (CBT), cognitive therapy (CT) and interpersonal therapy (IPT) have been well researched
Level B	Suggested	• If talk therapy is not feasible, a selective serotonic reuptake inhibitor (SSRI) may be considered • Bupropion may also be an option
Level C	May be considered	• Consider serotonin norepinephrine reuptake inhibitors (SNRIs), if SSRIs have been unsuccessful • Polypharmacy—augmenting bupropion with an SSRI
Major depressive disorder—moderate		
Level A	Recommended	• Combined medication and talk therapy is preferred starting point • If a combined approach is not available, talk therapy and pharmacotherapy are both first-line monotherapies
Level B	Suggested	• SNRIs, tricyclic antidepressants (TCAs), monoamine oxidase inhibitor (MAO-I) • Polypharmacy—augmenting with an additional SSRI or combining bupropion with an SSRI
Level C	May be considered	• Stimulants
Major depressive disorder—severe without psychotic features		
Level A	Recommended	• CBT, CT, IPT • SSRIs and SNRIs • Bupropion
Level B	Suggested	• Combined therapy—talk therapy with pharmaceutical intervention • Polypharmacy
Level C	May be considered	• Stimulant medication
Major depressive disorder—severe with psychotic features		
Level A	Recommended	• SSRI/SNRI augmented with aripiprazole
Level B	Suggested	• Combined CBT and pharmacotherapy • Electroconvulsive therapy (ECT) • TCAs
Level C	May be considered	• Other atypical antipsychotics

If primary care providers give reasonably positive expectations for therapy, treatment is more likely to be effective. Conversely, if a patient has an unrealistic expectation about how well or how fast an intervention will work, the patient is more likely to be disappointed. Aside from traditional therapeutic techniques, this effort of managing a patient's expectations may be one of the greatest contributions the clinician can make.

Illustrative Case Studies

Mrs. D, a 26-year-old female, came into the clinic reporting a depressed mood, weight gain, and loss of interest in pleasurable activities. She was also having difficulty concentrating at work and experienced feelings of worthlessness. She initially saw a psychologist for her intake appointment. Approximately half way through the intake she stopped the therapist (who had yet to offer an intervention) and told him "I have tried all of this therapy stuff and it doesn't work for me. I really just want to start meds." Mrs. D persisted in her request for medication, and so after completion of the intake and diagnostic interview the provider referred her to a prescribing psychologist.

The prescribing provider explained to Mrs. D that, while they could pursue a course of medication, there were numerous strategies that could be used to evaluate the effectiveness of the medicine, some of which could also be considered therapeutic interventions. She was agreeable to this, and so a course of escitalopram was started at 10 mg. During this same period, Mrs. D was asked to complete CT's ABC sheets, which related events to her beliefs and resulting emotional impact. She was also asked to engage in physical activities and rate the ease with which she was able to engage in these activities. Therapy subsequently focused on social outings and engaging in previously pleasurable activities, both as part of a course of therapy and to evaluate the impact that the medicine was having on her quality of life. The patient reported symptom remission within 8 weeks.

This case illustrates the benefits that can be earned by gaining "buy-in" from the patient, while acknowledging the patient's right to autonomy, and to participate voluntarily in the treatment planning. Recognizing her preference for medication while obtaining her agreement to participate in monitoring the results of treatment allowed for adding CBT methods that she would not have agreed to from the start, and which would have likely failed had her needs not been addressed and her agreement sought in all recommendations.

Mr. M was a 35-year-old male who had a history of prior depressive episodes and came to the clinic when he was having an additional bout of depression that was hindering his ability to engage in activities that he wanted to. Specifically, he had started to have difficulties at work and was also falling behind on academics (he was working full time and pursuing a Master's degree). He had been on sertraline previously with good results, and so we agreed to reinitiate this medicine and also start a course of CBT. Over the course of treatment he did not evidence improvement, and so sertraline was switched to venlafaxine, but he continued to struggle and to have a hard time completing even the most basic CBT homework. Given the unremitting severity of his condition, we agreed to initiate a trial of aripiprazole as an adjunct to the venlafaxine.

Over the course of the next 2 weeks his mood and energy levels improved dramatically, despite the medicine causing some fatigue in the hours after the patient took it. He began engaging in the therapy homework, as well as in his course work, and was also able to improve his performance at work. We agreed to withdraw the aripiprazole after 90 days, and he continued to do well and was able to evidence improvement through his involvement in sessions and through his use of CBT techniques.

References

Aberg-Wistedt, A., Agren, H., Ekselius, L., Bengston, F., & Akerblad, A. (2000). Sertraline versus paroxetine in major depression: Clinical outcome after six months of continuous therapy. *Journal of Clinical Psychopharmacology, 20,* 645–652.

American Psychiatric Association (2013). *Diagnostic and Statistical Manual of Mental Disorders* (5th ed.). Arlington, VA: American Psychiatric Association.

Barnett, J. E., & Neel, M. L. (2000). Must all psychologists study psychopharmacology? *Professional Psychology: Research and Practice, 31,* 619–627.

Bauer, M., Pfennig, A., Linden, M., Smolka, M. N., Neu, P., & Adli, M. (2009). Efficacy of an algorithm-guided treatment compared with treatment as usual: A randomized, controlled study of inpatients with depression. *Journal of Clinical Psychopharmacology, 29,* 327–333.

Bauer, M., Whybrow, P., Angst, J., Versiani, M., Möller, H. J., & WFSBP Task Force on Treatment Guidelines for Unipolar Depressive Disorders (2002). World Federation of Societies of Biological Psychiatry (WFSBP) guidelines for biological treatment of unipolar depressive disorders, Part 1: Acute and continuation treatment of major depressive disorder. *World Journal of Biological Psychiatry, 3,* 69–89.

Carlino, E., Pollo, A., & Benedeti, F. (2012). The placebo in practice: How to use it in clinical routine. *Supportive and Palliative Care, 6,* 220–225.

Colloca, L., & Miller, F. G. (2011). The nocebo effect and its relevance for clinical practice. *Psychosomatic Medicine, 73,* 598–603.

Cuijpers, P., Dekker, J., Hollon, S. D., & Andersson, G. (2009). Adding psychotherapy to pharmacotherapy in the treatment of depressive disorders in adults: a meta-analysis. *Journal of Clinical Psychiatry, 70,* 1219–1229.

Cuijpers, P., van Straten, A., Andersson, G., & van Oppen, P. (2008). Psychotherapy for depression in adults: a meta-analysis of comparative outcome studies. *Journal of Consulting and Clinical Psychology, 76,* 909–922.

Cuijpers, P., van Straten, A., Hollon, S. D., & Andersson, G. (2010). The contribution of active medication to combined treatments of psychotherapy and pharmacotherapy for adult depression: A meta-analysis. *Acta Psychiatrica Scandinavica, 121,* 415–423.

Dobson, K. S., Hollon, S. D., Dimidjian, S., Schmaling, K. B., Kohlenberg, R. J., Gallop, R. J., . . . & Gollan, J. K. (2008). randomized trial of behavioral activation, cognitive therapy, and antidepressant medication in the prevention of relapse and recurrence in major depression. *Journal of Consulting and Clinical Psychology, 76,* 568–577.

Frank, J. D., & Frank, J. (1993). *Persuasion and healing: A comparative study of psychotherapy.* Baltimore, MA: Johns Hopkins Press.

Gartlehner, G., Gaynes, B. N., Amick, H. R., Asher, G. N., Morgan, L. C., Coker-Schwimmer, E., . . . & Lohr, K. N. (2016). Comparative benefits and harms of antidepressant, psychological, complementary, and exercise treatments for major depression: An evidence report for a clinical practice guideline from the American College of Physicians. *Annals of Internal Medicine, 164,* 331–342.

Gloaguen, V., Cottraux, J., Cucherat, M., & Blackburn, I. M. (1998). A meta-analysis of the effects of cognitive therapy in depressed patients. *Journal of Affective Disorders, 49,* 59–72.

Hans, E., & Hiller, W. (2013). Effectiveness of and dropout from outpatient cognitive behavioral therapy for adult unipolar depression: A meta-analysis of nonrandomized effectiveness studies. *Journal of Consulting and Clinical Psychology, 81,* 75–88.

Hillhouse, T. M., & Porter, J. H. (2015). A brief history of the development of antidepressant drugs: From monoamines to glutamate. *Experimental and Clinical Psychopharmacology, 23*, 1–21.

Huhn, M., Tardy, M., Spineli, L. M., Kissling, W., Forstl, H., Pitschel-Walz, G., . . . & Leucht, S. (2014). Efficacy of pharmacotherapy and psychotherapy for adult psychiatric disorders: A systematic overview of meta-analyses. *JAMA Psychiatry, 71*, 706–715.

IsHak, W. W., Ha, K., Kapitanski, N., Bagot, K., Fathy, H., Swanson, B., Vilhauer, J., . . . & Rapaport, M., H. (2011). The impact of psychotherapy, pharmacotherapy, and their combination on the quality of life in depression. *Harvard Review Psychiatry, 19*, 277–289.

Keller, M., McCullough, J., Klein, D., Arnow, B., Dunner, D., . . . & Zajecka, J. (2000). A comparison of nefazodone, the cognitive behavioral-analysis system of psychotherapy, and their combination for the treatment of chronic depression. *New England Journal of Medicine, 342*, 1462–1470.

Kessler, R., Chiu, W., Demler, O., & Walters, E. (2005). Prevalence, severity, and comorbidity of twelve-month DSM-IV disorders in the national comorbidity survey replication (NCS-R). *Archives of General Psychiatry, 62*, 617–627.

Kessler, R. C., Petukhova, M., Sampson, N. A., Zaslavsky, A. M., & Wittchen, H. U. (2012). Twelve-month and lifetime prevalence and lifetime morbid risk of anxiety and mood disorders in the United States. *International Journal of Methods in Psychiatric Research, 21*, 169–184.

Kramer, U., Roten, Y., Perry, C., & Despland, J. (2013). Change in defense mechanisms and coping patterns during the course of a 2-year-long psychotherapy and psychoanalysis for recurrent depression: A pilot study of a randomized controlled trial. *Journal of Nervous and Mental Disease, 201*, 614–620.

Kroenke, K., West, S., & Swindle, R. (2001). Similar effectiveness of paroxetine, fluoxetine, and sertraline in primary care: A randomized trial. *JAMA, 286*, 2947–2955.

Lam, R. W., Lohn, S. L., Despiégel, N. (2010). Escitalopram versus serotonin noradrenaline reuptake inhibitors as second step treatment for patients with major depressive disorder: A pooled analysis. *International Clinical Psychopharmacology, 25*, 199–203.

Laska, K. M., Gurman, A. S., & Wampold, B. E. (2014). Expanding the lens of evidence-based practice in psychotherapy: A common factors perspective. *Psychotherapy, 51*, 467–481.

Lenox-Smith, A. J., & Jiang, Q. (2008). Venlafaxine extended release versus citalopram in patients with depression unresponsive to a selective serotonin reuptake inhibitor. *International Clinical Psychopharmacology, 23*, 113–119.

Lilienfeld, S. O. (2007). Psychological treatments that cause harm. *Perspectives on Psychological Science, 2*, 53–70.

Ludman, E. J., Simon, G. E., Tutty, S., & Von Korff, M. (2007). A randomized trial of telephone psychotherapy and pharmacotherapy for depression: Continuation and durability effects. *Journal of Consulting and Clinical Psychology, 75*, 257–266.

Management of Major Depressive Disorder Working Group (2016). *VA/DoD clinical practice guideline for the management of major depressive disorder, version 3.0—2016.* Washington, DC: US Government Printing Office.

Manber, R., Kraemer, H. C., Arnow, B. A., Triveldi, M. H., Rush, A. J., Thase, M. E., . . . & Keller, M. E. (2008). Faster remission of chronic depression with combined psychotherapy and medication than with each therapy alone. *Journal of Consulting and Clinical Psychology, 76*, 459–467.

Montgomery, S. A. (2001). A meta-analysis of the efficacy and tolerability of paroxetine versus tricyclic antidepressants in the treatment of major depression. *International Clinical Psychopharmacology, 16*, 169–178.

Montgomery, S. A., Baldwin, D. S., Blier, P., Fineberg, N. A., Kasper, S., Lader, M., . . . & Thase, M. E. (2007). Which antidepressants have demonstrated superior efficacy? A review of the evidence. *International Clinical Psychopharmacology, 22*, 323–329.

Muller, J. C., Pryor, W. W., Gibbons, J. E., & Orgain, E. S. (1955). Depression and anxiety occurring during rauwolfia therapy. *Journal of the American Medical Association, 159*, 836–839.

O'Donohue, W. T., & Engle, J. L. (2013). Errors in psychological practice: Devising a system to improve client safety and well-being. *Professional Psychology: Research and Practice, 44*, 314–323.

Papakostas, G. I., Thase, M. E., Fava, M., Nelson, J. C., & Shelton, R. C. (2007). Are antidepressant drugs that combine serotonergic and noradrenergic mechanisms of action more effective than the selective serotonin reuptake inhibitors in treating major depressive disorder? A meta-analysis or studies of newer agents. *Biological Psychiatry, 62*, 1217–1227.

Rizvi, S. J., Zaretsky, A., Schaffer, A., & Levitt, A. (2015). Is immediate CBT more beneficial than delayed CBT in treating depression?: A pilot study. *Journal of Psychiatric Practice, 21*, 107–113.

Rush, A. J., Fava, M., Wisniewski, S. R., Lavori, P. W., Trivedi, M. H., & Sackeim, H. A. (2004). Sequenced treatment alternatives to relieve depression (STAR*D) rationale and design. *Controlled Clinical Trials, 25*, 119–142.

Seligman, M. E. P. (1995). The effectiveness of psychotherapy: TheConsumer Reports study. *American Psychologist, 50*, 965–974.

Shaw, D. M., Camps, F. E., & Eccelston, E. G. (1967). 5-hydroxytryptamine in the hind-brain of depressive suicides. *British Journal of Psychiatry, 113*, 1407–1411.

Stahl, S. M., Grady, M. M., Moret, C., & Briley, M. (2005). SNRIs: Their pharmacology, clinical efficacy, and tolerability in comparison with other classes of antidepressants. *CNS Spectrum, 10*, 732–747.

Stulz, N., Thase, M. E., Klein, D. N., Manber, R., & Crits-Christoph, P. (2010). Differential effects of treatments for chronic depression: A latent growth model reanalysis. *Journal of Consulting and Clinical Psychology, 78*, 409–419.

Teri, L., Logsdon, R., Uomoto, J., & McCurry S. M. (1997). Behavioral treatment of depression in dementia patients: A controlled clinical trial. *Journals of Gerontology: Series B Psychological Sciences and Social Sciences, 52*, 159–166.

Thase, M. E., Greenhouse, J. B., Frank, E., Reynolds, C. F., Pilkonis, P. A., Hurley, K., . . . & Kupfer, D. J. (1997). Treatment of major depression with psychotherapy or psychotherapy-pharmacotherapy combinations. *Archives of General Psychiatry, 54*, 1009–1015.

Thase, M. E., Nierenberg, A. A., Vrijland, P., van Oers, H. J., Schutte, A., & Simmons, J. H. (2010). Remission with mirtazapine and selective serotonin reuptake inhibitors: A meta-analysis of individual patient data from 15 controlled trials of acute phase treatment of major depression. *International Clinical Psychopharmacology, 25*, 189–198.

Trivedi, M. H., Rush, A. J., Wisniewski, S. R., Nierenberg, A. A., Warden, D., & Ritz, L. (2006). Evaluation of outcomes with citalopram for depression using measurement-based care in STAR*D: Implications of clinical practice. *American Journal of Psychiatry, 163*, 28–40.

Wampold, B. E. (2001). *The great psychotherapy debate: Models, methods, and findings.* Mahwah, NJ: Lawrence Erlbaum.
Wampold, B. E., Minami, T., Baskin, T. W., & Callen Tierney, S. (2002). A Meta-(re)analysis of the effects of cognitive therapy versus "other therapies" for depression. *Journal of Affective Disorders, 68,* 159–165.
Wampold, B. E., Mondin, G. W., Moody, M., Stich, F., Benson, K., & Ahn, H. (1997). A meta-analysis of outcome studies comparing bona fide psychotherapies: Empirically, "All Must Have Prizes." *Psychological Bulletin, 122,* 203–215.
Weihs, K., & Wert, J. M. (2011). A primary care focus on the treatment of patients with major depressive disorder. *American Journal of the Medical Sciences, 342,* 324–330.
Willetts, J., Lippa, A., & Beer, B. (1999). Clinical development of citalopram. *Journal of Clinical Psychopharmacology, 19*(Suppl. 1), 36S–46S.
World Health Organization (2016). *Depression: Fact sheet.* Retrieved from http://www.who.int/mediacentre/factsheets/fs369/en/

4

Mood Disorders: Evidence-Based Integrated Biopsychosocial Treatment of Bipolar Disorder

Randon Welton and Brenda J. B. Roman

Careful observers have long recognized the signs, symptoms, and behaviors that we now classify as bipolar disorder. Soranus of Ephesus in the 1st century AD differentiated melancholia, which included "weeping without reason," dejection, and often a desire for death, from mania, which was characterized by fluctuating anger and merriment and "continual wakefulness." Aretaeus of Cappadocia in the 2nd century AD linked mania and melancholia as different stages of one disease (Goodwin & Jamison, 1990). Hermann Boerhaave, in the early 18th century, described melancholia, and reported that it occasionally resulted in "a wild Fury" called "Madness." While in a fit of "Madness," the patient "generally shews (sp) a great Strength of the Muscles, an incredible Wakefulness, a bearing to a wonder of Cold and Hunger, [and] frightful Fancies. . ." (Boerhaave & Delacoste, 1986).

By the mid-19th century both Falret and Baillarger began to discuss the cyclic nature of mania and melancholia (Goodwin & Jamison, 1990). Emil Kraepelin, at the end of the century, described maniacal-depressive insanity (circular stupor). This condition had discrete periods of depression and excitement. The depression consisted of prolonged bouts of being "low-spirited" with an impediment to drive and initiative. Depressed patients displayed decreased appetite, impaired cognition, and low energy. Maniacal excitement or "mania" resulted in a "joyous and exalted" frame of mind. These individuals became extremely talkative and were difficult to interrupt when speaking. Their thoughts were frequently disorganized and digressive. They often became disruptive and combative as they overindulged in pleasurable pursuits (Kraepelin, 1988 [1913]).

By 1952 the American Psychiatric Association's Diagnostic and Statistical Manual of Mental Disorders had a section for manic-depressive reactions. These patients had severe mood swings with a tendency toward remission and relapses. Their mania was described as "elation or irritability, with overtalkativeness, flight of ideas, and increased motor activity." Mania alternated with a "depression of mood and with mental and motor retardation and inhibition; in some cases there is much uneasiness and apprehension. Perplexity, stupor or agitation may be prominent symptoms" (American Psychiatric Association, 1952).

Currently, mental health professionals in the United States use, together with the International Classification of Diseases and Related Health Problems, 10th Revision (ICD-10) (World Health Organization, 2016), the Diagnostic and Statistical Manual of

Cognitive Behavioral Psychopharmacology: The Clinical Practice of Evidence-Based Biopsychosocial Integration, First Edition. Edited by Mark Dana Muse.

Mental Disorders, fifth edition (DSM-5) (American Psychiatric Association, 2013) for classifying mental illness. The section for bipolar and related disorders of the DSM-5 describes mania as consisting of periods of abnormally and persistently elevated, expansive, or irritable mood. This altered mood is accompanied by a combination of increased goal-directed activities, increased energy, inflated self-esteem, decreased need for sleep, increased talkativeness, flight of ideas, distractibility, or an excessive involvement in activities and risky behavior. If this episode lasts for 7 or more days and is accompanied by marked impairment in social or functional impairment, it is described as mania. If the episode lasts for at least 4 days but does not cause marked impairment, then it can be described as hypomania. Depressive episodes in bipolar disorder are diagnostically identical with major depressive disorder and consist of at least 2 weeks of depressed mood accompanied by a combination of anhedonia, altered sleep, altered appetite, decreased energy, impaired concentration, psychomotor retardation or agitation, feelings of worthless or guilt, impaired cognitive functioning, or thoughts of death. By convention, if a patient has had one manic episode they should be diagnosed with "bipolar I disorder." If they have had at least one hypomanic episode and one major depressive episode then they are diagnosed with "bipolar II disorder" (American Psychiatric Association, 2013). These criteria are consistent with the description of bipolar affective disorder found in the World Health Organization's ICD-10.

Bipolar I disorder is seen across the world in all cultures and socioeconomic classes. In a study of 11 countries, the 12-month prevalence of bipolar I disorder ranged from 0% to 0.6%. In the United States the 12-month prevalence is 0.6%. Bipolar I disorder seems to be slightly more common in men with a ratio of 1.1 to 1. In patients who go on to manifest bipolar I disorder, the first mood disturbance occurs at approximately 18 years of age, although there are a few who will not have the onset of the disease until their sixth or seventh decade of life. Almost everyone (~90%) who has had a manic episode will have recurrent mood episodes, and 60% of manic episodes immediately precede a major depressive episode. Many patients with bipolar disorders will return to normal functioning after the mood episode, but up to 30% will have continuing, severe impairment of occupational functioning (American Psychiatric Association, 2013).

Bipolar II disorder is recognized in 0.3% of adults over a 12-month period according to international studies, but it has a 0.8% 12-month prevalence in the United States. The mood disturbance in bipolar II disorder presents slightly later than bipolar I disorder with the average age of onset being the mid-20s. Patients with bipolar II disorder tend to have more episodes of mood disturbance during their life, but tend to return to normal functioning between episodes. Only 15% have evidence of functional impairment between episodes (American Psychiatric Association, 2013).

Suicide is a significant concern in both bipolar I and bipolar II disorders. The lifetime risk of suicide in individuals with any bipolar disorder is 15 times higher than the general population, and nearly one-fourth of all people who have committed suicide have a bipolar disorder diagnosis. Although the rate of attempted suicide is nearly equal in bipolar I and bipolar II disorders (36.3% and 32.4%, respectively), the lethality of attempts in bipolar II disorder seems higher (American Psychiatric Association, 2013). The frequent combination of a bipolar disorder and substance abuse further raises the risk of suicide.

Since the time of Kraepelin, bipolar disorders were noted to have severe episodes of depression and mania with fairly good resolution of symptoms in between episodes. This helped distinguish it from the persistent downward spiral of dementia praecox (schizophrenia). John Cade, an Australian psychiatrist, noted in the late 1940s that lithium calmed agitated psychotic patients (Cade, 1949), and later it was found that lithium was effective in reducing the symptoms of mania and minimizing reoccurrences (Schou, Juel-Nielsen, Stromgren, & Voldby, 1954). Lithium became available in 1970 for the treatment of bipolar disorder, and has been the gold standard ever since (Baldessarini & Tondo, 2000; International Consensus Group, 2008). Although psychotherapeutic treatments exist for depression, neither mania nor the psychosis that often accompanies mania are amenable to talk therapy. Traditionally, therefore, the research into treating bipolar disorders focused mostly on controlling acute mood symptoms using physical interventions such as medication or electroconvulsive treatments. Over the past 20 years, however, there has been increasing interest in the use of psychosocial interventions to augment psychopharmacology as well as its employment as an independent treatment to help ameliorate the suffering of the individual with bipolar disorder (Depp, Moore, Patterson, Lebowitz, & Jeste, 2008).

Diagnosis and Acute Management of Mania

Clinical Case

Paul is a 19-year-old college freshman who is brought to the emergency department by his roommate because "he isn't acting right." Paul states that he feels "great," and that his roommate is simply envious of his energy and "special powers." He does not understand why anyone is concerned about him, as "I got my paper done in just three hours for my business class, worked on a class project and got all of my studying done in record time." He does acknowledge that he is not concentrating as well on studies because his "mind is moving really fast." On examination, his affect is euphoric, his speech is pressured, and he has delusions of grandeur. He had three beers 24 h earlier, but denies illicit drug use or misuse of prescription medication. He has no prior psychiatric history, although he reports two periods in high school during which he was "down for a couple of weeks." His family history is positive for a maternal uncle with bipolar disorder and a grandfather who committed suicide. He is admitted for further evaluation, and is ultimately diagnosed with bipolar disorder, to which he responds, "I am not crazy like my Uncle." His parents are also distraught about the diagnosis of bipolar I disorder.

Psychoeducation

Psychoeducation should be included in all medical treatment as patients have a right to know their diagnosis, the risks of the treatment, alternative treatments, and why the treatment is likely to be helpful. Psychoeducation is, therefore, a part of the informed consent process. For patients with bipolar disorder, psychoeducation can be an extremely valuable psychosocial intervention. Psychoeducation early in the course of the illness can result in long-term benefits.

Psychoeducation is a cornerstone of several broader psychosocial strategies for bipolar disorder, including family focused therapy (FFT) and interpersonal and social rhythm therapy (IPSRT) (Otto, Reilly-Harrington, & Sachs, 2003; Smith, Jones, &

Simpson, 2010). In FFT, for example, the first seven sessions are educational and address topics such as the signs and symptoms of bipolar disorder, stress vulnerability, and relapse prevention (Smith et al., 2010). Although in these therapies psychoeducation is provided as a part of a larger package, it can be provided independently. Perry, Tarrier, Morriss, McCarthy, and Limb (1999) report a study in which 34 patients received individual psychoeducation to help them identify prodromal symptoms of depression and mania. During an average of nine meetings with their provider, the patients developed a personalized algorithm for self-monitoring and intervention at the early signs of relapse. This intervention led to a significant reduction in days of mania and time to relapse of mania, as well as a significant improvement in social functioning and employment. Javadpour, Hedayati, Dehbozorgi, & Azizi (2013) studied 108 patients seen for eight 50-min psychoeducation sessions, and then followed by monthly telephone contact for 18 months. Those receiving psychoeducation had lower rates of relapse and hospitalizations, and had significantly improved medication adherence and quality of life. Although individual psychoeducation may be helpful, it will probably not be as effective as more extensive, individual psychosocial interventions such as FFT or psychoeducation followed by cognitive-behavioral therapy (CBT) (Swartz & Swanson, 2014). Group psychoeducation also seems to be more successful than individual psychoeducation (Bond & Anderson, 2015).

Bauer, McBride, Chase, Sachs, and Shea (1998), in a 5-week, manualized psychoeducation group, covered bipolar disorder and treatment options (1 week), depression (2 weeks), and mania and hypomania (2 weeks). The groups focused on the common patterns of illness, and the group members discussed their individual warning signs and triggers for relapse. This intervention led to an increase in their knowledge about bipolar disorder and helpful coping strategies. Colom et al. (2003a) followed 25 patients after they received 20 90-min psychoeducation group sessions. The group discussions focused on illness awareness, treatment adherence, lifestyle regularity, and early detection of prodromal symptoms. By the end of 2 years, 92% of patients in the control group had relapsed and 36% had been hospitalized compared to only 60% and 8% in the intervention cohort. The consensus of the literature is that group psychoeducation for bipolar disorder leads to decreased recurrences of mood episodes, decreased time spent in relapses, and decreased frequency and duration of hospitalizations (Swartz & Swanson, 2014; Miziou et al., 2015). A systematic review of 16 studies (Bond & Anderson, 2015) found that psychoeducation was effective at preventing all types of mood relapse, and is most effective in preventing manic or hypomanic relapse. In addition to acquiring facts about their illness, many patients seem to benefit from the social support inherent in the group (Poole, Smith & Simpson, 2015). In a qualitative assessment of group psychoeducation, group members reported that they had acquired new knowledge about their illness or had a confirmation of things learned previously, but they also reported a decreased sense of shame and stigma about having a mental illness. Some also reported new insight into their illness and relapse triggers, and a decreased resistance to taking medications (Poole et al., 2015). To be covered later in the chapter, there is evidence that even fairly brief group psychoeducation significantly increased treatment adherence (Bond & Anderson, 2015; Eker & Harkin, 2012; Javadpour et al., 2012; Miziou et al., 2015).

As an aside, the potential appears to exist for using technology to help provide psychoeducation. A trial of psychoeducation, using in-person and then internet-based information, found that educating patients through didactics and vignettes on the internet was feasible and generally acceptable to patients. Patients who were more used to computer-based training were more likely to benefit from this approach (Poole, Simpson, & Smith, 2012).

Based on these studies and general treatment principles, psychoeducation should be provided over an extended period of time and preferably in a group format (Miziou et al., 2015). Several topics should be systematically addressed including:

- Review of bipolar disorder.
  - Diagnostic criteria—review the standard signs and symptoms used to diagnose bipolar disorders.
  - Etiology—discuss the biopsychosocial nature of bipolar disorder, including genetic and stress vulnerabilities.
  - Personalized diagnostic criteria—while depressed patients readily acknowledge that they are suffering, patients with mania and hypomania often resist the idea that they have a mental illness. Denial of their illness will likely decrease adherence to treatment plans. The provider should help the patient develop a life narrative that describes how their symptoms have caused them distress and problems. The provider can demonstrate that these are manifestations of the patient's bipolar disorder.
- Description of the course and prognosis of bipolar disorder.
  - Helping patients understand the fluctuating symptoms inherent in bipolar disorder may help them continue to follow treatment recommendations even when they are feeling well.
- Discussion of treatment options.
  - Reviewing the relative risks and benefits of a variety of treatments, including psychopharmacological, psychosocial, and complementary/alternative medicine options helps create acceptance of the proposed treatment options and increases the patient's participation in treatment decisions. Ideally, the patient will be able to explain to the provider why the chosen treatment option is the best choice for them (Otto et al., 2003).
- Vigilance for common co-morbid conditions.
  - Patients should be cautioned against excessive use of alcohol or other illicit substances. Signs and symptoms of anxiety disorder should also be reviewed.
- Development of self-management skills.
  - Help the patient develop a regular, healthy schedule of activities, including a healthy sleep schedule.
  - Patients should develop an understanding of the connection between stress, their behaviors, and relapse. They should be able to identify behaviors that make relapse more or less likely.
- Identification of warning signs of relapse.

  Patients and providers can develop self-monitoring strategies and action plans for dealing with concerning thoughts, emotions, and behaviors. They can create and even practice these with their therapist.

  (Smith et al., 2010; Swartz & Swanson, 2014)

Somatic Treatments for Acute Mania

Starting effective medications is of the utmost importance in controlling the devastating symptoms of mania. A recent systematic review and meta-analysis found that neither individual psychosocial interventions (three trials) nor group interventions (six trials) made an impact on symptoms of mania (Oud et al., 2016). On the other hand, for over a half of a century, lithium has been used to treat bipolar disorder. Lithium has been extensively studied, and has demonstrated efficacy in the treatment of acute mania. The use of lithium is complicated, however, by frequent side effects and significant toxicity that begins at doses only slightly higher than the therapeutic range. Valproate and carbamazepine, which were both developed for the prevention of seizures, have been found to be effective in the treatment of mania although they both have significant side effects. Collectively, these medications, along with lithium, are commonly referred to as "mood stabilizers," all of which have good data regarding treatment efficacy. There have been relatively few head-to-head trials of these medications in mania, and most of those have found that they are essentially equal in efficacy. Currently, there is insufficient evidence to say that any one mood stabilizer is more effective than the others. (Burgess et al., 2003; Emilien, Maloteaux, Seghers, & Charles, 1996; Ceron-Litvoc, Soares, Geddes, Litvoc, & de Lima 2009; Cipriani, Pretty, Hawton, & Geddes, 2005; Davis, Bartolucci, & Petty, 1999; Fountoulakis et al., 2012; Geddes, Burgess, Hawton, Jamison, & Goodwin, 2004; Grunze et al., 2009; Macritchie et al., 2003; Poolsup, Li Wan Po, & de Oliveira, 2003; The Management of Bipolar Disorder Working Group, 2010). Treatment with the mood stabilizers requires ongoing, routine monitoring of serum levels of the medication as well as other specific studies. Lithium requires periodic monitoring of renal and thyroid function. Patients on valproate will need their liver enzymes checked regularly, and prescribing carbamazepine necessitates checking blood cell counts.

Second-generation antipsychotic medications, such as aripiprazole, olanzapine, quetiapine, risperidone, and ziprasidone are effective in treating mania. Systematic reviews of second-generation antipsychotics for the treatment of mania have found them to be essentially equal in efficacy. While the potential side effects of the second-generation antipsychotics are very similar, several studies have noted weight gain to be more prominent with olanzapine (Fountoulakis et al., 2012; Fountoulakis, Vieta, & Schmidt, 2011; Gao & Calabrese, 2005; Jeste & Dolder, 2004; Ketter, Miller, Dell'Osso, & Wang, 2016; Perlis, Welge, Vornick, Hirschfeld, & Keck, 2006; The Management of Bipolar Disorder Working Group, 2010). The second-generation antipsychotic medications do not require blood levels of the active medication, but there is a requirement to monitor studies related to increased weight, blood glucose, and lipids (i.e., metabolic syndrome). Combinations of mood stabilizers and antipsychotic medications are indicated for the most severe manic episodes. The combination of an antipsychotic medication with a mood stabilizer increases the response rate by about 20% over the response rate to monotherapy with a mood stabilizer (The Management of Bipolar Disorder Working Group, 2010). The first-generation antipsychotic medication, haloperidol, has good evidence for its efficacy in controlling acute mania but does not have evidence supporting long-term use. It is also associated with increased risks of tardive dyskinesia compared to the second-generation antipsychotic medications (McIntyre, Brecher, Paulsson, Huizar, & Mullen, 2005; Smulevich et al., 2005; Vieta et al., 2005). The mood stabilizers and/or antipsychotic medications should be started soon after confirming the diagnosis as they may take several days to a week before their positive effects are noted.

Electroconvulsive therapy (ECT) remains a safe and effective treatment for severe mania (The Management of Bipolar Disorder Working Group, 2010). An older review found that 80% of patients with mania experienced remission or marked clinical improvement with ECT (Mukherjee, Sackeim, & Schnur, 1994). Because of the efficacy of psychopharmacology, ECT is typically not considered a first-line treatment for most patients with mania, but there are populations in which ECT may be recommended. These populations include patients with life-threatening conditions such as severe malnutrition, catatonia, or severe suicidality, pregnant patients, and patients who have not responded to medications (The Management of Bipolar Disorder Working Group, 2010).

Continuing Treatment

Clinical Case—Continued

Paul was started on lithium carbonate and quetiapine for his bipolar I disorder, and within 10 days showed considerable improvement. During his hospitalization and subsequent outpatient visits he was educated about the diagnostic criteria for bipolar disorder and its prognosis. His providers pointed out that some of Paul's recent experiences were manifestations of his bipolar disorder. Following discharge, Paul did well for 6 months, returning to school and receiving As and Bs in all of his classes, but he stopped taking his medication, as "I am well now. I have no need for medication, as I can control my moods." Another factor leading to his stopping his medications was the hospital team's insistence that he not drink alcohol while he takes medications. He was frustrated that he had not been able "to party with friends" so he stopped medication in order to go out on the weekends with his friends and "not feel like the loser who can't drink." He also acknowledges that he did not like the laboratory blood draws and the ten pound weight gain since being hospitalized.

Psychosocial Interventions for Treatment Adherence

Convincing patients to follow through with their mental health treatment plans is always difficult, but it is perhaps even more difficult in patients with bipolar disorder. Bipolar disorder is highly recurrent by nature, so patients must recognize the need to continue on their treatment indefinitely in order to prevent relapses. Patients who have had hypomanic experiences often remember them positively and do not wish to prevent them from recurring (Otto et al., 2003). Patients with mania may not recognize that they have an illness, and they may resist attempts by others to keep them on medications. Adherence is worsened by the fact that many of the medications effective in bipolar disorder have significant side effect profiles.

Table 4.1 provides a listing of some of the more common and troublesome side effects of the commonly used medications.

Adherence to treatment plans is a top priority in the management of a patient's bipolar disorder, but the understanding of adherence is changing over time. Traditionally,

Table 4.1 Side effects of medication for bipolar disorder. Adapted from The Management of Bipolar Disorder Working Group (–2010).

Category	Examples	Common and bothersome side effects (not an all-inclusive list)
Lithium	Lithium	Acne Alopecia Diabetes insipidus Electrocardiogram changes Gastrointestinal complaints (nausea, diarrhea) Hyperparathyroid Hypothyroidism Leukocytosis Mental status changes (impaired concentration and memory) Polyuria Rash Renal impairment Tremor Weight gain
Mood stabilizers (a.k.a. anticonvulsants)	Valproate Carbamazepine Lamotrigine	Agranulocytosis Alopecia (valproate acid) Aplastic anemia Ataxia Cognitive impairment Hepatotoxicity (valproate) Pancreatitis (valproate) Peripheral edema Rash Stephens–Johnson syndrome Tremor Visual changes Weight changes

adherence was defined as strict compliance with the physician's instructions. In a more collaborative medical setting, however, it consists of abiding by the treatment approach that the patient and provider develop following an open discussion. This helps shift adherence from being an "all-or-nothing" submission to the will of a paternalistic physician, to a shared decision making model (Berk et al., 2010).

Adherence to the treatment plan, however, goes far beyond patients taking their prescribed medication. Behavioral adherence consists of numerous actions unrelated to taking medications. These can include:

- attending scheduled appointments;
- participating in assigned homework;

- abstaining from alcohol and illicit drugs;
- maintaining regular lifestyle patterns (reasonable exercise, consistent sleep–wake cycles).

The vast majority of research has focused on medication adherence and very little has looked at behavioral adherence (Gaudiano, Weinstock, & Miller, 2008). Medication adherence includes taking the right amount of medication at the right times. Sometimes nonadherence to medications can be involuntary as in the cases of patients who forget or do not understand their medication regimen. Some patients may take only some of their medications or lower doses of the medications they have been prescribed (partial adherence). Patients may also take full doses of medications during some periods and then limit or stop medications at other times (irregular adherence) (Berk et al., 2010).

Accurately measuring adherence defies simple solutions. The most obvious method is self-report, with the provider asking directly or through questionnaires about the patient's medication-taking behavior. Patients, however, may be hesitant to report not taking their medications or may not accurately remember their use of medication. Blood levels can be monitored with some medications, such as lithium, valproate, and carbamazepine, but this only reveals how much medication the patient had been taking in the few days preceding the blood draw, and may not accurately reflect their use over time. Providers or family members can count the remaining pills from a prescription and calculate how many pills have been taken. This, however, does not account for pills that were disposed of rather than ingested. Finally, there are efforts to electronically monitor when pill bottles are opened and pills are removed. These are expensive and, again, they do not prevent patients from merely disposing of their pills. The most accurate assessments involve using several strategies to monitor the patient (Berk et al., 2010).

Estimates of nonadherence in patients with bipolar disorder range from 20% to 60%. Scott and Pope (2002), in a tightly controlled study, defined nonadherence as missing at least 30% of prescribed medications. By that definition 32% of patients were nonadherent in the past month and 50% were nonadherent at some point in the past 2 years. Increasing adherence to treatment is an important goal for clinicians. Nonadherence to medications is associated with increased rates of relapse and recurrences, hospitalizations, functional impairment, and suicide (Gaudiano et al., 2008; Sajatovic, Davies, & Hrouda, 2004).

Nonadherence is not distributed evenly among patients with bipolar disorders. There are several significant risk factors.

- Patient-related:
  - demographic—younger age, single, male, lower education level;
  - co-morbid conditions—substance use disorders, personality disorder, cognitive impairment (any source);
  - attitude toward illness—denial of illness or need for medication.
- Medication-related:
  - side effects of medication (concerns about dependence on medications or feared future side effects may be more important than actual, current side effects);
  - longer duration of treatment;
  - beliefs about the risks and benefits of medications.

- Provider-related:
  - poor therapeutic alliance with the patient;
  - decreased patient satisfaction with care.

(Depp et al., 2008; Gaudiano, et al., 2008; Sajatovic et al., 2004)

Efforts to increase adherence have included short-term and long-term interventions that either focus on adherence as the primary goal or as one of several studied outcomes. These approaches have had mixed but generally positive results. One review (Gaudiano et al., 2008) looked at 14 clinical trials that focused on increasing adherence. Of six trials of CBT, four increased adherence. Most of these trials included medication adherence as only one of many goals. These trials tended to be smaller in size, and the largest trial with 253 patients found no increase in adherence. Five trials looked at psychoeducation, which was mostly provided in an extended group format. Of those five trials, three improved medication adherence. Two trials of FFT also measured medication adherence as an outcome. One of them showed increased medication adherence at the 1-year follow up.

A more recent study examined four distinct modules for treating patients with bipolar disorder (Sajatovic et al., 2012). The modules included: psychoeducation related to bipolar disorder, modified motivational enhancement therapy, coaching on communication with providers, and coaching on medication routines. Patients were nonrandomly assigned to complete one to four of these modules based on a structured assessment. Each module had four weekly sessions and then two telephone follow up visits. The 43 patients included in the study all had a history of poor medication adherence. A total of 40 of the 43 patients went through at least three of the modules. Nonadherence was measured through self-report and pill counting, and indicated that at baseline these patients had not taken nearly half of their prescribed medication (48%) during the prior week. By the end of 6 months these patients were taking 75% of their prescribed medication. Benefits were gained from including family members and significant others in efforts to increase adherence, especially when it came to behavioral adherence such as attending appointments (Gaudiano et al., 2008; Sajatovic et al., 2004).

International studies have also demonstrated that psychoeducation can increase adherence. In addition to the Javadpour et al. study mentioned previously, a Turkish study of 71 patients (Eker & Harkin, 2012) found that six group sessions lasting 90–120 min resulted in a doubling of medication adherence in the treatment group (from 40% to 86.7%) over a 6-week period, while the control group showed a worsening of adherence (from 38.9% to 24.2%).

Although the data are limited and only somewhat positive, the best outcomes seem to arise from studies that targeted the patient's knowledge and attitudes toward their medications. Simply handing out sheets of information appears to be a largely unsuccessful intervention. All of the successful approaches have an interaction with a provider who emphasizes adherence (Sajatovic et al., 2004). The interventions should focus on the reasons that patients give for not continuing these medications. These include knowledge and attitude about illness and medications, their relationships with their providers, the stigma of having a mental illness, and social pressures about their illness and medications (Sajatovic et al., 2012).

Steps to increasing medication adherence include:

- *Increasing knowledge about the disorder*: Individuals who are highly adherent have a greater understanding of their illness' severity. Individuals should understand the natural course of their illness and the problems that can arise from not treating their illness. The provider can discuss the problems with stigma and social pressure that the patient is experiencing. It might also be helpful, with the patient's permission, to include family members and significant others in these discussions.
- *Addressing knowledge and attitude about medications*: Individuals are more likely to stay on medications when they understand the benefits of the medications and the risks of suddenly stopping their medications.
- *Increasing awareness of medication side effects*: Patients should have an understanding of the common and severe medication side effects. There should also be discussions about how they can manage side effects that arise.
- *Developing a positive therapeutic alliance*: All providers should focus on developing a warm, empathic bond with their patients, and collaborate with their patients to develop reasonable goals.
- *Emphasizing collaboration in developing the treatment plan*: Patients are more likely to comply with treatment recommendations when they fully understand the rationale behind the recommendations, and when they have played a role in creating their treatment plan.

(Berk et al., 2010; Gaudiano et al., 2008; Sajatovic, et al., 2004, 2012)

Bipolar Depression

Clinical Case—Continued

Paul reluctantly restarted and remained on lithium carbonate over the past year. In his regularly scheduled appointment with his clinician, he states that for the past 3 weeks he has been very depressed. He has not been attending class for the past week as "I don't feel like seeing anyone, and I really can't concentrate." He has not been going out with his friends and has little energy, despite sleeping at least 10 h a day. He has thoughts of death, but denies suicidal intent as "I would never hurt my family in that way. My grandfather's suicide really devastated my grandmother."

Somatic Treatments for Bipolar Depression

Treating bipolar depression creates several challenges for the provider. Many patients with bipolar disorder spend more time with a depressed mood than they do with mania or hypomania. Depression can be the most debilitating aspect of bipolar disorder and is associated with significant social and occupational dysfunction and suicide. No medications have been developed specifically for bipolar depression, and many of the ones that are currently used carry limitations because of side effects and failure of response.

Antidepressants, the mainstay for treating unipolar depression, increase the risk of switching the patient with bipolar depression into hypomania or mania. Their effectiveness for treating bipolar depression has also been questioned (Geddes & Miklowitz, 2013; Malhi et al., 2015; Sachs et al., 2007). In general, using antidepressant medications as monotherapy for bipolar depression is not recommended due to their lack of proven efficacy and an increased risk of adverse events (The Management of Bipolar Disorder Working Group, 2010). The data for valproate and carbamazepine in treating the depressed phase of bipolar disorder are weak to nonexistent (Baldassano, Hosey, & Coello, 2011; Davis et al., 2005; Ghaemi et al., 2007;). Mood stabilizers that have shown themselves to be useful in bipolar depression include lithium and lamotrigine. Lithium has a fair amount of evidence for effectiveness in the depressed phase of bipolar disorder, as well as preventing further depressed episodes (Baldassano et al., 2011; Suppes et al., 2008; Zornberg & Pope, 1993). An additional benefit of lithium is a reduction in suicidality (Cipriani et al., 2005; Goodwin et al., 2003). Lamotrigine is effective for the acute depressive phase in bipolar disorder, as well as preventing further depressive episodes (Calabrese et al., 2003; Goodwin et al., 2004; Suppes et al., 2008; Baldassano et al., 2011). Several second-generation antipsychotic medications have been found to be effective in treating the depressed phase of bipolar disorder. Olanzapine is better than placebo in the treatment of bipolar depression and additionally seems to prevent further episodes of depression (Baldassano et al., 2011; Gao & Calabrese, 2005). Quetiapine also has good evidence for treating and preventing depression in bipolar disorder (Cookson, Keck, Ketter, & Macfadden, 2007; Vieta, Calabrese, Goikolea, Raines, & Macfadden, 2007; Ketter et al., 2016; Suppes, Vieta, Liu, Brecher, & Paulsson, 2009). Lurasidone has also been approved for the treatment of bipolar depression (Loebel & Citrome, 2015). There is insufficient evidence from head-to-head trials to determine which medication is the most effective in bipolar depression.

Electroconvulsive treatment (ECT), although underutilized, effectively and rapidly treats bipolar depression. For patients without medical contraindications, ECT can be a life-saving intervention. It should be especially considered in patients with life-threatening conditions such as severe malnutrition, catatonia, or severe suicidality, pregnant patients, and patients who have not responded to medications (The Management of Bipolar Disorder Working Group, 2010). ECT can generate substantial reductions in symptomatology even in medication-resistant patients with bipolar depression and mixed mania (Ciapparelli et al., 2001). A multicenter comparison of ECT with algorithm-cased psychopharmacology in patients with treatment-resistant bipolar depression found that remission rates were similar (34.8% vs. 30.0%), but that response rates were significantly higher in the ECT group (73.9% vs. 35.0%) (Schoeyen et al., 2015).

Psychosocial Interventions for Bipolar Depression

The research into psychosocial interventions for bipolar depression has focused on using it as adjunctive treatment. Pharmacology remains essential for treating bipolar depression, but over the past 15 years researchers have studied the distinct benefits of adding psychosocial interventions. Both the British National Collaborating Centre for Mental Health (NCCMH) and the Royal Australian and New Zealand College of Psychiatrists recommend adding adjunctive psychosocial interventions to medication when treating bipolar depression (Malhi et al., 2015; NCCMH, 2014).

The NCCMH report included a review of seven studies of various individual therapies for bipolar depression (total $n = 637$). It found low quality evidence that they had a small effect on depression (ES = −0.23). Eight trials of various group psychotherapies for depression ($n = 423$) had very low quality evidence of a small effect (ES = −0.24). One study of extended family-based psychoeducation found low quality evidence for a medium effect on depressive symptoms (ES = −0.73). These results were confirmed in an independent systematic review and meta-analysis in 2016 (Oud et al., 2016).

Most of the studies treating bipolar depression used CBT. The results are generally positive. One of the early studies (Zaretsky, Segal, & Gemar, 1999) provided 20 sessions of CBT to 11 patients with bipolar disorder who were on medications, compared to 11 controls who were on medication but not receiving therapy. At the end of treatment those receiving CBT had fewer depressive symptoms. Miziou et al. (2015), however, reviewed 14 studies of CBT for bipolar disorder and reported only limited support for CBT as an adjunct to pharmacology during the acute phase of bipolar depression. Nonetheless, a meta-analysis of eight studies (Zaretsky, Rizvi, & Parikh, 2007) found that CBT was as effective for bipolar depression as it was for unipolar depression. Studies have also found that CBT has also been effective at decreasing residual depressive symptoms in patients who no longer meet criteria for a major depressive episode (Swartz & Swanson, 2014). CBT manuals have been published for the treatment of bipolar depression, but there is limited evidence as to their effectiveness (Swartz & Frank, 2001).

Interpersonal and social rhythm therapy (IPSRT) focuses on interpersonal themes such as minimizing distress related to grief, role transitions, role disputes, and interpersonal deficits. In addition, IPSRT emphasizes the connection between stressful life events and symptom relapse, and the importance of maintaining a stable routine. In a trial of depressed patients with bipolar II disorder, ISPRT was as effective as quetiapine in reducing depressive symptoms (Miziou et al., 2015). A very small study of ISPRT delivered in a group format found an improvement of depressive symptoms, but the study, which had only six people at follow up, is far too small to be conclusive (Hoberg, Ponto, Nelson, & Frye, 2013). The NCCMH meta-analysis concluded that the present evidence for ISPRT in bipolar depression is inconclusive (NCCMH, 2014).

FFT consists of 21 sessions provided over 9 months. It helps patients deal with critical or hostile family members. FFT includes components of psychoeducation, communication skills training, and problem solving skills training (Geddes & Miklowitz, 2013). FFT was also assessed by the NCCMH, which found that, based on one study, FFT had low quality evidence of a medium effect (ES = −0.40) in bipolar depression (NCCMH, 2014).

The largest single study of the psychosocial treatment of bipolar depression was the Systematic Treatment Enhancement Program for Bipolar Disorder (STEP-BD). This 15-site study looked at 293 patients with bipolar depression. Individual CBT, FFT, or ISPRT were compared to collaborative care. The active treatment arms included up to 30 sessions provided over 9 months. Patients were followed for 1 year, and at that time those in active treatment were significantly more likely to have recovered (64.4% vs. 51.5%). Patients receiving any of the three specific interventions improved more quickly. Although the recovery rate was greatest for FFT, there was no significant difference between the three active treatment arms (Miklowitz et al., 2007).

Maintenance Phase

Clinical Case—Continued

Paul's depression was stabilized by adding aripiprazole to the lithium carbonate. After a thorough discussion regarding side effect and efficacy profiles, he now understands the importance of medication adherence. He wants to know if there is anything else he can do to decrease his chances of relapse.

Medications for Relapse Prevention

As bipolar disorders are highly recurrent illnesses, comprehensive management should include a focus on the prevention of future episodes. After recovering from an acute mood episode, over one-third of patients with a bipolar disorder will have a relapse within a year, even if treated. Nearly 75% will have a recurrence within 5 years and most of those will have had multiple episodes during that time (Gitlin, Swendsen, Heller, & Hammen, 1995). Over 90% of those who have had a single manic episode will eventually go on to suffer another episode of mania or depression, and many will have several episodes per year (American Psychiatric Association, 2013). Continuing medication is therefore vital for these patients.

Lithium and lamotrigine are approved for preventing recurrences of mood episodes during the maintenance phase of treatment and seem to be more effective than valproate and carbamazepine in preventing relapses. Lamotrigine seems to be more effective in preventing recurrences of depressive episodes in particular. The second-generation antipsychotic medications may be less helpful during the maintenance phase. Olanzapine is effective as monotherapy for the maintenance phase of bipolar disorder (Cipriani, Reddell, & Geddes, 2009), although it appears to be more effective in preventing further manic/hypomanic episodes than in preventing depressive episodes. Quetiapine can be combined with lithium or valproate for the maintenance phase of bipolar disorder (Suppes et al., 2009; Vieta & Suppes, 2008). The data for aripiprazole are less robust in the maintenance phase of bipolar disorder than in the acute phase of mania (Keck et al., 2007, 2009). The exact choice of medication will depend on prior treatment response, co-morbid medical conditions, and potential side effect concerns, such as the weight gain that can be caused by lithium, the anticonvulsants, and most of the second-generation antipsychotic medications. Ultimately, the increased side effect profiles from combinations must be weighed against potential improvements for relapse prevention (Buoli, Serati, & Altamura, 2014). A common clinical recommendation is to maintain the patient on the same medication that controlled their acute symptoms.

Psychotherapy for Relapse Prevention

Numerous studies have demonstrated the benefits of augmenting psychopharmacology with psychotherapy for the prevention of recurrences (Geddes & Miklowitz, 2013; Oud et al., 2016). A meta-analysis of eight psychotherapy trials found that the addition of psychotherapy reduced relapses by 40% (Scott, Colom, & Vieta, 2007). A second meta-analysis of 10 studies, including many of the studies reported above, found a 26% decrease in relapse rates (Lam, Burbeck, Wright, & Pilling, 2009). These trials included group psychoeducation, cognitive therapy, ISPRT, and FFT. NCCMH, looking at seven trials of various individual therapies, found moderate evidence that they resulted in long-term reduction in risk of relapse, and that at least three studies demonstrated a reduction in rates of hospitalization. Group psychotherapy interventions were more successful in reducing relapses of depression than mania (NCCMH, 2014). A 2016 systematic review and meta-analysis of 55 trials found moderate-quality evidence that individual psychosocial interventions were associated with a 34% decrease in the risk of relapse at the end of treatment and a 26% reduction in risk at follow up. Group psychoeducation and family psychoeducation also reduced relapse rates (Oud et al., 2016).

The benefits of psychoeducation in relapse prevention have already been mentioned. Patients and their families can be instructed about the importance of accepting their illness, taking their medications as prescribed, and maintaining a regular lifestyle. Early warning signs of recurrence can be identified and strategies prepared for early intervention. A comparison of maintenance medication with usual care or individual psychoeducation lasting 7–12 sessions found that psychoeducation resulted in a 30% decrease in manic relapses, longer intervals to manic relapse, and improved social functioning over 18 months (Miklowitz, 2006). Overall, however, the benefits of individual psychoeducation seem less robust than interventions with more intensive treatment (e.g., CBT) or those provided in a group format (Swartz & Swanson, 2014).

A study of 121 patients who had been in remission for 6 months compared 21 structured psychoeducation group sessions to 21 unstructured support groups over a 2-year period (Colom et al., 2003b). The patients receiving structured psychoeducation groups had fewer relapses and had less time ill. Patients receiving a multicomponent intervention featuring structured group psychoeducation along with monthly telephone monitoring and a mechanism for providing feedback to providers were followed for 2 years. The intervention decreased mean mania scores and led to a decrease in the time with manic symptoms. The benefits were most noticeable in those who started the study with clinically significant mood symptoms (Simon, Ludman, Bauer, Unutzer, & Operskalski, 2006). A study of 92 patients on medications compared subjects on medication alone to subjects receiving medication plus family therapy or a group family intervention (Solomon, Keitner, Ryan, Kelley, & Miller, 2008). The group family therapy focused on psychoeducation and group support. After 28 months, only 5% of the patients in the multifamily group had been hospitalized compared to 31% of patients receiving family therapy and 38% of those on medications alone. All of these patients were prescribed medications throughout the course of the study, but the specifics of the medications such as name, dosage, or adherence to medication were not reported.

The NCCMH review mentioned earlier included three low quality trials of family psychoeducation. They concluded that the family psychoeducation was effective in reducing the risk of relapse (NCCMH, 2014). The Royal Australian and New Zealand Clinical Practice guidelines stated that psychoeducation has Level 1 evidence for relapse preventions (Malhi et al., 2015).

A trial of 14 sessions of cognitive therapy over a 6-month span followed by two booster sessions over the next 6 months resulted in fewer bipolar episodes, fewer days in bipolar episodes, fewer hospitalizations, and increased social functioning over the year of the study (Lam et al., 2003). When this group was followed for 30 months, the group receiving cognitive therapy had an overall increase in time to relapse and a decrease in days spent in a bipolar episode, but the effect on relapse prevention was lost (Lam, Hayward, Watkins, Wright, & Sham, 2005). Another trial followed 253 patients for 18 months (Scott et al., 2006). These patients received up to 22 CBT sessions. There were no differences in recurrence rates in the overall groups, but a *post hoc* analysis found that CBT was effective in preventing recurrences in those patients who started the study with less than 12 previous episodes. The Royal Australia and New Zealand Clinical Practice Guidelines rate CBT as having Level 1 evidence for relapse prevention (Malhi et al., 2015).

ISPRT is based on the idea that disruptions in life style such as sleep–wake cycles and significant social disruptions increase the risk of recurrence. ISPRT is intended to help patients with bipolar disorder lead more predictable lives and thereby lower the risk of recurrence (Frank et al., 1997). A total of 175 acutely ill patients with bipolar I disorder were followed for 2 years. Patients receiving ISPRT during the acute phase of their illness survived longer without a new affective episode than did those receiving intensive clinical management (Frank et al., 2005). The Royal Australia and New Zealand Clinical Practice Guidelines rate ISPRT as having Level 3 evidence for relapse prevention (Malhi et al., 2015), but a 2016 review found no benefit of ISPRT when compared to treatment as usual (Oud et al., 2016).

FFT interventions are based on findings that patients from families with high expressed emotions (e.g., criticism, hostility or overinvolvement) are at greater risk of relapse (Kim & Miklowitz, 2004). FFT is usually provided as 21 sessions over a 9-month period. Followed for 1 year, FFT resulted in a decrease in relapses and longer delays before relapse. These patients also showed a decrease in depressive symptoms compared to those who had received two family psychoeducation classes and follow up crisis management (Miklowitz et al., 2000). When that cohort was followed for another year, the FFT cohort still had fewer relapses and longer survival intervals. Subjects also showed decreases in mood disorder symptoms and improved adherence to their medication regimen (Miklowitz, George, Richards, Simoneau, & Suddath, 2003). In a separate study, FFT resulted in a 30% decrease in hospitalization and relapses (Geddes & Miklowitz, 2013). The Royal Australia and New Zealand Clinical Practice Guidelines rate FFT as having Level 2 evidence for relapse prevention (Malhi et al., 2015).

Summary

A diagnosis of bipolar disorder is often devastating for individuals and their family members. A portion of patients will continue to experience severe illness over the course of their lifetime; however, the majority of patients can do well with effective treatment. In addition to medications, psychotherapeutic strategies are powerful treatment tools which enhance the overall wellbeing of the suffering individual.

Table 4.2 presents our findings and our treatment recommendations.

Table 4.2 Integrative biopsychosocial intervention with bipolar disorders: Summary of best-practice recommendations by level of confidence derived from strength of evidence.

Mania		
Level A	Recommended	• Psychotherapy has not been proven to be effective in managing acute mania • Patients diagnosed with mania should be started on medications with proven efficacy – Carbamazepine, lithium, valproate – Second-generation antipsychotic medications including aripiprazole, olanzapine, quetiapine, risperidone, and ziprasidone • For severe mania, combinations of mood stabilizers and second-generation antipsychotic medications should be considered • Provide psychoeducation over an extended period (~6 months) covering: – Personalized diagnostic criteria – Course and prognosis of bipolar disorder – Treatment options – Common co-morbid conditions – Self-management skills – Identification of warning signs and symptoms of relapse
Level B	Suggested	• Provide psychoeducation in a group format • Electroconvulsive therapy should be considered for patients with severe mania accompanied by psychotic symptoms, significant suicidality, life-threatening malnutrition, or catatonia, and for those patients who fail to respond to medications
Level C	May be considered	• Electroconvulsive therapy should be considered for pregnant patients with mania
Adherence to treatment		
Level A	Recommended	• Assess and manage medication side effects • Assess adherence to medication prescriptions • Make adherence to treatment recommendations a persistent focus of therapy
Level B	Suggested	• Emphasize adherence to behavioral factors such as homework and attending appointments as well as adhering to medication recommendations • If the patient permits, include family members and significant others in discussions of adherence
Level C	May be considered	• Use a variety of methods to assess medication adherence • Specifically focus on: – Maintaining a positive therapeutic alliance – Utilizing a collaborative process to develop treatment recommendations and goals – Increasing patients' knowledge about the disorder – Increasing their knowledge about treatment options including side effects

(Continued)

Table 4.2 (Continued)

Bipolar depression		
Level A	Recommended	• Electroconvulsive therapy should be considered for severely depressed patients and for patients with severe mania accompanied by psychotic symptoms, significant suicidality, life-threatening malnutrition, or catatonia, and for those patients who fail to respond to medications • Traditional antidepressants should be avoided since they increase risk of switching to a manic or hypomanic mood
Level B	Suggested	• Start the patient on a medication with evidence of efficacy in bipolar depression – Lithium, lamotrigine, olanzapine, quetiapine, or lurasidone • Augment psychopharmacology with cognitive-behavioral therapy, family focused therapy, or interpersonal and social rhythm therapy
Level C	May be considered	• Consider augmenting a mood stabilizer or second-generation antipsychotic medication with an antidepressant
Maintenance treatment		
Level A	Recommended	• Continue the patient on medications that controlled their acute symptoms • Provide psychoeducation for relapse prevention focusing on: – The nature of bipolar disorder – The importance of maintaining a regular schedule – Taking medications as prescribed • Augment psychopharmacology with cognitive therapy
Level B	Suggested	• Provide psychoeducation or psychotherapy in a group format • Augment psychopharmacology with cognitive therapy or family focused therapy • Start a medication with proven efficacy in preventing affective episodes – Lithium, lamotrigine, olanzapine
Level C	May be considered	• Consider augmenting psychopharmacology with interpersonal and social rhythm therapy

References

American Psychiatric Association (1952). *Diagnostic and statistical manual of mental disorders*. Washington DC: American Psychiatric Association, Mental Hospital Service.

American Psychiatric Association (2013). American Psychiatric Association. (2013). *Diagnostic and statistical manual of mental disorders* (5th ed.). Washington, DC: American Psychiatric Association..

Baldassano, C. F., Hosey, A., & Coello, J. (2011). Bipolar depression: An evidence-based approach. *Current Psychiatry Reports, 13*, 483–487.

Baldessarini, R. J., & Tondo, L. (2000). Does lithium treatment still work? Evidence of stable responses over three decades. *Archives of General Psychiatry, 57*, 187–190.

Bauer, M. S., McBride, L., Chase, C., Sachs, G., & Shea, N. (1998). Manual-based group psychotherapy for bipolar disorder: A feasibility study. *Journal of Clinical Psychiatry, 59*, 449–455.

Berk, L., Hallam, K. T., Colom, F., Vieta, E., Hasty, M., Macneil, C., & Berk, M. (2010). Enhancing medication adherence in patients with bipolar disorder. *Human Psychopharmacology, 25*, 1–16.

Boerhaave, H., & and Delacoste, J. (1986). *Boerhaave's aphorisms concerning the knowledge and cure of diseases* (Special Edition for the Classics of Medicine Library ed.). Birmingham, AL: The Classics of Medicine Library.

Bond, K., & Anderson, I. M. (2015). Psychoeducation for relapse prevention in bipolar disorder: A systematic review of efficacy in randomized controlled trials. *Bipolar Disorders, 17*, 349–362.

Buoli, M., Serati, M., & Altamura, A. C. (2014). Is the combination of a mood stabilizer plus an antipsychotic more effective than mono-therapies in long-term treatment of bipolar disorder? A systematic review. *Journal of Affective Disorders, 152–154*, 12–18.

Burgess, S., Geddes, J., Hawton, K., Townsend, E., Jamison, K., & Goodwin, G. (2001). Lithium for maintenance treatment of mood disorders. *Cochrane Database of Systematic Reviews, 3*, CD003013.

Cade, J. F. (1949). Lithium salts in the treatment of psychotic excitement. *Medical Journal of Australia, 2*, 349–352.

Calabrese, J. R., Bowden, C. L., Sachs, G., Yatham, L. N., Behnke, K. M., Mehtonen, O. P., . . . & DeVeaugh-Geiss, J. (2003). A placebo-controlled 18-month trial of lamotrigine and lithium maintenance treatment in recently depressed patients with bipolar I disorder. J Lamictal 605 Study Group. *Clinical Psychiatry, 9*, 1013–1024.

Ceron-Litvoc, D., Soares, B. G., Geddes, J., Litvoc, J., & de Lima, M. S. (2009). Comparison of carbamazepine and lithium in treatment of bipolar disorder: A systematic review of randomized controlled trials. *Human Psychopharmacology, 24*, 19–28.

Ciapparelli, A., Dell'Osso, L., Tundo, A., Pini, S., Chiavacci, M. C., Di Sacco, A., & Cassano, G. B. (2001). Electroconvulsive therapy in medication-nonresponsive patients with mixed mania and bipolar depression. *Journal of Clinical Psychiatry, 7*, 552–555.

Cipriani, A., Pretty, H., Hawton, K., & Geddes, J. R. (2005). Lithium in the prevention of suicidal behavior and all- cause mortality in patients with mood disorders: A systematic review of randomized trials. *American Journal of Psychiatry, 162*, 1805–19.

Cipriani, A., Rendell, J., & Geddes, J. (2009). Olanzapine in long-term treatment for bipolar disorder. *Cochrane Database Systematics Review, Jan 21*(1), CD004367.

Colom, F., Vieta, E., Reinares, M., Martinez-Aran, A., Torrent, C., Goikolea, J. M., & Gasto, C. (2003a). Psychoeducation efficacy in bipolar disorders: Beyond compliance enhancement. *Journal of Clinical Psychiatry, 64*, 1101–1105.

Colom, F., Vieta, E., Martinez-Aran, A., Reinares, M., Goikolea, J. M., Benabarre, A., & Corominas, J. (2003b). A randomized trial on the efficacy of group psychoeducation in the prophylaxis of recurrences in bipolar patients whose disease is in remission. *Archives of General Psychiatry, 60*, 402–407.

Cookson, J., Keck, P. E., Jr., Ketter, T. A., & Macfadden, W. (2007). Number needed to treat and time to response/remission for quetiapine monotherapy efficacy in acute bipolar depression: Evidence from a large, randomized, placebo-controlled study. *International Clinical Psychopharmacology, 22*, 93–100.

Davis, L. L., Bartolucci, A., & Petty, F. (2005). Divalproex in the treatment of bipolar depression: A placebo-controlled study. *Journal of Affective Disorders, 85*, 259–66.

Depp, C. A., Moore, D. J., Patterson, T. L., Lebowitz, B. D., & Jeste, D. V. (2008). Psychosocial interventions and medication adherence in bipolar disorder. *Dialogues in Clinical Neuroscience, 10,* 239–250.

Eker, F., & Harkin, S. (2012). Effectiveness of six-week psychoeducation program on adherence of patients with bipolar affective disorder. *Journal of Affective Disorders, 138,* 409–416.

Emilien, G., Maloteaux, J. M., Seghers, A., & Charles, G. (1996). Lithium compared to valproic acid and carbamazepine in the treatment of mania: A statistical meta-analysis. *European Neuropsychopharmacology, 6,* 245–252.

Fountoulakis, K. N., Kasper, S., Andreassen, O., Blier, P., Okasha, A., Severus, E., . . . & Vieta, E. (2012). Efficacy of pharmacotherapy in bipolar disorder: A report by the WPA section on pharmacopsychiatry. *European Archives of Psychiatry and Clinical Neuroscience, 262,* S1–S48.

Fountoulakis, K. N., Vieta, E., & Schmidt, F. (2011). Aripiprazole monotherapy in the treatment of bipolar disorder: A meta-analysis. *Journal of Affective Disorders, 133,* 361–370.

Frank, E., Hlastala, S., Ritenour, A., Houck, P., Tu, X. M., Monk, T. H., . . . & Kupfer, D. J. (1997). Inducing lifestyle regularity in recovering bipolar disorder patients: Results from the maintenance therapies in bipolar disorder protocol. *Biological Psychiatry, 41,* 1165–1173.

Frank, E., Kupfer, D. J., Thase, M. E., Mallinger, A. G., Swartz, H. A., Fagiolini, A. M., & Monk, T. (2005). Two-year outcomes for interpersonal and social rhythm therapy in individuals with bipolar I disorder. *Archives of General Psychiatry, 62,* 996–1004.

Gao, K., & Calabrese, J. R. (2005). Newer treatment studies for bipolar depression. *Bipolar Disorders, 7,* 13–23.

Gaudiano, B. A., Weinstock, L. M., & Miller, I. W. (2011). Improving treatment adherence in patients with bipolar disorder and substance abuse: Rationale and initial development of a novel psychosocial approach. *Journal of Psychiatric Practice, 17,* 5–20.

Geddes, J. R., Burgess, S., Hawton, K., Jamison, K., & Goodwin, G. M. (2004). Long-term lithium therapy for bipolar disorder: Systematic review and meta-analysis of randomized controlled trials. *American Journal of Psychiatry, 161,* 217–222

Geddes, J. R., & Miklowitz, D. J. (2013). Treatment of bipolar disorder. *Lancet, 381,* 1672–1682.

Ghaemi, S. N., Gilmer, W. S., Goldberg, J. F., Zablotsky, B., Kelley, M. E., . . . & Dunn R. T. (2007). Divalproex in the treatment of acute bipolar depression: A preliminary double-blind, randomized, placebo-controlled pilot study. *Journal of Clinical Psychiatry, 68,* 1840–1844.

Gitlin, M. J., Swendsen, J., Heller, T. L., & Hammen, C. (1995). Relapse and impairment in bipolar disorder. *American Journal of Psychiatry, 152,* 1635–1640.

Goodwin, F. K., Fireman, B., Simon, G. E., Hunkeler, E. M., Lee, J., & Revicki, D. (2003). Suicide risk in bipolar disorder during treatment with lithium and divalproex. *JAMA, 290,* 1467–1473.

Goodwin, F. K., & Jamison, K. R. (1990). *Manic-depressive illness.* New York: Oxford University Press.

Goodwin, G. M., Bowden, C. L., Calabrese, J. R., Grunze, H., Kasper, S., White, R., . . . & Leadbetter, R. (2004). A pooled analysis of 2 placebo-controlled 18-month trials of lamotrigine and lithium maintenance in bipolar I disorder. *Journal of Clinical Psychiatry, 65,* 432–441.

Grunze, H., Vieta, E., Goodwin, G. M., Bowden, C., Licht, R. W., Möller, H. J., & Kasper, S. (2009). Guidelines for the biological treatment of bipolar disorders: Update 2009 on the treatment of acute mania. *World Journal of Biological Psychiatry, 10*, 85–116.

Hoberg, A. A., Ponto, J., Nelson, P. J., & Frye, M. A. (2013). Group interpersonal and social rhythm therapy for bipolar depression. *Perspectives in Psychiatric Care, 49*, 226–234.

International Consensus Group (2008). International Consensus Group on the evidence-based pharmacologic treatment of bipolar I and II depression. *Journal of Clinical Psychiatry, 69*, 1632–1646.

Javadpour, A., Hedayati, A., Dehbozorgi, G. R., & Azizi, A. (2013). The impact of a simple individual psycho-education program on quality of life, rate of relapse and medication adherence in bipolar disorder patients. *Asian Journal of Psychiatry, 6*, 208–213.

Jeste, D. V., & Dolder, C. R. (2004). Treatment of non-schizophrenic disorders: Focus on atypical antipsychotics. *Journal of Psychiatric Research, 38*, 73–103.

Keck, P. E. Jr., Calabrese, J. R., McIntyre, R. S., McQuade, R. D., Eudicone, J. M., . . . & Sanchez, R. (2007). Aripiprazole monotherapy for maintenance therapy in bipolar I disorder: A 100-week, double-blind study versus placebo. *Journal of Clinical Psychiatry, 68*, 1480–1491.

Keck, P. E., Orsulak, P. J., Cutler, A. J., Sanchez, R., Torbeyns, A., Marcus, R. N., . . . & Carson, W. H. (2009). Aripiprazole monotherapy in the treatment of acute bipolar I mania: A randomized, double- blind, placebo- and lithium-controlled study. *Journal of Affective Disorder, 112*, 36–49.

Ketter, T. A., Miller, S., Dell'Osso, B., & Wang, P. W. (2016). Treatment of bipolar disorder: Review of evidence regarding quetiapine and lithium. *Journal of Affective Disorders, 191*, 256–273.

Kim, E. Y., & Miklowitz, D. J. (2004). Expressed emotion as a predictor of outcome among bipolar patients undergoing family therapy. *Journal of Affective Disorders, 82*, 343–352.

Kraepelin, E. (1988 [1913]). In T. Johnstone (Ed.), *Lectures on clinical psychiatry* (3rd English ed.). Birmingham, AL: The Classics of Psychiatry and Behavioral Sciences Library.

Lam, D. H., Burbeck, R., Wright, K., & Pilling, S. (2009). Psychological therapies in bipolar disorder: The effect of illness history on relapse prevention: A systematic review. *Bipolar Disorders, 11*, 474–482.

Lam, D. H., Hayward, P., Watkins, E. R., Wright, K., & Sham, P. (2005). Relapse prevention in patients with bipolar disorder: Cognitive therapy outcome after 2 years. *American Journal of Psychiatry, 162*, 324–329.

Lam, D. H., Watkins, E. R., Hayward, P., Bright, J., Wright, K., Kerr, N., & Sham, P. (2003). A randomized controlled study of cognitive therapy for relapse prevention for bipolar affective disorder: Outcome of the first year. *Archives of General Psychiatry, 60*, 145–152.

Loebel, A., & Citrome, L. (2015). Lurasidone: A novel antipsychotic agent for the treatment of schizophrenia and bipolar depression. *British Journal of Psychology Bulletin, 39*, 237–241.

Macritchie, K., Geddes, J. R., Scott, J., Haslam, D., & Goodwin, G. (2003). Valproate for acute mood episodes in bipolar disorder. *Cochrane Database Systematics Review, 1*, CD004052.

Malhi, G. S., Bassett, D., Boyce, P., Bryant, R., Fitzgerald, P. B., Fritz, K., & Singh, A. B. (2015). Royal Australian and New Zealand College of Psychiatrists clinical practice guidelines for mood disorders. *The Australian and New Zealand Journal of Psychiatry, 49*, 1087–1206.

McIntyre, R. S., Brecher, M., Paulsson, B., Huizar, K., & Mullen, J. (2005). Quetiapine vs haloperidol as monotherapy for bipolar mania: A 12 week, double-blind, randomized, parallel-group, placebo-controlled trial. *European Neuropsychopharmacology, 15,* 573–585.

Miklowitz, D. J. (2006). A review of evidence-based psychosocial interventions for bipolar disorder. *Journal of Clinical Psychiatry, 67*(Suppl 11), 28–33.

Miklowitz, D. J., George, E. L., Richards, J. A., Simoneau, T. L., & Suddath, R. L. (2003). A randomized study of family-focused psychoeducation and pharmacotherapy in the outpatient management of bipolar disorder. *Archives of General Psychiatry, 60,* 904–912.

Miklowitz, D. J., Otto, M. W., Frank, E., Reilly-Harrington, N. A., Wisniewski, S. R., Kogan, J. N., . . . & Sachs, G. S. (2007). Psychosocial treatments for bipolar depression: A 1-year randomized trial from the systematic treatment enhancement program. *Archives of General Psychiatry, 64,* 419-426.

Miklowitz, D. J., Simoneau, T. L., George, E. L., Richards, J. A., Sachs-Ericsson, N., & Suddath, R. (2000). Family-focused treatment of bipolar disorder: 1-year effects of a psychoeducational program in conjunction with pharmacotherapy. *Biological Psychiatry, 48,* 582–592.

Miziou, S., Tsitsipa, E., Moysidou, S., Karavelas, V., Dimelis, D., Polyzoidou, V., & Fountoulakis, K. N. (2015). Psychosocial treatment and interventions for bipolar disorder: A systematic review. *Annals of General Psychiatry, 14,* 15–57.

Mukherjee, S., Sackeim, H.S., & Schnur, D.B. (1994). Electroconvulsive therapy for acute manic episodes: A review of 50 years' experience. *American Journal of Psychiatry, 151,* 169–176.

National Collaborating Centre for Mental Health (2014). *Bipolar disorder: The assessment and management of bipolar disorder in adults, children and young people in primary and secondary care.* London: The British Psychological Society and the Royal College of Psychiatrists.

Otto, M. W., Reilly-Harrington, N., & Sachs, G. S. (2003). Psychoeducational and cognitive-behavioral strategies in the management of bipolar disorder. *Journal of Affective Disorders, 73,* 171–181.

Oud, M., Mayo-Wilson, E., Braidwood, R., Schulte, P., Jones, S. H., Morriss, R., . . . & Kendall, T. (2016). Psychological interventions for adults with bipolar disorder: Systematic review and meta-analysis. *British Journal of Psychiatry, 208,* 213–222.

Perlis, R. H., Welge, J. A., Vornick, L. A., Hirschfeld, M. A., & Keck, P. E. (2006). Atypical antipsychotics in the treatment of mania: A meta-analysis of randomized, placebo controlled trials. *Journal of Clinical Psychiatry, 67,* 509–516.

Perry, A., Tarrier, N., Morriss, R., McCarthy, E., & Limb, K. (1999). Randomised controlled trial of efficacy of teaching patients with bipolar disorder to identify early symptoms of relapse and obtain treatment. *British Medical Journal (Clinical Research Ed.), 318,* 149–153.

Poole, R., Simpson, S. A., & Smith, D. J. (2012). Internet-based psychoeducation for bipolar disorder: A qualitative analysis of feasibility, acceptability and impact. *BMC Psychiatry, 12,* 139-244X-12-139.

Poole, R., Smith, D., & Simpson, S. (2015). Patients' perspectives of the feasibility, acceptability and impact of a group-based psychoeducation programme for bipolar disorder: A qualitative analysis. *BMC Psychiatry, 15,* 184-015-0556-0.

Poolsup, N., Li Wan Po, A., & de Oliveira, I. R. (2000). Systematic overview of lithium treatment in acute mania. *Journal of Clinical Pharmacy and Therapeutics, 25*, 139–56.

Sachs, G. S., Nierenberg, A. A., Calabrese, J. R., Marangell, L. B., Wisniewski, S. R., Gyulai, L., . . . & Thase, M. E. (2007). Effectiveness of adjunctive antidepressant treatment for bipolar depression. *New England Journal of Medicine, 356*, 1711–1722.

Sajatovic, M., Davies, M., & Hrouda, D. R. (2004). Enhancement of treatment adherence among patients with bipolar disorder. *Psychiatric Services (Washington, D.C.), 55*, 264–269.

Sajatovic, M., Levin, J., Tatsuoka, C., Micula-Gondek, W., Fuentes-Casiano, E., Bialko, C. S., & Cassidy, K. A. (2012). Six-month outcomes of customized adherence enhancement (CAE) therapy in bipolar disorder. *Bipolar Disorders, 14*, 291–300.

Schoeyen, H. K., Kessler, U., Andreassen, O. A., Austad, B. H., Bergsholm, P., Malt, U. F., . . . & Vaaler, A. (2015). Treatment-resistant bipolar depression: A randomized controlled trial of electroconvulsive therapy versus algorithm-based pharmacological treatment. *American Journal of Psychiatry, 172*, 41–51.

Schou, M., Juel-Nielsen, N., Stromgren, E., & Voldby, H. (1954). The treatment of manic psychoses by the administration of lithium salts. *Journal of Neurology, Neurosurgery and Psychiatry, 17*, 250–260.

Scott, J., Colom, F., & Vieta, E. (2007). A meta-analysis of relapse rates with adjunctive psychological therapies compared to usual psychiatric treatment for bipolar disorders. *International Journal of Neuropsychopharmacology/Official Scientific Journal of the Collegium Internationale Neuropsychopharmacologicum (CINP), 10*, 123–129.

Scott, J., Paykel, E., Morriss, R., Bentall, R., Kinderman, P., Johnson, T., . . . & Hayhurst, H. (2006). Cognitive-behavioural therapy for severe and recurrent bipolar disorders: Randomised controlled trial. *British Journal of Psychiatry: The Journal of Mental Science, 188*, 313–320.

Scott, J., & Pope, M. (2002). Nonadherence with mood stabilizers: Prevalence and predictors. *Journal of Clinical Psychiatry, 63*, 384–390.

Simon, G. E., Ludman, E. J., Bauer, M. S., Unützer, J., & Operskalski, B. (2006). Long-term effectiveness and cost of a systematic care program for bipolar disorder. *Archives of General Psychiatry, 63*, 500–508.

Smith, D., Jones, I., & Simpson, S. (2010). Psychoeducation for bipolar disorder. *Advances in Psychiatric Treatment, 16*, 147–154.

Smulevich, A. B., Khanna, S., Eerdekens, M., Karcher, K., Kramer, M., & Grossman, F. (2005). Acute and continuation risperidone monotherapy in bipolar mania: A 3-week placebo-controlled trial followed by a 9-week double-blind trial of risperidone and haloperidol. *European Neuropsychopharmacology, 15*, 75–84.

Solomon, D. A., Keitner, G. I., Ryan, C. E., Kelley, J., & Miller, I. W. (2008). Preventing recurrence of bipolar I mood episodes and hospitalizations: Family psychotherapy plus pharmacotherapy versus pharmacotherapy alone. *Bipolar Disorders, 10*, 798–805.

Suppes, T., Marangell, L. B., Bernstein, I., Kelly, D., Fischer, E. G., Zboyan, H. A., . . . & Gonzalez, R. (2008). A single blind comparison of lithium and lamotrigine for the treatment of bipolar II depression. *Journal of Affective Disorder, 111*, 334–343.

Suppes, T., Vieta, E., Liu, S., Brecher, M., & Paulsson, B. (2009). Maintenance treatment for patients with bipolar I disorder: Results from a North American study of quetiapine in combination with lithium or divalproex (trial 127). *American Journal of Psychiatry, 166*, 476–488.

Swartz, H. A., & Frank, E. (2001). Psychotherapy for bipolar depression: A phase-specific treatment strategy? *Bipolar Disorders, 3,* 11–22.

Swartz, H. A., & Swanson, J. (2014). Psychotherapy for bipolar disorder in adults: A review of the evidence. *Focus (American Psychiatric Publishing), 12,* 251–266.

The Management of Bipolar Disorder Working Group. (2010). VA/DoD clinical practice guideline for management of bipolar disorder in adults. Retrieved from https://www.healthquality.va.gov/bipolar/bd_306_sum.pdf. Department of Veterans Affairs and Department of Defense.

Vieta, E., Bourin, M., Sanchez, R., Marcus, R., Stock, E., McQuade, R., McQuade, R., . . . & Iwamoto, T.(2005). Effectiveness of aripiprazole v. haloperidol in acute bipolar mania: Double-blind, randomised, comparative 12-week trial. *British Journal of Psychiatry, 187,* 235–242.

WHO (2016) International Statistical Classification of Diseases and Related Health Problems, 10th Revision (http://apps.who.int/classifications/icd10/browse/2016/en). Geneva: World Health Organization.

Vieta, E., Calabrese, J. R., Goikolea, J. M., Raines, S., & Macfadden, W. (2007). Quetiapine monotherapy in the treatment of patients with bipolar I or II depression and a rapid-cycling disease course: A randomized, double-blind, placebo-controlled study. *Bipolar Disorders, 9,* 413–425.

Zaretsky, A. E., Rizvi, S., & Parikh, S. V. (2007). How well do psychosocial interventions work in bipolar disorder? *Canadian Journal of Psychiatry. Revue Canadienne De Psychiatrie, 52*(1), 14–21.

Zaretsky, A. E., Segal, Z. V., & Gemar, M. (1999). Cognitive therapy for bipolar depression: A pilot study. *Canadian Journal of Psychiatry. Revue Canadienne De Psychiatrie, 44,* 491–494.

Zornberg, G. L., & Pope, H. G. (1993). Treatment of depression in bipolar disorder: New directions for research. *Journal of Clinical Psychopharmacology, 6,* 397–408.

5

Mood Disorders: Evidence-Based Integrated Biopsychosocial Treatment of Dysthymia and Adjustment Disorder with Depression

Kevin McGuinness, Samuel Dutton, and Peter Smith

Dysthymic disorder and adjustment disorder with depression oftentimes lack the discrete, severe episodes that mark major depression and bipolar disorder. Dysthymic disorder, unlike adjustment disorder with depression, usually has a prolonged course. Both disorders, however, may be associated with identifiable triggers, environmental or cognitive, which distinguish them from other mood disorders that correspond more closely to biological rhythms, such as those found in mood swings attributed to major depressive disorders and bipolar disorders.

In ancient Greece the term "dysthymia" meant "bad temper" and was considered to be part of the concept of melancholy, a term derived from temperament or character. The concept of dysthymia experienced a renewed interest in the 19th century with a greater emphasis on the interplay of personality and objective stressors. In 1863, Karl Ludwig Kahlbaum used the term in referring to forms of melancholy that exhibit just one phase of attenuated depression. By 1860 the term "depression" appeared in medical dictionaries, and use of the term "melancholy" was increasingly circumscribed (Spanemberg & Juruena, 2004).

With the release of the psychodynamically oriented first edition of the Diagnostic and Statistical Manual of Mental Disorders, or DSM-I (American Psychiatric Association, 1952), "Depressive Reaction," a nonpsychotic form of depression, was viewed as a psychological defense mechanism and classified as a psychoneurotic disorder. Longitudinal studies of individuals with neurotic disorders showed evidence of periodic or constant adjustment difficulties. The DSM-I also included a diagnosis of adult situational reaction under the classification of Transient Situational Personality Disorders. A transient situational personality disorder was a precursor of today's adjustment disorder insofar as the clinical picture was one of superficial maladjustment to a difficult situation, and newly experienced environmental factors. When the DSM-II was released, the more severe form of depressive reaction was replaced by the term depressive neurosis and a new, more chronic and less severe depression appeared as neurasthenic neurosis (American Psychiatric Association, 1968). Also, adult situational reaction was replaced by adjustment reaction to adult life. According to the DSM-II, neurasthenic neurosis differs from depressive neurosis in the moderateness of the depression and in the chronicity of its course. It was not until 1980 that Dysthymic Disorder and Adjustment Disorder appeared in the

Cognitive Behavioral Psychopharmacology: The Clinical Practice of Evidence-Based Biopsychosocial Integration, First Edition. Edited by Mark Dana Muse.

DSM-III taxonomy (American Psychiatric Association, 1980); these diagnoses remained relatively intact through the DSM-IV-TR (American Psychiatric Association, 2000).

Over the years many hypotheses have been proposed to distinguish between major depressive disorder and dysthymic disorder, based on variables such as personality, stress, adversity in early development, and parental psychopathology. Until very recently, the conceptual distinction between major depressive disorder and chronic depressive disorders, with respect to these variables, has found little support from research. In 2000, however, Lizardi and Klein studied 97 adult outpatients with early-onset dysthymic disorder (45 adult outpatients with episodic major depressive disorder, 45 normal controls, and their first-degree relatives) with respect to early home environment and parental psychopathology. The study's authors reported that parental mood and personality disorders were strongly associated with early adversity. However, patients with dysthymic disorder continued to differ significantly from patients with episodic major depressive disorder and normal controls when parental psychopathology was isolated. Emphasizing early childhood adversity as well as objective and subjective stress, Riso, Miyatake, and Thase (2002) reported that the determinants of chronic depression are not qualitatively different from those of acute depression, but the chronicity of depression seems to implicate increased levels of childhood adversity, protracted environmental stress, and heightened stress reactivity. Nonetheless, McCullough et al. (2003) studied 681 outpatients with chronic major depression, double depression, recurrent major depression without full inter-episode recovery, and chronic major depression superimposed on antecedent dysthymia, and observed that, with respect to a broad range of demographic, clinical, psychosocial, family history, and treatment response variables, there were few differences distinguishing the subjects.

While Lizardi and Klein (2000), Riso et al. (2002), and McCullough et al. (2003) were studying psychosocial variables in their efforts to understand depressive illness, a parallel study of biological variables began to reaffirm the stress–depression association, as well as define a distinction between acute and chronic depression, and reunify physical and mental health in a manner that promised, in turn, to redefine the relationship between clinical psychopharmacology and cognitive-behavioral therapies (CBTs). In 1998, Maier and Watkins described a framework for understanding behavior, mood, and cognition in terms of bidirectional immune-to-brain communication (Maier & Watkins, 1998). Soon thereafter, Zorrilla et al. (2001) published a meta-analysis using more than 180 studies of the relationship of depression and objective stressors to immunological assays. The investigators reported that major depression and naturally occurring stressors shared multiple immune system effects. In 2004, Segerstrom and Miller, in a meta-analysis of more than 300 empirical articles spanning three decades, further described a relationship between psychological stress and parameters of the immune system in human participants (Segerstrom & Miller, 2004).

The psychopharmacology research of recent years has lent considerable support to the idea that maladaptation brackets dysthymia (Anisman et al., 2003; Hannestad, Dellagioia, & Bloch, 2011; Raison et al., 2006). In 2014, Vogelzangs et al. conducted a prospective study to answer the question of whether inflammatory and metabolic dysregulation might predict the 2-year course of depressive disorders among antidepressant users. Utilizing data from the *Netherlands Study of Depression and Anxiety* the authors studied 315 persons, aged 18–65 years, currently treated with antidepressants for depressive disorders. Measured at baseline were inflammatory factors such as C-reactive protein, interleukin-6 (IL-6), tumor-necrosis factor-α, and metabolic measures of waist circumference, triglycerides, high-density lipoprotein (HDL) cholesterol, blood pressure, and fasting glucose factors. Depression was deemed to be chronic if patients at 2-year follow up still met DSM-IV criteria for depression. The authors found that elevated IL-6, low HDL cholesterol, hypertriglyceridemia, and hyperglycemia were associated with the chronicity of depression in antidepressant users. Vogelzangs and colleagues concluded that elevations of these inflammatory and metabolic measures predict a poor course for depressive disorders, and that treatment of depression with anti-inflammatory medications and/or behavioral interventions might improve outcomes. In late 2015, Kiecolt-Glaser Derry, and Fagundes reported that physical inflammation and depression were inextricably linked via bidirectional reciprocity, mediated by cytokine activity. Nonetheless, neither Vogelzangs et al. (2014) nor Kiecolt-Glaser et al. (2015) distinguished between dysthymia and recurrent major depressive episodes.

Catecholamines, metabolic hormones, and various cytokines comprise some of the stress markers utilized in the studies cited above. That these are correlated with depression should not be surprising as depression is stressful, and it is not unreasonable to assume that dysthymia results in chronic impediment to daily adaptation and a consequent increased stress load to those under its influence. Should not such a chronic stress load be distinguishable from less chronic stressors? Might not acute depression be distinguished from chronic depression by measuring immune system stress markers?

Ho, Yen, Chen, Huang, and Liang (2017) addressed these questions to determine whether depression occurring as part of dysthymic disorder differs from major depression. Ho and colleagues analyzed the serum of 12 patients with dysthymic disorder, 12 with major depression, and a matched control group of 20 healthy volunteers. They concluded that the cytokine milieu in dysthymic disorder differed from that of subjects with major depression and that of healthy control group members.

If dysthymic disorder can be distinguished from major depression in terms of its chronic psychosocial and biochemical manifestations of stress, what can be said of more acute disorders of adjustment? Unlike dysthymic disorder, adjustment disorder with depression is not conceptualized as a disorder of mood, but as maladaptation to objective stressors; and, contrary to dysthymic disorder, it is characterized by a predictably shorter course. These differences are not only important to note in the differential diagnosis of depression, but are also of great import when treating the presenting condition; in particular, when considering the treatment of dysthymia and adjustment disorder with depression it is advisable to select treatments according to the targeted clinical outcome. With dysthymia, it may be that pharmacological treatment is necessary when symptom severity compromises safety over the long term, whereas the depression associated with adjustment disorder is expected, in most cases, to resolve spontaneously shortly after the psychosocial stressor is removed, and may not readily justify the use of pharmacological agents that require maintenance beyond the projected time for resolution. Nevertheless, given that there is no medication that confers on its own a greater adaptability to the world in which one lives, or changes on its own ingrained maladaptive cognitive styles, pharmacological treatment alone is rarely justified in the treatment of adjustment disorder or dysthymic disorder.

Dysthymia

Chronic depression comes in many forms, but even the minor forms of chronic depression such as dysthymic disorder cause psychological dysfunction with significant social impairment in occupational, interpersonal, and family life; and, over time, such "minor" depression may be debilitating as in the classic forms of major depression (Klein & Santiago, 2003). One of the difficulties differentiating a diagnosis of dysthymia from other forms of depressive disorder has been the high co-morbidity and concomitant impairment that many patients suffer along with this condition. In addition, patients with dysthymia tend not to identify their difficulties as a change from baseline functioning, as they frequently consider their mood disorder as their *normal*, and may identify their impaired functioning as part of their baseline functioning.

Dysthymic disorder is quite common. Klein and Santiago (2003) note that previous research identified over 6% of the US population as having experienced an episode of dysthymia at some point in their lives, and over 3% had experienced dysthymia in the past year. Its prevalence is reported by Sansone and Sansone (2009) to be 3–6% in the US general population, 7% in primary care, and up to 33% in outpatient mental health settings. There is an increased risk among women for dysthymia that is similar to the reported gender differences for major depression: the incidence is twice that found among men. Moreover, the presence of a chronic depression increases the risk of major depressive episodes, and, according to Keller et al. (1995), approximately 75% of persons with dysthymic disorder had reported a major depressive episode at some point in their lives. In prospective longitudinal studies, the rate exceeds 90% (Klein, Schwartz, Rose, & Leader, 2000). Conversely, approximately 25% of patients presenting with a major depressive episode have an antecedent dysthymic disorder. What is more, Cuijpers et al. (2010) report that 20% of all depressed individuals, and up to 47% of the patients treated in the mental health system, experience chronic depression.

According to Olfson (2002), the rate of outpatient treatment for depression increased by three-fold from a rate of 0.73 per 100 persons in 1987 to 2.33 per 100 persons in 1997. As the rate of utilization increased there was also a considerable change in the way various forms of depression were being treated. During the 10-year period documented by the authors there was a distinct decrease in the utilization of psychotherapy and a concomitant increase in the use of antidepressant medication. In particular, it was noted that the percentage of people using pharmacology increased from 37.3% to 74.5%. The increased use of pharmacologic treatment for depression is understandable given growing evidence demonstrating antidepressant medication to be superior to placebo in thousands of controlled clinical trials (Fournier et al., 2010), but other factors are also likely contributors to the apparent growing imbalance in favor of pharmacotherapy over psychotherapy, including cultural bias toward a biological disease model, research funding streams influenced by commercial marketing and other fiscal pressures, and researcher preference as influenced by academic and political fashion.

Pharmacotherapy with Dysthymia

Historically, research on dysthymia has not received the same attention as major depressive disorder and bipolar disorder. Dismissing, as scientifically unsupported lore, the viewpoint that dysthymia is best treated with psychotherapy, Howland (1991) reviewed the literature describing the pharmacologic treatment of the disorder. He concluded that the efficacy of monoamine oxidase inhibitors (MAOIs) and tricyclic antidepressants (TCAs) in the treatment of dysthymia was supported by substantial evidence. Interest in the psychopharmacology of dysthymia continued throughout the 1990s (Thase, 1998; Versiani, Nardi, & Figueria, 1998) and, as newer psychotropic agents were introduced, including the selective serotonin reuptake inhibitors (SSRIs), researchers observed that patients with dysthymia, relative to patients with major depressive disorder, tended to be less tolerant of side effects and more likely to drop out of long-term treatment (Versiani et al., 1998).

Toward the end of the 1990s, Ravindran et al. (1999) observed broad support for the use of psychotropic medications for the treatment of dysthymia. The beginning of the new millennium appeared to echo previous results of the past century as Arnow and Constantino (2003) reported their conclusion that psychopharmacological treatment for dysthymic disorder had relatively well-established efficacy. An example of such findings is the systematic review by de Lima and Hotopf (2003), which described 14 trials comparing the effectiveness of tricyclic antidepressants and SSRIs in the treatment of chronic depression and dysthymia. The randomized and quasi-randomized trials included in the study compared at least two active drugs for the treatment of dysthymia. All medications were found to be effective treatments. A later study by de Lima, Moncrieff, & Soares (2005) reviewed 15 randomized controlled studies comparing active drug versus placebo for treatment of patients with dysthymia. The authors concluded that pharmacotherapy across drug types was equally effective. In particular, they reported that when compared with placebo, and using stable remission in the absence of treatment response as the main outcome measure, there were similar results across drug classes, which included TCAs, SSRIs, MAOIs, sulpride, amineptine, and ritanserin. The main difference reported was an increase in side effects produced by tricyclic medications.

More recently, a meta-analysis published by Levkovitz, Tedeschini and Papakostas (2011) describing the use of antidepressants for the treatment of dysthymia included randomized double-blind placebo-controlled trials of antidepressants for treatment of either major depression or dysthymia. While 194 studies were found eligible for their meta-analysis, only 17 focused upon treatment of dysthymia. The authors concluded that the results for patients with dysthymia treated with pharmacotherapy were superior to those of patients diagnosed with major depressive disorder. They also found lower rates of placebo response in those patients being treated for dysthymia when compared with those who were being treated for major depression.

Von Wolff, Hölzel, Westphal, Härter, and Kriston (2013) published a study in which they compared the effectiveness and tolerability of both SSRIs and TCAs for the treatment of multiple forms of chronic depression, including dysthymia. The authors reviewed studies that included adults with a form of chronic depression (i.e., dysthymia, double depression, chronic major depression, or recurrent depression without complete remission). They focused upon those studies that included pharmacological treatment with either an SSRI or TCA, with a focus upon treating depressive symptoms. Twenty RCTs (22 comparisons, 2,772 participants) reported in 51 publications were included in the review. The authors found "similar results" for SSRIs and TCAs with regard to rates of response and remission, when compared to placebo. Treatment with TCAs, however, was associated with significantly higher dropout and adverse event rates.

The studies described above have issued from, and guided practice toward, a biological model, one that may have directly or indirectly created in patients and practitioners a bias that is by now quite culturally ingrained (McGuinness, 2014). Arguably, this cultural bias has incubated a growing placebo effect impacting new drug trials (Kaptchuk & Miller, 2015) and has spurred an increase in popularity of medicinal pills and medical procedures over prevention and behavior change (Dahl, 2015). It may also have an impact on the types of research, clinical practice, and public policy decisions that are made every day. Clinically, for example, it has been the authors' experience that primary care prescribers are better informed about published clinical guidelines than about the science or biases behind those guidelines. This state of affairs places considerable responsibility upon scientist-practitioners to continue to research alternative treatments, and to share with their colleagues information derived from evidence-based studies.

Increasingly, scientific research is more openly considering that "behavioral health" must refer to all behaviors impacting health, not just mental health; that any separation of mind and body is a scientifically unsupported and clinically distracting artifice. The research to date quite consistently supports the conclusion that whether treating episodic or chronic depression, antidepressant medications can be beneficial. Howland (1991), as we have seen, proceeded to study the effects of medications in part due to the lack of evidentiary support for psychotherapy as the best treatment for dysthymic disorder; yet, all of the drug–dysthymia research has not disproven the initial "lore" of the psychosocial management of depression.

Psychosocial Treatment of Dysthymia as a Stand-Alone or In Combination with Pharmacotherapy

Much of the available psychotherapy research classifies psychosocial interventions into modalities such as cognitive-behavioral therapies (CBT) (including problem solving therapy, referred to as PST), dynamic therapy, and interpersonal psychotherapy. While it is true that dysthymia has been relatively neglected in pharmacological studies, it is so much more the case in studies designed to test the effectiveness of psychotherapies in the treatment of dysthymia. Still, when taken together, pharmacological and psychotherapy studies have slowly accumulated an evidence base that promises to close the gap in our understanding of effective treatment approaches to dysthymia.

Studying the relationship between dysthymia and psychosocial variables, Hayden and Klein (2000) sought to identify the predictors of course and outcome in dysthymic disorder. Their 5-year prospective study of 86 outpatients with early-onset dysthymic disorder collected data at 30 and 60 months using the Longitudinal Interval Follow-Up Evaluation and the Hamilton Depression Rating Scale. The authors reported that family history of dysthymic disorder, poor childhood maternal and paternal relationships, childhood sexual abuse, cluster C personality features, neuroticism, history of anxiety disorders, and chronic stress predicted higher levels of depression at follow up. All of these predictive factors implicate psychosocial adaption in both the etiology and course of chronic depressions.

Ravindran et al. (1999) noted, in a review of studies investigating psychosocial treatment of dysthymia, that relatively few studies have investigated the effects of psychological or behavioral therapies in dysthymia as compared to major depressive disorder. Arnow and Constantino (2003) concluded in an early review of the efficacy of nonpharmacological treatment for dysthymia that 41% of psychotherapy patients met criteria for significant clinical improvement. They observed, however, that as of the publication of their article, they could find just three published studies that compared psychotherapy with pharmacotherapy, and which did not examine the efficacy of combining these modalities. Only one of the three studies examined the treatment of dysthymic disorder with cognitive therapy. That study by Dunner et al. (1996) examined the treatment of dysthymic patients for 16 weeks with either fluoxetine or cognitive psychotherapy. The authors reported that there was no statistically significant difference between the medication or psychotherapy groups.

As mentioned earlier, Ravindran et al. (1999) examined the effectiveness of pharmacologic treatment (sertraline) or group CBT for patients with dysthymia. They also tested the relative efficacy of drug treatment augmented by group cognitive therapy. Recognizing that clinical improvement may not correspond to functional improvement, the investigation assessed the impact of treatment on quality of life, coping styles, and stress perception. Subjects were 97 adult men and women between the ages of 21 and 54 years. Control subjects were primarily university and hospital staff. Prior to administration of treatment, each treatment group underwent a 1-week placebo washout, during which none of the patients was excluded due to early placebo response. Treatment started with 50 mg and increased bi-monthly with the dose at week eight being carried through week 12 at an average maximum does of 177.90 mg/day. Twenty-five of the patients receiving drug treatment also received group cognitive therapy, with 22 patients receiving no counseling services. Groups consisted of 7–10 patients with two therapists, and therapy consisted of 12 90-min sessions. Results showed a reduction of clinical symptoms/impairment by those subjects receiving sertraline therapy, whether or not they received group CBT. Group CBT alone did not reduce clinical symptoms of dysthymia any more effectively than placebo. However, although group CBT alone did not have as pronounced an effect on clinical symptoms as sertraline alone, when combined with sertraline, group CBT seemed to enhance performance on functionality measures.

In a paper described as a "non-systematic review of the literature of original studies complemented with data from meta-analyses and specialized textbooks" Powell, Abreu, Oliveira, and Sudak (2008, p. S73) and Abreu, Bitencourt, and Sudak (2012) reported that depressed patients who respond to CBT express a more durable response than patients treated with medication. Although the authors examined studies of patients with major depressive disorder, they considered the implications for patients with dysthymia. They concluded that "CBT in the treatment of depression is one of the therapeutic alternatives with the highest empirical evidence of efficacy, whether applied alone or in combination with pharmacotherapy" (p. S78). The authors also observed a relapse rate of 9–57% for patients across the depression types reviewed. In an earlier study Versiani et al. (1998) reported a relapse rate as high as 89.1% for antidepressant-treated dysthymia patients following discontinuation of pharmacotherapy. Powell et al. (2008) observed that cognitive therapies seemed to reduce the relapse rate of recurrent depression.

Von Wolff et al. (2012) compared the combination of pharmacotherapy and psychotherapy against pharmacotherapy alone with chronic depression (including, but not limited to dysthymia). Patients with a formal diagnosis of chronic depression, such as chronic major depression, dysthymia, double depression, or recurrent depression without remission were included in the meta-analysis. Psychotherapy modalities that were reported included brief supportive psychotherapy (SP), CBT, cognitive-behavioral analysis system of psychotherapy (CBASP), and interpersonal psychotherapy (IPT). Overall, 28 publications allowed for a total of nine comparisons across eight studies of a combined intervention versus pharmacotherapy alone. Out of these eight studies, five specified that participants met the criteria for dysthymia. Two of those studies included participants with double depression. Medications utilized in these five studies included sertraline, moclobemide, and amitriptyline/desipramine. Overall, the authors identified three factors that modified the treatment outcomes, including target disorder (major depression versus dysthymia), type of psychotherapy administered, and type of pharmacotherapy. Patients suffering from chronic major depression receiving combined therapies demonstrated greater treatment effects than similarly treated subjects with dysthymia; patients receiving pharmacotherapy combined with CBASP demonstrated greater treatment effects than patients receiving pharmacotherapy combined with IPT; and, the use of SSRIs resulted in a diminished "add-on effect" as compared with other medications included in the study, suggesting, perhaps, that SSRIs and psychotherapy may address overlapping symptoms. It was also observed that combined therapies had a significantly greater beneficial impact on quality of life scales included in the meta-analysis

Cuijpers et al. (2013) also attempted to compare the efficacy of psychotherapy and pharmacotherapy with dysthymia and other depressive and anxiety disorders. The overall effect size for all conditions indicated the difference between psychotherapy and pharmacotherapy at posttest for all 78 comparisons was .02; the difference was not significantly different than zero, and suggested equal efficacy across domains and modalities.

Von Wolff et al. (2013) addressed concerns related to specificity of treatment modalities. As such, they compared single treatments, rather than grouped treatments, during the acute treatment phase. They reported that for the acute treatment of dysthymic disorder, medication was the most effective treatment option and suggested that psychotherapies, such as CBASP, had also shown promise as an effective therapy. However, the distribution of psychotherapy types across diagnostic subtypes such as major depressive disorder or dysthymia (now subsumed under the umbrella of Persistent Depressive Disorder in DSM-5) confounded results and made interpretation somewhat ambiguous.

Recently, perhaps reflecting growing acceptance of the multifactorial nature of dysthymia, Ebrahimi Neshatdoost, Mousavi, Asadollahi, and Nasiri (2013) compared the efficacy of spiritual integrated psychotherapy (SIPT) and CBT on the intensity of depression symptoms and dysfunctional attitudes of patients with dysthymic disorder. The authors reported that SIPT and CBT were more effective than pharmacotherapy as measured by the Beck Depression Inventory (Beck, Ward, Mendelson, Mock, & Erbaugh, 1961) and the Dysfunctional Attitudes Scale (de Graaf, Roelofs, & Huibers, 2009; Weissman & Beck, 1999;). However, SIPT was found to be more effective in changing dysfunctional attitudes than CBT or medication.

Dysthymic disorder appears to have both biochemical and psychosocial components, which may interact, unlike other less chronic forms of depressive illness. It may combine characteristics of both episodic depression, as reflected in periodic symptomatic exacerbation or double depression, and chronic suboptimal psychosocial adaptability. Pharmacotherapy is clearly efficacious in the treatment of neurovegetative symptoms of acute or chronic depression. Likewise, psychotherapy is clearly efficacious in the treatment of psychosocial maladaptability presenting with recurrent acute or chronic forms of depression. The clinical decision to treat dysthymic disorder with pharmacotherapy, psychotherapy, or a combination must depend on a clinical assessment that considers symptom severity, chronicity, social adaptability, stress management strategies, age of onset, patterns of physical illness, and other factors. The accumulated evidence suggests that dysthymic disorder is associated with neurovegetative symptoms, psychosocial maladaptation, and biochemical changes requiring a comprehensive treatment approach. While psychotherapy alone may be considered adequate treatment for a given patient, it does not appear that pharmacotherapy alone can be generally justified, given the apparently ubiquitous association of dysthymia with psychosocial maladaptation, both before and after treatment with medication. Finally, while combined psychotherapeutic and pharmacotherapeutic interventions are preferred, the timing and duration of these therapies must be strategic, taking into consideration relative importance of long-term remission over shorter-term symptom relief.

The following case study is an apropos segue from our discussion of dysthymia to that of adjustment disorder with depression.

Case Study in Dysthymia

The patient is a 24-year-old female who described a 6-month period, ending approximately 2 years ago, which she experienced as a very "dark period" during which she had frequent suicidal thoughts, but formulated no intent or plan. Patient reported that during her dark period she visited a primary care physician who diagnosed a depression, without elaborating, and prescribed an SSRI. Patient described significant improvement while taking the SSRI, but there was no psychotherapy provided and inadequate medication management. The patient self-discontinued paroxetine when she felt better. More recently, the patient reported to a different primary care provider, based upon intuition that her mood was darkening once again. She described a history of poor decisions and generally poor social adaptability. The most prominent symptom was anxiety. The patient was diagnosed by her primary care provider with adjustment disorder with anxiety and referred to a psychologist for treatment. Upon presentation to the psychologist, the patient described diminished sleep, diminished concentration, intermittent sadness against a backdrop of chronic irritability, and variable, but generally diminished, energy. She was acutely fearful of a return to the depression of almost 2 years prior. The patient acknowledged chronic social maladjustment, chronically low self-esteem, and self-dislike. There was no identifiable precipitating event. There was no active suicidality.

In retrospect, this patient initially presented to a primary care clinic during a major depressive episode. At that time she described her symptoms as severe, including frequent suicidal ideation, and an acute onset. She left the 15-min appointment with a diagnosis of depression and a prescription for an SSRI. Two years later the patient presented with a less severe set of symptoms, no suicidality, and prominent anxiety. The patient described a series of objectively stressful life events, which were interpreted by the new provider as precipitant to the presenting symptoms. The new provider refrained from writing a prescription, given the lower severity of the symptoms presented. The new provider identified that the patient had poor coping skills with associated anxiety. This time the patient left the clinic with a diagnosis of adjustment disorder with anxiety; depression was not identified as prominent, and the patient was referred to a psychologist.

The psychologist's initial evaluation revealed a chronic depression/dysthymia with a history of at least one superimposed major depressive episode (double depression). The patient was diagnosed with dysthymic disorder. Her fear of a returning major depressive episode was associated with her acute anxiety symptoms. CBT/problem solving therapy was subsequently initiated and an SSRI was prescribed.

Adjustment Disorder with Depression

While adjustment disorders occupy a small fraction of the pages within DSM-5, in behavioral health practice they represent a much larger proportion of cases, and they are especially prevalent in the primary care environment (Blacker & Clare, 1988; Casey, Dillon, & Tyrer, 1984). Adjustment disorder prevalence increases with the severity of medical illness, so that hospitalized patients demonstrate even higher levels of this diagnosis, and contribute significantly to the demand for consult-liaison psychiatry/psychology (American Psychiatric Association, 2013). Despite its ubiquitous presence across treatment settings, the true prevalence of adjustment disorders has not been definitively determined because the largest epidemiological studies have not included this diagnostic category in their efforts: Neither the Epidemiological Catchment Area Study (Myers et al., 1984), nor the National Comorbidity Survey (Kessler et al., 2005), nor, indeed, the National Psychiatric Morbidity Survey (Jenkins et al., 2003) included adjustment disorders (Casey, 2009). Lack of comprehensive data notwithstanding, the DSM-5 makes the following statement:

> Adjustment disorders are common, although prevalence may vary widely as a function of the population studied and the assessment methods used. The percentage of individuals in outpatient mental health treatment with a principal diagnosis of an adjustment disorder ranges from approximately 5% to 20%. In a hospital psychiatric consultation setting, it is often the most common diagnosis, frequently reaching 50%. (American Psychiatric Association, 2013, p. 287).

Adjustment disorders occur in response to an identifiable stressor. They impair one or more functional life areas (e.g., work or relationships), or represent distress greater than expected for that stressor. The proviso is that the stress-related disturbance does not meet criteria for another mental health disorder, nor can it be an exacerbation of a preexisting diagnosis—it must be linked to the identified stressor. The stress-related disturbance must occur within 3 months of the onset of the stressor, and is expected to resolve within 6 months of the stressor itself. As long as these criteria are met, adjustment disorders can be co-morbid with other mental health disorders. In the DSM-5, adjustment disorders maintain the same subtypes as in previous editions of the DSM, but lose the specifier of being acute or chronic. However, the DSM-5 makes it clear that in some cases, adjustment disorders can be "continuous" or "persistent" (e.g., chronic pain) (American Psychiatric Association, 2013).

Adjustment disorders are associated with a higher risk of suicide than is generally appreciated. A study of an inpatient psychiatry unit found that, on admission, those with an adjustment disorder had higher rates of prior suicide attempts than patients without adjustment disorders, 96% vs. 79%, respectively (Kryzhanovskaya & Canterbury, 2001). Another study revealed that patients brought to an emergency room for suicide attempts were most likely to have had an adjustment disorder diagnosis (48%), with substance abuse (22%) and mood disorders (15%) occurring at lower rates (Schnyder & Valach, 1997). Na et al. (2013) demonstrated a higher risk of previous suicide attempts in adjustment disordered patients who displayed alexithymia, and specifically, with those who had difficulty describing their feelings. Difficulty describing feelings is one of five constructs assessed by the Toronto Alexithymia Scale (Taylor, 1994). Finally, the DSM-5 notes,

"Adjustment disorders are associated with an increased risk of suicide attempts and completed suicide" (American Psychiatric Association, 2013, p. 287).

Pharmacotherapy with Adjustment Disorders

Because adjustment disorders are often seen in primary care, they are frequently treated with psychotropic medication by general practitioners. The prevalence of adjustment disorders in primary care has been estimated to range from 11% to 18% (Blacker & Clare, 1988; Casey et al., 1984). In a separate investigation based on stricter criteria than previous studies, and using the Structured Clinical Interview for DSM-IV (SCID) (First, Spitzer, Gibbon, & Williams, 2002), Fernandez et al. (2012) found adjustment disorders in 3% of primary care patients. Of these patients, 37% were prescribed a psychotropic medication by their primary care provider. Those treated pharmacologically received an anxiolytic (e.g., benzodiazepine) in 71% of the cases, while 44% received an antidepressant, and 10% received a sedative-hypnotic (e.g., for insomnia). The study did not distinguish between adjustment disorders with different presentations (anxiety, depression, disturbance in behavior).

An earlier French study (Semaan et al., 2001) looked only at the subtype adjustment disorder with anxiety, and found it diagnosed in 1% of all primary care patients; the researchers determined that 74% of those diagnosed with adjustment disorder with anxiety were treated with medication. Of those treated with medication, 88% received anxiolytics, 14% received an antidepressant, and 11% received a sedative-hypnotic. In both the Fernandez et al. (2012) and Semaan, et al. (2001) studies, the psychotropic medication prescribed by primary care providers was heavily weighted toward benzodiazepines.

Apart from the primary care setting, adjustment disorders are common in outpatient psychiatry, and are frequently treated with psychotropic medication in that setting as well. The DSM-5 notes prevalence rates of adjustment disorders in outpatient mental health treatment of 5–20%. Past studies of adult psychiatric outpatient treatment support rates ranging from 5–21% and include Jones, Yates, Williams, Zhou, & Hardman (1999), Despland, Monod, & Ferrero (1995), and Andreasen and Wasek (1980). Shear et al. (2000) found adjustment disorders were the most frequent clinical diagnosis among seven outpatient psychiatry clinics, representing 35% of all diagnoses. In this study, when formal assessment criteria utilizing the SCID were subsequently applied to the original data, a much lower estimated rate of adjustment disorders was obtained, just 3%. This study provides important empirical evidence that adjustment disorders are far more frequently diagnosed and utilized in clinical practice than would be the case if strict diagnostic criteria were applied. Moreover, this discrepancy is quite large, accounting for a 32 percentage point difference. Clinicians were found in the Shear et al. (2000) study to underdiagnose major depressive disorder, and this missed disorder alone explained the majority of the 32-percentage point difference between clinician-diagnosed and SCID-diagnosed adjustment disorders.

In the world of consult-liaison psychiatry, where supporting psychosocial therapies are more easily accessed than in the primary care setting, Strain et al. (1998) found 77% of adjustment disorder patients were referred to therapy, and 12% were prescribed psychotropic medications. Of those who received medicine, 60% received antidepressants, 20% received anxiolytics, 10% received sedative-hypnotics, and 10% received antipsychotics. A comparison with the prescribing patterns of primary care yields an immediate difference: far fewer anxiolytics and far more antidepressants are prescribed for adjustment disorders in the behavioral health setting than within primary care. The prescribing of sedative-hypnotics for insomnia within psychiatry is consistent with such use in primary care (10% and 11%, respectively), while antipsychotic use represents more complex psychopharmacotherapy, commensurate with prescribing behavioral health practices. Possible rationales for antipsychotic use with adjustment disorders, with second-generation antipsychotics most often employed, can include efforts to augment antidepressant or anxiolytic effects (especially in treatment-resistant cases), reduce agitation/stabilize mood, address co-morbid personality disorder features, resolve insomnia, or a combination of these factors.

After an exhaustive search of the literature to date, which included accessing all relevant material at the National Library of Medicine, Bethesda, Maryland, we have concluded that there have been no significant randomized clinical trials of pharmacotherapy for adjustment disorder with depression, nor are there any treatment guidelines issued by the American Psychiatric Association or any European psychiatric organization. This finding is in stark contrast to dysthymia, which has accumulated a comparatively greater database for pharmacological studies over psychosocial ones, albeit with significant methodological limitations on the generalizability of results.

Without hard evidence to guide one's clinical choices, practice interventions must be guided by broader evidence. As noted above, primary care settings favor anxiolytics, while behavioral health settings favor antidepressants, many of which have anxiolytic properties. Despite the paucity of research, there are rational arguments for considering antidepressants over anxiolytics. In the authors' experience, anxiolytics in primary care are almost exclusively relatively short-acting benzodiazepines (e.g., alprazolam or lorazepam). While benzodiazepines can be effective with short-term anxiety, they are problematic for use beyond a 2–4-week window due to potential dependence, tolerance, withdrawal risks, and depressogenic contributions over time. Such drugs may also interfere with the therapeutic goal of empowering patients to manage their own mental health through concerted problem solving and behavioral changes. Even though adjustment disorders can be less severe than many of their Axis I relatives, they will invariably result in treatment longer than 2–4 weeks' duration. Despland et al. (1995) demonstrated an average treatment length of 8 months with psychotropic medications for adjustment disorders; and psychotherapy studies for adjustment disorder included in the *Cochrane Review* discussed below were typically 4–6 weeks (Arends et al., 2012). The extended pharmacological treatment of adjustment disorder beyond the 6-month expected remission prognosis may be due in part to practitioner unfamiliarity with the disorder, misdiagnosis of adjustment disorder where a more severe or chronic disorder exists (such as dysthymia or major depressive disorder), or failure to discontinue psychotropics postremission, etc.

Abuse and dependence risk associated with benzodiazepine use is particularly problematic in clients with substance abuse vulnerability. Benzodiazepines also pose pharmacodynamic issues that are obviated by the antidepressants. Anxiolytics used in primary care tend to have short half-lives, and thus will produce uneven effects throughout the day. This is in contrast to antidepressants, which provide more stable, continuous effects when taken as directed. A final caveat with the use of benzodiazepines to treat adjustment disorders is the common "discovery" by patients that their benzodiazepines can be used with good success for sleep. Such discovery has led many to begin to misuse these medications for sleep support without consulting the prescriber, adding additional complexity to their treatment. There are other pharmacological alternatives that can be considered when sleep is targeted as a separate treatment focus. Nonetheless, behavioral approaches, including sleep hygiene promotion, are generally indicated over pharmacological management of insomnia, and even more so in the case of adjustment disorders where the emphasis is on cognitive-behavioral adjustment to the triggering stressor.

Benzodiazepines are a poor choice for treatment of depressive symptoms, which characterize many adjustment disorders; they have no known efficacy for depression. In fact, there is some evidence that benzodiazepines may potentiate depressive symptoms, especially with long-term use (Ashton, 1986; Lader & Petursson, 1981). Benzodiazepines induce adverse cognitive effects on memory and concentration, which may be superimposed on memory and concentration problems already associated with ongoing depression. Adding to these concerns, a recent revision to existing black box warnings was issued by the Food and Drug Administration (FDA) for combining benzodiazepines with opioids, as such a "cocktail" increases risk of central respiratory depression (FDA, 2016).

In contrast, SSRIs are effective for both the depressive and anxiety symptoms that accompany the spectrum of adjustment disorders. They are relatively safe and can be used for long periods of time without the misuse, dependence, tolerance, and side effect issues of benzodiazepines. Serotonin–norepinephrine reuptake inhibitors (SNRIs) are an option in addition to SSRIs, as is bupropion, which is described as a norepinephrine–dopamine reuptake inhibitor (NDRI). However, bupropion can sometimes increase anxiety due to its activating properties via norepinephrine and dopamine, and might best be reserved for patients whose distress is confidently limited to depression without any anxiety.

Given that antidepressants hold a number of advantages over benzodiazepines, it is fair to ask whether there is any basis for choosing one antidepressant over another. Since there is no research on efficacy of treating adjustment disorders with medicines, broader evidence on the general efficacy of antidepressant medication with depressive disorders provides some guidance in selecting antidepressants for the treatment of adjustment disorder with depression. To the degree that depression experienced in adjustment disorders is on a continuum with depression experienced in major depressive disorder, allied research investigating the comparative effectiveness of different antidepressants with major depressive disorder may have value. As noted above, the fact that this overlap *de facto* exists is supported by Shear et al. (2000), who determined that a significant portion of clients initially diagnosed with adjustment disorder were more correctly rediagnosed with major depressive disorder when strict DSM criteria were applied.

Perhaps the most extensive attempt to answer the question of comparative efficacy of medicines for major depression was completed by the Cochrane Collaboration. Cipriani et al. (2009) examined 117 randomized controlled trials involving 25,928 participants from 1991 to 2007. There have been relatively few new antidepressants introduced since this very inclusive analysis. Cipriani et al. (2009) used multitreatment meta-analysis, which accounts for both direct and indirect comparisons of antidepressants used to treat depression. Essentially, the meta-analysis looked at studies that compared one antidepressant with another, and then considered in aggregate what statistical relationship best explained the efficacy of each antidepressant in comparison with all of the others. This is perhaps most easily conceptualized by Fig. 5.1.

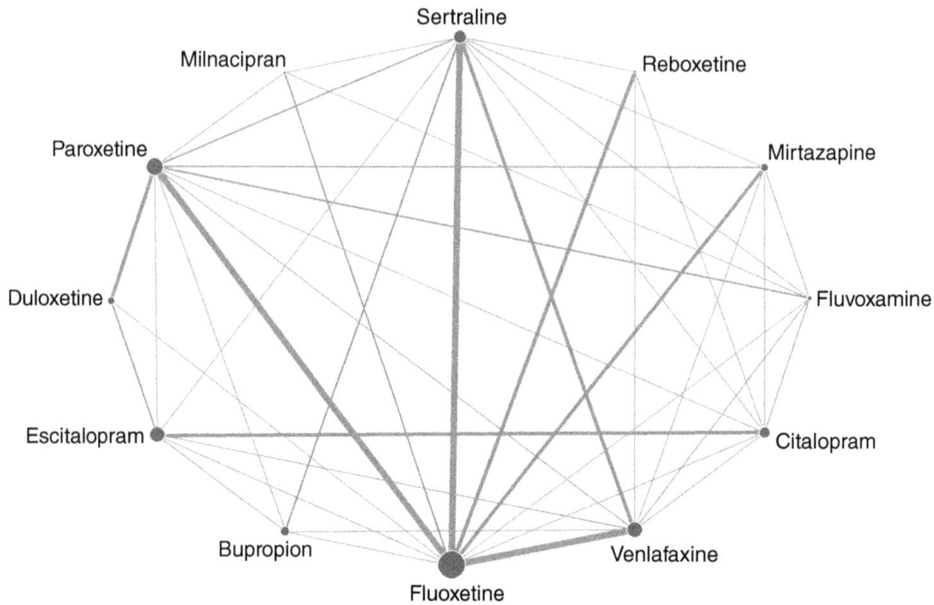

Figure 5.1 Network of eligible comparisons for the multiple-treatment meta-analysis for efficacy (response rate). The width of the lines is proportional to the number of trials comparing each pair of treatments, and the size of each node is proportional to the number of randomized participants (sample size). From Cipriani et al. (2009).

Cipriani et al. (2009) examined not just the efficacy of each antidepressant, but also the tolerability as measured by all-cause dropouts from each of the 117 studies. The study thus addresses the two questions most frequently posed by the prescribing clinician: How well does this medicine work, and how well will it be tolerated by my patient? Table 5.1, an adaptation from the study data, summarizes the results:

In reviewing this information, escitalopram is 1.32 times more likely than fluoxetine to be successful in treating depressive symptoms in clients with major depressive disorder. In addition, according to Cipriani et al. (2009), escitalopram has 84% the chance of fluoxetine to be discontinued for tolerability reasons. In order to view both efficacy and tolerability across medicines more easily, we have rearranged the data by taking the inverse of the tolerability column; this allows for easier comparison and shows that escitalopram is 1.19 times more likely to be tolerated than fluoxetine (Dutton, 2014). Since both efficacy and tolerability are important to clients, we calculated a final heuristic by multiplying efficacy and tolerability together, giving an indicator of the likelihood of success, and termed it the Success Index (Dutton, 2014, 2016). The antidepressants are thus ordered by the value of their Success Index in Table 5.1.

Psychosocial Treatment of Adjustment Disorders

The most sustained attempt to answer the question of which psychotherapies are effective in treating adjustment disorder-related depression was conducted in The

Table 5.1 Relative efficacy and tolerability of various antidepressant medications.[a]

		Odds ratio for		Success
Ranking	Antidepressant	Efficacy	Tolerability	Index
1	Escitalopram	1.32	1.19	1.57
2	Sertraline	1.25	1.14	1.43
3	Mirtazapine	1.37	0.97	1.33
4	Citalopram	1.10	1.11	1.22
5	Venlafaxine	1.28	0.94	1.21
6	Bupropion	1.08	1.12	1.20
7	Fluoxetine	1.00	1.00	1.00
8	Milnacipran[b]	1.01	0.97	0.98
9	Paroxetine	1.02	0.91	0.93
10	Duloxetine	0.99	0.84	0.83
11	Fluvoxamine	0.98	0.82	0.80
12	Reboxetine[b]	0.68	0.70	0.47

[a] Adapted from Cipriani et al. (2009).
[b] Note that two of these medicines are not approved for depression in the US market: milnacipran and reboxetine.

Netherlands, where investigators focused on stress related to work absences (van der Klink, Blonk, Schene, & Van Dijk, 2001). Continuing efforts led to the "Dutch Practice Guidelines for Managing Adjustment Disorders" (van der Klink & van Dijk, 2003), which addressed therapy choice. The primary conclusion of the Dutch study was that CBT, or a combination of CBT and relaxation training, were effective with adjustment disorders in general. The primary element of CBT involves restructuring problematic cognitions to develop a more productive point of view, which helps to create a starting point from which solutions become more apparent (van der Klink & van Dijk, 2003). About 10 years later, research in The Netherlands culminated with the *Cochrane Review*, "Interventions to facilitate return to work in adults with adjustment disorders" (Arends et al. 2012). For this review, nine randomized clinical trials were considered. In contrast to van der Klink & van Dijk (2001), the more rigorous review by Arends et al. (2012) did not support standard CBT as having a significant effect. However, the results did support PST, a form of CBT focused more directly on coping strategies than on symptomatic relief of depression, as an effective intervention. Arends and colleagues describe PST in terms of the following steps: (1) making an inventory of problems and/or opportunities; (2) brainstorming solutions; (3) writing down solutions and any support needed for these solutions, and assessing the applicability of these solutions; (4) discussing solutions and making an action plan; and (5) evaluating the action and implementation of solutions.

In line with their earlier studies, Arends et al. (2014) conducted a randomized controlled trial of PST and found it provided significantly greater improvement compared to the control group. Moreover, Arends et al. (2014) also attempted to determine which elements of PST were most significant. The primary conclusion was that, in addition to making an inventory of problems, clients who discussed solutions with their clinician and strategized how those solutions might be realized had significantly better outcomes that those who focused more exclusively on their problems. This somewhat self-evident finding highlights that problem-focused treatment in which the problem is examined is not as helpful as a solution-focused therapy that encourages patients to identify concrete practicable changes in their lives (Arends et al., 2014).

Combining Pharmacotherapy and Psychotherapy in Treating Adjustment Disorder with Depression

Psychotherapy is particularly indicated for the treatment of adjustment disorders due to the nature of the disorder: there is an identified stressor linked with both the onset and resolution of this condition, and problem solving approaches have been demonstrated to be helpful with such psychosocial factors by assisting the individual to adjust to them (Arends et al., 2012, 2014). Quite often, one expects psychotherapy to be effective and sufficient in resolving the symptom of depression associated with an adjustment disorder. In the case where this is not the outcome, medication may be added, and a combined approach pursued. When medication is used, antidepressants are recommended over benzodiazepines.

While there are no studies to guide optimal use of medication adjunctive to primary psychotherapy, the following factors are proposed, based on risks reviewed above and clinical experience. The greater the presence of these factors, the stronger the recommendation for combined treatment:

- *Degree of suicidality*: Expressed suicidal ideation and intent, past suicidal ideation and seriousness of past intent, and past self-harm behaviors can all be assessed. A caveat here, however, is the black box warning on increased suicidal thoughts associated with antidepressant medication.
- *Degree of functional impairment*: For example, when sleep or work are seriously impacted. Relationship or marital issues are also a common index stressor for adjustment disorders, and some clients request medications that can help reduce anger, irritability, and stress in the context of those relationships.
- *Degree of duration*: Some stressors can be long term, such as difficulties at a workplace, ongoing or chronic medical issues, or long-term relationship issues.
- *Severity of symptoms*: With more severe depressive and anxiety symptoms, one might expect criteria for major depression or generalized anxiety disorder might be met. Whether the condition is rediagnosed or not, severe symptoms of depression are suggestive of the need for adjunctive pharmacotherapy.
- *Lack of target gains in therapy*: *Ceteris paribus*, this may be correlated to personality features, as suggested above by Na et al. (2013). In any event, lack of therapeutic gains requires considering additional or alternative intervention.

The determination by the clinician to include medication in the treatment of adjustment disorder with depression is a complex one. The above factors are considered by the authors to be a starting place in that determination. The following case study is illustrative.

Case Study in Adjustment Disorder with Depression

A 22-year-old white male with 16 years of education presented to an outpatient clinic with depressed mood of 1 month in response to the breakup of a serious dating relationship of 9 months. He was having difficulty focusing at work, and left in the middle of his workday without prior planning to seek counseling help. He had no prior mental health history. His Patient Health Questionnaire-9 (Kroenke, Spitzer, & Williams, 2001) revealed depressive symptoms in the mild range (PHQ-9 = 12), with Item 9, "Thoughts that you would be better off dead or of hurting yourself in some way," endorsed at a 2 ("More than half the days"). On intake, he denied prior suicide attempts and expressed fleeting thoughts of hurting himself. His generalized anxiety disorder (GAD-)7 scale score (Kroenke, Spitzer, Williams, & Lowe, 2006) revealed generalized anxiety symptoms also in the mild range (GAD-7 = 9). He had no ongoing medical issues and vital signs were normal. He was not on any medicines. Sleep was mildly impaired with initial insomnia for up to an hour on some nights.

The patient was diagnosed with adjustment disorder with depressed mood. He was started in group therapy for cognitive restructuring of problematic thoughts. Tragically, 3 weeks later, after attending two group sessions, he took his own life.

In retrospect, it may be argued that major depressive disorder was a more accurate diagnosis, but as is often the case clinically, an identified stressor in the context of no prior mental health history with mild symptoms influenced the selection of the working diagnosis. It can be argued that the patient had two other indicators of more severe impact: he left unplanned in the middle of his workday to seek help, and he endorsed thoughts he might be better off dead "more days than not," perhaps unusual given a mild level of depressive symptoms. Despite the scarce evidence base, the treatment modality of group therapy, albeit with a cognitive approach, is not one that has any known efficacy for adjustment disorder with depressed mood.

While the patient's ultimate suicide may be surprising, the literature reviewed above supports the real presence of suicide risk with an adjustment disorder diagnosis. Hindsight is 20 20, but this patient may have been better served if a combination of individual PST and medication had been initiated at the outset of his treatment.

In summary, dysthymia and adjustment disorder with depression have received little research attention. Although they are often considered "minor" diagnoses in comparison with major depression and bipolar disorder, they impact significantly on patient health and wellbeing. Table 5.2 summarizes our findings with regard to the treatment of these two pernicious disorders.

Table 5.2 Integrative biopsychosocial intervention with dysthymia and adjustment disorder with depression: Summary of best-practice recommendations by level of confidence derived from strength of evidence.

Dysthymia		
Level A	Recommended	• Combination of cognitive-behavioral therapy (CBT) and pharmacotherapy, depending upon symptom severity and medication tolerance
Level B	Suggested	• None
Level C	May be considered	• Pharmacotherapy or psychotherapy alone Medication may not be tolerated due to side effects, adverse reactions, drug sensitivities, or other factors
Adjustment disorder with depression		
Level A	Recommended	• Problem solving therapy (PST)
Level B	Suggested	• None
Level C	May be considered	• Antidepressants, consider in the presence of more severe factors detailed above • CBT

References

Abreu, N., Bitencourt, V., & Sudak, D. (2012). Cognitive-behavioral therapy for depression in *Standard and Innovative Strategies in Cognitive Behavior Therapy.*

Andreasen, N. C., & Wasek, P. (1980). Adjustment disorders in adolescents and adults. *Archives of General Psychiatry, 37,* 1166–1170.

American Psychiatric Association (1952). *Diagnostic and statistical manual of mental disorders* (1st ed.). Washington, DC: American Psychiatric Association.

American Psychiatric Association (1968). *Diagnostic and statistical manual of mental disorders* (2nd ed.). Washington, DC: American Psychiatric Association.

American Psychiatric Association (1980). *Diagnostic and statistical manual of mental disorders* (3rd ed.). Washington, DC: American Psychiatric Association.

American Psychiatric Association (2000). *Diagnostic and statistical manual of mental disorders* (4th ed., text rev.). Washington, DC: American Psychiatric Association.

American Psychiatric Association. (2013). *Diagnostic and statistical manual of mental disorders* (5th ed.). Washington, DC: American Psychiatric Association.

Anisman, H., Ravindran, A. V., Griffiths, J., & Merali, Z. (1999). Endocrine and cytokine correlates of major depression and dysthymia with typical or atypical features. *Molecular Psychiatry, 4,* 182–188.

Arends, I., Bruinvels, D. J., Rebergen, D. S., Nieuwenhuijsen, K., Madan, I., Neumeyer-Gromen, A., . . . & Verbeek, J. H. (2012). Interventions to facilitate return to work in adults with adjustment disorders. *Cochrane Database of Systematic Reviews, 2012,* 1–114.

Arends, I., Bultmann, U., Nielsen, K., van Rhenen, W., de Boer, M. R., & van der Klink, J. J. L. (2014). Process evaluation of a problem solving intervention to prevent recurrent sickness absence in workers with common mental disorders. *Social Science and Medicine, 100*, 123–132.

Arnow, B., & Constantino, M. (2003). Effectiveness of psychotherapy and combination treatment for chronic depression. *Journal of Clinical Psychology, 59*, 893–905.

Ashton, C. H. (1986). Adverse effects of prolonged benzodiazepine use. *Adverse Drug Reaction Bulletin, 118*, 440–443.

Beck, A. T., Ward, C. H., Mendelson, M., Mock, J., & Erbaugh, J. (1961). An inventory for measuring depression. *Archives of General Psychiatry, 4*, 561–571.

Blacker, C. V., & Clare, A. W. (1988). The prevalence and treatment of depression in general practice.*Psychopharmacology, 95*(Suppl), S14–S17.

Casey, P. (2009). Adjustment disorder: Epidemiology, diagnosis, and treatment. *CNS Drugs, 23*, 927–938.

Casey, P., Dillon, S. & Tyrer, P. (1984). The diagnostic status of patients with conspicuous psychiatric morbidity in primary care. *Psychological Medicine, 14*, 673–681.

Cipriani, A., Furukawa, T. A., Salanti, G., Geddes, J. R., Higgins, J. P., Churchill, R., . . . & Barbui, C. (2009). Comparative efficacy and acceptability of 12 new-generation antidepressants: A multiple-treatments meta-analysis. *The Lancet, 373*, 746–758.

Cuijpers, P., van Straten, A., Schuurmans, J., van Oppen, P., Hollon, S., & Andersson, G. (2010). Psychotherapy for chronic major depression and dysthymia: A meta-analysis. *Clinical Psychology Review, 30*, 51–62.

Cuijpers, P., Sijbrandij, M., Koole, S., Andersson, G., Beekman, A., & Reynolds, C. (2013). The efficacy of psychotherapy and pharmacotherapy in treating depressive and anxiety disorders: a meta-analysis of direct comparisons. *World Psychiatry, 12*, 137–148.

Dahl, M. (2015). The placebo effect is getting stronger—But only in the U.S. Science of Us. *New York Magazine*, October 9. Retrieved from http://nymag.com/scienceofus/2015/10/placebo-effect-is-getting-stronger.html

de Graaf, L. E., Roelofs, J., and Huibers, M. J. H. (2009). Measuring dysfunctional attitudes in the general population: The Dysfunctional Attitude Scale (form A) Revised. *Cognitive Therapy and Research, 33*, 345–355.

De Lima, M., & Hotopf, M. (2003). Pharmacotherapy for dysthymia. *Cochrane Database of Systematic Reviews.*

De Lima, M., Moncrieff, J., & Soares, B. (2005). Drugs versus placebo for dysthymia. *Cochrane Database of Systematic Reviews.*

Despland, J. N., Monod, L., & Ferrero, F. (1995). Clinical relevance of adjustment disorder in DSM-III-R and DSM-IV. *Comprehensive Psychiatry, 36*, 454–460.

Dunner, D. L., Schmaling, K. B., Hendrickson, H., Becker, J., Lehman, A., & Bea, C. (1996). Cognitive therapy versus fluoxetine in the treatment of dysthymic disorder. *Depression, 4*, 34–41.

Dutton, S. S. (2014). Psychopharmacology for depression. In S. S. Dutton, & D. S. Shearer (Co-Chairs), Psychopharmacology for Depression and Integrated Psychopharmacology for Anxiety. Symposium at the Annual Convention of the American Psychological Association, Washington, DC.

Dutton, S. S. (2016). Depression treatment: Psychopharmacology and interdisciplinary aspects. Presentation at the Annual Convention of the American Psychological Association, Denver, CO.

Ebrahimi, A., Nasiri-Dehsorkhi, H., & Mousavi, S. G. (2015). Effectiveness of spiritually augmented psychotherapy on dysfunctional attitudes in patients with dysthymic disorder. *International Journal of Body, Mind and Culture.* Retrieved February 5, 2017, from http://ijbmc.org/index.php/ijbmc/article/view/23

Ebrahimi, A., Neshatdoost, H., Mousavi, S., Asadollahi, G., & Nasiri, H. (2013). Controlled randomized clinical trial of spirituality integrated psychotherapy, cognitive-behavioral therapy and medication intervention on depressive symptoms and dysfunctional attitudes in patients with dysthymic disorder. *Advanced Biomedical Research, 2*, 53.

Fernandez, A., Mendive, J. M., Salvador-Carulla, L., Rubio-Valera, M., Luciano, J. V., Pinto-Meza, A., . . . & Serrano-Blanco, A. (2012). Adjustment disorders in primary care: Prevalence, recognition and use of services. *British Journal of Psychiatry, 201*, 137–142.

First, M. B., Spitzer, R.L, Gibbon, M., & Williams, J. B. W. (2002). *Structured clinical interview for DSM-IV-TR axis i disorders, research version, patient edition* (SCID-I/P). New York: Biometrics Research, New York State Psychiatric Institute.

Fournier, J., DeRubeis, R., Hollon, S., Dimidjian, S., Amsterdam, J., Shelton, R., & Fawcett, J. (2010). Antidepressant drug effects and depression severity. *JAMA, 303*, 47.

Griffiths, J., Ravindran, A. V., Merali, Z., & Anisman, H. (2000). Dysthymia: A review of pharmacological and behavioral factors. *Molecular Psychiatry, 5*, 242–261.

Hannestad, J., Dellagioia, N., & Bloch, M. (2011). The effect of antidepressant medication treatment on serum levels of inflammatory cytokines: a meta-analysis. *Neuropsychopharmacology, 36*, 2452–2459.

Ho, P., Yen, C., Chen, C., Huang, S., & Liang, C. (2017). Changes in cytokine and chemokine expression distinguish dysthymic disorder from major depression and healthy controls. *Psychiatry Research, 248*, 20–27.

Howland, R. H. (1991). Pharmacotherapy of dysthymia. *Journal of Clinical Psychopharmacology, 11*, 83–92.

Jenkins, R., Lewis, G., Bebbington, P., Brugha, T., Farrell, M., Gill, B., & Meltzer, H. (2003). The National Psychiatric Morbidity Surveys of Great Britain—initial findings from the Household Survey. *International Review of Psychiatry, 15*, 29–42.

Jones, R., Yates, W., Williams, S., Zhou, M., & Hardman, L. (1999). Outcome for adjustment disorder with depressed mood: Comparison with other mood disorders. *Journal of Affective Disorders, 55*, 55–61.

Kaptchuk, T. J., & Miller, F. G. (2015). Placebo effects in medicine. *New England Journal of Medicine, 373*, 8–9.

Keller, M. B., Klein, N., Hirschfeld, R. M. A., Kocsis, J. H., McCullough, J. P., Miller, I., . . . & Marin, D. B. (1995). Results of the DSM-IV mood disorders field trial. *American Journal of Psychiatry, 152*, 843–849.

Kessler, R. C., Chiu, W., Demler, O., & Walters E. E. (2005). Prevalence, severity, and comorbidity of 12-month DSM-IV disorders in the National Comorbidity Survey Replication. *Archives of General Psychiatry, 62*, 617–627.

Kiecolt-Glaser, J., Derry, H., & Fagundes, C. (2015). Inflammation: Depression fans the flames and feasts on the heat. *American Journal of Psychiatry, 172*, 1075–1091.

Klein, D., & Santiago, N. (2003). Dysthymia and chronic depression: Introduction, classification, risk factors, and course. *Journal of Clinical Psychology, 59*, 807–816.

Klein, D. N., Schwartz, J. E., Rose, S. & Leader, J. B. (2000). Five-year course and outcome of dysthymic disorder: A prospective, naturalistic follow-up study. *American Journal of Psychiatry, 157*, 931–939.

Kroenke, K., Spitzer, R. L., & Williams, J. B. (2001). The PHQ-9. *Journal of General Internal Medicine, 16*, 606–613.

Kryzhanovskaya, L. & Canterbury, R. (2001). Suicidal behavior in patients with adjustment disorders. *Crisis: The Journal of Crisis Intervention and Suicide Prevention, 22*, 125–131.

Lader, M. H., & Petursson, H. (1981). Benzodiazepine derivatives—side-effects and dangers. *Biological Psychiatry, 16*, 1195–1221.

Levkovitz, Y., Tedeschini, E., & Papakostas, G. (2011). Efficacy of antidepressants for dysthymia. *Journal of Clinical Psychiatry, 72*, 509–514.

Lizardi, H., & Klein, D. N. (2000). Parental psychopathology and reports of the childhood home environment in adults with early-onset dysthymic disorder. *Journal of Nervous and Mental Disease, 188*, 63–70.

Maier, S. F., & Watkins, L. R. (1998). Cytokines for psychologists: Implications of bidirectional immune-to-brain communication for understanding behavior, mood, and cognition. *Psychological Review, 105*, 83–107.

McCullough, J. P., Klein, D. N., Borian, F. E., Howland, R. H., Riso, L. P., Keller, M. B., & Banks, P. L. (2003). Group comparisons of DSM-IV subtypes of chronic depression: validity of the distinctions, Part 2. [Abstract]. *Journal of Abnormal Psychology, 112.*

McGuinness, K. M. (2014). Institutional decision making: Empowering of health system and economic transformation. *American Psychologist, 69*, 817–827.

Myers, J. K., Weissman, M. M., Tischler, G. L., Holzer III, C. E., Leaf, P. J., Orvaschel, H., . . . & Stoltzman, R. (1984). Six-month prevalence of psychiatric disorders in three communities: 1980 to 1982. *Archives of General Psychiatry, 41*, 959–967.

Na, K., Oh, S., Jung, H., Lee, S., Kim, Y., Han, C., . . . & Kim, S. (2013). Alexithymia and low cooperativeness are associated with suicide attempts in male military personnel with adjustment disorder: A case–control study. *Psychiatry Research, 205*, 220–226.

Olfson, M. (2002). National trends in the outpatient treatment of depression. *JAMA, 287*, 203.

Powell, V. B., Abreu, N., Oliveira, I. R., & Sudak, D. (2008). Terapia cognitivo-comportamental da depressão. *Revista Brasileira De Psiquiatria, 30*, s78–s80.

Raison, C. L., Capuron, L., & Miller, A. H. (2006). Cytokines sing the blues: Inflammation and the pathogenesis of depression. *Trends in Immunology, 27*(1), 24–31. doi:10.1016/j.it.2005.11.006

Ravindran, A., Anisman, H., Merali, Z., Charbonneau, Y., Telner, J., Bialik, R. . . . & Griffiths, J. (1999). Treatment of primary dysthymia with group cognitive treatment of primary dysthymia with group cognitive therapy and pharmacotherapy: Clinical symptoms and functional impairments. *American Journal of Psychiatry, 156*, 1608–1617.

Riso, L. P., Miyatake, R. K., & Thase, M. E. (2002). The search for determinants of chronic depression: A review of six factors. *Journal of Affective Disorders, 70*, 103–115.

Sansone, R. A., & Sansone, L. A. (2009). Dysthymic disorder: Forlorn and overlooked? *Psychiatry (Edgmont), 6*, 46–51.

Schnyder, U., & Valach, L. (1997). Suicide attempters in a psychiatric emergency room population. *General Hospital Psychiatry, 19*, 119–129.

Segerstrom, S. C., & Miller, G. E. (2004). Psychological stress and the human immune system: A meta-analytic study of 30 years of inquiry. *Psychological Bulletin, 130*, 601–630.

Seligman, D. A., & Schmidt, K. (2001). The relationship of depression and stressors to immunological assays: A meta-analytic review. *Brain, Behavior, and Immunity, 15*, 199–226.

Semaan, W., Hergueta, T., Bloch, J., Charpak, Y., Duburcq, A., Le Guern, M., . . . & Rouillon, F. (2001). Cross-sectional study of the prevalence of adjustment disorder with anxiety in general practice. *Encephale, 27,* 238–244.

Shear, K. M., Greeno, C., Kang, J., Ludewig, D., Frank, E., Swartz, H., & Hanekamp, M. (2000). Diagnosis of non-psychotic patients in community clinics. *American Journal of Psychiatry, 157,* 581–587.

Spanemberg, L., & Juruena, M. F. (2004). Dysthymia: historical/nosological characteristics and its relationship with major depressive disorder. *Revista de Psiquiatria do Rio Grande do Sul, 26,* 300–311.

Spitzer, R. L., Kroenke, K., Williams, J. B., & Lowe, B. (2006). A brief measure for assessing generalized anxiety disorder. *Archives of Internal Medicine, 166,* 1092.

Strain, J. J., Smith, G. C., Hammer, J. S., McKenzie, D. P., Blumenfield, M., Muskin, P., . . . & Schleifer, S. S. (1998). Adjustment disorder: A multisite study of its utilization and interventions in the consultation-liaison psychiatry setting. *General Hospital Psychiatry, 20,* 139–149.

Taylor, G. J. (1994). The alexithymia construct: Conceptualization, validation and relationship with basic dimensions of personality. *New Trends in Experimental and Clinical Psychiatry, 10,* 61–74.

Thase, M. E. (1998). Antidepressant treatment of dysthymia and related chronic depressions [Abstract]. *Current Opinion in Psychiatry, 11,* 77–83.

van der Klink, J. J., Blonk, R. W. B., Schene, A. H., & Van Dijk, F. J. H. (2001). The benefits of interventions for work-related stress. *American Journal of Public Health, 91,* 270–276.

van der Klink, J. J., & Van Dijk, F. J. (2003). Dutch practice guidelines for managing adjustment disorders in occupational and primary health care. *Scandinavian Journal of Work, Environment and Health, 29,* 478–487.

Von Wolff, A., Hölzel, L., Westphal, A., Härter, M., & Kriston, L. (2013). Selective serotonin reuptake inhibitors and tricyclic antidepressants in the acute treatment of chronic depression and dysthymia: A systematic review and meta-analysis. *Journal of Affective Disorders, 144,* 7–15.

Versiani, M., Nardi, A., & Figueira, I. (1998). Pharmacotherapy of dysthymia: Review and new findings. *European Psychiatry, 13,* 203–209.

Vogelzangs, N., Beekman, A. T., Dortland, A. K., Schoevers, R. A., Giltay, E. J., Jonge, P. D., & Penninx, B. W. (2014). Inflammatory and metabolic dysregulation and the 2-year course of depressive disorders in antidepressant users. *Neuropsychopharmacology, 39,* 1624–1634.

Weissman, A. N., & Beck, A. T. (1978). Development and validation of the dysfunctional attitude scale. Paper presented at the Annual meeting of the Association for the Advanced Behavior Therapy, Chicago, IL, November.

Zorrilla, E. P., Luborsky, L., Mckay, J. R., Rosenthal, R., Houldin, A., Tax, A., . . . Schmidt, K. (2001). The relationship of depression and stressors to immunological assays: A meta-analytic review. *Brain, Behavior, and Immunity, 15,* 199–226.

6

Anxiety Disorders: Evidence-Based Integrated Biopsychosocial Treatment

Mark D. Muse and Stephen M. Stahl

There is little to no evidence that anxiety disorders exist as discrete conditions, unique from one another. On the contrary, there is good evidence that various anxiety disorders share symptoms in common such as heightened anxiety and fear, heightened stress reactivity to adverse stimuli, and elevated amygdala response to threat-relevant stimuli (Rauch & Drevets, 2009). Several factor analytic studies have found that specific phobia, panic disorder, and obsessive-compulsive disorder (OCD)[1] are highly co-morbid, and might be conceptualized as forming a "fear factor" stemming from perceived threat in the present, whereas generalized anxiety and posttraumatic stress[2] disorders might be said to form an "anxious" factor due to anticipated threat (Bienvenu, Wuyek, & Stein, 2010). Still, attempts to divide anxiety disorder into discrete nosologic subcategories are replete with overlap and duplication, reducing the discriminant validity in most cases. Moreover, the data available are insufficient to justify periodic reclassifications of the kind set out in the Diagnostic and Statistical Manual of Mental Disorders (DSM) revisions (Craske et al., 2009).

These limitations notwithstanding, a certain degree of differential diagnosing allows us to better review the evidence that has accumulated over the years on how best to address the manifest symptoms that accompany anxiety; such evidence has tended to be presented along the lines of the following "disorders": generalized anxiety, specific phobia, social anxiety, panic, posttraumatic stress, and obsession-compulsion.

While there is much overlap of symptoms among the conditions making up the anxiety disorders, one might divine the most salient symptom that best defines a particular disorder by simply referring to the name of the disorder. When classified in such a manner, the prevalence of the anxiety disorders are found to vary, as is indicated in Table 6.1.

A Brief History of the Treatment of Anxiety Disorders

One might arbitrarily pick the American Civil War as a starting point of the modern era's recognition and treatment of anxiety disorders if we consult Dr. Jacob Mendes Da Costa's *Medical Diagnoses*, first published in 1864, in which he coins the term "Irritable Heart/Soldier's Heart" (Da Costa, 1871; Paul, 1987) to refer to what might be diagnosed today as posttraumatic stress disorder (PTSD)-related somatoform sequela, including

Cognitive Behavioral Psychopharmacology: The Clinical Practice of Evidence-Based Biopsychosocial Integration, First Edition. Edited by Mark Dana Muse.

Table 6.1 Prevalence of anxiety disorders.[a]

Disorder	Prevalence (%)
Adult total anxiety disorder	29
Adolescent total anxiety disorder	25
Social anxiety disorder	10
Specific phobia disorder	6–12
Generalized anxiety disorder (GAD)	3–5
Panic disorder	2–5
Obsessive-compulsive disorder (OCD)	2–3
Posttraumatic stress disorder (PTSD)	1–10

[a] Table 6.1 (adapted from Kessler et al., 2005; Kessler, Ruscio, Shear, & Wiichen, 2010; Merikangas et al., 2010; Michael, Zetsche, & Margraf, 2007) represents estimates of the average ranges for lifetime occurrence in the western world. Prevalence for each disorder is relatively stable among western countries, except for the case of PTSD, where incidents are higher for the United States than for Europe, arguably influenced by returning American veterans from Vietnam, Iraq, and Afghanistan, and by decades of immigration from traumatized Central American, Asian, and African countries.

irregular heartbeat and chronic pain (Iribarren, Prolo, Neagos, & Chiappelli, 2005; Wood, 1941). The treatment for Soldier's Heart was, in its day, a curious integrative approach that combined opium with exercise and lifestyle change.

At the end of the 19th century and beginning of the 20th, the psychosocial treatment of anxiety bifurcated into the two seemingly irreconcilable paths of Pavlov's learning theory and Freud's psychodynamic theory. Pavlovian-inspired treatment of anxiety consisted in exposure-based behavioral approaches, pioneered by John B. Watson (Watson & Rayner, 1920), while psychiatry developed psychoanalysis (Freud, 1937). Pharmacotherapy of anxiety disorders first appeared in 1903 when Adolph von Baeyer issued the first hypnotic drug in the form of barbiturate. Barbiturates were used largely to address anxiety-related sleep disturbances, and the pharmacologic treatment of anxiety itself had to wait until the late 1950s when the tricyclic imipramine was observed to forestall panic attacks (Klein, 2002); subsequently, the development and marketing of meprobamate for generalized anxiety in 1955 under the trade name Miltown created the first blockbuster psychotropic drug (Tone, 2009). Later, in the 1960s, the benzodiazepines were employed to treat the entire spectrum of anxiety symptoms, and still more recently, starting in the late 1980s, the selective serotonin reuptake inhibitors (SSRIs) have become the first line of pharmacotherapy for anxiety disorders.

Psychosocial approaches to the treatment of emotional and mental distress in the 20th century were prolific;[3] yet, many of these psychotherapies have disappeared or have merged with others, and today, in the 21st century, we may identify four major psychotherapeutic approaches: psychodynamic, cognitive-behavioral, interpersonal, and supportive (humanistic-existential) therapies. While psychoanalysis has in some cases proved to be less effective in treating anxiety than cognitive-behavioral therapies (CBTs), psychodynamic therapy, as well as interpersonal therapy and supportive therapy have been shown in other cases to be as effective as cognitive-behavioral approaches[4] (Leichsenring et al. 2009; Tolin, 2010). Nonetheless, cognitive-behavioral approaches tend to be favored in evidence-based practice over the other psychosocial treatment options because more research has been conducted with cognitive-behavioral approaches (Muse, Morre, & Stahl, 2013) and more evidence-based recommendations are, consequently, available. Such recommendations include CBT as first-line treatment for all of the anxiety disorders, with particular indication for behavioral exposure/response prevention for OCD (Abramowitz, 1997), a strong cognitive component in CBT for social anxiety disorder (Feske & Chambless, 1995; Taylor, 1997), and the cognitive-behavioral use of desensitization and flooding with PTSD (Bradley, Greene, Russ, Dutra, & Westen, 2005). Of interest is the recent suggestion that a unified therapeutic approach (Barlow, Allen, & Choate, 2004; Barlow et al., 2010) that applies an integration of several therapeutic approaches for the treatment of all anxiety disorders is as effective as specific therapies directed at specific symptomatology. Although recent in its inception, some evidence has been presented to support this view (Farchione et al., 2012).

Psychopharmacology has also evolved, and the number of agents used in the pharmacotherapy treatment of anxiety has increased considerably, although many patients with anxiety disorders fail to respond adequately to these pharmacologic agents (Ravindran & Stein, 2010), even to those agents considered first line (Koen & Stein, 2011). Without exception, the SSRIs are considered first-line treatment for all of the anxiety disorders (Western Australian Psychotropic Drugs Committee, 2008; Koen & Stein, 2011) because of well documented evidence to support their efficacy as well as for their low side effect profile. Olfson Marcus, Wan, and Geissler (2004) confirmed in a review of the literature that an increase in antidepressant use for the treatment of anxiety disorders has displaced the use of anxiolytics. One serotonin–norepinephrine reuptake inhibitor (SNRI), venlafaxine, is also considered first line in the treatment of GAD. Generalized anxiety notwithstanding, SNRIs are generally considered second line for the rest of the anxiety disorders due to their relative paucity of evidence when compared with SSRIs in the treatment of anxiety. The evidence supporting the use of benzodiazepines in the treatment of GAD, social anxiety, and panic disorder is solid, but the potential for abuse makes this agent a second choice. Tricyclic antidepressants (TCAs) also have accumulated substantial evidence attesting to their efficacy in the treatment of all of the anxiety disorders with the exception of social anxiety,[5] but their multiple side effects, including cardiotoxicity, anticholinergic effects, and risk of overdose make them a second-line treatment option. The one exception here might be the largely serotonergic tricyclic clomipramine, which initially appeared to be somewhat more effective in the treatment of OCD than the SSRIs, although this impression has since been questioned (Koen & Stein, 2011). Pregabalin and buspirone, but especially pregabalin, are supported enough by evidence to warrant their inclusion as second-line treatments for GAD, while a host of other agents may be considered third line due to scarcity of evidence; these include valproate, mirtazapine, bupropion, and quetiapine (Roy-Byrne & Cowley, 2007). A case apart is D-cycloserine, which is an N-methyl-D-aspartate (NMDA) receptor partial agonist that enhances the extinction of learned fear in exposure therapy for anxiety disorders. Little is known of the mechanisms that promote loss of fear with D-cycloserine (Baker, McNally, & Richardson, 2012), but its effectiveness in augmenting therapeutic effects of exposure therapy for many of the anxiety disorders appears to be increasingly established (Davis, Ressler, Rothbaum, & Richardson, 2006). Here, it is worthwhile noting that a large pool of "cognitive enhancers" besides D-cycloserine (yohimbine, cortisol, L-dopa, oxytocin, neuropeptides Y and S, and opioids) have been identified as facilitating therapeutic extinction (Singewald, Schmuckermair, Whittle, Holmes, & Ressler, 2015), which leaves the unanswered question of whether these specific agents enhance learning through unique mechanisms of action, or whether there is a common factor (Muse & Moore, 2012), such as the mode in which they are employed just prior to or during exposure, that enhances new learning across the various agents.

Integrating Biopsychosocial Treatments of Anxiety Disorders

Muse et al. (2013) previously summarized indications and cautions in the integrated treatment of anxiety as follows: (1) psychosocial approaches are favored over pharmacotherapy for the majority of anxiety disorders. (2) When used, pharmacological interventions are mainly adjunctive and supportive of psychotherapy. (3) There are several specific instances where pharmacotherapy of anxiety may be contraindicated due to its tendency to interfere with the therapeutic goal of patient-generated management of response to anxiety symptoms. (4) Monotherapy is generally preferred to combination therapy because of cost, reduced exposure to side effects, and limited data supporting the superiority of a combined approach over judiciously assigned monotherapy.

With these previous observations serving as a general orientation, we extend here evidence-based best-practice indications for the integrated treatment of anxiety to each of the major anxiety diagnoses.

Generalized Anxiety Disorders

Hidalgo, Tupler, and Davidson (2007) reviewed medications for their respective effectiveness in the treatment of GAD and concluded that the largest effect sizes on anxiety symptoms were achieved with the calcium channel blocker pregabalin, followed by the antihistamine hydroxyzine and the SNRI venlafaxine, with multiple benzodiazepines and SSRIs lagging somewhat behind. Buspirone performed no better than placebo, while the homeopathic Kava-Kava performed worse than placebo. These results were valid for adults as well as adolescents and children; however, the effect sizes were significantly higher for adolescent and children than adults, indicating that anxiolytics in general tend to have a greater impact on the younger population.

While the SSRIs continue to be recommended widely as first-line pharmacotherapy for GAD, if not for their overall effectiveness then in large part due to evidence of their relative safe use in comparison with the tricyclics and benzodiazepines, pregabalin, a molecule that is structurally analogous to gamma-aminobutyric acid (GABA) and thought to bind to the alpha-2-delta subunit of the voltage-gated calcium channels, resulting in increased levels of neuronal GABA and a concomitant inhibition of the release of excitatory neurotransmitters such as glutamate and noradrenaline (Koen & Stein, 2011), might deserve greater research and clinical attention.

It is not uncommon to read that CBT takes priority over other psychosocial therapies in the treatment of anxiety disorders, including GAD (Craske, 2015), but it is more difficult to find the evidence that indicates CBT is more effective than other psychotherapeutic approaches. CBT has certainly been more researched than other therapies and has been found to be more effective than placebo in most cases; however, it is uncommon to see a head-to-head controlled study where CBT has been compared in effectiveness to other psychotherapies in the treatment of GAD. One exception is a study conducted by Leichsenring et al. (2009), in which CBT was compared to short-term psychodynamic psychotherapy. In this randomized controlled study, both CBT and short-term psychodynamic psychotherapy yielded stable improvements, with no significant differences in outcome found between treatments with regard to the primary outcome measure.

Adding other psychosocial components to CBT does not appear to improve the effectiveness of CBT in the case of emotional-focused/interpersonal approaches (Newman et al., 2011), whereas a separate attempt to augment CBT with mindfulness found this combined approach effective, but the design did not allow for separating the effects of one approach from the other (Hayes-Skelton, Roemer, & Orsillo, 2013).

The treatment of GAD with pharmacotherapy alone is replete with difficulties (Comaty & Advocat, 2012), including mixed clinical results, higher rates of dropout (Mitte, 2005a), difficulty in maintaining gains, and potential for abuse and discontinuation syndrome. Because psychotherapy has proved to be as effective as pharmacotherapy, to work as fast or faster, and to have improved remission rates with fewer side effects, it should be considered the treatment of choice with this form of anxiety disorder. For example, a meta-analysis of 35 studies showed CBT to be more effective in the treatment of GAD in the long term than pharmacologic treatment, and while both treatments reduce anxiety, CBT is more effective in reducing depression associated with GAD (Gould, Otto, Pollack, & Yap, 1997). Mitte (2005a) found in a meta-analysis of CBT vs. drugs for the management of GAD that both approaches were equivalent in effectiveness. Nonetheless, when considering issues such as drug side effects the American Psychological Association (2012) concluded in a meta-analysis that the overall evidence supported CBT as the first line of treatment for GAD, while Gould et al. (1997), in a preliminary meta-analysis, observed greater relapse in GAD symptoms with discontinuation of pharmacology than termination from CBT. Power et al. (1990) conducted a randomized clinical trial in which they concluded that combined treatment is more effective in early stages of GAD treatment. Hoffman, Sawyer, Korte, and Smits (2009) concluded in their meta-analysis of all major medications used in the treatment of GAD in combination with CBT that pharmacotherapy is more helpful in early-stage treatment of GAD.

Based on a benefit vs. side effect equation, the first-line treatment for GAD should be psychotherapeutic, and CBT is a reasonable first choice. Switching to another, perhaps psychodynamic, psychosocial approach appears to be indicated when CBT proves ineffective for any given patient. Adding to or augmenting CBT with further cognitive or behavioral approaches does not find much support in the literature. Psychopharmacology, because of its potential for unwanted side effects, may be best considered second line, with SSRIs being the first choice among psychotropics; the possibility of switching out of the SSRIs to a different class of medication (pregabalin, hydroxyzine, venlafaxine, benzodiazepines) should be seriously entertained if the patient fails to respond to one or more SSRIs. Combined psychotherapy–pharmacotherapy may be considered if the patient has not responded to psychotherapy alone, and wishes to augment therapy with medication. Here, it is appropriate to quote the National Institute for Health and Clinical Excellence's (NICE, 2011) best-practice recommendation for GAD: "Base the choice of treatment on the person's preference as there is no evidence that either mode of treatment (individual high-intensity psychological intervention or drug treatment) is better."

Specific Phobias

Extrapolating from randomized clinical trials, Isaac Marks and colleagues concluded nearly a half century ago (Marks, Viswanathan, Lipsedge, & Gardner, 1972) that there is limited value for pharmacotherapy (benzodiazepines) in exposure to specific phobias. Sartory (1983), in a review of several randomized controlled trials (RCTs), equally concludes that benzodiazepines are of little use, and should be discontinued before treating a specific phobia. Zitrin, Klein, Woerner, and Ross (1983) found no difference in an RCT between placebo and the antidepressant imipramine in treating specific phobia with adults without a psychosocial component. Fryer conducted a review of the evidence as it pertained to anxiolytics and antidepressants in the latter half of the 1980s (Fyer, 1987) and found that no pharmacological agent proved effective in treating simple phobia at that time. Finally, Choy Fyer, and Lipsitz (2007) concluded in a meta-analysis spanning from 1960–2005 that medications have not been shown to be generally effective with phobias, with the exception of adjunctive D-cycloserine.

In a comparison among psychotherapeutic approaches for the treatment of phobias, Wolitzky-Taylor, Horowitz, Powers, and Telch (2008) performed a meta-analysis of 33 randomized treatment studies and concluded that exposure, especially *in vivo* exposure, is the most effective treatment among CBT techniques for simple phobia, although the difference between *in vivo* and alternative modes of exposure were no longer present at follow up. Curiously, while CBT outperformed placebo conditions, Wolitzky-Taylor and colleagues also found evidence for improvement in phobia with placebo alone. Silverman et al. (1999) observed in a randomized clinical trial of 104 children aged 6–16 that not only were two different exposure techniques effective in reducing phobia in children, but the control condition of providing educational support was equally as effective. Choy et al. (2007) confirmed the superiority of *in vivo* exposure for the treatment of specific phobias in adults, but this meta-analysis also found high dropout and low treatment acceptance to be unwanted side effects, while systematic desensitization and virtual reality techniques provided moderate effect size but greater compliance. In the Choy study, cognitive therapy was found to be most helpful with claustrophobia. Zlomke (2008) reviewed studies involving one-session, prolonged exposure in the treatment of specific phobias, and found the approach to be generally effective. Nonetheless, concerns over the tolerance of many patients to this intense form of therapy makes it a less overall recommended approach.

Spiegel and Bruce (1997) reviewed attempts to combine benzodiazepines with behavioral therapy, and report that, while benzodiazepine-based monotherapy for phobia (agoraphobia) provides no lasting relief once the drug is withdrawn, its combination with behavioral therapy may facilitate learning during exposure if it is used only during the exposure trials, and not continuously. The primary benefit of combining benzodiazepines in the initial stages of exposure is to reduce discomfort and to enhance compliance and tolerance to the exposure method (Hafner & Marks, 1976). Concern over transferring learning from exposure with benzodiazepines to real life situations without the medication is based on interference of benzodiazepines with memory consolidation (Barbee, Black, & Todorov, 1992), as well as concerns over state-dependent learning (Colpaert & Koek, 1995; Overton, 1964; Reus, Weingartner, & Post, 1979; Spiegel et al., 1993). Interference of memory consolidation appears to be dose-related, and appears not to be a major problem at lower doses, while state-dependent learning concerns are obviated by using the benzodiazepines only in initial trials as an agent to enhance compliance with patients who are highly anxious and apprehensive but are able to continue on without the benzodiazepines in subsequent exposures. The concerns of state-dependent learning have been difficult to isolate and test, although there appears to be some evidence to suggest that state-dependent learning interference may affect generalization to real life learning in a dose-dependent manner (Bouton, Kennedy, & Rosengard, 1990): fear extinction during exposure with higher doses of diazepam is associated with greater recurrence of the initial fear response once the drug is removed, while greater sustained reduction in the fear response in the absence of the drug is observed in subjects who were exposed to fear stimuli with lower doses of benzodiazepines.

Combining pharmacotherapy and psychotherapy was further studied in a meta-analysis by Norberg, Krystal, and Tolin (2008), who compared D-cycloserine's effectiveness when paired with exposure therapy in specific phobia. Forty-four articles were identified from 1998 through 2007 in which D-cycloserine augmented fear extinction when administered with exposure techniques. It proved to be more effective when administered a limited number of times and when given immediately before or after extinction training/exposure therapy.

The recent hopeful results of combining D-cycloserine with exposure therapy notwithstanding, if there were one diagnosis among the anxiety disorders where one is tempted to state categorically that medications have no place, it would be with specific phobias. However, this would be an overstatement as there are circumstances in which the use of a short acting anxiolytic may facilitate exposure therapy by increasing compliance, such as in the case study presented at the end of this chapter. There are also circumstances, such as with one-time dental procedures or blood extractions when a single dose of a benzodiazepine may facilitate completing the procedure, although one-session imaginal exposure has proved to be equally as effective in dental phobia (Thom, Sartory, & Johren, 2000) as has one-session muscle tension training to offset parasympathetic blood pressure drop in the case of blood-injury phobia (Ost & Sterner, 1987; Ost, Sterner, & Fellenius, 1989). Nonetheless, a sole dose of benzodiazepines to overcome phobic avoidance in a single exposure situation comes close to constituting monopharmacotherapy, and illustrates the difficulty in taking an absolute stance on any condition/treatment pairing. What would appear to be evident, however, is that anxiety-relieving medications prescribed on a continuous basis, such as SSRIs, are not generally indicated with specific phobias.

Social Anxiety Disorder

Pharmacotherapy and psychosocial treatment of social anxiety disorder have not been as effective as with other anxiety disorders to date, and dropout rate with the first medication selected is high (Baldwin et al., 2009). This first medication is usually an SSRI as this class of medication is considered first line (Bandelow, Seidler-Brandler, Becker, Wedekind, & Ruther, 2007; Hedges, Brown, Shwalb, Godfrey, & Larcher, 2007). There is no evidence that one SSRI is more efficacious in treating social anxiety disorder, although their respective side effect profiles are different and should be weighed in the initial selection (Hansen et al., 2008). Additionally, there is evidence that SNRIs can be as effective as SSRIs (Ipser, Kariuki, & Stein, 2008). Federoff and Taylor (2001) also found in a meta-analysis that high potency benzodiazepines are as effective as SSRIs in social phobia, and can be dispensed when the patient is facing truly phobic settings. In this vein, Sareen and Stein (2000) have suggested that beta blockers are more effective with discrete performance anxiety than with generalized social anxiety. Liebowitz et al. (1988), however, found in a randomized comparative trial that phenelzine, a monoamine oxidase (MAO) inhibitor, was more effective in treating social anxiety disorder than the cardioselective β-adrenergic blocker atenolol. The Liebowitz et al. study concluded that "pathological social anxiety is due to a chronic biological overreactivity that is modifiable by drug therapy." While this view reflects the thinking at the end of the 20th century, evidence since supports the view that social phobia is a conditioned response that is amenable to relearning through CBT. For example, Mayo-Wilson et al. (2014) conducted a recent meta-analysis that spanned the period between 1988 and 2013, and concluded that individual CBT is associated with large effect sizes and low risk of side effects, and should be regarded as the best intervention for the initial treatment of social anxiety disorder. For patients not amenable to CBT, the SSRIs show the most consistent evidence of benefits among pharmacotherapies.

CBT is as effective as medication in the treatment of social anxiety disorder (Heimberg 2002), although CBT, across all anxiety disorders, is least effective with social anxiety disorder (Norton & Price, 2007). When treating with CBT, social anxiety appears to respond well to a group treatment modality (Camart, Andre, Trybou, & Bourdel, 2006; Heimberg & Becker, 2002; McEvoy & Perini, 2009), although group CBT has not always lived up to expectation (Foa, 2006; Hope, Heimberg, & Bruch, 1995; Juster & Heimberg, 1995). One study, however (Otto et al., 2000), investigated the relative efficacy of clonazepam vs. exposure within a CBT group, and found that the two treatment modalities produced significant and similar improvement. Few studies have been done to test social anxiety response to psychosocial approaches other than cognitive-behavioral, but one large RCT study (Leichsenring et al., 2013) recently found that CBT and psychodynamic therapy were significantly superior to a wait list for both remission and response. Nonetheless, CBT proved to be significantly superior to psychodynamic therapy for remission, but not for initial response.

Combination therapy for social anxiety disorder has shown more promise with cognitive enhancing agents during behavioral training than the use of antidepressant or anxiolytic drugs. Clark et al. (2003) discovered no advantage in a placebo-controlled RCT of combining CBT with fluoxetine in the treatment of social anxiety. Contrary to traditional combinations of full regime pharmacotherapy with psychotherapy, several studies have suggested that punctually adding an enhancing drug at critical moments of behavioral therapy may promote new learning. Guastella et al. (2009), in a randomized clinical trial, showed that oxytocin enhances treatment for social anxiety, and in a separate RCT, Guastella, et al. (2008) found D-cycloserine before exposure therapy enhanced social anxiety treatment. Hoffman, Meuret and Smits (2006) also showed that D-cycloserine is more effective than placebo as an adjunct to exposure in social phobia, and Heimberg et al. (2002) found that the beta blocker propranolol enhances social skills training.

The treatment of social anxiety disorder is often challenging to the clinician because, although equally responsive to pharmacotherapy and psychosocial therapy, it tends to be in general less responsive to treatment than the other anxiety disorders. Monotherapy is the treatment of choice, unless a cognitive enhancer is added during exposure phases of behavioral treatment. Given the equal efficacy of pharmacotherapy and psychosocial therapy, and the relative lower side effects of CBT, CBT, either individual or group, is recommended as the initial therapeutic intervention, to be switched to psychodynamic psychotherapy or pharmacotherapy if the patient is resistant or unresponsive to CBT. Finally, few pharmacological studies have been undertaken with children in treatment for anxiety disorders, and still fewer studies have focused on childhood social anxiety disorder (Beidel, Ferrell, Alfano, & Yeganeh, 2001). In regards to psychosocial approaches, little attention has been given to developmental considerations when recommending psychosocial treatment for this age group.

Panic Disorder

Bakker et al. (2002) performed a meta-analysis and concluded that TCAs are as effective as SSRIs in treating panic, but the comparative side effect profiles of the two classes of medication argue in favor of SSRIs. Mitte (2005b) conducted a meta-analysis of various pharmacological treatments of panic disorder and discovered that benzodiazepines can be as effective as SSRIs and TCAs in alleviating panic, but their potential for abuse, and the need for increased dosing to overcome tolerance, relegate the benzodiazepines to a second-line alternative. Batelaan, Van Balkom, and Stein (2012), in a review of evidence-based studies, conclude that there is evidence that SSRIs and venlafaxine are effective in managing panic as long as therapy is maintained. Batelaan and colleagues also found evidence that the temporary co-administration of benzodiazepines with antidepressants is justified in otherwise resistant cases. The American Psychiatric Association (2009) has acknowledged SSRIs, TCAs, and benzodiazepines as effective in the treatment of panic, and has suggested that the agent used might be selected by side effect profile. Bakker, van Balkom, and Stein (2005) reviewed numerous studies to conclude that SSRIs, based in part on their lighter side effect profile, are first-line pharmacologic treatment for panic; yet, evidence of the plausibility of antidepressants for the treatment of panic disorder is predicated on studies that do not usually compare such compounds to effective psychosocial therapy outcomes, but merely against placebo controls (Serretti et al., 2011). An exception is a study by Black, Wesner, Bowers, and Gabel (1993) that showed a superior response to fluvoxamine over cognitive therapy in the treatment of panic disorder. In contrast, Clark et al. (1994) found that cognitive therapy was superior to both relaxation training and imipramine at the end of treatment, as well as upon a 15-month follow up.

The effectiveness of cognitive-behavioral treatment of panic disorder and agoraphobia is well documented, with remission rates around 80% with follow up at 1 year (Clark and Ehlers, 1993; Elkins & Moore, 2011; Margraf, Barlow, Clark, & Telch, 1993). McHugh, Smits, and Otto (2009) recently showed that individual CBT is effective in managing panic, while Gould, Otto, and Pollack (1995) found in a meta-analysis that group CBT is effective with panic disorder and more effective than pharmacotherapy. Marks et al. (1993) found exposure therapy to be twice as effective as alprazolam. Bakker et al. (1998), in a quantitative review of previous studies, concluded that gradual exposure rather than implosion is most effective with the treatment of panic. Psychodynamic therapy has developed a theoretical model to explain panic disorder (Shear, Cooper, Klerman, Busch, & Shapiro, 1993), and an open trial pilot study by Milrod and colleagues (2000) initially found this approach effective in treating and retaining patients. Milrod et al. (2007) further found in a randomized clinical trial that psychodynamic therapy can be effective with panic disorder, although this approach was not tested head-to-head with CBT. Perhaps the most salient finding in the series of Milrod studies is the very low dropout rate of 7% (Busch & Milrod, 2008). Panic-focused psychodynamic therapy (Busch & Milrod, 2009) has accumulated sufficient evidence to be considered as an alternative for those patients who are noncompliant with the rigors of CBT.

Combining pharmacology with psychotherapy in the treatment of panic has not yielded positive results. Indeed, pharmacotherapy concurrent with psychotherapy interferes with CBT's prolonged therapeutic result (Barlow, Gorman, & Shear, 2000), and may also interfere with psychodynamic psychotherapy of panic disorder (Merra, Godeas, & Persico, 1993). Marks et al. (1993) observed in a randomized clinical trial that greater relapse was associated with combined treatment of CBT with benzodiazepines for panic, and Furukawa, Watanabe, and Churchill (2006) concluded in a meta-analysis that a combination of antidepressants with CBT was initially superior to monotherapy, only later to observe that the original advantage was lost after discontinuation of the antidepressant. Spiegel and Bruce (1997), in a systematic review of RCTs, found that anxiolytic drugs retard exposure effects, while Woods, Barlow, Gorman, and Shear (1998), in a multisite clinical trials protocol, observed greater relapse for TCA, with or without CBT, and concluded that patients did better without concurrent use of antidepressant medication while in psychotherapy for panic disorder with mild to moderate agoraphobia. These findings are contradictory to the position of the World Council on Anxiety, which recommends combined, integrated treatment for panic disorders; however, this recommendation appears to have been arrived upon without taking into consideration the evidence to the contrary. Rather, the recommendation appears to follow earlier assumptions that if CBT and pharmacotherapy are effective then combining the two "may provide the best treatment" (Pollack et al., 2003).

In conclusion, pharmacotherapy is effective in the short run for controlling symptoms of panic, but tends to lose its effectiveness upon the discontinuation of medicine; whether anxiolytics or antidepressants, symptoms of panic are temporarily ameliorated (Williams, Richardson, & Galovski, 2014), but often reemergence upon discontinuation. Moreover, these same medications tend to interfere with new learning during psychotherapy. On the other hand, psychosocial treatments, especially CBT and psychodynamic therapy, are effective in treating panic and in preventing relapse.

Posttraumatic stress disorder

Williams and colleagues (2014) point out that while pharmacotherapy can be beneficial it rarely provides complete remission of PTSD. Indeed, a variety of medications have been shown to provide adjunctive benefit in reducing PTSD symptoms, but the consensus is that at this time there is no clear drug treatment for PTSD. Ipser and Stein (2012) noted in a review that the quality of studies in the area of psychopharmacology with PTSD is poor, and that such studies yield conflicting results. For example, Stein, Iper, and Seedat (2009), in a Cochrane review, found PTSD to be effectively treated by SSRIs, while the Institute of Medicine (2007) concluded in its own review that the data do not show that SSRIs are effective treatment for PTSD. Hageman, Andersen, and Jorgensen (2001), on the other hand, conclude in their review of previous studies that SSRIs should be considered first-line treatment, whereas TCAs and MAOIs should be relegated to second line for safety reasons. Yehuda (2002) holds the opinion that benzodiazepines have little place in the treatment of PTSD, and Braun, Greenburg, Dasberg, and Lerer (1990), in an RCT, concluded that alprazolam failed to improve PTSD symptoms. Gelpin, Bonne, Peri, Brandes, and Shalev (2002) conclude in a perspective study that benzodiazepines are not useful with PTSD treatment. Krystal et al. (2011) in a multisite RCT found that risperidone was not effective for SSRI nonresponders suffering from PTSD. On the other hand, there is mounting evidence that prazosin may provide some relief from PTSD-related nightmares. Raskin et al. (2003, 2007) demonstrated in several placebo-controlled trials that PTSD-related nightmares were reduced with prazosin in combat veterans. Taylor et al. (2008) also found in a placebo-controlled study that trauma-related nightmares were reduced in civilians taking prazosin, and Benedek, Friedman, Zatzick, and Ursano (2009), in reviewing the evidence, concluded that prazosin may serve to augment SSRIs in PTSD treatment.

Although the NICE study (2011) recommends trauma-focused CBT and eye movement desensitization and reprocessing (EMDR) for the treatment of PTSD, based largely on their respective effectiveness over wait lists, Benish, Imel, and Walpold (2008), in a meta-analysis concluded that trauma-focused psychotherapies were no more effective than other psychotherapies in the treatment of PTSD. The Benish et al. study has been challenged by some (Ehlers et al., 2010) and defended by others (Wampold et al., 2010). Nonetheless, meta-analyses of different trauma-focused treatments for PTSD have consistently found no difference among the efficacy of these treatments (Bisson & Andrews, 2007; Bisson, Roberts, Andrew, Cooper, & Lewis, 2013). Bisson et al. (2013) found in a meta-analysis, however, weak evidence that trauma focused therapies may be better than other psychotherapies in the treatment of chronic PTSD, and Steenkamp, Litz, Hoge, and Marmar (2015) found in a meta-analysis that trauma-focused interventions showed marginal superior results when compared to active control conditions, but noted that nonresponse rates were high and many patients continue to have symptoms. Guillis et al. (2013) in a systematic review found that several psychotherapies are effective in treating PTSD in children and adolescents, while no single psychotherapy stood out as better than the others. Bradley et al. (2005), again in a meta-analysis, concluded that multiple psychotherapies are highly effective in mitigating PTSD, but residual PTSD symptoms persist beyond treatment. Apart from high dropout rates for exposure therapy with the PTSD population (Rothbaum et al., 2006), a caveat for the use of exposure with this population is that immediate debriefing, especially single-session debriefing, after a trauma may be harmful for PTSD patients (Bisson, 2007; Van Emmerik, Kamphuis, Hulsbosch, & Emmelkamp, 2002). Finally, the incorporation of mindfulness approaches, perhaps as a group therapy adjunct to individual psychotherapy, appears to offer benefits in the treatment of PTSD (Polusny et al., 2015). In a random clinical trial study, Polusny and colleagues demonstrated that group administered mindfulness-based stress reduction for PTSD veterans resulted in a greater decrease in PTSD symptom severity when compared with an active control condition.

Choi, Rothbaum, Gerardi, and Ressler (2009) and Hetrick, Purcell, Garner, and Parslow (2010) concluded in two separate meta-analyses that combined pharmacotherapy with psychotherapy in the treatment of PTSD yields mixed results. In the few cases when medication has been found to be useful in the treatment of PTSD, it is as an add-on to psychosocial treatment, such as in the case of sertraline, which was found in a pilot study by Otto et al. (2003) to augment CBT, or in the case of Schneier et al. (2011), who determined in an RCT that sequencing paroxetine after prolonged exposure therapy resulted in enhanced results. Cognitive enhancers have shown promise as an add-on to CBT, and Singewald et al. (2015) have concluded in an extensive review that preclinical and clinical evidence indicate that D-cycloserine, yohimbine, cortisol, and L-dopa, when given as adjuncts to CBT exposure-extinction therapy, promote greater treatment efficacy. At the same time, Singewald and colleagues found that using anxiolytics such as benzodiazepines as adjuncts can undermine long-term treatment success. When pharmacotherapy has proved to be useful in the treatment of PTSD it is not employed as a continuous treatment, but punctually, to enhance the psychosocial work being done. Muse (1984) presented a case study in which sodium amytal (Gray, 1970) was used to induce trance during exposure therapy with PTSD. The patient was administered the drug only during multiple sessions of intense *in vitro* exposure, and a complete remission was achieved with the severe PTSD symptoms that had resisted traditional exposure monotherapy.

To summarize, monotherapy with medication is not indicated with PTSD since there is no drug treatment at this time for this disorder. Medications may play an adjunctive role in the case of PTSD. While psychotherapies in general are helpful in treating PTSD, no particular therapy has emerged as more effective than others. CBT and trauma-focused therapies are equally effective. Combined pharmacotherapy and psychosocial therapies have not yielded better results than psychotherapy alone. Monotherapy with a psychosocial approach is recommended, with medication used only adjunctively to treat specific symptoms such as sleep disorder in the case of prazosin. Indeed, avoiding potential side effects of benzodiazepines, antipsychotics, and antidepressants is advised.

Obsessive-Compulsive Disorder

It would be ingenuous to say one anxiety disorder is more serious than another; still, OCD is distinguished as having a comparatively high incidence of suicide (Ankelakis, et al., 2015; Kamath, Reddy, & Kandavel, 2007). Although OCD responds to both pharmacological and psychosocial therapies, symptoms typically persist at moderate levels even after following an adequate course of treatment (Eddy, Dutra, Bradley, & Westen, 2004), while the more severe cases tend to be resistant to both pharmacotherapy and psychosocial treatment, and therefore pose a special challenge to the clinician.

Pharmacologic approaches have not proved to be as effective as CBT in reducing compulsions, and research on the effectiveness of pharmacotherapy with other OCD symptoms has provided mixed results. SSRIs are consensually considered first line, but are oftentimes augmented with other medications to enhance effectiveness in lowering anxiety and reducing obsessions. Denys, de Geus, van Megen, and Westenberg (2004) concluded in an RCT that quetiapine may be added to SSRIs when SSRIs are not effective; yet, Kordon et al. (2008), in a separate RCT, concluded that augmentation of SSRI treatment with quetiapine in severe OCD had no additional effect. Ackerman and Greenland (2002) found in a meta-analysis that clomipramine is superior to placebo in treatment of OCD. Abramowitz and Jacoby (2013), in a review of the literature, found that the TCA clomipramine is better than SSRIs in ameliorating OCD symptoms, while there is no difference among the various SSRIs' efficacy with OCD. Shearer et al. (2014) reviewed the evidence thus far and offered the opinion that clomipramine's slight advantage over SSRIs may pale when weighing the possible side effects of Torsades de Pointes and Q-T prolongation. Kellner (2010) notes that several studies which initially indicated that higher dosing of the SSRIs afforded better response rates have not been replicated, and no significant effect sizes were observed between different dosing ranges in a double-blind placebo-controlled study (Ninan et al., 2006). Bandelow et al. (2007) found in a review conducted for the World Federation of Societies of Biological Psychiatry (WFSBP) that there was weak evidence that the antipsychotics haloperidol, olanzapine, and quetiapine were more effective when combined with SSRI than SSRI monotherapy in treatment-resistant cases of OCD. Notwithstanding the WFSBP guidelines, evidence is still inconclusive for the efficacy of olanzapine (Bloch et al., 2006), and further meta-analyses and RCTs have failed to show unequivocal results for quetiapine (Denys et al., 2004; Fineberg et al., 2006; Kordon et al., 2008). Simpson et al. (2013) found that adding CBT to SSRIs was more effective than augmenting SSRIs with risperidone for the treatment of resistant OCD. Apart from the mixed results of antidepressants, with or without antipsychotic augmentation, in treating OCD, Hollander, Kaplan, and Stahl (2003) found clonazepam no better than placebo in an RCT, while recent interest in glutamatergic-based cognitive enhancing agents such as memantine, amantadine, and D-cycloserine as augmentation therapy or combined therapies with CBT (Hoffman, Pollack, & Otto, 2006) is still in the developmental stage.

CBT has become first line among psychosocial approaches in the treatment of OCD due to a substantial body of research data attesting to its efficacy, and Simpson and Liebowitz (2011) have argued in a review of six studies comparing psychotherapy to medication that CBT can be more effective than SSRIs when employed by skilled clinicians. What is more, Warren and Thomas (2001) demonstrated that research findings are applicable to the clinical setting in establishing that clinical treatment outcome of CBT with OCD clients was comparable to results obtained in RCTs. Strict behavioral therapy in the form of exposure and response prevention proved effective with OCD in the 1980s (Emmelkamp, 1982; Marks, 1987) and a cognitive component was added in the 1990s (van Oppen et al., 1994). One of the first meta-analyses of CBT in the treatment of OCD was conducted by Abramowitz (1998), in which the effectiveness of 16 outcome trials using the Maudsley Obsessive-Compulsion Inventory demonstrated substantial improvement posttreatment, and stable change at a 5-month follow up. Fisher and Wells (2004) used the Yale–Brown Obsessive Compulsive Scale to measure therapeutic change, and found that exposure and response prevention were the most effective treatments among psychosocial interventions, demonstrating a 50–60% recovery rate. When a stricter asymptomatic criterion was applied, exposure–response prevention was equivalent to cognitive therapy with full recovery rate at 25%. Rosa-Alcazar, Sanchez-Meca, Gomez-Conesa, and Marin-Martinez (2008) found in a meta-analysis of 19 studies conducted between 1980 and 2006 that effect size was similar for exposure–response prevention alone, cognitive restructuring alone, and a combination of exposure–response prevention with cognitive restructuring. Therapist-guided exposure was better than self-exposure, and *in vivo* exposure combined with exposure in imagination was better than exposure *in vivo* alone. At least one study (Wilhelm et al., 2009) suggests that cognitive therapy that targets misinterpretations associated with beliefs, without a behavioral exposure–response prevention (ERP) component, is effective in reducing OCD symptoms. The authors of the Wilhelm study suggest that cognitive therapy may be an alternative to CBT and/or SSRI therapy when the patient develops side effects to medication or finds exposure therapy too invasive. Anderson and Rees(2007), in a controlled trial, found that group exposure/response prevention is effective, although individual treatment affords quicker results. Fals-Stewart, Marks, and Schafer (1993) found in a randomized clinical trial that exposure–response prevention was superior to the relaxation–control group, while group therapy is nearly as effective as individual therapy for OCD. Franklin, Abramowitz, Foa, Levitt, and Kozak (2000), in a clinical open label study, established the dropout rate to exposure therapy was 10% with OCD. Other studies have found the dropout rate to be higher, however, and Vogel, Stiles, and Gotestam (2004) observed in a controlled study that adding a cognitive component reduced dropout rates to exposure techniques in OCD treatment. Several other psychosocial therapies have proved to be effective in treating OCD, and include group therapy and family treatment interventions (Van Noppen & Steketee, 2004).

Combining pharmacotherapy with CBT does not find support in evidence-based studies. While pharmacotherapy benefits from adding a CBT component, CBT is not enhanced by adding pharmacotherapy (Franklin et al., 2011). The one exception to this rule is Eddy et al. (2004), who found in a meta-analysis that OCD treated with CBT is more effective when combined with pharmacotherapy, and clomipramine was found to be the most effective among pharmacologic agents. Marks, Stern, Mawson, Cobb, and McDonald (1980) had previously opined that OCD is best treated with *in vivo* exposure, but clomipramine may be useful with co-morbid depression. Foe et al. (2005), however, concluded in an RCT that OCD is best treated alone with exposure + response prevention, while the addition of clomipramine is not justified. Simpson et al. (2008) found in an RCT that SSRI nonresponder OCD patients improved after adding CBT, and van Balkom et al. (1998) concluded from an RCT that combination therapy is not justified with SSRIs: adding SSRIs does not improve CBT outcome. Antony and Swinson (2001), in a review of the literature, found that the data do not support combined treatment for OCD over monotherapy; yet, the American Psychiatric Association (2007) has offered the guideline that OCD is best treated with exposure, but residual symptoms may benefit from medications. Simpson et al. (2011) reviewed the evidence to date and conclude that both CBT and SSRIs are effective with OCD, but combined there is no added advantage. Finally, as with nearly all of the anxiety disorders, Wilhelm et al. (2008) have found evidence that D-cycloserine may augment behavior therapy in the initial stages of treatment.

In summary, SSRIs form the first-line pharmacological treatment of OCD although they do not offer an adequate response in many cases. Data are equivocal as to whether increasing dose, switching to another medication, or augmenting SSRIs with neuroleptics increase response in a significant or reliable fashion. On the other hand, CBT has proved to be effective in the treatment of OCD, and may best stand alone since there is little evidence to suggest that augmenting CBT with pharmacotherapy provides any real advantage.

Final Conclusions and Discussion

Over 20 years ago, Wolfe and Maser (1994) observed in relation to anxiety disorders such as agoraphobia and panic that "there is a pervasive belief—with little empirical data to support it—that combined treatment regimens are superior to other treatments administered alone." Our survey of evidence-based integrated care in the treatment of anxiety confirms the suspicions of Wolfe and Maser, and leads us to the conclusion that the preferred mode of therapy is not combined, but, indeed, monotherapy involving psychosocial interventions; this is our conclusion because the evidence to date points us in that direction. The discerning use of medication has a role in managing certain anxiety disorders, but clearly it is a secondary role in most cases. The scientist-practitioner must go where the evidence leads, and in the case of anxiety disorders the data suggest that integrative care should incorporate psychosocial interventions as first line in the treatment of most cases of anxiety while combining pharmacotherapy with psychosocial approaches only in those cases that warrant the exception.

Table 6.2 summarizes our research findings and conclusions.

Finally, Table 6.3 presents a summary of our practice recommendations.

Table 6.2 State of research and derived conclusions on integrative biopsychosocial intervention with anxiety disorders.

Research:

A) There is long-standing confirmation of the effectiveness of behavioral approaches in the treatment of all of the anxiety disorders. More research on other psychosocial approaches is needed
   1) Such research would ideally compare different psychosocial therapies, rather than simply show superiority over placebo

B) Much more research is needed with the child and adolescent population to show benefits and adverse reactions to pharmacotherapy in anxiety disorders

Conclusions:

A) Monotherapy is generally indicated over combination therapy for the anxiety disorders

B) Psychosocial therapy is the treatment of choice for the great majority of anxiety disorders. When cognitive-behavioral therapy (CBT) is not successful, switching to another psychotherapy, especially psychodynamic psychotherapy, is indicated

C) Switching to pharmacotherapy may be considered when one or more psychosocial therapies have proved ineffective

D) Augmenting psychosocial therapy with medication for a combined treatment regimen is not recommended. However, the use of an enhancer such as D-cycloserine when the anxiety condition is unresponsive to CBT alone is worthy of consideration

Table 6.3 Integrative biopsychosocial intervention with anxiety disorders: Summary of best-practice recommendations by level of confidence derived from strength of evidence.

Generalized anxiety disorder		
Level A	Recommended	• The first-line treatment for generalized anxiety disorder (GAD) should be psychotherapeutic, and cognitive-behavioral therapy (CBT) is a reasonable first choice
Level B	Suggested	• Switching to another psychosocial approach such as psychodynamic, interpersonal or supportive therapy appears to be indicated when CBT proves ineffective for any given patient
Level C	May be considered	• Psychopharmacology may be best considered second line, with selective serotonin reuptake inhibitors (SSRIs) being the first choice • Switching out of the SSRIs to a different class of medication (pregabalin, hydroxyzine, venlafaxine, benzodiazepines) should be seriously entertained if the patient fails to respond to one or more SSRIs
Specific phobias		
Level A	Recommended	• First-line treatment for simple phobias should be CBT, with exposure techniques emphasized • No psychotropic medication is recommended on a continuous basis for the treatment of phobias
Level B	Suggested	• Combining benzodiazepine to increase compliance in the initial phase of exposure therapy may be considered when the patient is unable to proceed with exposure therapy alone. In such cases, the dose should be an amount that allows compliance while mitigating fear and anxiety minimally
Level C	May be considered	• D-cycloserine as an augmenting agent in enhancing the effects of exposure therapy in the treatment of certain fears shows promise
Social anxiety disorder		
Level A	Recommended	• Social anxiety disorder is more resistant to treatment than other anxiety disorders, and it responds about equally well to pharmacological and psychosocial treatment • SSRIs are considered first-line pharmacological treatment of social anxiety disorder, whereas benzodiazepines or beta blockers may provide effective *pro re nata* coverage for performance anxiety • CBT is recommended as a first-line psychosocial treatment, with a group therapy approach particularly indicated
Level B	Suggested	• There is no advantage to combining CBT with SSRIs in the treatment of social anxiety disorder
Level C	May be considered	• Psychodynamic therapy has been proved to be effective, although less so than CBT, and should be considered if the patient is unresponsive to CBT or prefers a different approach to CBT
Panic disorder		
Level A	Recommended	• CBT is the treatment of choice for panic disorder. Psychodynamic therapy should be considered for those patients unable to tolerate CBT for panic disorder

Table 6.3 (Continued)

Level B	Suggested	• Pharmacotherapy as monotherapy does not tend to maintain gains during follow up
Level C	May be considered	• Combination therapy is contraindicated in the treatment of panic disorder as pharmacotherapy interferes with CBT
Posttraumatic stress disorder		
Level A	Recommended	• Monotherapy with medication is not indicated with PTSD since there is no drug treatment at this time for this disorder. Medications play an adjunctive role only in the management of PTSD
Level B	Suggested	• While psychotherapies in general are helpful in treating PTSD, no particular therapy has emerged as more effective than others. CBT and trauma-focused therapies are equally effective
Level C	May be considered	• Combined pharmacotherapy and psychosocial therapies have not yielded better results than psychotherapy alone • Monotherapy with a psychosocial approach is recommended, with medication used only adjunctively to treat specific symptoms such as sleep disorder in the case of prazosin • Avoiding potential side effects of benzodiazepines, antipsychotics, and antidepressants is advised • There is expert opinion in support of trauma-based CBT and eye movement desensitization and reprocessing (EMDR) in the treatment of PTSD
Obsessive-compulsive disorder		
Level A	Recommended	• CBT is the treatment of choice, and should be prescribed as a monotherapy since combining it with pharmacotherapy provides no real advantage
Level B	Suggested	• SSRIs are the medication of choice when pharmacotherapy is selected
Level C	May be considered	• Adding CBT may improve the results of SSRIs

Illustrative Case Study in the Clinical Practice of Biopsychosocial Integration with Anxiety

Monica, a 23-year-old who was overwhelmed by her immigration to the US, did not want to leave her country of origin, but she did so for the future of her husband. She found the transition hard, and felt that she was unprepared for the language barrier and the demands of keeping house. In Bolivia she was a shop manager, and she had domestic help with housekeeping. She found it hard to fit into the American culture, and she had virtually no friends and was isolated at home. Within a few months of her immigration, she became completely housebound when not accompanied by her husband to the supermarket or to doctors' appointments.

Once in treatment, Monica was resistant to try any in vivo exposure, and so she was initially assigned to covert imagined exposure, which followed a hierarchy from stepping outside of her house by herself to catching a bus on her own to the market. Her anxiety was extremely

(Continued)

high and she was unable to transition from in vitro *exposure to* in vivo *without the aid of medication to lower her anxiety. We avoided the SSRIs, and used instead the benzodiazepine alprazolam, front-loading during the initial attempts at each step in her* in vivo *hierarchy, and completely withdrawing the benzodiazepine during the last two* in vivo *exposures before proceeding to the next step of the hierarchy. We role played each step initially with relaxation training and* in vitro *desensitization, but later finished each* in vitro *hierarchical step without relaxation until a subject units of distress (SUDs) score of < 2/10 was achieved on two consecutive trials; then, her therapy was transferred to* in vivo *with the use of benzodiazepine, initially accompanied by her husband, and eventually alone, without alprazolam or husband.*

She achieved a SUDs score below 2 on each step of her in vivo *hierarchy before proceeding to the next step. In a period of 5 months of weekly therapy sessions and daily homework assignments, she was able to leave the house on her own, catch a bus, interview for a job, and finally begin working. Not surprisingly, her secondary depression disappeared and her attitude toward her new host country became far more positive as she gradually reached a higher level of autonomy than she had experienced in her native country.*

Notes

1 OCD is no longer considered to be a pure anxiety disorder in the DSM-V. There is considerable controversy as to where it should be classified (Stein et al., 2010).

2 Although PTSD has recently been reconceptualized as a trauma and stress-related disorder in the DSM-V (American Psychiatric Association, 2013), it is included here as an anxiety disorder since much of the research reviewed was carried out under the traditional classification of this disorder.

3 Crits-Christoph and Connolly-Gibbons (2010) estimate that the history of psychotherapy includes more than 250 schools or approaches.

4 Of interest has been recent evidence pointing to the equivalence of computer-based vs. face-to-face cognitive behavioral therapy for anxiety (Cuijpers & Marks, 2009).

5 Social anxiety is particularly resistant to pharmacotherapy, with up to 50% of patients not responding to initial medication management (Van Ameringen, Mancini, Pipe, & Bennett, 2004); few of these patients benefit from switching to a different pharmacologic agent.

References

Abramowitz, J. (1997). Effectiveness of psychological and pharmacological treatments for obsessive-compulsive disorder: A quantitative review. *Journal of Consulting and Clinical Psychology, 65*, 44–52.

Abramowitz, J. (1998). Does cognitive-behavioral therapy cure obsessive-compulsive behavior? A meta-analytic evaluation of clinical significance. *Behavior Therapy, 29*, 339–355.

Abramowitz, J., & Jacoby, R. (2013). Obsessive compulsive disorder. In S. Stahl, & B Moore (Eds.), *Anxiety disorders: A guide for integrating psychopharmacology and psychotherapy* (pp. 133–154). New York: Routledge.

Ackerman, D., & Greenland, S. (2002). Multivariate meta-analysis of controlled drug studies for obsessive-compulsive disorder. *Journal of Clinical Psychopharmacology, 22*, 309–317.

American Psychiatric Association (2007). *Practice guideline for the treatment of patients with obsessive-compulsive disorder*. Arlington, VA: American Psychiatric Association.

American Psychiatric Association (2009). *Practice guideline for the treatment of patients with panic disorder* (2nd ed.). Washington, DC: American Psychiatric Association.

American Psychological Association (2012). Website on research-supported psychological treatments. Retrieved from https://www.div12.org/psychological-treatments/

American Psychiatric Association (2013). *Diagnostic and statistical manual of mental disorders* (5th ed.). Arlington, VA: American Psychiatric Association.

Anderson, R., & Rees, C. (2007). Group versus individual cognitive-behavioural treatment of obsessive-compulsive disorder: A controlled trial. *Behaviour Research and Therapy, 45*, 123–137.

Angelakis, I., Gooding, P., Tarrier, N., et al. (2015). Suicidality in obsessive compulsive disorder (OCD): A systematic review and meta-analysis. *Psychological Review, 39*, 1–15.

Antony, M., & Swinson, R. (2001). Comparative and combined treatments for obsessive-compulsive disorder. In M. Sammons, & N. Schmidt (Eds.), *Combined treatments for mental disorders: A guide to psychological and pharmacological interventions* (pp. 53–80). Washington, DC: American Psychological Association.

Baker, K., McNally, G., & Richardson, R. (2012). D-cycloserine does not facilitate fear extinction by reducing conditioned stimulus processing or promoting conditioned inhibition to contextual cues. *Learning Memory, 19*, 461–469.

Bakker, A., van Balkom, A., Spinhoven, P., Blaauw, B, & van Dyck, R.. (1998). Follow-up on the treatment of panic disorder with or without agoraphobia: A quantitative review. *Journal of Nervous and Mental Diseases, 186*, 414–419.

Bakker, A., van Balkom, A., & Spinhoven, P. (2002). SSRIs vs. TCAs in the treatment of panic disorder: A meta-analysis. *Acta Psychiatrica Scandinavica, 106*, 163–167.

Bakker, A., van Balkom, & Stein, D. (2005). Evidence-based pharmacotherapy of panic disorder. *International Journal of Neuropsychopharmacology, 8*, 473–482.

Baldwin, D., Stein, D., Dolberg, O., & Bandelow, B. (2009). How long should a trial of escitalopram treatment be in patients with major depressive disorder, generalized anxiety disorder or social anxiety disorder? An exploration of the randomized controlled trial database. *Humanistic Psychopharmacology, 24*, 269–275.

Bandelow, B., Seidler-Brandler, U., Becker, A., Wedekind, D., & Ruther, E. (2007). Meta-analysis of randomized controlled comparisons of psychopharmacological and psychological treatments of anxiety disorders. *World Journal of Biological Psychiatry, 8*, 175–187.

Barbee, J., Black, F., & Todorov, A. (1992). Differential effects of alprazolam and buspirone upon acquisition, retention, and retrieval processes in memory. *Journal of Neuropsychiatry, 4*, 308–314.

Barlow, D., Farchione, T., Fairholme, C., Ellard, K., Boisseau, C., Allen, L., & May, E. (2010). *Unified protocol for transdiagnostic treatment of emotional disorders*. Oxford: Oxford University Press.

Barlow, D., Gorman, J., & Shear, M. (2000) Cognitive-behavioral therapy, imipramine, or their combination for panic disorder: A randomized controlled trial. *JAMA, 283*, 2529–2450.

Barlow, T., Allen, L., & Choate, M. (2004). Towards a unified treatment of emotional disorders. *Behaviour Therapy, 35,* 205–230.

Beidel, D., Ferrell, C. Alfano, C., & Yeganeh, R. (2001). The treatment of childhood social anxiety disorder. *Psychiatric Clinics of North America, 24,* 831–846.

Benedek, D., Friedman, M., Zatzick, D., & Ursano, R. (2009). Guideline watch: Practice guidelines for the treatment of patients with acute stress disorder and posttraumatic stress disorder. *Focus: The Journal of Lifelong Learning in Psychiatry, 7,* 204–213.

Benish, S., Imel, Z., & Walpold, B. (2008). The relative efficacy of bona fide psychotherapies for treating post-traumatic stress disorder: A meta-analysis of direct comparisons. *Clinical Psychology Review, 28,* 1281.

Batelaan, N., Van Balkom, A., & Stein, D. (2012). Evidence-based pharmacotherapy of panic disorder: An update. *International Journal of Neuropsychopharmacology, 15,* 403–415.

Bienvenu, J., Wuyek, L., & Stein, M. (2010). Anxiety disorders diagnosis: Some history and controversies. In M. Stein, & T. Steckler (Eds.), *Behavioral neurobiology of anxiety and its treatment* (pp. 3–19). New York: Springer.

Bisson, J. (2007). Post-traumatic stress disorder. *Occupational Medicine, 57,* 399–403.

Bisson, J., & Andrews, M. (2007). Psychological treatments of post-traumatic stress disorder (PTSD). The Cochrane Library 2007, Issue 3. Retrieved from www .thecochranelibrary.com

Bisson, J., Roberts, N., Andrew, M., Cooper, R., & Lewis, C. (2013). Psychological therapies for chronic post-traumatic stress disorder (PTSD) in adults. *Cochrane Database Systematic Review, December 13.* Retrieved from www.thecochranelibrary.com

Black, D., Wesner, R., Bowers, W., & Gabel (1993). A comparison of fluvoxamine, cognitive therapy, and placebo in the treatment of panic disorder. *Archives of General Psychiatry, 50,* 44–50.

Bloch, M., Landeros-Weisenberger, A.,Kelmendi, B., Coric, V., Bracken, M., & Leckman, J. (2006). A systematic review: antipsychotic augmentation with treatment refractory obsessive-compulsive disorder. *Molecular Psychiatry, 11,* 622–632.

Bradley, R., Greene, J., Russ, E., Dutra, L., & Westen, D. (2005). A multi-dimensional meta-analysis of psychotherapy for PTSD. *American Journal of Psychiatry, 162,* 214–227.

Braun, P., Greenburg, D., Dasberg, H., & Lerer, B. (1990). Core symptoms of PTSD unimproved by alprazolam treatment. *Journal of Clinical Psychiatry, 51,* 236–238.

Bouton, M., Kennedy, F., & Rosengard, C. (1990). State-dependent fear extinction with two benzodiazepines tranquilizers. *Behavioral Neuroscience, 104,* 44–55.

Busch, F., & Milrod, B. (2008). Panic-focused psychodynamic psychotherapy. *Psychiatry Times, February 1.*

Busch, F., & Milrod, B. (2009). Psychodynamic treatment of panic disorder: Clinical and research assessment. In R. Levy, & J. Ablon (Eds.), *Handbook of evidence-based psychodynamic psychotherapy* (pp. 29–34). New York: Humana Press.

Camart, N., Andre, C., Trybou, V., & Bourdel, M. (2006). Short-term effects of cognitive-behavioral group therapy in social phobia: Evaluation of sixty patients. *L'Encephale, 32,* 1011-1018.

Choi, D., Rothbaum, B., Gerardi, M., & Ressler, K.. (2009). Pharmacological enhancement of behavioral therapy: Focus on postraumatic stress disorder. In M. Stein, & T. Steckler (Eds.), *Behavioral neurobiology of anxiety and its treatment: Current topics in behavioral neurosciences* (pp. 280–295). Heidelberg: Springer.

Choy, Y., Fyer, A., & Lipsitz, J. (2007). Treatment of specific phobia in adults. *Clinical Psychology Review, 27,* 266–286.

Clark, D., & Ehlers, A. (1993). An overview of the cognitive theory and treatment of panic disorder. *Applied and Preventive Psychology, 2,* 131–139.

Clark, D., Ehlers, A., McManus, F., Hackman, A., Fennel, M., Campbell, H., Flower, T., . . . & Louis, B. (2003). Cognitive therapy versus fluoxetine in generalized social phobia: A randomized placebo controlled trial. *Journal of Consulting and Clinical Psychology, 71,* 1058–1067.

Clark, D., Salkovskis, P., Hackmann, A., Middleton, H., Anastasiades, P., & Gelder, M.. (1994). A comparison of cognitive therapy, applied relaxation and imipramine in the treatment of panic disorder. *British Journal of Psychiatry, 164,* 759–769.

Colpaert, F., & Koek, W. (1995). Empirical evidence that the state dependence and drug discrimination paradigms can generate different outcomes, *Psychopharmacology, 120,* 272–279.

Comaty, J., & Advokat, C. (2012). Generalized anxiety disorder. In S. Moore & B. Stahl (Eds.), *Clinical handbook of anxiety disorders: Psychopharmacology and psychotherapy practice* (pp. 97–113). Abingdon: Routledge.

Craske, M. (2015). *Psychotherapy for generalized anxiety disorder.* Retrieved from http//:www.uptodate.com

Craske, M., Rauch, S., Ursano, M., Prenoveau, J., Pine, D., & Zinbarg, R. (2009). What is anxiety disorder? *Depression and Anxiety, 26,* 1066–1085.

Crits-Christoph, P., & Connolly-Gibbons, M. (2010). Psychotherapy. In I. Weiner, & W. Craighead (Eds.), *Corsini's encyclopedia of psychology.* Hoboken, NJ: Wiley.

Cuijpers, P., Marks, I., van Straten, A., Cavanagh, K., Geg, L., & Andersson, G. (2009). Computer-aided psychotherapy for anxiety disorder: A meta-analytic review. *Cognitive-Behavioral Therapy, 38,* 66–82.

Da Costa, J. (1871). An irritable heart; a clinical study of a form of functional cardiac disorder and its consequences. *American Journal of the Medical Sciences, 61,* 18–52.

Davis, M., Ressler, K., Rothbaum, B., & Richardson, R. (2006). Effects of D-cycloserine on extinction: Translation from preclinical to clinical work. *Biological Psychiatry, 60,* 369–375.

Denys, D. de Geus, F., van Megen, H., & Westenberg, H. (2004). A double-blind, randomized, placebo-controlled trial of quetiapine addition in patients with obsessive-compulsive disorder refractory to serotonin reuptake inhibitors. *Journal of Clinical Psychiatry, 65,* 1040–1048.

Eddy, K., Dutra, L., Bradley, R., & Westen, D. (2004). A multidimensional meta-analysis of psychotherapy and pharmacotherapy for obsessive-compulsive disorder. *Clinical Psychology Review, 24,* 1011–1030.

Ehlers, A., Bisson, J., Clark, D., Creamer, M., Pilling, S., Richards, D., . . . &Yule, W. (2010). Do all psychological treatments really work the same in posttraumatic stress disorder? *Clinical Psychology Review, 30,* 269–276.

Elkins, S., & Moore, T. (2011). A time-series study of the treatment of panic disorder. *Clinical Case Studies, 10,* 3 22.

Emmelkamp, P. (1982). *Phobic and obsessive compulsive disorder: Theory, research and practice.* New York: Plenum Press.

Farchione, T., Fairholme, C., Ellard, K., Boisseau, C., Thompson-Hollands, J., Carl, J., . . . & Barlow, D.. (2012). Unified protocol for transdiagnostic treatment of emotional disorder: A randomized controlled trial. *Behavioral Therapy, 43,* 666–678.

Fals-Stewart, W., Marks, A., & Schafer, J. (1993). A comparison of behavioral group therapy and individual behavior therapy in treating obsessive-compulsive disorder. *Journal of Nervous and Mental Diseases, 181,* 189–193.

Federoff, I., & Taylor, S. (2001). Psychological and pharmacological treatments of social phobia: A meta-analysis. *Journal of Clinical Psychopharmacology, 21,* 311–324.

Feske, U., & Chambless, D. (1995). Cognitive behavioral versus exposure only treatment for social phobia: A meta-analysis. *Behavior Therapy, 26,* 695–720.

Feyer, A. (1987). Simple phobia. *Modern Problems in Pharmacopsychiatry, 22,* 174–192.

Fineberg, N., Stein, D., Premkumar, P., Carey, P., Sivakumaran, T., Vythilingum, B., . . . & Denys, D. (2006). Adjunctive quetiapine for serotonin reuptake inhibitor-resistant obsessive-compulsive disorder: A meta-analysis of randomized controlled treatment trials. *International Clinical Psychopharmacology, 21,* 337–343.

Fisher, P., & Wells, A. (2004). How effective are cognitive and behavioral treatments for obsessive-compulsive disorder? A clinical significance analysis. *Behaviour Research and Therapy, 43,* 1543–1558.

Foa, E. (2006). Social anxiety disorder treatments: Psychosocial therapies. *Clinical Psychiatry, 67,* 27–30.

Foe, E., Liebowitz, M., Kozak, M., Davies, S., Campeas, R., Franklin, M., . . . & Tu, X. (2005). Randomized, placebo controlled trial of exposure and ritual prevention, clomipramine, and their combination in the treatment of obsessive-compulsive disorder. *American Journal of Psychiatry, 162,* 151–161.

Franklin, M., Abramowitz, J., Foa, E., Levitt, J., & Kozak, M. (2000). Effectiveness of exposure and ritual prevention for obsessive-compulsive disorder: Randomized compared with nonrandomized samples. *Journal of Consulting and Clinical Psychology, 68,* 594–602.

Franklin, M., Sapyta, J., Freeman, J., Khanna, M., Compton, S., Almirall, D., . . . & March, J. (2011). Cognitive behavior therapy augmentation of pharmacotherapy in pediatric obsessive-compulsive disorder: The Pediatric OCD Treatment Study II (POTS II) randomized controlled trial. *Journal of the American Medical Association, 306,* 1224–1232.

Freud, S. (1937). *Studies in hysteria.* New York: Nervous and Mental Disease Publishing.

Furukawa, T., Watanabe, N., & Churchill, R. (2006). Psychotherapy plus antidepressant for panic disorder with or without agoraphobia. *British journal of Psychiatry, 188,* 305–312.

Gelpin, E., Bonne, O., Peri, T., Brandes, D., & Shalev, A. (2002). Treatment of recent trauma survivors with benzodiazepines: A prospective study. *Journal of Clinical Psychiatry, 57,* 390–394.

Gillies, D., Taylor, F., Gray, C., et al. (2012). Psychological therapies for the treatment of post-traumatic stress disorder in children and adolescents *Cochrane Database Systematic Review, Dec 12.*

Gillies, D., Taylor, F., Gray, C., O'Brien, L., & D'Abrew, N. (2013). Psychological therapies for the treatment of post-traumatic stress disorder in children and adolescents (Review). *Evidence Based Child Health, 8,* 1004–1116.

Gould, R., Otto, M., & Pollack, M. (1995). A meta-analysis of treatment outcome for panic disorder. *Clinical Psychology Review, 15,* 819–844.

Gould, R., Otto, M., Pollack, M., & Yap, L. (1997). Cognitive behavioral and pharmacological treatment of generalized anxiety disorder: A preliminary meta-analysis. *Behavior Therapy, 28,* 285–305.

Gray, J. A. (1970). Sodium amobarbital, the hippocampal theta rhythm and the partial reinforcement extinction effect. *Psychological Review, 77*, 465–480.
Guastella, A., Rischardson, R., Lovibond, P., Rapee, R., Gaston, J., Mitchell, P., . . . & Dadds, M. (2008). A randomized controlled trial of D-cycloserine enhancement of exposure therapy for social anxiety disorder. *Biological Psychiatry, 63*, 544–549.
Guastella, A., Howard, A., Dadds, M., et al. (2009). A randomized controlled trial of intranasal oxytocin as an adjunct to exposure therapy for social anxiety disorder. *Psychoneuroendocrinology, 34*, 917–923.
Hansen, R., Gaynes, B., & Gartlehner, G., et al. (2008). Efficacy and tolerability of second-generation antidepressants in social anxiety disorder. *International Journal of Clinical Psychopharmacology, 23*, 170–179.
Hafner J., & Marks I. (1976). Exposure in vivo of agoraphobics: Contributions of diazepam, group exposure, and anxiety evocation. *Psychological Medicine, 6*, 71–88.
Hageman, I., Andersen, H., & Jorgensen, M. (2001). Post-traumatic stress disorder: A review of psychobiology and pharmacology. *Acta Psychiatrica Scandinavica, 104*, 411–422.
Hayes-Skelton, S., Roemer, L., & Orsillo, S. (2013). Randomized clinical trial comparing an acceptance based behavior therapy to applied relaxation for generalized anxiety disorder. *Journal of Consulting and Clinical Psychology, 81*, 761–773.
Hedges, D., Brown, B., Shwalb, D., Godfrey, K., & Larcher, M.. (2007). The efficacy of selective serotonin reuptake inhibitors in adult social anxiety disorder: A meta-analysis of double-bind, placebo controlled trials. *Journal of Psychopharmacology, 21*, 102–111.
Heimberg, R. (2002). Cognitive-behavioral therapy for social anxiety disorder: Current status and future directions. *Society for Biological Psychiatry, 51*, 101–108.
Heimberg, R., & Becker, R. (2002). *Cognitive-behavioral group therapy for social phobia: basic mechanisms and clinical strategies*. New York: Guilford Press.
Hetrick, S., Purcell, R., Garner, B., & Parslow, R. (2010). Combined pharmacotherapy and psychological therapies for post-traumatic stress disorder (PTSD). *Cochrane Database Systematic Review, July 7*(7), CD007316. doi:10.1002/14651858.CD007316.pub2
Hidalgo, R., Tupler, L., & Davidson, J. (2007). An effect-size analysis of pharmacologic treatments for generalized anxiety disorder. *Journal of Psychopharmacology, 21*, 864–872.
Hoffmann, S., Meuret, A., & Smits, J. (2006). Augmentation of exposure therapy with D-cycloserine for social anxiety. *Archives of General Psychiatry, 63*, 298–304.
Hoffman, S., Pollack, M., & Otto, M. (2006). Augmentation treatment of psychotherapy for anxiety disorders with D-cycloserine. *CNS Drug Reviews, 12*, 208–217.
Hoffman, S., Sawyer, M., Korte, K., & Smits, J. (2009). Is it beneficial to add pharmacotherapy to CBT when treating anxiety disorders? A meta-analytic review. *International Journal of Cognitive Therapy, 2*, 160–175.
Hollander, E., Kaplan, A, & Stahl, S. (2003). A double-blind, placebo controlled trial of clonazepam in obsessive-compulsive disorder. *World Journal of Biological Psychiatry, 4*, 30–34.
Hope, D., Heimberg, R., & Bruch, M. (1995). Dismantling cognitive-behavioral group therapy for social phobia. *Behaviour Research and Therapy, 33*, 637–650.
IOM, Institute of Medicine (2007). *Treatment of PTSD: Assessment of the evidence.* Washington, DC: National Academies Press.
Ipser, J., Kariuki, C., & Stein, D. (2008). Pharmacotherapy for social anxiety disorder: A systematic review. *Expert Review Neurotherapeutics, 8*, 235–257.

Ipser, J. & Stein, D. (2012). Evidence-based pharmacotherapy of posttraumatic stress disorder. *International Journal of Neuropsychopharmacology, 15,* 825–840.

Iribarren, J., Prolo, P., Neagos, N., & Chiappelli, F. (2005). Post-traumatic stress disorder: Evidence-based research for the third millennium. *Evidence Based Complement Alternative Medicine, 2,* 503–512.

Juster, H., & Heimberg, R. (1995). Social phobia: Longitudinal course and long-term outcome of cognitive-behavioral treatment. *Psychiatric Clinics of North America, 18,* 821–842.

Kamath, P., Reddy, Y., & Kandavel, T. (2007). Suicidal behavior in obsessive-compulsive disorder. *Journal of Clinical Psychiatry, 68,* 1741–1750.

Kellner, M. (2010). Drug treatment of obsessive-compulsive disorder. *Dialogues in Clinical Neuroscience, 12,* 1887–197.

Kessler, R., Berglund, P., Demler, O., Jin, R., Merikangas, K., & Walters, E. (2005). Lifetime prevalence and age-of-onset distributions of DSM-IV disorders in the National Comorbidity Survey Replication. *Archives of General Psychiatry, 62,* 617–627.

Kessler, R., Ruscio, A., Shear, K., & Wiichen, H.-U. (2010). Epidemiology of anxiety disorders. In M. Stein, & T. Steckler (Eds.), *Behavioral neurobiology of anxiety and its treatment* (pp. 21–35). New York: Springer.

Klein, D. (2002). Historical aspects of anxiety. *Dialogues in Clinical Neuroscience, 4,* 295–304.

Koen, N., & Stein, D. (2011). Pharmacotherapy of anxiety disorders: A critical review. *Dialogues in Clinical Neuroscience, 13,* 423–437.

Kordon, A., Wahl, K., Koch, N., Zurowski, B., Anlauf, A., Vielhaber, K., . . . & Kahl, K.. (2008). Quetiapine addition to serotonin reuptake inhibitors in patients with severe obsessive-compulsive disorder: A double-blind, randomized, placebo-controlled study. *Journal of Clinical Psychopharmacology, 28,* 550–554.

Krystal, J., Rosenheck, R., Cramer, J., Vesicchio, J., Jones, K., Vertrees, J., . . . & Stock, C. (2011). Adjunctive risperidone treatment for antidepressant-resistant symptoms of chronic military service-related PTSD: A randomized trial. *Journal of the American Medical Association, 306,* 493–502.

Leichsenring F., Salzer S., Jaeger, U., Kachele, H., Kreische, R., Leweke, F., . . . & Leibing, E. (2009). Short-term psychodynamic psychotherapy and cognitive-behavioral therapy in generalized anxiety disorder: A randomized, controlled trial. *American Journal of Psychiatry, 166,* 875–881.

Leichsenring, F., Salzer, S., Beutel, M., Herpertz, S., Hiller, W., Hoyer, J., . . . & Leibing, E. (2013). Psychodynamic therapy and cognitive-behavioral therapy in social anxiety disorder: A multicenter randomized controlled trial. *American Journal of Psychiatry, 170,* 759–767.

Liebowitz, M., Gorman, J., Fyer, A., Campeas, R., Levin, A., Sandberg, D., . . . & Goetz, D. (1988). Pharmacotherapy of social phobia: An interim report of a placebo-controlled comparison of phenelzine and atenolol. *Clinical Journal of Psychiatry, 49,* 252–257.

Margraf, J., Barlow, D., Clark, D., & Telch, M. (1993). Psychological treatment of panic: Work in progress on outcome, active ingredients, and follow-up. *Behaviour Research and Therapy, 31,* 1–8.

Marks, I. (1987). *Fears, phobias, and rituals. panic, anxiety, and their disorders.* New York: Oxford University Press.

Marks, I., Stern, R., Mawson, D., Cobb, J., & McDonald, R. (1980). Clomipramine and exposure for obsessive compulsive rituals. *British Journal of Psychiatry, 136*, 1025.

Marks, I., Swinson, R., Basoglu, M., Kuch, K., Noshivani, H., O'Sullivan, G., . . . & Sengun, S.. (1993). Alprazolam and exposure alone and combined in panic disorder with agoraphobia: A controlled study in London and Toronto. *British Journal of Psychiatry, 162*, 776–787.

Marks, I., Viswanathan, R., Lipsedge, M., & Gardner, R. (1972). Enhanced relief of phobias by flooding during waning diazepam effect. *British Journal of Psychiatry, 121*, 493–505.

Mayo-Wilson, E., Dias, S., Mavranezouli, I., Kew, K., Clark, D., Ades, A., . . . & Pilling, S. (2014). Psychological and pharmacological interventions for social anxiety disorder in adults: A systematic review and network meta-analysis. *Lancet Psychiatry, 1*, 368–376.

McEvoy, P., & Perini, S. (2009). Cognitive behavioral group therapy for social phobia with and without attention training: A controlled study. *Journal of Anxiety Disorders, 23*, 519–528.

McHugh, R., Smits, J., & Otto, M. (2009). Empirically supported treatments for panic disorder. *Psychiatric Clinics of North America, 32*, 593–610.

Merikangas, K., He, J., Burstein, M., Swanson, S., Avenevoli, S., Cui, L., . . . & Swendsen, J. (2010). Lifetime prevalence of mental disorders in U.S. adolescents: results from the National Comorbidity Survey Replication—Adolescent Supplement (NCS-A). *Journal of the American Academy of Child and Adolescent Psychiatry, 49*, 980–989.

Merra, S., Godeas L., & Persico, G. (1993). Integrated therapy in panic attack disorders. *Minerva Psichiatrica, 3*, 121–124.

Michael, T., Zetsche, U., & Margraf, J. (2007). Epidemiology of anxiety disorders. *Epidemiology and Psychopharmacology, 6*(4), 136–142.

Milrod, B., Busch, F., Leon, A., Shapiro, T., Aronson, A., Roiphe, J., . . . & Shear, M. (2000). Open trial of psychodynamic psychotherapy for panic disorder: A pilot study. *American Journal of Psychiatry, 157*, 1878–1880.

Milrod, B., Leon, A., Busch, F., Rudden, M., Schwalberg, M., Clarkin, J., . . . & Shear, M. (2007). A randomized controlled clinical trial of psychoanalytic psychotherapy for panic disorder. *American Journal of Psychiatry, 164*, 265–272.

Mitte, K. (2005a). A meta-analysis of cognitive-behavioral treatments of generalized anxiety disorder: A comparison with pharmacotherapy. *Psychological Bulletin, 131*, 785–795.

Mitte, K. (2005b). A meta-analysis of the efficacy of psycho- and pharmacotherapy in panic disorder with or without agoraphobia. *Journal of Affective Disorders, 88*, 27–85.

Muse, M. (1984). Narcosynthesis in the treatment of posttraumatic chronic pain. *Rehabilitation Psychology, 29*, 113–118.

Muse, M., & Moore, B. (2012). Integrating clinical psychopharmacology within the practice of medical psychology. In M. Muse, & B. Moore (Eds). *Handbook of clinical psychopharmacology for psychologists* (pp. 17–43). Hoboken, NJ: Wiley.

Muse, M., Moore, B., & Stahl, S. (2013). Benefits and challenges of integrated treatment. In S. Stahl, & B. Moore (Eds.), *Clinical handbook of anxiety disorders: Psychopharmacology and psychotherapy practice* (pp. 3–24). Abingdon: Routledge.

National Institute for Health and Clinical Excellence (NICE) (2011). *Generalised anxiety disorder and panic disorder (with or without agoraphobia) in adults: Management in primary, secondary and community care.* Retrieved from www.nice.org.uk

Newman, M., Castonguay, L., Borkovec, T., Aaron, F., Boswell, J., Szkodny, L., . . . & Norberg, S. (2011). A randomized controlled trial of cognitive-behavioral therapy for generalized anxiety disorder with integrated techniques from emotion-focused and interpersonal therapies. *Journal of Consulting and Clinical Psychology, 79*, 171–181.

Ninan, P., Koran, L., Kiev, A., Davidson, J., Rasmussen, S., Zajecka, J., . . . & Austin, C.. (2006). High-dose sertraline strategy for non-responders to acute treatment for obsessive-compulsive disorder: A multi-center double-bind trial. *Journal of Clinical Psychiatry, 67*, 15–22.

Norberg, M., Krystal, J., & Tolin, D. (2008). A meta-analysis of D-cycloserine and the facilitation of fear extinction and exposure therapy. *Biological Psychiatry, 63*, 1118–1126.

Norton, P., & Price, E. (2007). A meta-analytic view of adult cognitive behavioral treatment outcome across the anxiety disorders. *Journal of Nervous and Mental Diseases, 195*, 521–531.

Olfson, M., Marcus, S., Wan, G., & Geissler, E. (2004). National trends in the outpatient treatment of anxiety disorders. *Journal of Clinical Psychiatry, 65*, 1166–1173.

Ost, L., & Sterner, U. (1987). Applied tension: A specific behavioral method for treatment of blood phobia. *Behaviour Research and Therapy, 25*, 25–29.

Ost, L., Sterner, U., & Fellenius, J. (1989). Applied tension, applied relaxation, and the combination in the treatment of blood phobia. *Behaviour Research and Treatment, 27*, 109–121.

Otto, M., Hinton, D., Korbly, N., Chea, A., Gershuny, B., & Pollack, M. (2003). Treatment of pharmacotherapy-refractory posttraumatic stress disorder among Cambodian refugees: A pilot study of combining treatment with cognitive-behavior therapy vs. sertraline alone. *Behavioral Research and Therapy, 41*, 1271–1276.

Otto, M., Pollack, M, Gould, R., Worthington, J. J., McArdle, E. T., & Rosenbaum, J. F. (2000). A comparison of the efficacy of clonazepam and cognitive-behavioral group therapy for the treatment of social phobia. *Journal of Anxiety Disorders, 14*, 345–358.

Overton, D. (1964). State-dependent or "dissociated" learning produced with pentobarbital. *Journal of Comparative and Physiological Psychology, 57*, 3–12.

Paul, O. (1987). Da Costa's syndrome or neurocirculatory asthenia. *British Heart Journal, 58*, 306–315.

Pollack, M., Allgulander, C., Bandelow, B., Cassano, B., Greist, J., Hollander, E., . . . & Swinson, R. (2003). WCA recommendations for the long-term treatment of panic disorder. *CNS Spectrums, 8*, 17–30.

Polusny, M., Erbes, C., Thuras, P., Moran, A., Lamberty, G., Collins, R., . . . & Lim, K.. (2015). Mindfulness-based stress reduction for posttraumatic stress disorder among veterans: A randomized clinical trial. *Journal of the American Medical Association, 314*, 456–465.

Power, K., Simpson, R., Swanson, V., & Wallace, L. (1990). A controlled comparison of cognitive behavior therapy, diazepam, and placebo, alone and in combination, for the treatment of generalized anxiety disorder. *Journal of Anxiety Disorders, 4*, 267–292.

Raskind, M., Peskind, E., Hoff, D., Hart, D., Holmes, Warren, D., . . . & McFall, M. (2007). A parallel group placebo controlled study of prazosin for trauma nightmares and sleep disturbance in combat veterans with posttraumatic stress disorder. *Biological Psychiatry, 61*, 928–934.

Raskind, M., Peskind, E., Kanter, E., Petrie, E., Radant, A., Thompson, E., . . . & McFall, M. (2003). Reduction of nightmares and other PTSD symptoms in combat veterans by prazosin: A placebo-controlled study. *American Journal of Psychiatry, 160*, 371–373.

Rauch, S., & Drevets, W. (2009). Neuroimagining and neuroanatomy of stress-induced and fear circuitry disorders. In A. Charney (Ed.) *Stress-induced and fear circuitry disorders* (pp. 226–231) Arlington, VA: American Psychiatric Association.

Ravindran, L., & Stein, M. (2010). The pharmacologic treatment of anxiety disorders: A review of progress. *Journal of Clinical Psychiatry, 71*, 839–854.

Reus, V., Weingartner, H, & Post, R. (1979). Clinical implications of state-dependent learning. *American Journal of Psychiatry, 136*, 927–931.

Rosa-Alcazar, A., Sanchez-Meca, J., Gomez-Conesa, A., & Marin-Martinez, F. (2008). Psychological treatment of obsessive-compulsive disorder: A meta-analysis. *Clinical Psychology Review, 28*, 1310–1325.

Rothbaum, B., Cahill, S., Foa, S., Davidson, J., Compton, J., Connor, K., . . . & Hahn, C. (2006). Augmentation of sertraline with prolonged exposure in the treatment of posttraumatic stress disorder. *Journal of Traumatic Stress, 1*, 625–638.

Roy-Byrne, P., & Cowley, D. (2007). Pharmacological treatments of panic disorder, generalized anxiety disorder, specific phobia, and social anxiety disorder. In P. Nathan, & J. Gorman (Eds.), *A guide to treatments that work* (pp. 395–431). New York: Oxford University Press.

Sareen, J., & Stein, M. (2000). A review of the epidemiology and approaches to the treatment of social anxiety. *Drugs, 59*, 494–509.

Sartory, G. (1983). Benzodiazepines and behavioural treatment of phobic anxiety. *Behavioral Psychotherapy, 11*, 204–217.

Schneier, F., Neria, Y., Pavlicova, M., Hembree, E., Suh, E. Amsel, L., & Marshal, R. (2011). Combined prolonged exposure therapy and paroxetine for PTSD related to the World Trade Center attack: A randomized controlled trial. *American Journal of Psychiatry, 169*, 80–88.

Serretti, A., Chiesa, A., Calati, R., Giampaolo, P., Bellodi, L., & De Rochi, D. (2011). Novel antidepressants and panic disorder: Evidence beyond current guidelines. *Neuropsychobiology, 63*, 1–7.

Shear, M., Cooper, A., Klerman, G., Busch, F., & Shapiro, T. (1993). A psychodynamic model of panic disorder. *American Journal of Psychiatry, 150*, 850–866.

Shearer, D., Brown, C., Harmon, C., & Moore, B. (2014). Integrating psychopharmacology and psychotherapy in anxiety disorders. In I. Reis de Oliveira (Ed.), *Integrating psychotherapy and psychopharmacology: A handbook for clinicians* (pp. 125–147). New York: Routledge.

Silverman, W., Kurtines, W., Ginsburg, G., Weems, C., Rabian, B., & Serafini, L. (1999). Contingency management, self-control, and educational support in the treatment of childhood phobic disorders. A randomized clinical trial. *Journal of Consulting and Clinical Psychology, 67*, 675–687.

Simpson, H., Foa, E., Liebowitz, M., Ledley, D., Huppert, J., Cahil, S., . . . & Petkova, E. (2008). A randomized, controlled trial of cognitive-behavioral therapy for augmenting pharmacotherapy in obsessive-compulsive disorder. *American Journal of Psychiatry, 165*, 621 630.

Simpson, H., Foa, E., Liebowitz, M., Huppert, J., Cahill, S , Maher, J., . . . & Campea, R. (2013). Cognitive-behavioral therapy vs risperidone for augmenting serotonin reuptake inhibitors in obsessive-compulsive disorder: A randomized clinical trial. *JAMA Psychiatry, September 11*.

Simpson, H., & Liebowitz, M. (2011). Combining pharmacotherapy and cognitive-behavioral therapy in the treatment of OCD. In J. Abramowitz, & A. Houts (Eds.),

Concepts and controversies in obsessive-compulsive disorder (pp. 359–376). New York: Springer.
Singewald, N., Schmuckermair, C., Whittle, N., Holmes, A., & Ressler, K. (2015). Pharmacology of cognitive enhancers for exposure-based therapy of fear, anxiety and trauma-related disorders. *Pharmacology and Therapeutics, 149,* 150–190.
Spiegel, D., & Bruce, T. (1997). Benzodiazepines and exposure-based cognitive behavior therapies for panic disorder: Conclusions from combined treatment trials. *American Journal of Psychiatry, 154,* 773–781.
Spiegel, D., Roth, M., Weissman, M., Lovori, P., Gorman, J., Rush, J., & Ballenger, J. (1993). Comment of the London/Toronto study of alprazolam and exposure in panic disorder with agoraphobia. *British Journal of Psychiatry, 162,* 788–789.
Steenkamp, M., Litz, B., Hoge, C., & Marmar, C. (2015). Psychotherapy for military-related PTSD: A review of randomized clinical trials. *Journal of the American Medical Association, 314,* 489–500.
Stein, D., Fineberg, N., Bienvu, O., Denys, D., Lochner, C., Nestadt, G., . . . & Phillips, K. (2010). Should OCD be classified as an anxiety disorder in DSM-V? *Depression and Anxiety, 27,* 495–506.
Stein, D., Iper, J., & Seedat, S. (2009). Pharmacotherapy for posttraumatic stress disorder (PTSD). *The Cochrane Library: Cochrane Database Systematic Review, 4,* CD002795.
Taylor, F., Martin, P., Thompson, C., Williams, J., Mellman, M., Gross, C., . . . & Raskind, M. (2008). Prazosin effects on objective sleep measures and clinical symptoms in civilian trauma posttraumatic stress disorder: A placebo controlled study. *Biological Psychiatry, 63,* 629–632.
Taylor, S., Woody, S., Koch, W., McLean, P., Paterson, R., & Anderson, K. (1997). Cognitive restructuring in the treatment of social phobia. *Behavior Modification, 21,* 487–511.
Thom, A., Sartory, G., & Johren, P. (2000). Comparison between one-session psychological treatment and benzodiazepine in dental phobia. *Journal of Consulting and Clinical Psychology, 68,* 378–387.
Tolin, D. (2010). Is cognitive-behavioral therapy more effective than other therapies? A meta-analytic review. *Clinical Psychology Review, 30,* 710–720.
Tone, A. (2009). *"The Fashionable Pill." The Age of Anxiety: A History of America's Turbulent Affair with Tranquilizers.* New York: Basic Books.
Van Ameringen, M., Mancini, C., Pipe, B., & Bennett, M. (2004). Optimizing treatment in social phobia: A review of treatment resistance. *CNS Spectrums, 9,* 753–762.
van Balkom, A., de Hann, E. van Oppen, P., Spinhoven, P., Hoogduin, K., & van Dyck, R. (1998). Cognitive and behavioral therapies alone versus in combination with fluvoxamine in the treatment for obsessive-compulsive disorder, *Journal of Nervous and Mental Disorders, 186,* 492–499.
Van Emmerik, A., Kamphuis, J., Hulsbosch, A., & Emmelkamp, P. (2002). Single session debriefing after psychological trauma: A meta-analysis. *The Lancet, 360,* 766–771.
Van Noppen, B., & Steketee, G. (2004). Individual, group and multifamily cognitive-behavioral treatments. In Pato & Zohar (Eds.), *Current treatments of obsessive-compulsive disorders* (2nd ed.) (pp. 133–172). Washington, DC: American Psychiatric Publishing.
Van Oppen, P., de Haan, E., van Balkom, A., Spinhoven, P., Hoogduin, K., & van Dyck, R. (1994). Cogntivie therapy and exposure in vivo in the treatment of obsessive compulsive disorder. *Behavior Research and Therapy, 33,* 379–390.

Vogel, P., Stiles, T., & Gotestam, K. (2004). Adding cognitive therapy elements to exposure therapy for obsessive-compulsive disorder: A controlled study. *Behavioural and Cognitive Psychotherapy, 32,* 275–290.

Wampold, B., Imel, Z., Laska, K., Benish, S., Miller, S., Flückinger, C., . . . & Budge, S. (2010). Determining what works in the treatment of PTSD. *Clinical Psychology Review, 30,* 923–933.

Warren, R., & Thomas, J. (2001). Cognitive-behavior therapy of obsessive-compulsive disorder in private practice: An effectiveness study. *Journal of Anxiety Disorders, 15,* 277–285.

Watson, J., & Rayner, R. (1920). Conditioned emotional reactions. *Journal of Experimental Psychology, 3,* 1–14.

Western Australian Psychotropic Drugs Committee (2008). *Anxiety disorders drug treatment guidelines.* WATAG.

Wilhelm, S., Bulmann, U, Tolin, D., Meunier, S., Pearlson, G., Reese, H., . . . & Rauch, S. (2008). Augmentation of behavioral therapy with d-cycloserine for obsessive-compulsive disorder. *American Journal of Psychiatry, 165,* 335–341.

Wilhelm, S., Steketee, G., Fama, J., Bulmann, U., Teachman, B., & Golan, E. (2009). Modular cognitive therapy of obsessive -compulsive disorder: A wait-list controlled trial. *Journal of Cognitive Psychotherapy, 23,* 294–305.

Williams, A., Richardson, G., & Galovski, T. (2014). Posttraumatic stress disorder. In S. Stahl & B. Moore (Eds.), *Anxiety disorders: A guide for integrating psychopharmacology and psychotherapy* (pp. 176–200) New York: Routledge.

Wolfe, B., & Maser, J. (1994). Origins and overview of the consensus development conference on the treatment of panic disorder. In B. Wolfe, & J. Maser (Eds.), *Treatment of panic disorder: A consensus development conference* (pp. 3–16). Washington, DC: American Psychiatric Press.

Wolitzky-Taylor, K., Horowitz, J., Powers, M., & Telch, M. (2008). Psychological approaches in the treatment of specific phobias: A meta-analysis. *Clinical Psychology Review, 28,* 1021–1037.

Wood, P. (1941). Da Costa's syndrome (or effort syndrome). Lecture I. *Lectures to the Royal College of Physicians of London. British Medical Journal, 4194,* 767–772.

Woods, S., Barlow, D., Gorman, J., & Shear, K. (1998). Follow-up results six months after discontinuation of all treatment. In D. Barlow (Ed.), Results from the multi-center clinical trial on the treatment of panic disorder: Cognitive behavioral treatment versus imipramine versus their combination. Symposium presented at the 32nd Annual Convention of the Association for Advancement of Behavior Therapy, Washington, DC.

Yehuda, R. (2002). Post-traumatic stress disorder. *New England Journal of Medicine, 246,* 108–114.

Zitrin, C., Klein, D.,Woerner, M., & Ross, D. (1983). Treatment of phobias: Comparison of imipramine hydrochloride and placebo. *Archives of General Psychiatry, 40,* 125–138.

Zlomke, K. (2008). One-session treatment of specific phobias: A detailed description and review of treatment efficacy. *Behavior Therapy, 39,* 207–223.

7

Personality Disorders: Evidence-Based Integrated Biopsychosocial Treatment of Borderline Personality Disorder

Donald Black, Joel Paris, and Charles Schulz

Personality disorders are characterized by the presence of an enduring pattern of inner experience and behavior that, according to the Diagnostic and Statistical Manual of Mental Disorders, Fifth Edition (DSM-5), "deviates markedly from the expectations of the individual's culture, is pervasive and inflexible, has an onset in adulthood, is stable over time, and leads to distress or impairment" (American Psychiatric Association, 2013, p. 645). As a general rule, personality disorders are not limited to episodes of illness, but reflect the individual's long-term adjustment. In the DSM-5, these 10 disorders are divided among three "clusters," based on shared phenomenology and diagnostic criteria. Cluster A ("eccentric cluster") consists of paranoid, schizoid, and schizotypal personality disorders, Cluster B ("dramatic cluster") consists of borderline, antisocial, histrionic, and narcissistic personality disorders, and Cluster C ("anxious cluster") consists of avoidant, dependent, and obsessive-compulsive personality disorders. Few individuals have a "pure" case in which they meet criteria for a single personality disorder. Those with mixtures of traits, but who do not meet full criteria, are diagnosed with either a specified or unspecified personality disorder.

From 10% to 15% of the general population meet criteria for a personality disorder, and rates are especially high in psychiatric samples and in special populations such as offenders and substance abusers (Torgersen, 2014). Younger persons are at higher risk for a personality disorder than older individuals, because prevalence diminishes with advancing age. Personality disorders typically have an onset in adolescence or early adulthood, with some being more frequent in men (e.g., antisocial personality disorder), while others are more frequent in women (e.g., borderline personality disorder (BPD). Personality disorders are associated with impaired social, interpersonal, and occupational functioning, as reflected by high rates of unemployment, homelessness, divorce and separation, domestic violence, and substance misuse. As a group, individuals with personality disorders are at high risk for early death from suicide, accidents, or homicide.

Some personality disorders have a natural process of recovery (e.g., borderline and antisocial personality disorders), while others are less likely to show improvement (e.g., schizotypal personality disorder). With BPD, follow up studies show that about 90% of patients in their 20s no longer meet diagnostic criteria by middle age and most have improved functioning (Paris, 2003, 2012). Prospective studies have documented even more rapid symptomatic improvement in some cases (Gunderson & Links, 2012).

Cognitive Behavioral Psychopharmacology: The Clinical Practice of Evidence-Based Biopsychosocial Integration, First Edition. Edited by Mark Dana Muse.

On the other hand, naturalistic studies indicate that people previously diagnosed with BPD who no longer meet formal criteria often remain impaired in overall vocational and interpersonal functioning (Zanarini, Frankenburg, Reich, & Fitzmaurice, 2012). BPD is also associated with a high utilization of healthcare resources, as these patients frequently present to emergency rooms and clinics with overdoses and deliberate self-harm, and are frequently admitted to hospitals (Forman, Berk, Henriques, Brown, & Beck, 2004; Hull, Yeomans, Clarkin, Li, & Goodman, 1996; Zanarini, Frankenburg, Khera, & Bleichmar, 2001).

The diagnosis of a personality disorder requires a comprehensive personal and social history combined with a careful mental status examination. Structured interviews and self-report assessments are helpful, although rarely used outside of research settings (Kolb & Gunderson, 1980; Zanarini et al., 2010). Many clinicians are reluctant to diagnose personality disorders, a problem well documented with BPD that is linked to stigma (Black, Allen, McCormick, & Blum, 2011). Despite these concerns, clinicians should know that the lack of recognition will not make the problem go away, and that ignoring the diagnosis also deprives patients of the opportunity to engage in an evidence-based treatment.

This chapter is focused on the treatment of BPD because it is the best researched of the personality disorders, supported by a data base that has accumulated in the past 25–40 years (Bateman & Krawitz, 2013). There is now good evidence supporting the efficacy and effectiveness of a number of psychotherapies for BPD. This literature is sufficiently mature that several clinical guidelines have been published using meta-analyses to determine the strength of the evidence in recommending their use. No guideline finds sufficient support for making clear comparisons among the various psychotherapies. At the same time, headway has been made in researching psychopharmacologic approaches. While many studies have been conducted with different agents, the results are decidedly mixed and clinical guidelines have recommended caution in their use. For these reasons, psychotherapy remains the treatment mainstay for this challenging patient population. While there has been some effort to examine the combination of psychotropic medication with psychotherapy, and early results are encouraging, the body of literature is insufficient to make recommendations.

Psychopharmacologic Treatment of BPD

The psychopharmacologic treatment of psychiatric patients began in earnest in the 1950s and 1960s, with the development of antidepressants, antipsychotics, and various tranquillizers (Klein, 1968). The initial focus of treatment was placed on patients with psychotic, mood, or anxiety disorders. The federal government assumed an active role in this process as the National Institute of Mental Health established a branch to objectively assess psychiatric treatment, usually in academic settings with an emphasis on randomized and controlled designs. By the late 1970s and early 1980s, interest in using psychotropic medication began to include BPD, spurred in part by the emergence of diagnostic criteria developed by Gunderson and Singer (1975), later adapted and included in the DSM-III (American Psychiatric Association, 1980), and research validating the disorder.

The goal of these early studies was to identify potential medications for BPD. While no psychotropics have been approved by the US Food and Drug Administration (FDA) to treat BPD, and treatment guidelines have not encouraged their use (National Institute for Health and Care Excellence (NICE), 2009), research, nonetheless, shows that these patients are often prescribed medication. In both academic and community settings, up to 100% of BPD patients have been prescribed medication, most typically antidepressants, antipsychotics, mood stabilizers, stimulants, or sedative-hypnotics (Black, Allen, McCormick, & Blum, 2011; Zanarini, Frankenburg, Reich, Conkey, & Fitzmaurice, 2015). The variety of medication classes prescribed should be seen as a reflection of the varied symptom domains that prescribing mental health providers are attempting to treat (e.g., anger/irritability, suicidality, mood instability). Additionally, it is not uncommon for patients to be prescribed multiple psychotropic medications, a practice often referred to as "polypharmacy." In some studies, the mean number of psychotropic medications taken by patients was more than three, and there is little evidence that the number of medications is associated with patient severity (Black, Allen, McCormick, & Blum, 2011). While this often-derided practice may not enhance patient outcomes, it is clearly associated with greater expense and more adverse effects.

Antipsychotic Medications

Antipsychotics were among the first medications used to treat BPD, perhaps reflecting their association with an earlier diagnosis used in these patients that implied they straddled the border between neurosis and psychosis ("pseudoneurotic schizophrenia"). In an early report, Brinkley Beitman, and Friedel (1979) described five cases of borderline patients who all appeared to benefit from low doses of traditional antipsychotics. This was followed by a report in which thiothixene and haloperidol were compared in a mixed sample of patients with either BPD or schizotypal personality disorder, each medication associated with a reduction in symptoms (Serban & Segal, 1984). They reported improvement in depression, anxiety, derealization, paranoid ideation, and global functioning. Because there was no placebo control, it was difficult to understand the full impact of medication. Further, in this and other early trials, it was not uncommon to recruit mixed groups of BPD and schizotypal patients.

Several better designed studies followed. Goldberg et al. (1986) reported the results of a randomized controlled trial (RCT) in which thiothixene was compared to placebo in patients with BPD or schizotypal personality disorder. Thiothixene was superior to placebo in the treatment of psychotic-like symptoms including illusions and ideas of reference, but also in self-rated obsessive-compulsive and phobic symptoms. Another RCT (Soloff et al., 1986) compared haloperidol to the tricyclic antidepressant amitriptyline and a placebo. Haloperidol outperformed amitriptyline and placebo on overall symptom severity, self-rated depression, anger and hostility, schizotypal symptoms, psychoticism, and impulsive behavior. Haloperidol was equal to amitriptyline for depressive symptoms.

Following these studies, Cowdry and Gardner (1988) designed a complicated crossover study to explore medications from four different pharmacologic classes (alprazolam, tranylcypromine, carbamazepine, trifluoperazine). Sixteen subjects were outpatients who serially received each medication in random order. Despite relatively poor completion rates, there were several important findings. Each medication was associated with improvement, except alprazolam, a benzodiazepine tranquillizer, which led to increased behavioral dyscontrol. Trifluoperazine led to improvement in anxiety and suicidality, while tranylcypromine was associated with improvement in depressive symptoms, and carbamazepine led to improved behavioral control. Because of this study, it has been generally assumed that benzodiazepines should be avoided in persons with BPD due to the possibility of behavioral disinhibition.

On the heels of these reports, was an open study of thioridazine, a sedating antipsychotic, tested in outpatients with BPD over 12 weeks. Thioridazine led to reductions in self-rated depression (Teicher et al., 1989). An additional study comparing haloperidol and the monoamine oxidase inhibitor phenelzine produced interesting results (Soloff et al., 1993). Of interest was that haloperidol was not better than placebo, yet phenelzine outperformed placebo. This trial led to a lessening of enthusiasm for low-dose antipsychotics.

Atypical antipsychotics emerged in the 1990s and were associated with fewer extrapyramidal side effects (i.e., movement disorders) than the earlier generation of antipsychotics. Because of positive trials in mood disorder patients, interest developed in using these medications to treat BPD. In the first study to be reported, Schulz, Camlin, Berry, and Jesberger (1999) reported a reduction in symptoms in 11 patients with BPD and co-morbid dysthymia taking olanzapine. There were significant reductions in measures of psychoticism, depression, interpersonal sensitivity, and anger.

Two RCTs of risperidone were conducted. In the first, significant reductions on a number of scales were found in the risperidone groups, but similar reductions were seen with placebo (Schulz, Camlin, Berry, & Friedman, 1998). At the same time, a European study reported an advantage of risperidone overall, and specifically for aggression and depressive symptoms (Rocca, Marchiaro, Cocuzza, & Bogetto, 2002).

Two pilot RCTs of olanzapine were conducted. In the first study (Bogenschutz and George, 2004), 40 subjects were randomized to olanzapine or placebo. Olanzapine was superior to placebo on global BPD symptoms. Zanarini and Frankenberg (2001) also reported an RCT finding in which the drug outperformed placebo in 28 women. Of great interest was the design of testing the subjects for 6 months. Over this time period, women assigned to olanzapine had greater improvement of interpersonal sensitivity, anger and hostility, anxiety and paranoia but not depression.

In view of these positive studies, the manufacturers of olanzapine designed two large RCTs with a combined sample of over 700 subjects with the goal of seeking US FDA approval for BPD. Of the first, olanzapine did no better than placebo (Schulz et al., 2008). In the other, olanzapine outperformed placebo for global BPD symptoms of anger, paranoid ideation, suicidal behavior, and irritability. A single-blind 6-month extension showed continued effectiveness (Zanarini et al., 2012; Zanarini, Frankenburg, Reich, & Fitzmaurice, 2011). Importantly, in the earlier trial (Schulz et al., 2008), there was statistically significant advantage of olanzapine compared to placebo during the trial, except for the final rating ($p = .062$). Because of the mixed results, the drug could not be approved.

Quetiapine is another atypical antipsychotic medication that has shown promise, and is currently approved for the treatment of schizophrenia and bipolar disorder. Open studies have suggested effectiveness for the drug in terms of global symptoms, depression, anger/irritability, paranoia, and dissociation (Adityanjee et al., 2008; Perella, Carrus, Costa, & Schifano, 2007). Following on the heels of these reports, Black et al. (2014) tested two fixed doses (150 mg, 300 mg) of a long-acting form of the drug in 95 subjects. Quetiapine at 150 mg daily was effective in treating global BPD symptoms, affective disturbance, and interpersonal relationships compared to placebo. As there were subsequent discussions about domains within medication trials, Lee, Allen, Black, Zanarini, and Schulz (2016) later analyzed the Black et al. findings and found significant improvements in self-reported interpersonal sensitivity, depression, and hostility.

Aripiprazole has also been tested in BPD patients. An RCT that included 52 subjects showed significant changes in many self-reported domains including aggressiveness/hostility, phobic anxiety, paranoid thinking, psychoticism, and various forms of anger (Nickel et al., 2006). This study made a further contribution to the field by examining the longer-term use of aripiprazole versus placebo over 18 months; the authors noted significant differences across time in the rating scales (Nickel, Loew, & Pedrosa, 2007) assessing depression, anxiety, anger, and other symptoms. Of note, the subjects did not gain weight during the 18-month study.

The long-acting injectable antipsychotic paliperidone palmitate was tested in a group of BPD patients. In this series, 10 patients were treated over 12 weeks and had objective ratings. The authors noted a statistically significant reduction in rating scales of symptoms and functions. They found that patients tended to gain weight, and several developed galactorrhea (Palomares, Montes, Diaz-Marsa, & Carrasco, 2015).

Clozapine, used to treat schizophrenia, requires complete blood count due to the possibility of developing a blood dyscrasia. Because of its value in treating refractory schizophrenia and its use in treatment-refractory cases, it has also been tried in patients with BPD. Frankenberg and Zanarini (1993) collected a series of BPD patients with co-morbid psychiatric illness and noted significant improvement in BPD symptoms. In Milan, Italy, Benedetti, Sforzini, Columbo, Maffei, and Smeraldi (1998) collected a case series of BPD patients who received low-dose clozapine. The authors note significant response with a reduction of impulsivity and affective instability.

Antidepressant Medications

Because of the association of BPD with depressed mood and suicidality, it made sense to many investigators to test antidepressant medication. In an early RCT, Soloff et al. (1986) reported that the tricyclic antidepressant amitriptyline was no better than placebo. These investigators later reported that the monoamine oxidase inhibitor phenelzine produced benefit (Soloff et al., 1993).

After the selective serotonin reuptake inhibitor fluoxetine became available in the late 1980s, Cornelius, Soloff, Perel, and Urich (1991) reported that five depressed BPD patients benefitted, particularly with depressive and impulsive symptoms. Markovitz, Calabrese, Schulz, and Meltzer (1991) reported a reduction in self-injury and Symptom Checklist-90-Revised subscales in a case series of 22 patients treated for 12 weeks. These two studies were followed by an RCT (Salzman et al., 1995) that showed a reduction in anger, noting that this was a significant problem in these patients. Since these early studies, subsequent trials have been disappointing. An RCT conducted by Zanarini et al. (2004) compared fluoxetine, olanzapine, and the combination. In this trial, fluoxetine did not perform as well as the other treatment cells, even though the authors noted that fluoxetine led to improvement in impulsive aggression and depression.

Anticonvulsants

As noted earlier, Cowdry and Gardner (1988) compared four different medications, including carbamazepine, mainly used in psychiatry as a mood stabilizer, and the drug was noted to significantly reduce behavioral dyscontrol. Another mood stabilizer, divalproex, was used to treat a broad group of subjects with impulsive aggression, including many with BPD (Hollander et al., 2003). Further studies by Hollander and colleagues (Hollander, Swann, Coccaro, Jiang, & Smith, 2005) illustrated the reduction of impulsivity and aggression in patients with BPD or other impulsive personality disorders. Further, Frankenberg and Zanarini (2002) illustrated the use of the anticonvulsant when the patients had both bipolar II disorder and BPD.

Lamotrigine is another anticonvulsant that has been tried in BPD. In a case series, Pinto and Akiskal (1998) reported that three of eight patients improved in their global functioning. Tritt et al. (2005) reported the first RCT of lamotrigine in BPD patients and, using the State-Trait Anger Expression Inventory (STAXI), patients had significant improvement. An 18-month extension revealed significant ongoing improvement (Lieberich, Nickel, Tritt, & Pedrosa, 2008). Reich et al. (2009) conducted an RCT using lamotrigine and found improvement for affective instability and impulsivity. Because of the potential for serious skin rash, dosing needs to be done carefully and patients and family informed about side effects.

Topiramate has also been examined in the treatment of BPD. In a series of studies, Nickel et al. (2004, 2005) conducted RCTs first in women and then in men. In these studies, BPD patients had significant improvement in anger, as well as improvement in interpersonal sensitivity, somatization, anxiety, hostility, and phobic anxiety. Regarding side effects, the investigators noted the subjects on the topiramate assignment had statistically significant weight loss compared to placebo. However, all of these studies of anticonvulsants in BPD need replication in larger samples.

Lithium Carbonate

An early study of subjects with DSM-II "emotionally unstable character disorder" showed positive results from lithium carbonate, first introduced in 1970 as a treatment for bipolar disorder (Rifkin, Quitkin, Carrillo, Blumberg, & Klein, 1972). Goldberg (1989) confirmed these positive results, but apart from these studies there have been no additional trials of lithium in BPD.

And of final interest, the supplement omega-3 fatty acid was given to BPD patients in an RCT conducted by Zanarini and Frankenberg (2003). Omega-3 fatty acid had a statistically significant advantage in the amelioration of aggression and depressive symptoms.

Benzodiazepines

As indicated earlier, Cowdry and Gardner (1988) tested four medications in 16 subjects with BPD using a cross-over design. Alprazolam was associated with increased symptomatology. Because of this study some experts have warned against treating BPD patients with benzodiazepines, yet surveys show that these medications are still widely prescribed (Knappich, Horz-Sagstetter, Schwerthoffer, Leucht, & Rentrop, 2014).

Summary of Findings from Psychopharmacological Trials

Despite nearly 40 years of clinical trial experience, researchers have yet to identify a pharmacologic treatment of choice for BPD. The pace of drug trials has appeared to slow, yet surveys show that medications are widely prescribed to BPD patients. Of the many classes of medications used in individuals with BPD, atypical antipsychotics have been the most extensively studied, and each of the agents has supportive data including aripiprazole, risperidone, quetiapine, and olanzapine. Yet, there remain concerns with small sample sizes, high attrition rates, variable outcome measures, and sample heterogeneity. In view of these concerns, the NICE (2009) guidelines concluded:

- There is evidence that psychotropic medication treats depression, anxiety, hostility, and impulsivity.
- There is no evidence that medications alter the fundamental nature of BPD.
- There is concern for the potential of substantial weight gain and/or the development of *tardive dyskinesia.*
- Finally, psychotropic medication should be directed at the co-morbid disorder.

A Cochrane review (Lieb, Vollm, Rucker, Timmer, & Stoffers, 2010) concluded that research findings tended to suggest benefit from second-generation antipsychotics, mood stabilizers, and omega-3 fatty acid, but cautioned that most effect estimates were based on single studies. In summary, they found that current findings are not sufficiently robust to make clear recommendations.

A meta-analysis that included data from RCTs and open-label studies led to more positive conclusions. Vita, De Peri, and Sacchetti (2011) report that evidence suggests that mood stabilizers and antipsychotics may be effective in treating affective dysregulation and impulsive behavior; that antipsychotics are effective in reducing cognitive-perceptual symptoms; that antidepressants are effective in treating affective dysregulation, but no other symptoms; and that placebo arms in RCTs showed significant improvement in symptoms as well. Finally, there were no differences in dropout rates between subjects on medication and those on placebo.

Psychosocial Treatments of BPD

In an early report, Stern (1938) described a group of "borderline" patients for whom standard forms of treatment were unsuccessful. While psychoanalysis was standard at the time, today's BPD patients require an approach different because they often do not respond to many forms of psychotherapy that are effective for other disorders, and they may require more specific interventions (NICE, 2009; Stoffers et al., 2012).

Psychodynamic Therapies

Psychoanalysts have long been interested in treating BPD. Past studies showed that when BPD patients were offered open-ended psychodynamic therapy, most dropped out within a few months (Skodol, Buckley, & Charles, 1983). Thus, therapists with this orientation adapted their methods, most particularly by increasing their activity (Gunderson & Links, 2012).

Cognitive-Behavioral Therapies

Dialectical behavior therapy (DBT) is mindfulness and acceptance-based behavior treatment that derives from cognitive-behavioral therapy (CBT) (Linehan, 1993). The 1-year long program is considered comprehensive because it combines weekly group therapy with weekly individual therapy that is conducted by a DBT-trained therapist. Designed to target emotional dysregulation, DBT also addresses impulsive behaviors and targets disturbed relationships. Behavioral analysis is used to help patients understand and change the chain of internal and external events that lead to self-injury and overdoses. DBT emphasizes empathic responses to distress that help validate the individual's inner experiences.

DBT was the subject of the first RCT that targeted BPD patients (Linehan, Armstrong, Suarez, Allmon, & Heard, 1991). DBT was compared to "treatment as usual" (TAU), defined as what an individual receives in the community, such as medication, psychotherapy, and case management. After a year of treatment, the sample receiving DBT was less likely to engage in self-harm, and spent less time in the hospital. The gap narrowed at 1-year follow up, but patients receiving DBT continued to show better functioning than the others (Linehan, Heard, & Armstrong, 1993). DBT is also effective in BPD patients with co-morbid substance abuse (Harned et al., 2008; Linehan et al., 1999, 2002; Verhuel et al., 2003).

In the first RCT (Linehan et al., 1991), 83% of patients treated with DBT stayed in therapy for the full year, a remarkable finding in a patient population known for high dropout rates. In a meta-analysis of 14 studies of DBT of 12 months or more, Barnicot, Katsakou, Marougka, and Priebe (2011) showed a mean retention rate of 70%, although findings varied greatly among studies. A second RCT (Linehan et al., 2006) showed DBT to be superior to treatment by community experts, although this time the advantage of DBT was narrower. The significant outcomes that differentiated the groups were treatment retention, suicide attempts, hospitalization for suicide ideation, medical risk, psychiatric emergency department visits, and differences in psychiatric hospitalization, although there were no differences in the frequency of self-harm. A more recent study (Linehan et al., 2015) showed that the skills training component of DBT was an important ingredient of DBT outcomes. The Linehan studies noted that 70% of the subjects were on medication at the time of the clinical trials, and there was an initial decrease in medication use after completing DBT. Medication use among this group, however, increased in the year following DBT.

Of note, studies of DBT have used small samples, and results may have been affected by selection biases (Bohus et al., 2004). For example, not every BPD patient will enter a clinical trial. On the other hand, DBT has been shown to be effective in nonacademic public health settings, for example, in the US (American Psychiatric Association, 1998); UK (Feigenbaum et al., 2012; Priebe et al., 2012), Ireland (Blennerhassett, Bamford, Whelan, Jamieson, & O'Raghaileigh, 2009), New Zealand (Brassington & Krawitz, 2006), and Australia (Pasieczny & Connor, 2011). Unfortunately, we do not know the long-term outcome of DBT, and thus we do not know whether DBT-treated samples maintain their gains and continue to improve, or whether they relapse.

Linehan (1993) had suggested that a full course of DBT could take several years, so that only the first stage (in which suicide, other life-threatening behavior, and self-harm behaviors are targeted priorities) has been formally tested. DBT is resource-intensive, which has limited its dissemination. In the US, DBT is not widely available because of its expense. Where DBT is available, there are often long waiting lists. To improve access one needs to determine whether DBT can be shortened and/or streamlined without losing efficacy (Paris, 2013).

While DBT is the most widely known psychological treatment, the question is whether it has specific effects that are superior to other treatments. This issue was addressed in a comparison of DBT and "general psychiatric management" (GPM), which found equal effectiveness at the end of 1 year of treatment and a 2-year follow up (McMain, Guimond, Streiner, Cardish, & Links, 2012). This raises the question of whether the mechanisms of change are specific to this method.

Linehan developed DBT after concluding that individual CBT was ineffective for BPD. But one form of CBT has been subjected to a clinical trial. Davidson et al. (2006; Davidson, Tyrer, Norrie, Palmer, & Tyrer, 2010) found that manualized CBT plus TAU was superior to TAU after a mean of 27 sessions, suggesting that briefer therapies can be effective.

Systems Training for Emotional Predictability and Problem Solving

Systems Training for Emotional Predictability and Problem Solving (STEPPS) is the best example to date of a brief CBT intervention (Blum et al., 2008; Blum, Pfohl, St. John, Monahan, & Black, 2002). This adjunctive program provides 20 weekly sessions of psychoeducation and skills training in a group format, and is designed as an add-on to TAU. Its relatively low cost and brief format makes it accessible. The program has been supported by RCTs conducted in the US (Blum et al., 2008) and The Netherlands (Bos, van Wel, Appelo, & Verbraak, 2010, 2011), including one in a "real-world" setting (Bos et al., 2011). The program has been shown to reduce BPD-related symptoms, depression, negative affectivity, impulsiveness, and emergency room visits. The program has become widespread in the UK and The Netherlands (Black & Blum, 2017), and it is the only program apart from DBT that has been used in correctional settings (Black, Blum, McCormick, & Allen, 2013). Due to its short length and low cost, STEPPS may have a special role in treating offenders who are often discharged from prison abruptly or transferred to other facilities. In naturalistic studies, it has been shown to boost mood and reduce borderline symptoms in offenders, and to also reduce disciplinary infractions and administrative segregation days.

Mentalization-Based Therapy

Mentalization-based therapy (MBT) is an 18-month comprehensive program that is based on the theory that BPD patients should learn to "mentalize," that is, explore their minds by experiencing and observing emotions and thoughts in self and others (Bateman & Fonagy, 2004). The first RCT was carried out in a partial hospitalization program (Bateman & Fonagy, 1999, 2001), and the second in an outpatient setting (Bateman & Fonagy, 2009). The first study found MBT to be statistically significantly superior to TAU, and the second study showed it superior to structured clinical management (SCM), although differences in the latter study were limited to those with the most severe presentations and symptoms (Bateman & Fonagy, 2013). The partial hospital sample had an improvement in symptoms that remained stable after 8 years (Bateman & Fonagy, 2008), a rare example of long-term follow up of an RCT. A replication in another center found MBT and "supportive psychotherapy" to be equally effective (Jørgensen et al., 2013). Finally, one should consider whether the elements of MBT can be applied in other ways. As MBT is a resource-intensive treatment, can dismantling research explore whether MBT or any of its elements can be used in less resource-intensive ways?

Transference-Focused Psychotherapy

Transference-focused psychotherapy (TFP) aims to correct distortions in the patient's perception of significant others by pointing out how they effect a transference relationship with the therapist (Yeomans, Clarkin, & Kernberg, 2015). TFP is strongly psychodynamic, but does not put as much emphasis on the past as does classical psychoanalysis. In a comparative trial of TFP and DBT, the outcome was similar (Clarkin, Levy, Lenzenweger, & Kernberg, 2007). There is also one trial showing superiority to therapy by community psychotherapists (Doering et al., 2010).

Conversational Model

The conversational model uses the therapy relationship, mediated through conversation to promote cohesion of the "self" and has been shown in an RCT to be equally effective to DBT on suicide and self-harm, although DBT outperformed on depression (Walton, Bendit, Carter, Baker, & Lewin, 2016).

Schema-Focused Therapy

Schema focused therapy (SFT) is a cognitive and psychodynamic therapy hybrid that focuses on maladaptive schema derived from adverse experiences in childhood (Young, 1999). Thus far, it has been supported by a comparative trial with TFP (Giesen-Bloo & Arntz, 2007; Giesen-Bloo et al., 2006). One problem with SFT related to treatment access is that it is resource-intensive and is designed to last as long as 3 years.

Cognitive Analytical Therapy

Cognitive analytical therapy combines concepts from cognitive and psychodynamic therapy creating a narrative of collaborative causal understanding and a transforming narrative. It has been shown to be effective in adolescents with BPD traits (Chanen et al., 2008).

Generalist Treatments and Supportive Care

Good psychiatric management (GPM) (formerly referred to as "general psychiatric management") integrates supportive psychodynamically informed therapy with a pharmacological algorithm. McMain and colleagues (2009, 2012) demonstrated GPM to be equally effective to DBT. Gunderson and Links have adapted the model (2014), which has yet to have published research data. Good clinical care is an individual therapy that is informed by clinical "common sense" and some principles of CBT that have been shown to be equally effective to cognitive analytical therapy (Chanen et al., 2008). Structured clinical management is a manualized treatment based on competencies that many generalist mental health clinicians already have, thus requiring only a small amount of training and no additional specialist supervision, and it has been shown to be nearly as effective as MBT, with MBT outperforming only for those with the severest BPD conditions (Bateman & Fonagy, 2013). Supportive psychotherapy (Rockland, 1992) provides empathic listening and validation of emotions, and was found in one study to be equally effective to DBT and TFP (Clarkin et al., 2007), and in another study equally effective to MBT (Jørgensen et al., 2013)

Summary of Published Data on Psychological Treatment of BPD

At least 26 published RCTs compare the effectiveness of BPD treatments that comprise 12 different treatment models, with DBT having the most published studies (16) followed by several treatments with one to three published studies. This in no way indicates that DBT is therefore a superior treatment *per se*; rather, the sheer weight of DBT publications of efficiency/effectiveness mean that DBT is the BPD treatment model most named by major relevant professional organizations.

Table 7.1 provides a synopsis of research-indicated effectiveness of various treatment strategies used in the treatment of BPD.

Table 7.2 presents a comparison of duration of RCTs among lengthy treatment approaches.

Table 7.1 Treatment efficacy/effectiveness research—randomized controlled trials.

Treatment model	Interpretation of data	Comment
Cognitive-behavioral therapies		
DBT		
Linehan et al. (1991)	DBT > TAU	First RCT of efficacy for BPD. Therapists rated for DBT adherence
Linehan et al. (1999)	DBT > TAU	First DBT replication. Therapists rated for DBT adherence
Koons et al. (2001)	DBT > TAU	First replication outside Linehan research group. Therapists rated for DBT adherence
Linehan et al. (2002)	DBT > 12 step program + comprehensive validation for people with BPD + substance use	Small numbers; retention rate lower in DBT arm (67% vs. 100%). Therapists rated for DBT adherence
Verhuel et al. (2003)	DBT > TAU	First replication in Europe; DBT therapists *not* rated for adherence
Linehan et al. (2006)	DBT > TBE	DBT > TBE on self-introject, a rating used to measure "deep" structural change (Bedics et al., 2012). DBT therapists rated for DBT adherence
Clarkin et al. (2007)	DBT = TFP = SP	Supportive psychotherapy based on experience and knowledge of psychoanalytical treatments. DBT therapists *not* rated for adherence
McMain et al. (2009, 2012)	DBT = GPM	67% of GPM clinicians were psychiatrists. DBT therapists rated for DBT adherence
Carter et al. (2010)	DBT > TAU but not for self-harm and hospital days	DBT therapists not intensively trained. DBT therapists *not* rated for DBT adherence

(Continued)

Table 7.1 (Continued)

Treatment model	Interpretation of data	Comment
Pasieczny & Connor (2011)	DBT > TAU while on DBT waitlist (*nonrandomized* controlled trial)	Routine Australian public mental health service. DBT therapists rated for DBT adherence using local adherence scale. DBT therapists with more intensive training achieved better client outcomes. Six-month study and clients who received more treatment after 6 months did better
Priebe et al. (2012); Barnicot, Savill, Bhatti, and Priebe(2014)	DBT > TAU	"Real-world" UK public mental health service. Therapists rated for DBT adherence using local adherence rather than Linehan adherence ratings
Feigenbaum et al. (2012)	DBT slightly > TAU (appears to be high quality TAU)	"Real-world" UK public mental health service. DBT therapists *not* rated for DBT adherence
Pistorello, Fruzzetti, Maclane, Gallop, & Iverson (2012)	DBT > optimized psychodynamic psychotherapy	Study population had three or more BPD traits + suicidal. DBT therapists rated as close to but not quite adherent
Mehlum et al. (2014)	DBT-A > EUC	First DBT for adolescents RCT; DBT therapists rated for adherence
Linehan et al. (2015)	Full DBT > DBT skills + case management > individual DBT + activities group	DBT therapists rated for adherence
Walton et al. (2016)	DBT = conversational model; DBT outperformed on depression	"Real-world" public mental health service. DBT therapists rated for adherence
STEPPS		
Blum et al. (2008)	STEPPS > TAU	20 weeks
Bos et al. (2010)	STEPPS > TAU	20 weeks
Bos et al. (2011)	STEPPS > TAU	20 weeks. "Real-world" sample
CBT		
Davidson et al. (2006, 2010)	CBT + TAU > TAU	"Real-world" sample
Psychodynamic therapies		
MBT		
Bateman & Fonagy (1999, 2001, 2008)	MBT > TAU	MBT was day treatment
Bateman & Fonagy (2009); Bateman & Fonagy (2013)	MBT > SCM when severest included, MBT = SCM when severest excluded	MBT was outpatient treatment
Jørgensen et al. (2013)	MBT = SP (Denmark)	MBT was outpatient treatment; MBT substantially more intensive (4-fold dose)
TFP		
Clarkin et al. (2007)	TFP = DBT = SP (see above)	Supportive psychotherapy based on experience and knowledge of psychoanalytical treatments. DBT therapists *not* rated for adherence

Table 7.1 (Continued)

Treatment model	Interpretation of data	Comment
Doering et al. (2010)	TFP > community psychotherapists	Self-harming did not change in either group
Giesen-Bloo et al. (2006)	SFT > TFP which was also effective	Doubts raised (Yeomans, 2007) and refuted (Giesen-Bloo, 2007) about TFP adherence
Conversational model		
Walton et al. (2016)	Conversational model = DBT, although DBT outperformed on depression	"Real-world" public mental health service. DBT therapists rated for adherence
Cognitive/psychodynamic therapies		
SFT		
Giesen-Bloo et al. (2006)	SFT > TFP	Doubts raised (Yeomans, 2007) and refuted (Giesen-Bloo, 2007) about TFP adherence
Cognitive analytical therapy		
Chanen et al. (2008)	CAT = GCC	Adolescents with at least two BPD criteria. 24 sessions
Generalist treatments		
GPM		
McMain et al. (2009, 2012)	GPM = DBT	67% of GPM clinicians were psychiatrists
SCM		
Bateman & Fonagy (2009, 2013)	SCM = MBT when data excluded for most severe	SCM provided by generalist mental health clinician
GCC		
Chanen et al. (2008)	GCC = CAT	Adolescents with at least two BPD criteria. 24 sessions
SP		
Clarkin et al. (2007)	SP (USA) = DBT = TFP	SP based on experience and knowledge of psychoanalytical treatments
Jørgensen et al. (2013)	SP (Denmark) = MBT	SP delivered by experienced psychodynamic clinicians
High quality TAU		
Feigenbaum et al. (2012)	TAU (appears to be high quality) nearly = DBT (see above)	"Real-world" UK public mental health service. DBT therapists *not* rated for DBT adherence

DBT, dialectical behavior therapy; EUC, enhanced usual care; CAT, cognitive analytical therapy; GCC, good clinical care; GPM, good psychiatric management; MBT, mentalization-based therapy; OPT, other specialized psychotherapeutic treatments; SCM, structured clinical management; SFT, schema-focused therapy; SP, supportive psychotherapy; STEPPS, systems training for emotional predictability and problem solving; TBE, treatment by experts; TFP, transference-focused psychotherapy.

Table 7.2 Treatment efficacy/effectiveness research (RCT): Treatment duration.

Author	Treatment duration
Behavioral	
DBT	
Linehan et al. (1991)	12 months
Linehan et al. (1999)	12 months and 4-month follow up
Koons et al. (2001)	6 months
Linehan et al. (2002)	12 months and 4-month follow up
Van den Bosch et al. (2005); Verhuel et al. (2003)	12 months and 6-month follow up
Linehan et al. (2006)	12 months and 12-month follow up
Clarkin et al. (2007)	12 months
McMain et al. (2009, 2012)	12 months and 24-month follow up
Carter et al. (2010)	6 months
Pasieczny & Connor (2011)	6–12 months
Barnicot et al. (2014); Priebe et al. (2012)	12 months and 6-month follow up
Feigenbaum et al. (2012)	12 months
Pistorello et al. (2012)	7–12 months and 6–11-month follow up
Linehan et al. (2015)	12 months and 12-month follow up
Walton et al. (2016)	14 months
STEPPS	
Blum et al. (2008)	20 weeks and 12-month follow up
Bos et al. (2010)	20 weeks and 6-month follow up
Bos et al. (2011)	20 weeks and 6-month follow up
CBT	
Davidson et al. (2006, 2010)	12 months
Psychodynamic treatments	
MBT	
Bateman & Fonagy (1999, 2001, 2008)	18 months and 5-year follow-up
Bateman & Fonagy (2009)	18 months
Jørgensen et al. (2013)	24 months
TFP	
Clarkin et al. (2007)	12 months
Doering et al. (2010)	12 months
Giesen-Bloo et al. (2006)	36 months
Conversational model	
Walton et al. (2016)	14 months

Table 7.2 (Continued)

Author	Treatment duration
Cognitive/psychodynamic therapies	
SFP	
Giesen-Bloo et al. (2006).	12 months
CAT	
Chanen et al. (2008)	24 sessions and 24-month follow up
Generalist treatments	
GPM	
McMain et al. (2009)	12 months and 24-month follow up
SCM	
Bateman & Fonagy (2009)	18 months
SP	
Clarkin et al. (2007)	12 months
Jørgensen et al. (2013)	24 months
GCC	
Chanen et al. (2008)	24 sessions and 24-month follow up
High quality TAU	
Feigenbaum et al. (2012)	12 months

DBT, dialectical behavior therapy; CAT, cognitive analytical therapy; CBT, cognitive behavioral therapy; GCC, good clinical care; GPM, good psychiatric management; MBT, mentalization-based therapy; SCM, structured clinical management; SFP, schema focused therapy; SP, supportive psychotherapy; STEPPS, systems training for emotional predictability and problem solving; TFP, transference-focused psychotherapy; TAU, treatment as usual.

Shorter Therapies for BPD

Now that there is clear evidence of the efficiency and effectiveness of BPD treatment, attention is turning to treatments that might be of shorter duration or more cost efficient, and such attention has turned to dismantling studies that might help in the dissemination of evidence-based treatments. Table 7.3 reports on six 20-week or less treatments. STEPPS, described earlier, is a 20-week adjunctive treatment with good evidence of efficacy and effectiveness (Blum et al., 2008; Bos et al., 2010, 2011). Soler et al. (2009) reported on the successful use of a 13-week adapted DBT skills group in an RCT. Soler et al. (2012), in a nonrandomized controlled trial, showed that the mindfulness module of DBT skills (DBT-M) delivered as 8 × 2 h group sessions, when used as an adjunct to GPM, improved attention and impulsivity compared to GPM alone. Elices et al. (2016) showed DBT mindfulness outperformed DBT interpersonal effectiveness with large effect sizes in a 2.5 h × 10 weeks group. Morton, Snowdon, Gopold, and

Guyner (2012) found a 12 × 2 h/week acceptance and commitment group therapy program plus TAU to outperform TAU in a public mental health service. Andreasson et al. (2016) demonstrated "collaborative assessment and management of suicidality" (CAMS) to be equally effective as a shortened adapted version of standard comprehensive DBT in a 16-week study. Another example of explorations to shorten treatments without losing efficacy, though not included in Table 7.3, is a study by Andion et al. (2012) reporting on a DBT adaptation designed to decrease the costs of treatment delivery by having the DBT individual therapist also deliver the DBT skills component.

Role of Acute Mental Health Unit Hospitalization

Because patients with BPD can be chronically suicidal, some approaches to therapy focus on this problem almost exclusively (Paris, 2006), resulting in what may be unnecessary hospitalization (Hull et al., 1998) when suicide prevention may, in many cases, be handled within ongoing outpatient therapy. The value of acute mental health hospital admission for this population has never been empirically demonstrated. While one in 10 patients with BPD will eventually complete suicide, mortality usually occurs late in the course of illness, when patients are out of treatment (Black, Blum, Pfohl, & Hale, 2004). Also, the peak of risk occurs not in young patients, but in those who fail to recover and are older than 30.

Hospitalization can sometimes produce negative effects associated with regression (Dawson & MacMillan, 1993). It is our opinion that acute mental health hospitalization in general needs to be only occasionally used, and then for a brief period (days) where risks of not hospitalizing the patient outweigh risks of hospitalizing for short-term

Table 7.3 Treatment efficacy/effectiveness research (RCT) on shorter treatments of 16 weeks or less duration.

Author	Comment
Andreasson et al. (2016)	CAMS = shortened adapted "DBT" in 16-week study
Blum et al. (2008); Bos et al. (2010, 2011)	STEPPS; 20 weeks
Elices et al. (2016)	DBT mindfulness skills > DBT interpersonal effectiveness skills (large effect sizes): 8 × 2.5 h
Morton et al. (2012)	ACT + TAU > TAU. 12 × 2 h addon to TAU. Public mental health service
Soler et al. (2009)	DBT group skills training > standard group therapy; 13 weeks × 2 h/week
Soler et al. (2012)	DBT-M of 8 × 2 h as add-on to GPM > GPM in nonrandomized controlled trial

ACT, acceptance and commitment therapy; CAMS collaborative assessment and management of suicidality; DBT, dialectical behavior therapy; DBT-M, dialectical behavior therapy-mindfulness; STEPPS, Systems training for emotional predictability and problem solving; TAU, treatment as usual.

antisuicide prevention, psychosis and, rarely, for providing a break for a hard-working community clinician. Unfortunately, the American Psychiatric Association guidelines for the treatment of borderline personality disorder (Oldham et al., 2001) recommended hospitalization for acute suicidal risk without elaboration of the complexities and possible disadvantages of such a broad statement.

When available, day treatment is an evidence-based alternative to full admission. MBT trials (Bales et al., 2012, 2015; Bateman & Fonagy, 1999) suggest that BPD patients can be managed effectively in this way. Most of the published evidence-based studies of BPD have taken place in the community or outpatient setting, where therapists and patients focus on learning in real-life contexts how to solve their problems (Krawitz & Jackson, 2008).

Integrating Medication and Psychotherapy

With many disorders, it is clear that certain types of patients respond better when medication and psychotherapy are combined (Black, 2006). For example, research shows that when major depression or obsessive-compulsive disorder are treated with a combination of medication and psychotherapy, outcomes are improved. Whether BPD patients similarly benefit from combined treatment has not been fully tested, yet there are clues that suggest that patients may benefit from the combination of treatments. The first investigation (Simpson et al., 2004) compared the combination of the antidepressant fluoxetine and DBT, but combined therapy was no better than DBT alone. Solar et al. (2005) subsequently conducted an RCT of olanzapine or placebo plus DBT in 50 subjects. There was statistical improvement in the DBT plus olanzapine cell, and also fewer dropouts. Linehan, McDavid, Brown, Sayres, and Gallup (2008) reported results of a similar study also showing the superiority of combined treatment, though not for anger dyscontrol.

Future Directions

The treatment of BPD has made significant strides as the number of psychotherapies has expanded, and researchers have explored the use of multiple medication classes. These advances were made possible by the development of diagnostic criteria (Gunderson & Singer, 1975) that paved the way to the application of structured interviews and objective measurement of patient symptoms that have helped harmonize subject assessment (Zanarini et al., 2010).

Where do we go from here? With psychotherapy, future research should begin to test models that integrate what is considered the best ideas from different programs, thereby drawing on some of the most fertile areas as we continue exploring better treatments (Paris, 2015). Meta-analyses of outcome research show that common factors generally account for twice as much change as specific techniques from different models (Lambert & Barley, 2002; Steering Committee, 2009; Wampold, 2001). Few differences have emerged in most of the few head-to-head studies of evidence-based BPD treatments that have been conducted. Livesley, Dimaggio, and Clarkin (2015) have described how the basic principles of all psychotherapy, as well as the best elements of the various programs, could be woven into a coherent whole. One example is the use of mindfulness in DBT and mentalizing in MBT, with both concepts having much in common. Linehan's concept of "radical acceptance," in which patients, as well as being encouraged to change that which can be changed, are also encouraged to move to a place of accepting that which cannot be changed, including their past experiences. This concept is well understood in the addiction treatment field and psychodynamic treatments, albeit using different language.

Researchers also must investigate the length of treatment programs. Currently, there has been no research comparing longer treatments (e.g., DBT) with briefer treatments (e.g., STEPPS). Clearly, longer treatments are more resource intensive, and are more prone to dropouts, thereby compromising program integrity and contributing to poorer outcomes. Next, we need more data regarding which patients can be successfully treated by generalists rather than specialist BPD clinicians, because the field would benefit from knowing which programs are best for treating which type of patient. Should patients receive a less intensive treatment such as GPM or STEPPS *before* referral to a comprehensive program such as DBT or schema-focused therapy? These are all questions worth researching, considering that the cost effectiveness of programs must be a priority at a time when resources are limited.

Additional research is needed to better determine the role of medication in treating BPD. Psychopharmacologists should continue to test different agents in an effort to identify effective medications that treat the entire BPD syndrome. The best candidates thus far are the atypical antipsychotics, but their many side effects will reduce their acceptability to many patients. Similar to dismantling research with the psychotherapies, it may be that different agents are best at treating specific symptom domains, and those associations need to be explored. If true, prescribing more than one medication could be helpful in selected patients, though this needs to be based on empirical data, not anecdote. Finally, the combination of medication and psychotherapy should be carefully studied. With some programs, such as STEPPS or GPM, the use of medication is compatible with the program, whereas some programs actively discourage the use of medication (e.g., DBT, MBT). Rather than placing prescribers and therapists at odds, perhaps both types of treatment providers may eventually conclude that these treatments are complementary and not antagonistic.

Conclusions

The historical treatment of patients with BPD reflects the paradigms that have shaped mental health treatments. When psychoanalysis was a central model, modified versions of analytic therapy were used for people with BPD. As cognitive therapy became popular, methods were developed to specifically target cognitions in people with BPD and, as third-wave mindfulness and acceptance-based behavioral therapies emerged, these targeted behaviors (including thoughts, emotions, and actions) in people with BPD were further identified. As psychiatric treatments have been increasingly dominated by pharmacological interventions, drugs from all classes have been used to treat BPD. At present, there is much stronger evidence for the effectiveness of psychotherapy in BPD than there is for medication. The main reasons psychological therapies are not more widely used, in our opinion, is the difficulty with getting information to funders and clinicians on the effectiveness of BPD psychotherapy treatments, including generalist psychotherapy treatments. It is our belief, based upon the evidence we have provided here, that a stepped-care model enables resources to be used more efficiently, providing generalist treatment for most patients, while reserving more expensive specialist programs for those with greatest severity.

In this chapter, we have outlined evidence of the treatability of BPD by psychopharmacological approaches, psychotherapy, and combined medication and psychotherapy. Fortunately, evidence-based BPD treatments are cost-effective (Brazier et al., 2006; Brettschneider, Riedel-Heller, & König, 2014). Thus far, five different generalist treatments have been found to be effective (GPM, SCM, GCC, supportive psychotherapy, and high quality TAU), and these treatments can be carried out as part of routine generalist mental health treatment, which would make effective evidence-based treatment available to all BPD clients attending mental health services, as is the case for other mental health conditions such as anxiety, depression, schizophrenia, and bipolar affective disorder.

Apart from the most severe and most at risk, BPD patients could generally be referred to a specialist BPD service *only* after having first received an evidence-based treatment carried out by generalist mental health clinicians. Bateman and Fonagy (2013) have shown that a generalist BPD treatment (SCM) had similar outcomes to the specialist BPD treatment (MBT), when those with greatest severity were excluded from the data analysis; whereas the specialist treatment outperformed for people with greatest severity (defined by having more Axis II conditions and greater subjective experience of distress). What this suggests to us is the value of a stepped care model, with generalist treatment provided to all, and with the more expensive specialist model saved for those with the severest conditions or when generalist treatment has been ineffective.

At present, the following conclusions are justified:

- BPD is a treatable condition.
- Many psychosocial treatments have been shown to be efficacious, but none has been shown superior to another. DBT has by far the largest number of published studies.
- Psychotropic medication is widely prescribed for BPD patients despite the absence of an FDA indication. Many agents show promise, with atypical antipsychotics having the largest body of supportive data.
- The treatment of BPD should receive funding and treatment commensurate with the high morbidity and mortality of the condition. Currently this is not happening on a widespread basis.
- Information is not reaching funders and clinicians about the availability of evidence-based BPD treatments and their cost-effectiveness. Stigma and discrimination surrounding BPD are largely based on misinformation (Black et al., 2011; Sheehan, Nieweglowski, & Corrigan, 2016).

We summarize our findings and recommendations in Table 7.4.

Table 7.4 Integrative biopsychosocial intervention with borderline personality disorder: Summary of best-practice recommendations by level of confidence derived from strength of evidence.

Borderline personality disorder		
Level A	Recommended	• Psychotherapy is first-line treatment of BPD. No given psychosocial approach, however, has proved more effective than other approaches. While DBT and MBT have proved effective interventions with BPD, STEPPS is a much shorter intervention with similar effectiveness • No medication is indicated for the treatment of BPD, *per se*, and benzodiazapines in particular should be avoided with this patient population
Level B	Suggested	• Antipsychotic medications, including aripiprazole, risperidone, quetiapine and olanzapine, have showed mixed results, and maybe helpful with the management of certain co-occurring symptoms such as anger • Acute hospitalization for suicide prevention is overused in this population, and might be replaced in many cases with intensive outpatient attention or hospital-based day treatment
Level C	May be considered	• Combined treatment of psychosocial therapy with antipsychotic medication may provide an advantage with some patients • Mood stabilizers, and omega-3 fatty acid may be considered on an individual basis • Referral to specialists might best be reserved for severe BPD or when generalists' initial interventions prove insufficient

References

Adityanjee, R. A., Brown, E., Thuras, P., Lee, S, & Schulz, S. C. (2008). Quetiapine in patients with borderline personality disorder: An open-label trial. *Annals of Clinical Psychiatry, 20*, 219–226.

American Psychiatric Association (1998). Gold award: Integrating dialectical behavior therapy into a community mental health program. *Psychiatric Services, 49*, 1138–1340.

American Psychiatric Association (1980). *Diagnostic and statistical manual of mental disorders* (3rd ed.). Washington, DC: American Psychiatric Press.

American Psychiatric Association (2013). *Diagnostic and statistical manual of mental disorders* (5th ed.). Arlington, VA: American Psychiatric Association.

Andion, A., Ferrer, M., Matali, J., Gancedo, B., Calvo, N., Barral, C., . . . & Casas, M. (2012). Effectiveness of combined individual and group dialectical behavior therapy compared to only individual dialectical behavior therapy: A preliminary study. *Psychotherapy, 49*, 241–250.

Andreasson, K., Krogh, J., Wenneberg, C., Jessen, H. K. L., Krakauer, K., Gluud, C., . . . & Nordentoft, M. (2016). Effectiveness of dialectical behavior therapy versus collaborative assessment and management of suicidality treatment for reduction of self-harm in adults with borderline personality disorder traits and disorder—a randomized observer-blinded clinical trial. *Depression and Anxiety, 33*, 520–530.

Bales, D., van Beek, N., Smits, M., Willemsen, S., Busschbach, J. J. V., Verhuel, R., & Andrea, H. (2012). Treatment outcome of 18-month, day hospital mentalization-based treatment (MBT) in patients with severe borderline personality disorder in the Netherlands. *Journal of Personality Disorders, 26*, 568–582.

Bales, D. L., Timman, R., Andrea, H., Busschbach, J. J. V., Verhuel, R., & Kamphuis, J. H. (2015). Effectiveness of day hospital Mentalization-based treatment for patients with severe borderline personality disorder: A matched control. *Clinical Psychology and Psychotherapy, 22*, 409–417.

Barnicot, K., Katsakou, C., Marougka, S., & Priebe, S. (2011). Treatment completion in psychotherapy for borderline personality disorder: A systematic review and meta-analysis. *Acta Psychiatrica Scandinavica, 123*, 327–338.

Barnicot, K., Savill, M., Bhatti, N., & Priebe, S. (2014). A pragmatic randomized controlled trial of dialectical behavior therapy: Effects on hospitalization and post-treatment follow-up. *Psychotherapy and Psychosomatics, 83*, 192–193.

Bateman, A., & Fonagy, P. (1999). Effectiveness of partial hospitalization in the treatment of borderline personality disorder: A randomized controlled trial. *American Journal of Psychiatry, 156*, 1563–156933.

Bateman, A., & Fonagy, P. (2001). Treatment of borderline personality disorder with psychoanalytically oriented partial hospitalization: An 18-month follow-up. *American Journal of Psychiatry, 158*, 36–42.

Bateman, A., & Fonagy, P. (2004). *Psychotherapy for borderline personality disorder: Mentalization based treatment*. Oxford: Oxford University Press.

Bateman, A., & Fonagy, P. (2008). 8-year follow-up of patients treated for borderline personality disorder: Mentalization-based treatment versus treatment as usual. *American Journal of Psychiatry, 165*, 631–638.

Bateman, A., & Fonagy, P. (2009). Randomized controlled trial of outpatient mentalization-based treatment versus structured clinical management for borderline personality disorder. *American Journal of Psychiatry, 166*, 1355–1364.

Bateman, A., & Fonagy, P. (2013). Impact of clinical severity on outcomes of mentalisation-based treatment for borderline personality disorder. *British Journal of Psychiatry, 203*, 221–227.

Bateman, A., & Krawitz, R. (2013). *Borderline personality disorder: An evidence-based guide for generalist mental health professionals*. New York: Springer.

Bedics, J., Atkins, D., Comtois, K., & Lineham, M. (2012). Treatment differences in the therapeutic relationship and introject during a 2-year randomized controlled trial of dialectical behavior therapy versus nonbehavioral psychotherapy experts for borderline personality disorder. *Journal of Consulting Psychology, 80*, 66–77.

Benedetti, F., Sforzini, L., Columbo, C., Maffei, C., & Smeraldi, C. (1998). Low-dose clozapine in acute and continuation treatment for severe borderline personality disorder. *Journal of Clinical Psychiatry, 59*, 103–107.

Black, D. W. (2006). Efficacy of combined pharmacotherapy and psychotherapy versus monotherapy in the treatment of anxiety disorders. *CNS Spectrums, 11*(Suppl 12), 29–33.

Black, D. W., Allen, J., McCormick, B., & Blum, N. (2011). Treatment received by persons with BPD participating in a randomized clinical trial of the Systems Training for Emotional Predictability and Problem Solving programme. *Personality and Mental Health, 5*, 159–168.

Black, D. W., & Blum, N. (Eds.) (2017). *Systems training for emotional predictability and problem solving: The STEPPS treatment model for persons with borderline personality disorder*. New York: Oxford University Press.

Black, D. W., Blum, N., McCormick, B., & Allen, J. (2013). STEPPS group treatment program for borderline offenders. *Journal of Nervous and Mental Disease, 201*, 124–129.

Black, D. W., Blum, N., Pfohl, B., & Hale, N. (2004). Suicidal behavior in borderline personality disorder: Prevalence, risk factors, prediction and prevention. *Journal of Personality Disorders, 18*, 226–239.

Black, D. W., Pfohl, B., Blum, N., McCormick, B., Allen, J., North, C. S., . . . & Zimmerman, M. (2011). Attitudes toward borderline personality disorder: A survey of 706 mental health clinicians. *CNS Spectrums, 16*, 67–74.

Black, D. W., Zanarini, M. C., Romine, A., Shaw, M., Allen, J., & Schulz, S. C. (2014). Comparison of low and moderate dosages of extended-release quetiapine in borderline personality disorder: A randomized, double-blind, placebo-controlled trial. *American Journal of Psychiatry, 171*, 1174–1182.

Blennerhassett, R., Bamford, L., Whelan, A., Jamieson, S., & O'Raghaileigh, J. W. (2009). Dialectical behaviour therapy in an Irish community mental health setting. *Irish Journal of Psychological Medicine, 26*, 59–63.

Blum, N., Pfohl, B., St. John, D., Monahan, P., & Black, D. W. (2002). STEPPS: A cognitive-behavioral systems-based group treatment for outpatients with borderline personality disorder—a preliminary report. *Comprehensive Psychiatry, 43*, 301–310

Blum, N., St. John, D., Pfohl, B., Stuart, S., McCormick, B., Allen, J., . . . & Black, D. W. (2008). Systems training for emotional predictability and problem solving (STEPPS) for outpatients with borderline personality disorder: A randomized controlled trial and 1-year follow-up. *American Journal of Psychiatry, 165*, 468–478.

Bogenschutz, M. P., & George, N. H.(2004). Olanzapine versus placebo in the treatment of borderline personality disorder. *Journal of Clinical Psychiatry, 65*, 104–109.

Bohus, M., Haaf, B., Simms, T., Limberger, M. F., Schmahl, C,. Unckel, C., . . . & Linehan, M. M. (2004). Effectiveness of inpatient dialectical behavioral therapy for borderline personality disorder: A controlled trial. *Behaviour Research and Therapy, 42*, 487–499.

Bos, E. H., van Wel, E. B., Appelo, M. T., & Verbraak, M. J. (2010). A randomized controlled trial of a Dutch version of systems training for emotional predictability and problem solving for borderline personality disorder. *Journal of Nervous and Mental Disease, 198*, 299–304.

Bos, E. H., van Wel, E. B., Appelo, M. T., & Verbraak, M. J. (2011). Effectiveness of training for emotional predictability and problem solving (STEPPS) for borderline personality disorder in a "real-world" sample: Moderation by diagnosis severity? *Psychotherapy and Psychosomatics, 80*, 173–181.

Brassington, J., & Krawitz, R. (2006). Australasian dialectical behaviour therapy pilot outcome study: Effectiveness, utility and feasibility. *Australasian Psychiatry, 14*, 313–319.

Brazier, J., Tumur, I., Holmes, M., Ferriter, M., Parry, G., Dent-Brown, K., & Paisley, S. (2006). Psychological therapies including dialectical behavior therapy for borderline personality disorder: A systematic review and preliminary economic evaluation. *Health Technology Assessment, 10*, 1–138.

Brettschneider, C., Riedel-Heller, S., & König, H.-H. (2014). A systematic review of economic evaluations of treatments for borderline personality disorder. *PLoS One, 9*, e107748.

Brinkley, J. R., Beitman, B. D., & Friedel, R. O. (1979). Low-dose neruoleptic regimens in the treatment of borderline patients. *Archives of General Psychiatry, 65*, 319–326.
Carter, G. L., Willcox, C. H., Lewin T. J., Conrad, A. M., & Bendit, N. (2010). Hunter DBT project: Randomly controlled trial of dialectical behavior therapy in women with borderline personality disorder. *Australian and New Zealand Journal of Psychiatry, 44*, 162–173.
Chanen, A. M., Jackson, H. J., McCutcheon, L. K., Jovev, M., Dudgeon, P., Yuen, H. P., . . . & McGorry, P. D. (2008). Early intervention for adolescents with borderline personality disorder using cognitive analytic therapy: A randomised controlled trial. *British Journal of Psychiatry, 193*, 477–484.
Clarkin, J. F., Levy, K. N., Lenzenweger, M. F., & Kernberg, O. F. (2007). Evaluating three treatments for borderline personality disorder: A multi-wave study. *American Journal of Psychiatry, 164*, 1–8.
Cornelius, J. R., Soloff, P., Perel, J. M., & Urich, R. F. (1991). A preliminary trial of fluoxetine in refractory borderline patients. *Journal of Clinical Psychopharmacology, 11*, 116–120.
Cowdry, R. W., & Gardner, D. L. (1988). Pharmacotherapy of borderline personality disorder. Alprazolam, carbamezepine, trifluoperazine, and tranylcypromine. *Archives of General Psychiatry, 45*, 111–9.
Davidson, K., Norrie, J., Tyrer, P., Gumley, A., Tata, P., Murray, H., & Palmer, S. (2006). The effectiveness of cognitive behavior therapy for borderline personality disorder: Results from the borderline personality disorder study of cognitive therapy (BOSCOT) trial. *Journal of Personality Disorders, 20*, 450–465.
Davidson, K. M., Tyrer, P., Norrie, J., Palmer, S. J., & Tyrer, P. (2010): Cognitive therapy v. usual treatment for borderline personality disorder: Prospective 6-year follow-up. *British Journal of Psychiatry, 197*, 456–462.
Dawson, D., & MacMillan, H. L. (1993). *Relationship management of the borderline patient: From understanding to treatment.* New York: Brunner/Mazel
Doering, D., Horz, S., Rentrop, M., Fischer-Kern, M., Schuster, P., Benecke, C., . . . & Buchheim, P. (2010). Transference-focused psychotherapy v. treatment by community psychotherapists for borderline personality disorder: Randomized controlled trial. *British Journal of Psychiatry, 196*, 389–395.
Elices, M., Pascaul, J. C., Portella, M. J., Feliu-Soler, A., Martin-Blanco, A., Carmona, C., & Soler, J. (2016). Impact of mindfulness training on borderline personality disorder: A randomized trial. *Mindfulness, 7*, 584–595.
Feigenbaum, J. D., Fonagy, P., Pilling, S., Jones, A., Wildgoose, A., & Bebbington, P. E. (2012). A real-world study of the effectiveness of DBT in the UK National Health Service. *British Journal of Clinical Psychology, 51*, 121–141.
Forman, E. M., Berk M. S., Henriques, G. R., Brown, G. K., & Beck, A. T. (2004). History of multiple suicide attempts as a behavioral marker of severe psychopathology. *American Journal of Psychiatry, 161*, 437–443.
Frankenburg, F. R., & Zanarini, M. C. (1993). Clozapine treatment of borderline patients: A preliminary study. *Comprehensive Psychiatry, 34*, 402–405.
Frankenburg, F. R., & Zanarini, M. C. (2002). Divalproex sodium treatment of women with borderline personality disorder and bipolar II disorder: A double-blind placebo-controlled pilot study. *Journal of Clinical Psychiatry, 63*, 442–446.
Giesen-Bloo, J., & Arntz, A. (2007). Questions concerning the randomized trial of schema-focused therapy vs transference-focused psychotherapy: In reply. *Archives of General Psychiatry, 64*, 610–611.

Giesen-Bloo, J., van Dyck, R., Spinhoven, P., van Tilburg, W., Dirksen, C., van Asselt, T., . . . & Arntz A. (2006). Outpatient psychotherapy for borderline personality disorder: Randomized trial of schema-focused therapy vs transference-focused psychotherapy. *Archives of General Psychiatry, 63*, 649–658.

Goldberg, S. C. (1989). Prediction of change in borderline personality disorder. *Psychopharmacology Bulletin, 25*, 550–555.

Goldberg, S. C., Schulz, S. C., Schulz, P. M., Resnick, R. J., Hamer, R. M., & Friedel, R. O. (1986). Borderline schizotypal personality disorders treated with low-dose thiothixene vs. placebo. *Archives of General Psychiatry, 43*, 680–686.

Gunderson, J. G., & Links, P. R. (2012). *Borderline personality disorder: A clinical guide* (2nd ed.).Washington, DC: American Psychiatric Publishing.

Gunderson, J. G, & Links, P. R. (2014). *Handbook of good psychiatric management for borderline personality disorder*. Washington DC: American Psychiatric Publishing.

Gunderson, J. G., & Singer, M. T. (1975). Defining borderline patients: An overview. *American Journal of Psychiatry, 132*, 1–10.

Harned, M. S., Chapman, A. L., Dexter-Mazza, E. T., Murray, A., Comtois, K. A., & Linehan, M. M. (2008). Treating co-occurring Axis I disorders in recurrently suicidal women with borderline personality disorder: A 2-year randomized trial of dialectical behavior therapy versus community treatment by experts. *Journal of Consulting and Clinical Psychology, 76*, 1068–1075.

Hollander, E., Tracy, K. A., Swann, A. C., Coccaro, E. F., McElroy, S. L., Woznaik, P., . . . & Nemeroff, C.B. (2003). Divalproex in the treatment of impulsive aggression: Efficacy in cluster B personality disorders. *Neuropsychopharmacology, 28*, 1186–1197.

Hollander, E., Swann, A. C., Coccaro, E. F., Jiang, P., & Smith, T. B. (2005). Impact of trait impulsivity and state aggression on divalproex versus placebo response in borderline personality disorder. *American Journal of Psychiatry, 162*, 621–624.

Hull, J. W., Yeomans, F., Clarkin, J., Li, C., & Goodman, G. (1996). Factors associated with multiple hospitalizations of patients with borderline personality disorder. *Psychiatric Services, 47*, 638–641.

Jørgensen, C. R., Freund, C., Boye, R., Jordet, H., Andersen, D., & Kjolbye, D. (2013). Outcome of mentalization-based and supportive psychotherapy in patients with borderline personality disorder: A randomized trial. *Acta Psychiatrica Scandinavica, 127*, 305–317.

Klein, D. F. (1968). Psychiatric diagnosis and typology of clinical drug effects. *Psychopharmacology, 13*, 359–386.

Knappich, M., Horz-Sagstetter, S., Schwerthoffer, D., Leucht, S., & Rentrop, M. (2014). Pharmacotherapy in the treatment of patients with borderline personality disorder: Results of a survey among psychiatrists in private practices. *International Clinical Psychopharmacology, 29*, 224–228.

Kolb, J. E., & Gunderson, J. G. (1980). Diagnosing borderline patients with a semistructured interview. *Archives of General Psychiatry, 37*, 37–41.

Koons, C. R., Robins, C. J., Bishop, G. K., Morse, J. Q., Tweed, J. L., Lynch, T. R., . . . & Bastian, L. A. (2001). Efficacy of dialectical behavior therapy with borderline women veterans: A randomized controlled trial. *Behavior Therapy, 32*, 371–390.

Krawitz, R., & Jackson, W. (2008). *Borderline personality disorder: The facts*. New York: Oxford University Press.

Lambert, M. J., & Barley, D. E. (2002). Research summary on the therapeutic relationship and psychotherapy. In J. C. Norcross (Ed.), *Psychotherapy relationships that work* (pp. 17–32). Oxford: Oxford University Press.

Lee, S. S., Allen, J., Black, D. W., Zanarini, M. C., & Schulz, S. C. (2016). Quetiapine's effect on the SCL-90-R domains in patients with borderline personality disorder. *Annals of Clinical Psychiatry, 28,* 4–10.

Lieb, K., Vollm, B., Rucker, G., Timmer, A., & Stoffers, J. M. (2010). Pharmacotherapy for borderline personality disorder: Cochrane systematic review of randomised trials. *British Journal of Psychiatry, 196,* 4–12.

Lieberich, P., Nickel, M. K., Tritt, K., & Pedrosa, G. F. (2008). Lamotrigine treatment of aggression in female borderline patients. *Journal of Psychopharmacology, 19,* 805–808.

Linehan, M. M. (1993). *Dialectical behavioral therapy of borderline personality disorder.* New York: Guilford.

Linehan, M. M., Armstrong, H. E., Suarez, A., Allmon, D., & Heard, H. (1991). Cognitive behavioral treatment of chronically parasuicidal borderline patients. *Archives of General Psychiatry, 48,* 1060–1064.

Linehan, M. M., Comtois, K. A., Murray, A. M., Brown, M. Z., Gallop, R. J., & Heard, H. L. (2006). Two-year randomized controlled trial and follow-up of dialectical behavior therapy vs therapy by experts for suicidal behaviors and borderline personality disorder. *Archives of General Psychiatry, 63,* 757–766.

Linehan, M. M., Dimeff, L., Reynolds, S. K., Comtois, K. A., Welch, S. S., Heagerty, P., & Kivlahan, D. R. (2002). Dialectical behavior therapy versus comprehensive validation therapy plus 12-step for the treatment of opioid dependent women meeting criteria for borderline personality disorder. *Drug and Alcohol Dependence, 67,* 13–26.

Linehan, M. M., Heard, H. L., & Armstrong, H. E. (1993). Naturalistic follow-up of a behavioral treatment of chronically parasuicidal borderline clients. *Archives of General Psychiatry, 50,* 1971–1974.

Linehan, M. M., Korslund, K. E., Harned, M. S., Gallop, R. J., Lungu, A., Neacsiu, A. D., . . . & Murray-Gregory, A. M. (2015). Dialectical behavior therapy for high suicide risk in individuals with borderline personality disorder: A randomized clinical trial and component analysis. *JAMA Psychiatry, 72,* 475–482.

Linehan, M. M., McDavid, J. D., Brown, M. Z., Sayres, J. H. R., & Gallup, R. J. (2008). Olanzapine plus dialectical behavior therapy for women with high irratability who met criteria for borderline personality disorder. A double-blind, placebo-controlled pilor study. *Journal of Clinical Psychiatry, 69,* 999–1005.

Linehan, M. M., Schmidt, H. 3rd, Dimeff, L. A. Craft, J. C., Kanter, J., & Comtois, K. A. (1999). Dialectical behavior therapy for patients with borderline personality disorder and drug-dependence. *American Journal of Addictions, 8,* 279–292.

Livesley, W. J., Dimaggio, G., & Clarkin, J. F. (2015). *Integrated treatment for personality disorder: A modular approach.* New York: Guilford Press.

Markovitz, P. J., Calabrese, J. R., Schulz, S. C., & Meltzer, H. Y. (1991). Fluoxetine in the treatment of borderline and schizotypal personality disorders. *American Journal of Psychiatry, 148,* 1064–1067.

McMain, S. F., Guimond, T., Streiner, D. L., Cardish, R. J., & Links, P. S. (2012). Dialectical behavior therapy compared with general psychiatric management for borderline

personality disorder: Clinical outcomes and functioning over a 2-year follow-up. *American Journal of Psychiatry, 69*, 650–661.
McMain, S. F., Links, P., Gnam, W. H., Guimond, T., Cardish, R. J., Korman, L. & Streiner, D. L. (2009). A randomized trial of dialectical behavior therapy versus general psychiatric management for borderline personality disorder. *American Journal of Psychiatry, 166*, 1365–1374
Mehlum, L., Tørmoen, A. J., Ramberg, M., Haga, E., Diep, L. M., Laberg, S., . . . & Grøholt, B. (2014). Dialectical behavior therapy for adolescents with repeated suicidal and self-harming behavior: A randomized controlled trial. *Journal of the American Academy of Child and Adolescent Psychiatry, 53*, 1082–1091.
Morton, J., Snowdon, S., Gopold, M., & Guyner, E. (2012). Acceptance and commitment therapy group treatment for symptoms of borderline personality disorder: A public sector pilot study. *Cognitive and Behavioral Practice, 19*, 527–544.
National Institute for Health and Care Excellence (2009). Borderline personality disorder: Recognition and management. *NICE guidelines.* Retrieved from https://www.nice.org.uk/guidance/CG78/
Nickel, M. K., Loew, T. H., & Pedrosa, G. F. (2007). Aripiprazole in treatment of borderline patients, part II: An 18-month follow-up. *Psychopharmacology, 191*, 1023–1026.
Nickel, M. K., Muehlbacher, M., Nickel, C., Kettler, C., Pedrosa, G. F., Bachler, E., . . . & Kaplan, P. (2006). Aripiprazole in the treatment of patients with borderline personality disorder: A double-blind, placebo-controlled study. *American Journal of Psychiatry, 163*, 833–8.
Nickel, M. K., Nickel, C., Kaplan, P., Lahmann, C., Muhlbacher, M., Tritt, K., . . . & Lowe, T. (2005). Treatment of aggression with topiramate in male borderline patients: A double-blind, placebo-controlled study. *Biological Psychiatry, 57*, 495–499.
Nickel, M. K., Nickel, C., Mitterlehner, F. O., Tritt, K., Lahmann, C., Leiberich, P., . . . & Lowe, T. (2004). Topiramate treatment of aggression in female borderline personality disorder patients: A double-blind, placebo-controlled study. *Journal of Clinical Psychiatry, 65*, 1515–1519.
Oldham, J. M., Gabbard, G. O., Goin, M. K., Gunderson, J., Soloff, P., Spiegel, D., . . . & Phillips, K.A. (2001). Practice guideline for the treatment of borderline personality disorder. *American Journal of Psychiatry, 158*, S1–S52.
Palomares, N., Montes, A., Diaz-Marsa, M., & Carrasco, J. (2015). Effectiveness of long-acting paliperidone palmitate in borderline personality disorder. *International Clinics of Psychopharmacology, 30*, 338–341.
Paris, J. (2003). *Personality disorders over time.* Washington DC: American Psychiatric Publishing.
Paris, J. (2006). *Half in love with death.* Mahwah, NJ: Lawrence Erlbaum.
Paris, J. (2012). The outcome of borderline personality disorder: Good for most but not for all patients. *American Journal of Psychiatry, 169*, 445–446.
Paris, J. (2013). Stepped care for patients with borderline personality disorder. *Psychiatric Services, 64*, 1035–1037.
Paris, J. (2015). Applying the principles of psychotherapy integration to the treatment of borderline personality disorder. *Journal of Psychotherapy Integration, 25*, 13–19.
Pasieczny, N., & Connor, J. (2011). The effectiveness of dialectical behavior therapy in routine public mental health settings: An Australian controlled trial. *Behavior Research and Therapy, 49*, 4–10.

Perella, C., Carrus, D., Costa, E., & Schifano, F. (2007). Quetiapine for the treatment of borderline personality disorder: An open-label study. *Progress in Neuro-Psychopharmacology and Biological Psychiatry, 31*, 158–163.
Pinto, O. C., & Akiskal H. S. (1998). Lamotrigine as a promising approach to borderline personality: An open case series without concurrent DSM-IV major mood disorder. *Journal of Affective Disorders, 51*, 333–343.
Pistorello, J., Fruzzetti, A. E., Maclane, C., Gallop, R., & Iverson, K. M. (2012). Dialectical behavior therapy (DBT) applied to college students: A randomized clinical trial. *Journal of Consulting and Clinical Psychology, 80*, 982–994.
Priebe, S., Bhatti, N., Barnicot, K., Bremner, S., Gaglia, A., Katsakou, C., . . . & Zinkler, M. (2012). Effectiveness and cost-effectiveness of dialectical behavior therapy for self-harming patients with personality disorder: A pragmatic randomized controlled trial. *Psychotherapy and Psychosomatics, 81*, 356–365.
Reich, D. B., Zanarini, M. C., & Bieri, K. A. (2009). A preliminary study of lamotrigine in the treatment of affective instability in borderline personality disorder. *International Clinical Psychopharmacology, 24*, 270–275.
Rifkin, A., Quitkin, F., Carrillo, C., Blumberg, A. G., & Klein, D. F. (1972). Lithium carbonate in emotionally unstable character disorder. *Archives of General Psychiatry, 27*, 519–23.
Rocca, P., Marchiaro, L., Cocuzza, E., & Bogetto, F. (2002). Treatment of borderline personality disorder with risperidonne. *Journal of Clinical Psychiatry, 63*, 241–244.
Rockland, L. H. (1992). *Supportive therapy for borderline patients*. New York: Guilford.
Salzman, C., Wolfson, A. N., Schatzberg, A., Looper, J., Henke, R., Albanese, M., . . . & Miyawaki, E. (1995). Effect of fluoxetine on anger in sypmptomatic volunteers with borderline personality disorder. *Journal of Clinical Psychopharmacology, 15*, 23–29.
Schulz, S. C., Camlin, K. L., Berry, S., & Friedman, L. (1998). Risperidone for borderline personality disorder: A double-blind study. *37th Annual Meeting of the American College of Neuropsychopharmacology*, San Juan, PR, December 14–18.
Schulz, S. C., Camlin, K. L., Berry, S. A., & Jesberger, J. A. (1999). Olanzapine safety and efficacy in patients with borderline personality disorder and comorbid dysthymia. *Biological Psychiatry, 46*, 1429–1435.
Schulz, S. C., Zanarini, M. C., Bateman, A., Bohus, M., Detke, H. C., Trzaskoma, Q., . . . & Corya, S. (2008). Olanzapine for the treatment of borderline personality disorder: Variable dose 12-week randomized double-blind placebo-controlled study. *British Journal of Psychiatry, 193*, 584–592.
Serban, G., & Segal, S. (1994). Response of borderline and schizotypal patients to small doses of thiothixene and haloperidol. *American Journal of Psychiatry, 141*, 1455–1458.
Sheehan, L., Nieweglowski, K., & Corrigan, P. (2016). The stigma of personality disorders. *Current Psychiatry Reports, 18*, 11–19.
Simpson, E. B., Yen, S., Costello, E., Rosen, K., Begin, A., Pistorello, J., & Pearlstein, T. (2004). Combined dialectical behavior therapy and fluoxetine in the treatment of borderline personality disorder. *Journal of Clinical Psychiatry, 65*, 379–385.
Skodol, A. E., Buckley, P., & Charles, E. (1983). Is there a characteristic pattern in the treatment history of clinic outpatients with borderline personality? *Journal of Nervous and Mental Disease, 171*, 405–410
Soler, J., Pascual, J. C., Campins, J., Barrachina, J., Puigdemont, D., Alvarez, E., & Pérez, V. (2005). Double-blind, placebo-controlled study of dialectical behavior therapy plus

olanzapine for borderline personality disorder. *American Journal of Psychiatry, 162*, 1221–1224.

Soler, J., Trujols, J., Pascaul, J. C., Tais, T., Cebria, A., Barrachina, J., . . . & Perez, V. (2009). Dialectical behavior therapy skills training compared to standard group therapy in borderline personality disorder. *Behaviour Research and Therapy, 47*, 353–358.

Soler, J., Valdeperez, A., Feliu-Soler, A., Pascaul, J. C., Portella, M. J., Martin-Blanco, A., . . . & Perez V. (2012). Effects of the dialectical behavior therapy-mindfulness module on attention in patients with borderline personality disorder. *Behaviour Research and Therapy, 50*, 150–157.

Soloff, P. H., Cornelius, J., George, A., Nathan, S., Perel, J. M., & Ulrich, R. F. (1993). Efficacy of phenelzine and haloperidol in borderline personality disorder. *Archives of General Psychiatry, 50*, 377–385.

Soloff, P. H., George, A., Nathan, R. S., Schulz, P. M., Ulrich, R. F., & Perel, J. M. (1986). Progress in pharmacotherapy of borderline disorders. A double-blind study of amitriptyline, haloperidol, and placebo. *Archives of General Psychiatry, 43*, 691–697.

Steering Committee (2002). Empirically supported therapy relationships: Conclusions and recommendations of the Division 29 Task Force. In J. C. Norcross (Ed.), *Psychotherapy relationships that work* (pp. 441–443). Oxford: Oxford University Press.

Stern, A. (1938). Psychoanalytic investigation of and therapy in the borderline group of neuroses. *Psychoanalytic Quarterly, 7*, 467–489.

Stoffers, J. M., Völlm, B. A., Rücker, G., Timmer, A., Huband, N., & Lieb, K. (2012). Psychological therapies for people with borderline personality disorder. *Cochrane Database of Systematic Reviews, 8*. Art. No.: CD005652. doi:10.1002/14651858.CD005652.pub2.

Substance Abuse and Mental Health Administration (2011). *Report to Congress on borderline personality disorder.* Retrieved from http://store.samhsa.gov/shin/content/SMA11-4644/SMA11-4644.pdf

Teicher, M. H., Glod, C. A., Aaronson, S. T., Gunter, P. A., Schatzberg, A. F., & Cole, J. O. (1989). Open assessment of the safety and efficacy of thioridazine in the treatment of patients with borderline personality disorder. *Psychopharmacol Bulletin, 25*, 535–549.

Torgersen, S. (2014). Prevalence, sociodemographics, and functional impairment. In J. M. Oldham, A. E. Skodal, & D. S. Bender (Eds.), *American Psychiatric Publishing textbook of personality disorders* (pp. 109–129). Washington DC: American Psychiatric Publishing.

Tritt, K., Nickel, C., Lahmann, C., Lieberich, P. K., Rother, W. K., Loew, T. H., & Nickel, M. K. (2005). Lamotrigine treatment of aggression in female borderline-patients: A randomized, double-blind, placebo-controlled study. *Journal of Psychopharmacology, 19*, 287–291.

Van den Bosch, L. M. C., Koeter, M. W. J., Stijnen, T., Verhuel, R., & van den Brink, W. (2005). Sustained efficacy of dialectical behaviour therapy for borderline personality disorder. *Behavior Research and Therapy, 43*, 1231–1241.

Verhuel, R., van den Bosch, L. M. C., Koeter, M. W. J., Ridder, M. A. J., Stijnen, T., & van den Brink, W. (2003). Dialectical behavior therapy for women with borderline personality disorder. *British Journal of Psychiatry, 182*, 135–140.

Vita, A., De Peri, L., & Sacchetti, E. (2011). Antipsychotics, antidepressants, anticonvulsants, and placebo on the symptom dimensions of borderline personality disorder: A meta-analysis of randomized controlled and open-label trials. *Journal of Clinical Psychopharmacology, 31*, 613–624.

Walton, C., Bendit, N., Baker, A., Carter, G., & Lewin, T. (2016). Dialectical behaviour therapy and the conversational model in the treatment of borderline personality disorder: A randomised clinical trial in a public sector mental health service. *Paper presented at the 8th World Congress of Behavior and Cognitive Therapies*, Melbourne, *Australia.*

Wampold, B. E. (2001). *The great psychotherapy debate: Models, methods, and findings.* Mahwah, NJ: Erlbaum Associates.

Yeomans, F. (2007). Questions concerning the randomized trial of schema-focused therapy vs transference-focused psychotherapy. *Archives of General Psychiatry, 64*, 609–610.

Yeomans, F. E., Clarkin, J. F., & Kernberg, O. F. (2015). *Transference-focused psychotherapy for borderline personality disorder: A clinical guide.* Washington, DC: American Psychiatric Publishing.

Young, J. E. (1999). *Cognitive therapy for personality disorders: A schema focused approach* (3rd ed.). Sarasota, FL: Professional Resource Press.

Zanarini, M. C., & Frankenburg, F. R. (2001). Olanzapine for the treatment of female borderline personality disorder patients: A double-blind, placebo-controlled pilot study. *Journal of Clinical Psychiatry, 62*, 849–854.

Zanarini, M. C., Frankenburg, F. R., Khera, G. S., & Bleichmar, J. (2001). Treatment histories of borderline inpatients. *Comprehensive Psychiatry, 42*, 144–150.

Zanarini, M. C., Frankenburg, F. R., Reich, D. B., Conkey, L. C., & Fitzmaurice, G. M. (2015). Rates of psychiatric treatment reported by patients with borderline personality disorder and other personality disorders 16 years of prospective follow-up. *Psychiatric Services, 66*, 15–20.

Zanarini, M. C., Frankenburg, F., Reich, B., & Fitzmaurice, G. (2012). Attainment and stability of sustained symptomatic remission and recovery among borderline patients and Axis II comparison subjects: A 16-year prospective follow-up study. *American Journal of Psychiatry, 169*, 476–483.

Zanarini, M. C., Schulz, S. C., Detke, H. C., Tanaka, Y., Zhao, F., Lin, D., . . . & Corya, S. (2011). A dose comparison of olanzapine for the treatment of borderline personality disorder: A 12-week randomized, double-blind, placebo-controlled study. *Journal of Clinical Psychiatry, 72*, 1353–1365.

Zanarini, M. C., Schulz, S. C., Detke, H., Zhao, F., Lin, D., Pritchard, M., . . .& Corya, S. (2012). Open-label treatment with olanzapine for patients with borderline personality disorder. *Journal of Clinical Psychopharmacology, 32*, 398–402.

Zanarini, M. C., Stanley, B., Black, D. W., Markowitz, J. C., Goodman, M., Pilkonis, P., . . . & Sanislow, C. (2010). Methodological considerations for treatment trials for persons with borderline personality disorder. *Annals of Clinical Psychiatry, 22*, 75–83.

8

Sleep Disorders: Evidence-Based Integrated Biopsychosocial Treatment of Insomnia

Taylor Bos and Helene A. Emsellem

Difficulties obtaining the proper quantity and quality of sleep are part of the human condition. Consequently, the search for effective treatments to induce or maintain sleep has been ongoing for the past two centuries (López-Muñoz, Ucha-Udabe, & Alamo, 2005). Although significant evidence supports the efficacy of several pharmacologic agents and nonpharmacologic interventions, there are relatively few studies examining integrated treatment approaches.

Insomnia as a disorder is characterized by difficulty initiating and/or maintaining sleep that causes significant distress and daytime impairment. In order to meet the diagnostic criteria for insomnia, patients must report some difficulty initiating or maintaining sleep and must experience clinically significant distress or impairment in functioning. These sleep complaints must occur at least three times per week and cannot be explained by an inadequate sleep opportunity or by the presence of another sleep disorder. The International Classification of Sleep Disorders, Third Edition (ICSD-3; American Academy of Sleep Medicine, 2014), the Diagnostic and Statistical Manual of Mental Disorders, Fifth Edition (DSM-5; American Psychiatric Association, 2013), and the International Statistical Classification of Diseases and Related Health Problems, 10th Edition (ICD-10; World Health Organization, 1993) categorize insomnia complaints that have been ongoing for 3 months or more as chronic insomnia, while insomnia occurring for less than 3 months is termed acute insomnia. “Other insomnia” is a subtype reserved for patients who experience clinically significant insomnia symptoms, but do not meet full criteria for either chronic or acute insomnia.

While the ICSD-2 and the DSM-IV-TR listed numerous independent subtypes of primary insomnia (e.g., psychophysiological insomnia, idiopathic insomnia, paradoxical insomnia), the current editions of both publications have condensed all forms of insomnia that are not better explained by a coincident medical, psychiatric, or substance use disorder into a single term: “primary insomnia.” Furthermore, both manuals direct that a diagnosis of insomnia should be made regardless of whether the insomnia was primary (occurring independently) or secondary (occurring as a consequence or symptom of another medical or psychiatric condition).

The above considerations reflect important changes in thought regarding the diagnosis and treatment of insomnia. First, specific pathophysiologies for subtypes of

Cognitive Behavioral Psychopharmacology: The Clinical Practice of Evidence-Based Biopsychosocial Integration, First Edition. Edited by Mark Dana Muse.

insomnia have not been discovered, which has led to a consensus to assess and treat insomnia consistently, regardless of root cause or presentation. Second, there has been a realization that insomnia needs to be evaluated and treated even if the disorder presents co-morbidly with other disorders. Substantial evidence shows that insomnia serves as a risk factor for relapse in patients treated for a co-morbid mood or anxiety disorder. *Therefore, the treatment of insomnia should not be delayed or regarded as secondary when treating patients with co-morbidities.*

Insomnia is a highly prevalent and debilitating disease affecting approximately 30% of the population (Roth, 2007), and it is one that is associated with significant impairments to an individual's quality of life. Patients with severe insomnia report greater loss of function due to pain, emotional effects, and mental health issues than patients with congestive heart failure, and insomnia patients report more physical sequelae than patients with depression (Katz & McHorney, 2002). Insomnia causes significant daytime impairments, perhaps the greatest of which is a 2.5 to 4.5 times increased incidence of accidents (Balter & Uhlenhuth, 1992). Patients with insomnia are more likely than good sleepers to report decreased job performance and absenteeism, and accrue 60% higher healthcare expenditures. An estimated 40% of patients with insomnia have a co-morbid psychiatric disorder (most commonly depression), and approximately 75% to 90% have an increased risk for a co-morbid medical disorder (Roth, 2007).

Modern conceptualizations of insomnia are derived from Arthur Spielman's 3P model for the assessment of the disorder, which posits that insomnia is initiated and maintained by a set of predisposing, precipitating, and perpetuating factors. Predisposing factors precede the onset of insomnia and are usually trait-like qualities (e.g., genetic risk, high state anxiety) that lower the threshold that facilitate stressors' ability to trigger insomnia. Precipitating factors are the particular events or stressors that initiate insomnia. Perpetuating factors are any features that support or maintain the insomnia over time, regardless of its origins; perpetuating factors typically serve as the best targets for treatment (Spielman, 1986).

Several models of insomnia have followed Spielman's 3P model, implicating multiple processes at various levels of analysis (e.g., genetic risk, neurotransmitters and hormones, homeostatic sleep drive and circadian rhythms, physiologic hyperarousal, maladaptive behavioral coping strategies, dysfunctional beliefs about sleep, etc.) in the development and maintenance of the disorder. Despite evidence for several of these mechanisms, the underlying pathophysiology of insomnia is not comprehensively understood.[1] Nonetheless, two core themes appear in several of these models: persistent hyperarousal and behaviors interfering with sleep maintenance. Both can be viewed as perpetuating factors and, consequently, may become targets for treatment.

Hyperarousal, long thought to be at the root of insomnia, may be the result of several processes. It can result from a sensitivity of wake-promoting neurotransmitter activity in the "bottom-up" reticular activating system and limbic networks, or "top-down" neocortex cognitive systems. These pathways involve a host of neurotransmitters, including acetylcholine, norepinephrine, serotonin, histamine, and orexin/hypocretin. Hyperarousal could also result from a decreased sensitivity of sleep-promoting systems mediated by gamma-aminobutyric acid (GABA), galanin, and melatonin activity (Levenson, Kay, & Buysse, 2015). Accordingly, these systems have served as targets for pharmacological treatment of insomnia.

In contrast, cognitive models of insomnia view the disorder as resulting from learned behaviors that interfere with sleep onset or maintenance. For example, some life stressor may cause insomnia acutely due to increased stress at sleep onset accompanied by frequent nighttime awakenings. If this pattern persists, the patient may develop dysfunctional beliefs and sleep-related anxiety leading to increased attention to sleep-related threats. This, in turn, further leads to an increase in the perceived severity of the sleep disturbance, which can perpetuate and maintain insomnia. Cognitive-behavioral therapy for insomnia (CBT-i) attempts to alter dysfunctional beliefs about sleep, and implement new behaviors to reduce sleep-related anxiety while increasing sleep efficiency.

Historical Treatments for Insomnia

Many substances have been used over the course of human history to induce sleepiness, but the first clinical treatment for insomnia came about in the 1800s with the discovery of the sedative-hypnotic and anticonvulsant properties of liquid solutions of bromide salts, which became the most widely used sedatives in the 19th century. Though effective sedatives, bromide use was associated with a host of adverse effects, largely resulting from high toxicity, including neurological and gastrointestinal disorders, irritability, hallucinations, deliria, and lethargy. Additionally, they had a long half-life and could accumulate in tissue. Bromides were phased out of use in the first part of the 20th century with the advent of barbiturates (López-Muñoz, 2005).

Barbital, the first barbiturate available on the market, was synthesized by Conrad and Guthzeit in 1881. Through small modifications of the barbituric acid molecule, over 2,500 different barbiturates were synthesized, about 50 of which were employed clinically (López-Muñoz, 2014). The popularity of barbiturates peaked in the 1930s and 1940s; the production of barbiturates in the United States increased by 400% from 1933 to 1936. This massive rise in popularity continued in spite of evidence of the potential for barbiturates to cause dependence as early as 1882; however, reliable data regarding dependence were not available until the 1950s. Furthermore, deaths by barbiturate overdose became a frequent occurrence, in part due to the small therapeutic margin of these agents. Despite these dangers, barbiturate use was common until the commercialization of the first benzodiazepine, chlordiazepoxide, in 1960 (López-Muñoz, 2014). Today, barbiturates are still used, but in very specific circumstances, such as phenobarbital in the management of epilepsy, and pentobarbital can be used to induce sleep for anesthesia. As sedative-hypnotics, barbiturates were largely replaced by benzodiazepines and other more recently developed drugs, and therefore will not be included in this chapter's review of current treatments for insomnia.

Concurrent with the synthesis of the first benzodiazepines, the cognitive revolution spurred interest into research and implementation of cognitive-behavioral therapies (CBTs) for various psychological disorders. This would eventually result in the creation of cognitive-behavioral therapy for insomnia.

Pharmacologic Treatments for Insomnia

Benzodiazepines

Following 1960, benzodiazepines replaced barbiturates as the most widely used sedative-hypnotic, and they experienced similar popularity well into the 1990s. Benzodiazepines achieve their effects through enhancing GABAergic transmission, resulting in sedative-hypnotic, anxiolytic, anticonvulsant, and muscle relaxant properties. Several meta-analyses have documented the efficacy of benzodiazepines over placebo in improving selected objective and subjective variables of sleep quality. Buscemi et al. (2007) found that, compared to placebo, benzodiazepines produced a significant reduction in sleep onset latency and wake after sleep onset, as well as significant improvements in sleep efficiency and total sleep time, assessed both by sleep diary and polysomnography. Similar results for objective and subjective sleep onset latency and sleep efficiency were shown by Holbrook, Crowther, Lotter, Cheng, and King (2000). A recent meta-analysis found that benzodiazepines produced significant improvements of moderate or large effect size in all measures, both objectively and subjectively, except for subjective total sleep time (Winkler, Auer, Doering, & Rief, 2014).

The evidence consistently demonstrates the efficacy of benzodiazepines in treating insomnia; however, several issues should be considered before clinical administration. First, the majority of studies included in these meta-analyses were funded by private sources. Therefore, there may be an increased bias to publish significant results over nonsignificant findings, and the pooled estimates of efficacy may be overestimations. Furthermore, few studies assessed change in daytime functioning or quality of life as a result of treatment. Given that insomnia is a disorder characterized by nighttime sleep disturbance as well as disturbances in daytime functioning, daytime function should be assessed in insomnia treatment trials (Buscemi et al., 2007).

Second, benzodiazepines carry with them a number of safety concerns, especially with long-term use. The majority of randomized controlled trials (RCTs) have a short treatment duration (≤ 4 weeks; Buscemi et al., 2007) in otherwise healthy adults with limited follow up data. Even in the absence of long-term studies, however, benzodiazepines are still associated with significantly more adverse events than placebo or than their cousin "Z-drugs" (discussed in the following section). Most common adverse effects included somnolence, headache, dizziness, nausea, and fatigue (Buscemi et al., 2007).

Despite a lack of data assessing the safety of long-term benzodiazepine use, some have argued that sedative-hypnotics should be considered as treatments for chronic insomnia (Shahid, Chung, Phillipson, & Shapiro, 2012). However, long-term benzodiazepine use has been shown to result in significant cognitive impairments as assessed by neuropsychological testing over 12 cognitive domains including processing speed, attention/concentration, working memory, and problem solving (Barker, Greenwood, Jackson, & Crowe, 2004a). These effects may persist for up to 6 months after the discontinuation of treatment (Barker, Greenwood, Jackson, & Crowe, 2004b) and such cognitive impairments may occur more frequently in the elderly (Paterniti, Dufouil, & Alperovitch, 2006). Benzodiazepines also have the potential to produce withdrawal symptoms. Of patients treated continuously with sedative-benzodiazepines, 5% of those treated for less than 8 months and 43% of those treated for more than 8 months experienced withdrawal symptoms (Rickels, Case, Downing, & Winokur, 1983). Nevertheless, these effects can be attenuated by tapering the dosage gradually (Busto et al., 1986). Most alarmingly, a recent study by de Gage and Colleagues (2012) and replicated by Shash et al. (2015) found that new use of benzodiazepines was associated with an increased incidence of dementia (hazard ratio = 1.60, 95% CI [1.08, 2.38]. Notwithstanding the de Gage and Shash studies, a more recent study found that although the risk of dementia was slightly higher for individuals with minimal benzodiazepine exposure, there was no increased risk in the group with the highest level of exposure. The authors cited this as evidence against a causal association between benzodiazepine use and dementia (Gray et al., 2016). More research is needed to evaluate this potential relationship.

A third concern with the research on the use of benzodiazepines in the treatment of insomnia is that, although meta-analytic techniques show statistically significant improvements in most sleep variables, the results may not be clinically significant. Pooled estimates of the improvement in sleep onset latency assessed by polysomnography ranged from 4.2 to 10.0 min. Improvements in objective total sleep time ranged from 32.7 to 61.8 min (Buscemi et al., 2007; Holbrook et al., 2000). Given the safety concerns noted above, clinicians must assess whether these improvements are worth the risks, or whether alternative treatments are more appropriate.

Benzodiazepine Receptor Agonists ("Z-drugs")

In the late 1980s and 1990s, a new class of drugs with similar therapeutic properties to benzodiazepines emerged in the treatment of insomnia. Benzodiazepine receptor agonists, colloquially known as "Z-drugs" (due to the fact that many drugs in this class begin with the letter "Z") have demonstrated similar efficacy in treating insomnia as the benzodiazepines, but with significantly fewer safety concerns and little to no evidence for the development of tolerance. Some meta analyses find that that Z-drugs have therapeutic effects that are marginally lower than those of benzodiazepines, but these differences are not always statistically significant (Buscemi et al., 2007; Winkler et al., 2014). Confounding the literature is the fact that there is at least a 50% placebo response rate in clinical trials assessing the efficacy of medications for insomnia. A meta-analysis of data submitted to the Food and Drug Administration (FDA) examining the effectiveness of Z-drugs and their associated placebo responses found that both effects were small and of limited clinical significance. However, the combined Z-drug/placebo effect produced a significant treatment response (Huedo-Medina, Kirsch, Middlemass, Klonizakis, & Siriwardena, 2013).

Intermittent, long-term zolpidem use (10 mg 3–5 nights per week over 12 weeks) has been shown as an effective treatment for chronic insomnia compared to placebo: subjects in the active treatment group experienced a 42% decrease in sleep latency, a 52% reduction in the number of awakenings, a 55% decrease in wake after sleep onset, and a 27% increase in total sleep time across the 12-week period of intermittent zolpidem use. Furthermore, there was no evidence of rebound insomnia on the nights that patients did not take zolpidem (Perlis, McCall, Krystal, & Walsh, 2004). Nonnightly use of sleep medications represents a possible treatment strategy that would reduce the costs compared to nightly use.

Regarding the comparative efficacy of specific Z-drugs and benzodiazepines, a review and meta-analysis (Dündar et al., 2004) found few consistent differences between treatments. The noticed differences in efficacy reflected differences in pharmacokinetics. For example, zaleplon produces a shorter sleep latency, but also a shorter duration of sleep when compared to zolpidem. This is unsurprising given zaleplon is more rapidly absorbed and has a shorter half-life than its counterpart. In general, drugs with the longest half-life produce the greatest impairments in daytime functioning (e.g., nitrazepam).

A primary advantage of Z-drugs over benzodiazepines is their improved safety profile. Z-drugs typically have a more rapid onset (≤ 30 min) and a shorter half-life (1–7 h) than benzodiazepines. In an open label trial of zaleplon in older adults, doses of 5 and

10 mg were shown to be both effective and safe for periods of 6–12 months (Ancoli-Israel et al., 2005). Similarly, a long-term trial of zolpidem extended-release showed a good safety profile for 12.5 mg doses administered 3–7 nights per week for 6 months (Krystal, Erman, Zammit, Soubrane, & Roth, 2007). Despite these findings, a recent increase in the frequency of Z-drug-related complications prompted cause for new concern. In January of 2013, the FDA released a statement advising lowering the dosage of zolpidem in women due to residual daytime effects and evidence for the slower rate of metabolism of the drug in women compared to men. An alarming review of the clinical and forensic toxicology of Z-drugs concluded that they had few advantages over benzodiazepines, noting that adverse Z-drug effects are more likely with therapeutic polydrug use and overdose with co-ingested psychoactive substances (Gunja, 2013). However, given that Z-drugs exhibit shorter half-lives compared to benzodiazepines, do not produce active metabolites, and do not inhibit rapid eye movement (REM) sleep, this position may be overstated.

Melatonin And Melatonin Agonists

Melatonin activity represents another potential target for inducing sleepiness. The two-process model of sleep regulation theorizes that sleep is modulated by two independent processes: a wake-dependent process whereby greater brain use during wakefulness increases the need for sleep (process S), and a wake-independent circadian process that generates sleep propensity based on the influences of exogenous light, melatonin, and social factors on the suprachiasmatic nuclei of the hypothalamus (process C) (Levenson et al., 2015). Although endogenous melatonin production is dependent on exposure to light sources (natural or artificial), exogenous melatonin is available as an over-the-counter supplement.

Despite its theoretical attraction, melatonin has only limited efficacy and effectiveness in the treatment of insomnia, with no large-scale placebo-controlled cohort studies available. Two meta-analyses (Brzezinski et al., 2005; Ferracioli-Oda, Qawasmi, & Bloch, 2013) examined the effects of melatonin in sleep disorders and concluded that melatonin significantly reduces sleep onset latency and increases total sleep time and sleep efficiency. These effects are smaller than other pharmacological treatments for insomnia and may not be clinically significant; pooled estimates for the reduction of sleep onset latency ranged from 4.0 to 7.6 min, and increases in total sleep time ranged from 8.25 to 12.8 min. A different research team conducted two meta-analyses (Buscemi et al., 2005, 2006) that specifically focused on the efficacy of melatonin in treating primary or secondary sleep disorders (sleep problems associated with medical, neurological, or substance use disorders). Although they found statistically significant improvements in sleep variables, they nonetheless determined that melatonin was not effective in treating sleep disorders due to the small effect size. Of note, melatonin appeared to be most effective in patients with delayed sleep phase syndrome (a disorder related to circadian misalignment).

Ramelteon, a selective melatonin receptor agonist approved by the FDA for the treatment of insomnia, is an available alternative to melatonin. Two separate meta-analyses (Liu & Wang, 2012; Kuriyama, Honda, & Hayashino, 2014) have found ramelteon reduced subjective sleep latency and improved subjective sleep quality. Although there was no noted improvement in subjective total sleep time, objective measures of all three variables showed some improvement with ramelteon treatment. Similar to exogenous melatonin, these modest effects may not be clinically relevant.

Ramelteon and melatonin may still have some clinical use on account of their benign side effect profiles. Neither substance demonstrates a higher risk ratio of any frequent adverse events compared to controls (Liu & Wang, 2012; Ferracioli-Oda et al., 2013). Kuriyama et al. (2014) noted that the only significant side effect associated with ramelteon use was somnolence. Consequently, either agent may be reasonable for cases of mild insomnia in patients with health complications or concurrent medications that may interact with other sedative-hypnotics.

Orexin/Hypocretin Antagonists

The newest addition to the armamentarium for insomnia are the orexin/hypocretin receptor antagonists. Orexin/hypocretin neurons of the lateral hypothalamus project to areas of the brain stem and hypothalamus that promote and maintain arousal. Antagonism of these centers can reduce arousal that opposes the inhibitory actions in the sleep-promoting pathways of the brain (Levenson et al., 2015). Suvorexant is currently the only such agent approved by the FDA for the treatment of insomnia. Suvorexant appears efficacious and generally well tolerated. Results from two separate 3-month RCTs comparing various dosages of suvorexant to placebo in nonelderly and elderly adults (Citrome, 2014; Herring et al., 2016) found significant, dose-dependent effects from baseline over 3 months on subjective total sleep time (15 or 20 mg, 55.3 min; 30 or 40 mg, 61.4 min), subjective wake time after sleep onset (15 or 20 mg, −34.5 min; 30 or 40 mg, −37.6 min), subjective sleep latency (15 or 20 mg, −24.9 min; 30 or 40 mg, −29.8 min), and both objective total sleep time (15 or 20 mg, −48.0 min; 30 or 40 mg, −50.9 min) and objective sleep latency (15 or 20 mg, −32.2 min; 30 or 40 mg, −34.0 min), assessed by polysomnography. These effect sizes are on a par with those demonstrated by benzodiazepines.

A 1-year trial of suvorexant reported that, though generally well tolerated, suvorexant was associated with significantly more adverse events than placebo. The most common adverse events associated with suvorexant included somnolence (13.2%), fatigue (6.5%), dry mouth (5.0%), dysnepsia (1.9%), and peripheral edema (1.7%; Michelson et al., 2013). Somnolence was most prominent in the 30 and 40 mg doses. Additional safety trials have been conducted to assess suvorexant's effect on next-morning driving performance, memory and balance, middle of the night safety in elderly subjects, and potential for rebound and withdrawal following discontinuation. Impaired driving performance was seen in some adults after taking either a 20 or a 40 mg dose. Additionally, four subjects taking suvorexant prematurely discontinued their driving tasks due to excessive somnolence. One of four trials of healthy nonelderly adults found a significant impairment in verbal recall following a single dose of suvorexant 40 mg. A small study assessing the safety of suvorexant in elderly adults in the middle of the night found that suvorexant produced less impairment than zolpidem 5 mg, which served as an active control (Citrome, 2014). Considering these safety concerns, the FDA decided in 2013 to approve suvorexant only at doses of 10, 15, and 20 mg. Despite the dose restrictions, suvorexant has demonstrated efficacy at lower doses and represents a new option in the treatment of insomnia.

Other Pharmacological Agents Used to Treat Insomnia

Several other agents are consistently prescribed off-label to treat insomnia due to their sleep-promoting effects. Relevant agents include various antidepressants, atypical antipsychotics, and antihistamines. Current American Academy of Sleep Medicine (AASM) Clinical Guidelines for Insomnia (2008) state that such medications may only be suitable for patients with co-morbid insomnia who would benefit from the primary action of these drugs. However, given that insomnia frequently occurs co-morbid with, and may help to maintain, other disorders, the following alternative treatments may be considered when determining the best pharmacologic intervention for a specific patient.

Antidepressants

Depression and insomnia frequently co-occur; the diagnostic criteria for depression includes sleep disturbance as a possible symptom (DSM-5, 2013; ICD-10, 1993). Although there is not substantial literature detailing the use of antidepressants in insomnia, many agents are used to treat both conditions simultaneously. Meta-analyses comparing the efficacy of benzodiazepines, Z-drugs, and antidepressants (Buscemi, 2007; Winkler et al., 2014) show that antidepressants as a class are efficacious in the treatment of insomnia, but to a lesser extent than the other drug classes.

Of the tricyclic antidepressants (TCAs), both amytriptyline and trimipramine have been shown to improve both sleep and mood in RCTs, and to show less disruption of REM sleep than other TCAs (Scharf, Hirschowitz, Zemlan, Lichstein, & Woods, 1986; Shipley et al., 1985; Ware, Brown, Moorad, & Pittard, 1989). Doxepin has shown efficacy in the treatment of sleep maintenance insomnia and has been approved by the FDA for that use (McCall & McCall, 2012). However, TCAs possess significant side effect profiles including the potential for lethal overdose.

Paradoxically, the selective serotonin reuptake inhibitors generally have sleep disruptive side effects documented by polysomnography, yet many patients report improvements in sleep, perhaps as a consequence of their improved mood (Jindal & Thase, 2004).

Trazodone, nefazodone, and mirtazapine are FDA-approved antidepressants that have shown some efficacy at relieving insomnia. Patients taking trazodone experience significantly fewer nighttime awakenings and demonstrate longer slow wave sleep; however, it may also be associated with cognitive and motor impairments (Roth, McCall, & Liguori, 2011). Similarly, mirtazapine reduces sleep latency and increases slow wave sleep and sleep efficiency in normal sleepers, as well as reduced sleep latency and increased total sleep time in patients with insomnia (Aslan, Isik, & Cosar, 2002; Ruigt, Kemp, Groenhout, & Kamphuisen, 1990). Nefazadone also improves sleep-related variables assessed by polysomnography (Rush et al., 1998), but usage is currently extremely limited due to a black box warning regarding liver failure.

Treatment of co-morbid insomnia and depression can be simplified with the administration of a single sedative antidepressant agent. However, there are occasions when these agents are ineffective or a patient presents with insomnia as a consequence of an activating antidepressant. In these cases, a combination of an antidepressant and a sedative-hypnotic may present the best course of action (Jindal & Thase, 2004). More research on polypharmacy for insomnia and depression is needed in order to development specific guidelines regarding safe and effective combinations. One RCT has shown efficacy for a combination of escitalopram and zolpidem ER for treating patients with insomnia and major depressive disorder (Fava et al., 2011). Also, a meta-analysis of insomnia and somnolence associated with second-generation antidepressants (Alberti, Chiesa, Andrisano, & Serretti, 2015) concluded that a combination of antidepressant with a sleep-enhancing agent may be an option for treating the two disorders of depression and insomnia, concurrently.

Atypical Antipsychotics

Quetiapine has shown promise in the treatment of insomnia. In a trial of healthy subjects, quetiapine significantly reduced sleep onset latency and improved sleep continuity, although it did give rise to significant periodic limb movements with doses of 100 mg (Cohrs et al., 2004). A small placebo-controlled trial of quetiapine found that both subjective and objective sleep variables, most notably total sleep time and sleep continuity, were improved in patients with dementia or mild cognitive impairment (Singer, 2011). A recent review found that quetiapine may show efficacy in treating sleep disturbance in patients with a variety of disorders, including autism, generalized anxiety disorder, and depression (McCall & McCall, 2012).

Anticonvulsants

Gabapentin and pregabalin are related drugs that are GABA analogues that interfere with the influx of calcium at nerve terminals. Both have been found to increase slow wave sleep in healthy adults (Foldvary-Schaefer et al., 2002; Hindmarch, Dawson, & Stanley, 2005). Gabapentin has been investigated as a sedative-hypnotic in alcoholism because it shows no significant abuse potential (Furieri & Nakamura-Placios, 2007). Both also have been shown to improve scores on self-report measures of sleep disturbance during treatment of fibromyalgia (Arnold et al., 2007, 2008), neuropathic pain associated with HIV (Hahn et al., 2004), varicella zoster virus (Rice, Maton, & Group1UK, 2001), and diabetes mellitus (Backonja, 1999; Freeman, Durso-Decruz, & Emir, 2008).

Antihistamines

Histamine is involved in the wake-promoting systems of the brain such as the tuberomammillary nucleus of the posterior hypothalamus (Levenson et al., 2015). Consequently, antagonism of histamine produces drowsiness, leading many people suffering from insomnia to use over-the-counter antihistamines for treatment. While the availability and low cost make the appeal of antihistamines clear, evidence for their efficacy in the treatment of insomnia is mixed or negative (Monti & Monti, 2000). Triprolidine, brompheniramine, and mepyramine have no effect on total sleep time or wake after sleep onset, but do increase latency to REM sleep and decrease REM sleep time. As a result, these medications cause significant daytime sleepiness and impairment in daytime functioning (Nicholson, Pascoe, & Stone, 1985). Promethazine, appears to increase stage 2 sleep time while increasing latency to REM sleep and decreasing REM sleep time. Results regarding its effect on total sleep time are mixed (Adam & Oswald, 1986; Risberg, Risberg, & Ingvar, 1975). Diphenhydramine produced no improvements in subjective or objective sleep variables, but did impair psychomotor performance the next day (Saletu, Grünberger, Krupka, & Schuster, 1987). Traditionally believed to be the ideal sedative medication for elderly patients, diphenhydramine has been shown to significantly increase the incidence of falls in this population (Finkle, Adams, Greenland, & Melmon, 2002). In addition to the questionable efficacy of these drugs, there is also the potential to develop acute tolerance to the sedative effects of antihistamines. Therefore, the use of antihistamines for the treatment of insomnia should be discouraged in favor of one of the aforementioned available therapeutic agents (Monti & Monti, 2000).

The available literature regarding pharmacological treatments for insomnia shows that benzodiazepines, Z-drugs, and the new orexin/hypocretin antagonists produce the largest effects across multiple sleep variables. However, the side effect profiles of each drug and the characteristics of the individual patient should be considered before deciding between the available treatments. Melatonin and ramelteon, though they produce minimal clinical effects, are by far the most benign of the available medications. Additionally, other drug classes with sedating properties or a combination of multiple drugs should be considered cautiously if the patient presents with a co-morbid condition. In general, antihistamines are not effective in the treatment of insomnia and should be discouraged.

Psychosocial Therapy for Insomnia

CBT, a combination of cognitive strategies designed to restructure dysfunctional beliefs and behavioral strategies to address and alter maladaptive behaviors, has become the standard psychological intervention for a multitude of psychiatric disorders. It should be remembered that CBT typically refers to a family of interventions that combine cognitive and behavioral techniques, not a specific manualized treatment for a disorder. CBT-i is no different. While there are several evidence-based, manualized treatments available for insomnia (see Edinger & Carney, 2015 for an example), most treatments comprise some combination of the following techniques: cognitive therapy, paradoxical intent, stimulus control, sleep restriction, sleep hygiene, and relaxation. Consequently, the literature typically examines the efficacy of CBT-i as a packaged treatment. However, there have been some trials of individual treatments, and several of these studies provide evidence for the efficacy of each component of CBT-i.

Sleep Hygiene

The goal of sleep hygiene is to change environmental and behavioral factors to promote sleep. Specific recommendations could include avoiding long naps during the day as well as avoiding light sources around bedtime, limiting caffeine and alcohol intake, or making the bedroom more comfortable and conducive to sleep. Sleep hygiene is often considered the minimum intervention for insomnia because it produces little effect on sleep on its own (Morin & Benca, 2012). Specific filtering of blue light using orange lens glasses before bedtime has been shown to help counteract light's inhibitory effect on melatonin production, and to help cue the brain that it is evening and time to go to sleep (Burkhart & Phelps, 2009; Sasseville, Paquet, Sévigny, & Hébert, 2006). This technique can be useful for shift-workers and individuals who must use light-emitting devices near bedtime. Furthermore, exercise has also been long regarded as beneficial to obtaining a good night's sleep, and is associated with better quality sleep (Ancoli-Israel, 2001). Historically, sleep experts have recommended a 4-h window between exercise and bedtime, however recent research has shown that this is not necessary (Flausino, Da Silva Prado, Queiroz, Tufik, & Mello, 2011). Sleep hygiene is often used as a comparison group in trials assessing the efficacy of other interventions for insomnia; however it is also a component of most CBT-i treatments (Trauer, Qian, Doyle, Rajaratnam, & Cunnington, 2015).

Paradoxical Intention

Given that patients experience a high degree of sleep-anticipatory anxiety that interferes with their ability to fall asleep and stay asleep, paradoxical intention is a cognitive technique that attempts to alleviate that anxiety by instructing patients to stay awake as long as possible. It is thought that by removing the urgency in the need to fall asleep, anxiety will diminish and the patient will actually fall asleep faster. Sleep onset insomniacs treated with paradoxical intention exhibit significant decrease in sleep effort and sleep performance anxiety relative to a wait list control condition (Broomfield & Espie, 2003). In the Broomfield and Espie study, although treatment did not produce objective reductions in sleep onset latency, there was a trend toward a significant decrease in subjective sleep onset latency in patients treated with paradoxical intention.

Cognitive Therapy

The goal of cognitive therapy for insomnia is to identify, challenge, and replace specific dysfunctional beliefs about sleep. Altering these thoughts should reduce sleep-anticipatory anxiety and decrease the frequency of maladaptive sleep rituals, or eliminate them altogether. Examples of dysfunctional beliefs about sleep may involve unrealistic expectations of sleep, exaggerated consequences of sleep deprivation, or erroneous beliefs about sleep need (Trauer et al., 2015). Using an enhanced cognitive therapy for insomnia that targeted unhelpful beliefs about sleep, sleep-related or sleep-interfering worry, attentional bias and monitoring for sleep-related threat, and misperception of sleep, Harvey et al. (2014) found at posttreatment that cognitive therapy led to significant reductions in scores on the Insomnia Severity Index (ISI mean difference pre- to posttreatment = −8.21, SD = −1.94) with 63% of patients experiencing reductions of at least 8 points and 52% meeting criteria for remission of symptoms at 6-month follow up. Cognitive therapy also produced significant improvements in subjective sleep onset latency, wake after sleep onset, total sleep time, and sleep efficiency.

Relaxation

Relaxation techniques are designed to decrease stress and arousal in order to facilitate sleep onset. Several methods of teaching relaxation exist such as meditation, yoga, progressive muscle relaxation, and biofeedback training. Progressive muscle relaxation has been shown to significantly improve sleep quality and reduce waking up after sleep onset (Means, Lichstein, Epperson, & Johnson, 2000). However, in the Means et al. study there was no improvement in daytime functioning. There are mixed results for progressive muscle relaxation improving sleep onset latency (Lichstein & Riedel, 1994; Means et al., 2000).

Some have attempted to enhance the effects of relaxation with electromyogram (EMG) biofeedback by giving patients information about their muscle activity. Interestingly, although EMG biofeedback coupled with progressive muscle relaxation does lead to significant reductions in subjective sleep onset latency, these results were not significantly different from a group that received EMG biofeedback alone. It is possible that giving patients a feeling of control over their tension and anxiety is enough to produce a small effect on subjective sleep variables (Nicassio, Boylan, & McCabe, 1982).

Stimulus Control

Issues with sleep onset and maintenance can be a result of learned maladaptive behaviors regarding nighttime awakenings in the context of the bedroom. For example, if a patient who wakes in the middle of the night decides to surf the internet on his or her phone until tired, the patient has now learned to associate bed with stimulating material. Stimulus control aims to restrict behaviors in the bedroom to sleep and sex. Therefore, patients are instructed not to go to bed until tired and to leave the bedroom if they awake in the night and feel like they cannot go back to sleep. Stimulus control has been shown to be more effective than both placebo and relaxation in improving sleep parameters (Espie, Lindsay, Brooks, Hood, & Turvey, 1989), and a review of psychological treatments for insomnia found that it had considerable evidence (Morin et al., 2006).

Sleep Restriction

Sleep restriction is a behavioral technique that attempts to improve a patient's sleep efficiency by restricting their time in bed. For example, if a patient is in bed nightly from 10:00 pm to 6:00 am, but reports (either by self-report or actigraphy) that they only sleep 5 h per night, then their sleep time would be restricted to the 5 h prior to their wake time, 1:00 am to 6:00 am As their sleep efficiency improved, time in bed would gradually be increased to a normal duration of about 8 h. Sleep restriction has been shown to lead to highly significant improvements in sleep efficiency over time, and is more effective than placebo or relaxation in improving subjective sleep variables (Lichstein et al., 2001).

Using the same rationale, a group of researchers developed intensive sleep retraining (ISR), a condensed behavioral treatment to decrease sleep onset latency and increase sleep efficiency through intensive training of proper sleep habits (Harris, Lack, Kemp, Wright, & Bootzin, 2012). In this 25-h protocol, patients are required to restrict their sleep on the night before treatment to 5 h. Patients were then seen at the sleep laboratory on the following night for a series of 50 nap trials at 30-min intervals. In each trial, patients were allowed 20 min to initiate sleep. If sleep was not initiated by that time, the trial was discontinued and the patient remained awake for the next 10 min until the start of the next trial. If the patient was able to fall asleep, they were allowed to sleep for 3 consecutive min prior to being awakened. ISR produced significant improvements in scores on the Pittsburgh Sleep Quality Index (PSQI, Cohen's $d = 0.97$), Dysfunctional Beliefs about Sleep scale (DBAS, Cohen's $d = 0.79$), as well as ratings of daytime impairment (Cohen's $d = 0.57$) and sleep self-efficacy (Cohen's $d = 1.10$). These effects were durable in a 6-month follow up, and the effect was significantly improved if ISR was combined with stimulus control therapy (Harris et al., 2012).

In summary, the evidence for the efficacy of CBT-i is robust. A recent meta-analysis by Okajima, Komada, and Inoue (2011) showed that CBT-i produced significant improvements in subjective measures of sleep onset latency, total sleep time, total wake time, wake after sleep onset, early morning awakenings, and sleep efficiency as well as objective measures of sleep onset, latency and sleep efficiency. All effect sizes were medium to large. Another meta-analysis by Trauer et al. (2015) confirmed these finding with regard to sleep onset latency, wake after sleep onset, and sleep efficiency. These effects were durable even 6 to 12 months posttreatment. Furthermore, separate meta-analyses have shown that CBT-i is comparably efficacious in both middle-aged adults and older adults of 55+ years of age (Irwin, Cole, & Nicassio, 2006), is an effective treatment for insomnia in patients with both medical and psychological co-morbidity (Wu, Appleman, Salazar, & Wong, 2015), and is implementable in both group (Koffel,

Koffel, & Gehrman, 2015) and via online formats (Seyffert et al., 2016; Zachariae, Lyby, Ritterband, & O'Toole, 2015).

Integrating Biopsychosocial Treatments for Insomnia

Both pharmacologic agents and nonpharmacologic interventions are efficacious in the treatment of insomnia, but does either approach show incremental efficacy over the other, or does the combination of the two approaches produce the best results? Several RCTs have compared CBT-i to benzodiazepines or Z-drugs, or to a combination of the two drugs.

In a trial comparing CBT-i, temazepam, and the combination of the two, Wu, Bao, Zhang, Deng, and Long (2006) found that all three treatment groups showed marked improvements over placebo. Temazepam was the most efficacious immediately post-treatment, but CBT showed superiority at 3-month follow up that was durable at an 8-month follow up as well. Combined treatment showed no improvement over CBT alone, and both the combined treatment and temazepam groups were returning to their pretreatment impairment at the 8-month follow up. Similar results regarding CBT, temazepam, and combination therapy were found by Morin, Colecchi, Stone, Sood, and Brink (1999). A study comparing CBT, zolpidem, and combination treatment found CBT was the most effective treatment with durable treatment gains at 12-month follow up. The combination group showed similar stability of results, but the effect size was not as large (Jacobs, Pace-Schott, Stickgold, & Otto, 2004). Studies examining the comparative efficacy of CBT and zopiclone (no combination group) revealed superiority of CBT, especially at 6-month follow up (Omvik et al., 2008; Sivertsen et al., 2006).

In general, CBT is more efficacious than either medication or a combination of the two. One explanation for the superiority of CBT over combination therapy is that, similar to combined treatment for panic disorder, medication interferes with long-term treatment gains provided by CBT alone. This may be due to an attribution of treatment gains to the effect of medication rather than CBT. However, Morin et al. (2009) have suggested that optimizing treatment for insomnia requires testing new treatment algorithms or combinations of treatments (e.g., intermittent long-term use of sedative-hypnotics, use of CBT booster sessions at various intervals, etc.).

Small pilot studies have been conducted to examine combinations of sequenced therapy regimens of zolpidem and CBT (Vallières, Morin, & Guay, 2005; Vallières, Morin, Guay, Bastien, & LeBlanc, 2004). Improvements in sleep variables occurred at different times depending on the sequence used. In general, sleep improvements were most likely to occur following the introduction of CBT. Sequences including a combined treatment phase followed by CBT alone showed the greatest efficacy, although differences between treatment groups were marginal.

Morin and colleagues (2009) extended this research by examining the added value of medication or maintenance sessions of CBT over acute CBT treatment. Subjects were assigned to one of four groups: (1) 6-week acute treatment with CBT followed by monthly sessions of CBT for 6 months, (2) 6-week acute treatment with CBT alone, (3) 6-week acute treatment with CBT and nightly zolpidem 10 mg followed by monthly sessions of CBT for 6 months, and (4) 6-week acute treatment with CBT and nightly zolpidem 10 mg followed by extended CBT and zolpidem 10 mg as needed.

All conditions were effective in the treatment of persistent insomnia. The addition of zolpidem to CBT during the acute phase of treatment produced some modest improvement in total sleep time, but these were of questionable clinical significance. CBT booster sessions did not significantly improve outcomes compared to acute CBT treatment alone. Long-term outcomes were best for subjects receiving a combination of CBT and zolpidem in the acute phase followed by CBT booster sessions and discontinuation of zolpidem (Morin et al., 2009). Although the addition of zolpidem to CBT produced minimal improvements in sleep variables, the possibility that it increased compliance with CBT should not be overlooked. A recent review of the integration of CBT and pharmacotherapy in the treatment of insomnia discusses the current knowledge on best combinations and sequencing for patients with insomnia alone or with co-morbid psychiatric illnesses (Sudak, Kloss, & Zamzow, 2014). Despite these preliminary results, recent clinical practice guidelines developed by the American College of Physicians (ACP) concludes that there is insufficient evidence for the incremental value of CBT over pharmacotherapy or for combination treatment. The ACP recommends that all adult patients receive CBT-i as the initial treatment for chronic insomnia disorder and medication should be considered only for patients for whom CBT-i alone was unsuccessful, following a discussion of the benefits, harms, and costs of short-term medication use (Qaseem, Kansagara, Forciea, Cooke, & Denberg, 2016).

Final Conclusions and Discussion

A review of the literature yields substantial evidence for the efficacy of numerous pharmacological and psychological interventions in the treatment of insomnia. However, there is less evidence comparing the treatment modalities to each other, very few inter-drug comparison studies, and still less examining the comparative efficacy of combined treatment approaches. Generally, the literature supports the long-term superiority of CBT over pharmacologic intervention. While patients receiving CBT may not experience as rapid treatment gains as those treated with medications, the treatment effect continues to grow after the end of therapy and is maintained 1 to 2 years after the termination of therapy. CBT is also effective in both nonelderly and elderly subjects, as well as those with other co-morbidities for whom certain medications may be contraindicated. Lastly, CBT is flexible enough to be delivered in group form or via the internet, making it a readily available therapy.

This is not to say that pharmacotherapy has no place in the treatment of insomnia. In cases of acute insomnia, the early judicious use of pharmacologic agents could avert the development of chronic insomnia and could be an easier and equally efficacious treatment compared to CBT administered over several weeks. Equally important to keep in mind in the judicious use of pharmacotherapy is the observation that some patients may be better treated with a single agent to address multiple issues (i.e., antidepressants for patients with depression and insomnia).

We summarize our findings in Table 8.1, and provide treatment recommendations.

Additionally, research provides evidence that sequenced treatment strategies may provide a synergetic result in the treatment of insomnia, while the use of medication

Table 8.1 Integrative biopsychosocial intervention with insomnia: Summary of best-practice recommendations by level of confidence derived from strength of evidence.

Practice guidelines for insomnia		
Level A	Recommended	• CBT-i techniques should be considered first-line treatment due to the durability of treatment gains and lack of adverse effects associated with such treatment
Level B	Suggested	• Of the medications for insomnia benzodiazepines, Z-drugs, and orexin/hypocretin antagonists appear to have the greatest efficacy. However, all of these drugs may cause significant side effects and interact with other medications • Antihistamines have no place in the efficacious management of insomnia
Level C	May be considered	• Historically, integrated treatments utilizing both CBT-i and medication have shown no advantage over CBT-i alone. Recent evidence has indicated that combination therapy may be superior if the treatments are sequenced appropriately • Preliminary findings support combinations in which initial use of medication may avert patients discontinuing prior to the end of CBT-i

early in treatment may reduce attrition and increase further treatment compliance with CBT-i interventions that provide long-term results. It remains the task of the clinician to consider this research as well as individual patient variables, including patient preference, when determining the optimal therapeutic approach.

Table 8.2 summarizes our impressions of the research in the field, and our final conclusions.

Table 8.2 Final observations on research and treatment of insomnia.

Research:

A) There are numerous pharmacological and nonpharmacological interventions that have shown efficacy in the treatment of insomnia relative to placebo
B) Generally, research has shown that while medication can lead to more rapid alleviation of symptoms, CBT leads to longer lasting treatment gains
C) More research is needed to make specific comparisons between different pharmacological interventions, comparing pharmacological interventions to CBT, and examining the efficacy of different sequences of treatment combinations

Conclusions:

A) Integrated CBT-i with pharmacotherapy with proper sequencing may be the optimal treatment for insomnia, but more research is needed to confirm these results
B) Pharmacotherapy leads to faster alleviation of symptoms but is typically associated with adverse effects and return of symptoms upon discontinuation of medications
C) CBT-i leads to treatment effects similar to medication over a longer period of time and these effects are longer lasting. Supplementing CBT-i with medication can lead to better treatment compliance in the early stages of therapy

Illustrative Case Study in the Clinical Practice of Biopsychosocial Integration with Insomnia

Sara is a 38-year-old woman (BMI: 24.2) who presents with difficulty initiating sleep at night and associated daytime tiredness. She had a history of depression 5 years ago that was successfully treated with sertraline 75 mg. She successfully weaned off of medications after 2 years of treatment. She did well until 6 months ago when a series of stressors, including increased work demands and caretaking for her aunt with Alzheimer's disease, led to difficulty with sleep.

Prior to the stressors, she had a regular sleep–wake pattern, sleeping from 11:00 pm to 6:15 am on weekdays with a wake time of 7:30 am on weekends. Starting 6 months ago, however, she began to experience difficulty falling asleep. She would get in bed and worry about the issues that she was grappling with. She became concerned about the lack of sleep and compensated for her lack of sleep by moving her bedtime earlier and earlier in the hope of allocating more time for sleep. Eventually, the work problems improved and she set up a care system for her aunt limiting the patient's responsibilities to the evenings a few days a week. Despite dealing with her stressors, the problems initiating sleep nevertheless persisted.

Now she is in bed from 9:45 pm to 6:15 pm and finds that she is nearly panicked getting into bed worrying about the negative impact that insufficient sleep will have on her performance the next day. She has greater difficulty falling asleep, estimating that she is not falling asleep until after 12:30 pm. Once asleep she is able to sleep through the night and would like to be able to sleep in later in the mornings as she is exhausted when her alarm awakens her. She has maintained her consistent weekday wake time, primarily due to her work schedule. She has had anxiety around stressful events in the past, but now believes that her sleep problems are the principle cause of her anxiety. She does not report any physiological symptoms such as heart palpitations, restless legs, shortness of breath, or instances of gasping for air during the night, nor is she sleepy while driving. She does feel that her job performance has suffered because she is exhausted and has difficulty focusing at work.

Past medical history is notable for depression, anxiety, and asthma. The patient does not feel that she is depressed currently, and her anxiety primarily revolves around her difficulty obtaining adequate sleep. Her asthma is rarely an issue. Family history is notable for anxiety in her mother and her sister and depression in her father. Sara is a nonsmoker. She drinks two or three alcoholic beverages per week. She has noted that it is often easier for her to fall asleep after drinking a glass of wine; however, she does not regularly drink immediately before bed and does not report using alcohol for sleep. She used to exercise 3 h per week, but has felt too tired to exercise for the past 2–3 months.

Physical examination was unremarkable. Current medications include birth control pills and a rescue inhaler for asthma.

Sara's primary complaint is increased difficulty initiating sleep, a resultant foreshortened total sleep time, and daytime exhaustion. The problem has evolved in the setting of a fairly regimented sleep–wake schedule, indicating no evidence of an underlying circadian rhythm disorder. Furthermore, the sleep difficulty is not better explained by a concurrent sleep disorder or medical condition, such as restless leg syndrome or obstructive sleep apnea. Given that the sleep onset difficulties have been present for 6 months, chronic insomnia is an appropriate diagnosis. Sara's history of depression and anxiety are predisposing factors that made her vulnerable to sleep difficulties. The stressors at work and the demands of caretaking for her aunt served as precipitating factors that led to sleep onset difficulty. In an attempt to compensate for her sleep difficulties, Sara moved her bedtime up from 11:00 pm over a period of weeks increasingly earlier to 9:45 pm. Unfortunately, this served as a perpetuating factor and had the unintended consequence of increasing her sleep-anticipatory anxiety and her difficulty initiating sleep. It should be noted that the stressors that served as precipitating factors for the insomnia no longer appear to bother Sara as much as her anxiety specifically regarding her sleep, which has replaced the original stressors. Such an association can be conditioned over time when a patient is in bed but cannot sleep because of stress. Once the stress is gone, the bed and the nighttime environment have become conditioned stimuli for sleep-anticipatory anxiety.

The first step in Sara's treatment included a thorough assessment of her sleep pattern with sleep logs. Sleep logs are self-report records regarding the night's sleep that patients complete retrospectively each morning (see Fig. 8.1 for Sara's pretreatment sleep log). At a minimum, patients should indicate what time they got into bed, the estimated sleep onset time, when they awoke in the morning, and any interruptions throughout the night that they can recall in the morning. A graph format simplifies the information for review.

If the patient reports difficulty maintaining a sleep log, actigraphy is a potential alternative that objectively reports much of the same information (see Fig. 8.2 for Sara's treatment actigraph output). While the patient is completing sleep logs, it is reasonable to initiate behavioral strategies to address the insomnia. In Sara's case, restricting her time in bed to much closer to the time she is actually falling asleep is a first critical step. She was advised to delay getting in bed until 12:30 am and maintain her 6:15 am wake-up time. She was counseled in basic sleep hygiene and stimulus control principles, using the bed only for sleep, creating a consistently relaxing wind-down bedtime routine to separate daytime activity from night, and including limiting light exposure near bedtime.[2]

Sara returned after 2 weeks with the sleep log in Fig. 8.3. She reported difficulty staying awake until midnight, but found that she was so tired that she typically fell asleep by 12:45 am. Given her improved sleep efficiency, she was instructed to move the bedtime back to 12:15 am with the plan to gradually inch the bedtime back toward 11:00 pm, contingent upon a continued sleep latency of 20–30 min maximum and a good sleep efficiency. The addition of cognitive strategies to help the patient manage any negative thinking surrounding sleep and its outcome was helpful, and an online CBT-i was recommended to supplement other treatment efforts.

In instances where patients report inability to restrict their sleep time, the use of medication to manage anticipatory anxiety may be appropriate and necessary. Absent a clear indication for an anxiolytic medication, the addition of 5 mg of zolpidem at bedtime may be helpful in some situations and could increase compliance with concurrent nonpharmacologic interventions. Additionally, a regular exercise program should be encouraged for its positive effect on sleep latency and duration, reinforcing effect on the timing of the circadian rhythm, and to facilitate endorphin release benefit on mood and cardiovascular conditioning. Meeting physical activity guidelines has been shown to be associated with less frequent feelings of daytime sleepiness and difficulty concentrating (Loprinzi & Cardinal, 2011).

In Sara's case, she responded well to treatment. Over the ensuing 8 weeks, she was able to gradually move her sleep onset time back to 11:00 pm, allowing for 7.25 h of sleep opportunity, while maintaining her regular routine. In Sara's circumstance, the insomnia was clearly triggered by a cascade of stressors. Educating her about these stressors when her circadian rhythm is entrained could allow her to recognize and properly address such triggers in the future and avoid future episodes of insomnia. It may be appropriate to prescribe 5 mg zolpidem as needed to help address the sleep disruptive effects of future stressors proactively. Sara was very engaged in the treatment plan and was empowered by her ability to manage the insomnia. Less insightful patients may be frustrated by these strategies, and augmenting CBT-i with zolpidem can be particularly helpful to increase compliance with the behavioral aspects of therapy.

(Continued)

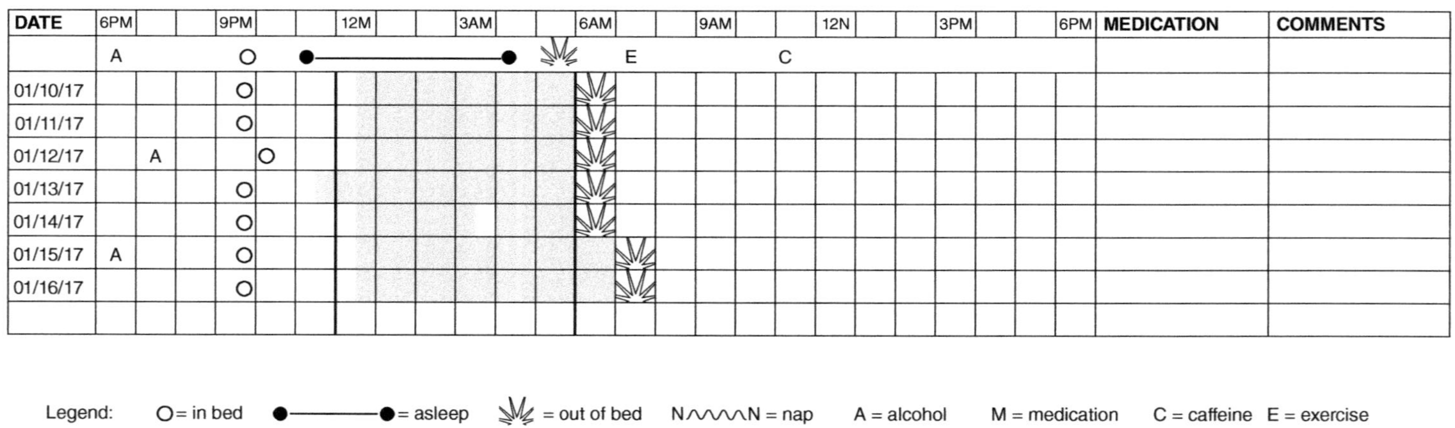

Figure 8.1 Sara's sleep log before treatment demonstrating an elongated sleep latency.

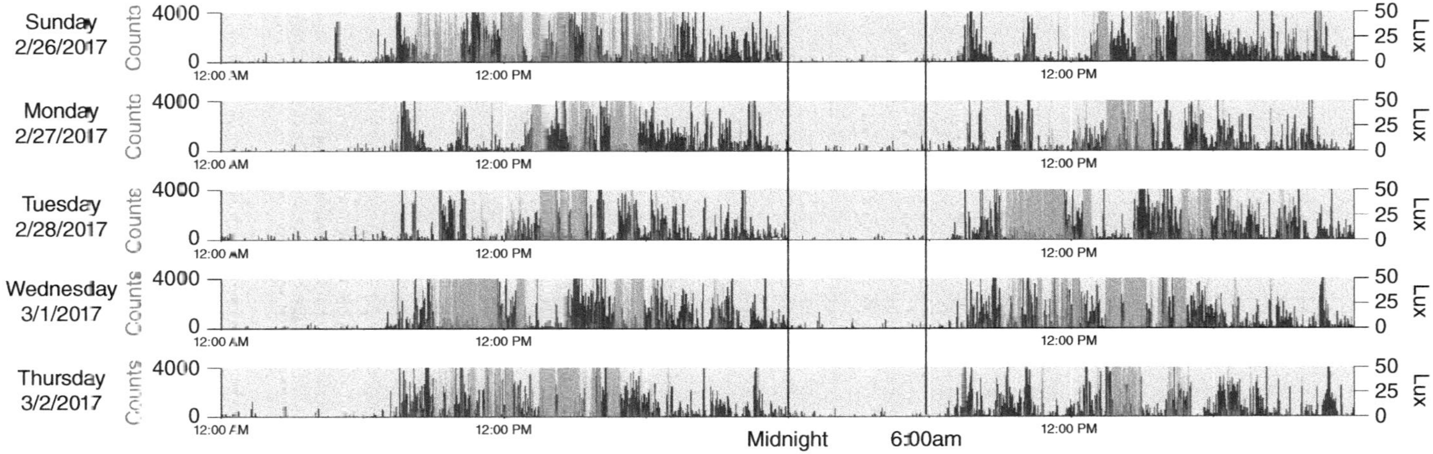

Figure 8.2 Sara's actigraph data during treatment. Her bed time has been restricted in order to maximize her sleep efficiency. The actigram is generated from a wrist-worn device and plots the presence and absence of activity over several days. The actigraph output shown here represents regular activity with darker shading and reduced levels of activity with lighter shading. The period from midnight to 6:00 am corresponds to sleep, with much less motor activity.

(Continued)

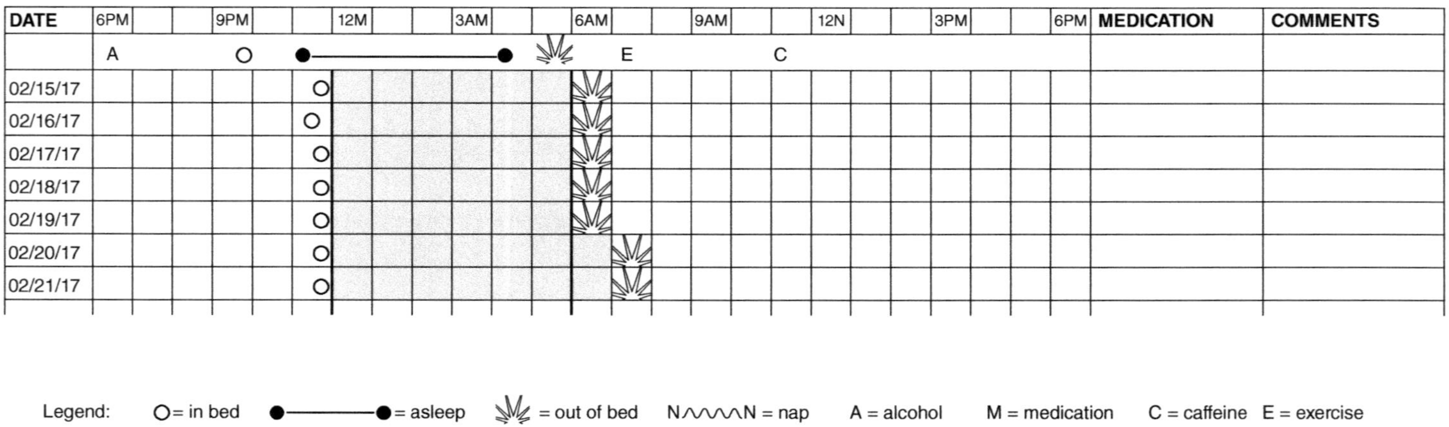

Figure 8.3 Sleep log mirroring the actigraph output in Fig. 8.2.

Notes

1 For a review of current thinking on the pathophysiology of insomnia, see Levenson, Kay, and Buysse (2015).
2 Note that when using sleep restriction, patients should be strongly cautioned against driving if sleepy the following day.

References

Adam, K., & Oswald, I. (1986). The hypnotic effects of an antihistamine: Promethazine. *British Journal of Clinical Pharmacology, 22,* 715–717.

Alberti, S., Chiesa, A., Andrisano, C., & Serretti, A. (2015). Insomnia and somnolence associated with second-generation antidepressants during the treatment of major depression: A meta-analysis. *Journal of Clinical Psychopharmacology, 35,* 296–303.

American Academy of Sleep Medicine (2014). *International classification of sleep disorders—third edition (ICSD-3).* Darien, IL: American Academy of Sleep Medicine.

American Psychiatric Association (2013). *Diagnostic and statistical manual of mental disorders (DSM-5®).* Arlington, VA: American Psychiatric Association.

Ancoli-Israel, S. (2001). "Sleep is not tangible" or what the Hebrew tradition has to say about sleep. *Psychosomatic Medicine, 63,* 778–787.

Ancoli-Israel, S., Richardson, G. S., Mangano, R. M., Jenkins, L., Hall, P., & Jones, W. S. (2005). Long-term use of sedative hypnotics in older patients with insomnia. *Sleep Medicine, 6,* 107–113.

Arnold, L. M., Goldenberg, D. L., Stanford, S. B., Lalonde, J. K., Sandhu, H. S., Keck, P. E., . . . & Hudson, J. I. (2007). Gabapentin in the treatment of fibromyalgia: A randomized, double-blind, placebo-controlled, multicenter trial. *Arthritis and Rheumatism, 56,* 1336–1344.

Arnold, L. M., Russell, I. J., Diri, E. W., Duan, W. R., Young, J. P., Sharma, U., . . . & Haig, G. (2008). A 14-week, randomized, double-blinded, placebo-controlled monotherapy trial of pregabalin in patients with fibromyalgia. *The Journal of Pain, 9,* 792–805.

Aslan, S., Isik, E., & Cosar, B. (2002). The effects of mirtazapine on sleep: A placebo controlled, double-blind study in young healthy volunteers. *Sleep, 25,* 677–679.

Backonja, M. M. (1999). Gabapentin monotherapy for the symptomatic treatment of painful neuropathy: A multicenter, double-blind, placebo-controlled trial in patients with diabetes mellitus1. *Epilepsia, 40,* s57–s59.

Balter, M. B., & Uhlenhuth, E. H. (1992). New epidemiologic findings about insomnia and its treatment. *Journal of Clinical Psychiatry, 53,* 34–39.

Barker, M. J., Greenwood, K. M., Jackson, M., & Crowe, S. F. (2004). Cognitive effects of long-term benzodiazepine use. *CNS Drugs, 18,* 37–48.

Barker, M. J., Greenwood, K. M., Jackson, M., & Crowe, S. F. (2004). Persistence of cognitive effects after withdrawal from long-term benzodiazepine use: A meta-analysis. *Archives of Clinical Neuropsychology, 19,* 437–454.

Broomfield, N. M., & Espie, C. A. (2003). Initial insomnia and paradoxical intention: An experimental investigation of putative mechanisms using subjective and actigraphic measurement of sleep. *Behavioural and Cognitive Psychotherapy, 31,* 313–324.

Brzezinski, A., Vangel, M. G., Wurtman, R. J., Norrie, G., Zhdanova, I., Ben-Shushan, A., & Ford, I. (2005). Effects of exogenous melatonin on sleep: A meta-analysis. *Sleep Medicine Reviews, 9*, 41–50.

Burkhart, K., & Phelps, J. R. (2009). Amber lenses to block blue light and improve sleep: A randomized trial. *Chronobiology International, 26*, 1602–1612.

Buscemi, N., Vandermeer, B., Hooton, N., Pandya, R., Tjosvold, L., Hartling, L., . . . & Vohra, S. (2005). The efficacy and safety of exogenous melatonin for primary sleep disorders. *Journal of General Internal Medicine, 20*, 1151–1158.

Buscemi, N., Vandermeer, B., Hooton, N., Pandya, R., Tjosvold, L., Hartling, L., . . . & Baker, G. (2006). Efficacy and safety of exogenous melatonin for secondary sleep disorders and sleep disorders accompanying sleep restriction: Meta-analysis. *BMJ, 332*, 385–393.

Buscemi, N., Vandermeer, B., Friesen, C., Bialy, L., Tubman, M., Ospina, M., . . . & Witmans, M. (2007). The efficacy and safety of drug treatments for chronic insomnia in adults: A meta-analysis of RCTs. *Journal of General Internal Medicine, 22*, 1335–1350.

Busto, U., Sellers, E. M., Naranjo, C. A., Cappell, H., Sanchez-Craig, M., & Sykora, K. (1986). Withdrawal reaction after long-term therapeutic use of benzodiazepines. *New England Journal of Medicine, 315*, 854–859.

Citrome, L. (2014). Suvorexant for insomnia: A systematic review of the efficacy and safety profile for this newly approved hypnotic—what is the number needed to treat, number needed to harm and likelihood to be helped or harmed? *International Journal of Clinical Practice, 68*, 1429–1441.

Cohrs, S., Rodenbeck, A., Guan, Z., Pohlmann, K., Jordan, W., Meier, A., & Rüther, E. (2004). Sleep-promoting properties of quetiapine in healthy subjects. *Psychopharmacology, 174*, 421–429.

de Gage, S. B., Bégaud, B., Bazin, F., Verdoux, H., Dartigues, J. F., Pérès, K., . . . & Pariente, A. (2012). Benzodiazepine use and risk of dementia: Prospective population based study. *British Medical Journal, 345*, e6231.

Dündar, Y., Dodd, S., Strobl, J., Boland, A., Dickson, R., & Walley, T. (2004). Comparative efficacy of newer hypnotic drugs for the short-term management of insomnia: A systematic review and meta-analysis. *Human Psychopharmacology: Clinical and Experimental, 19*, 305–322.

Edinger, J. D., & Carney, C. E. (2015) *Overcoming insomnia: Workbook* (2nd ed.). New York: Oxford University Press.

Espie, C. A., Lindsay, W. R., Brooks, D. N., Hood, E. M., & Turvey, T. (1989). A controlled comparative investigation of psychological treatments for chronic sleep-onset insomnia. *Behaviour Research and Therapy, 27*, 79–88.

Fava, M., Asnis, G. M., Shrivastava, R. K., Lydiard, B., Bastani, B., Sheehan, D. V., & Roth, T. (2010). Improved insomnia symptoms and sleep-related next-day functioning in patients with comorbid major depressive disorder and insomnia following concomitant zolpidem extended-release 12.5 mg and escitalopram treatment: A randomized controlled trial. *Journal of Clinical Psychiatry, 72*, 1–478.

Ferracioli-Oda, E., Qawasmi, A., & Bloch, M. H. (2013). Meta-analysis: Melatonin for the treatment of primary sleep disorders. *PLoS One, 8*, e63773.

Finkle, W. D., Adams, J. L., Greenland, S., & Melmon, K. L. (2002). Increased risk of serious injury following an initial prescription for diphenhydramine. *Annals of Allergy, Asthma and Immunology, 89*, 244–250.

Flausino, N. H., Da Silva Prado, J. M., Queiroz, S. S., Tufik, S., & Mello, M. T. (2012). Physical exercise performed before bedtime improves the sleep pattern of healthy young good sleepers. *Psychophysiology, 49*, 186–192.

Freeman, R., Durso-DeCruz, E., & Emir, B. (2008). Efficacy, safety, and tolerability of pregabalin treatment for painful diabetic peripheral neuropathy: Findings from seven randomized, controlled trials across a range of doses. *Diabetes Care, 31*, 1448–1454.

Foldvary-Schaefer, N., De Leon Sanchez, I., Karafa, M., Mascha, E., Dinner, D., & Morris, H. H. (2002). Gabapentin increases slow-wave sleep in normal adults. *Epilepsia, 43*, 1493–1497.

Furieri, F. A., & Nakamura-Palacios, E. M. (2007). Gabapentin reduces alcohol consumption and craving: a randomized, double-blind, placebo-controlled trial. *Journal of Clinical Psychiatry, 68*, 1691–1700.

Gunja, N. (2013). The clinical and forensic toxicology of Z-drugs. *Journal of Medical Toxicology, 9*, 155–162.

Gray, S. L., Dublin, S., Yu, O., Walker, R., Anderson, M., Hubbard, R. A., . . . & Larson, E. B. (2016). Benzodiazepine use and risk of incident dementia or cognitive decline: Prospective population based study. *British Medical Journal, 352*, i90.

Hahn, K., Arendt, G., Braun, J. S., von Giesen, H. J., Husstedt, I. W., Maschke, M., . . . & German Neuro-AIDS Working Group. (2004). A placebo-controlled trial of gabapentin for painful HIV-associated sensory neuropathies. *Journal of Neurology, 251*, 1260–1266.

Harris, J., Lack, L., Kemp, K., Wright, H., & Bootzin, R. (2012). A randomized controlled trial of intensive sleep retraining (ISR): A brief conditioning treatment for chronic insomnia. *Sleep, 35*, 49–60.

Harvey, A. G., Bélanger, L., Talbot, L., Eidelman, P., Beaulieu-Bonneau, S., Fortier-Brochu, É., . . . & Mérette, C. (2014). Comparative efficacy of behavior therapy, cognitive therapy, and cognitive behavior therapy for chronic insomnia: A randomized controlled trial. *Journal of Consulting and Clinical Psychology, 82*, 670–683.

Herring, W. J., Connor, K. M., Ivgy-May, N., Snyder, E., Liu, K., Snavely, D. B., . . . & Sangal, R. B. (2016). Suvorexant in patients with insomnia: Results from two 3-month randomized controlled clinical trials. *Biological Psychiatry, 79*, 136–148.

Hindmarch, I., Dawson, J., & Stanley, N. (2005). A double-blind study in healthy volunteers to assess the effects on sleep of pregabalin compared with alprazolam and placebo. *Sleep, 28*, 187–193.

Holbrook, A. M., Crowther, R., Lotter, A., Cheng, C., & King, D. (2000). Meta-analysis of benzodiazepine use in the treatment of insomnia. *Canadian Medical Association Journal, 162*, 225–233.

Huedo-Medina, T. B., Kirsch, I., Middlemass, J., Klonizakis, M., & Siriwardena, A. N. (2012). Effectiveness of non-benzodiazepine hypnotics in treatment of adult insomnia: Meta-analysis of data submitted to the Food and Drug Administration. *British Medical Journal, 345*, e8343.

Irwin, M. R., Cole, J. C., & Nicassio, P. M. (2006). Comparative meta-analysis of behavioral interventions for insomnia and their efficacy in middle-aged adults and in older adults 55+ years of age. *Health Psychology, 25*, 3–14.

Jacobs, G. D., Pace-Schott, E. F., Stickgold, R., & Otto, M. W. (2004). Cognitive behavior therapy and pharmacotherapy for insomnia: A randomized controlled trial and direct comparison. *Archives of Internal Medicine, 164*, 1888–1896.

Jindal, R. D., & Thase, M. E. (2004). Treatment of insomnia associated with clinical depression. *Sleep Medicine Reviews, 8*, 19–30.

Katz, D. A., & McHorney, C. A. (2002). The relationship between insomnia and health-related quality of life in patients with chronic illness. *Journal of Family Practice, 51*(3), 229–236.

Koffel, E. A., Koffel, J. B., & Gehrman, P. R. (2015). A meta-analysis of group cognitive behavioral therapy for insomnia. *Sleep Medicine Reviews, 19*, 6–16.

Krystal, A. D., Erman, M., Zammit, G. K., Soubrane, C., & Roth, T. (2008). Long-term efficacy and safety of zolpidem extended-release 12.5 mg, administered 3 to 7 nights per week for 24 weeks, in patients with chronic primary insomnia: A 6-month, randomized, double-blind, placebo-controlled, parallel-group, multicenter study. *Sleep, 31*, 79–90.

Kuriyama, A., Honda, M., & Hayashino, Y. (2014). Ramelteon for the treatment of insomnia in adults: A systematic review and meta-analysis. *Sleep Medicine, 15*, 385–392.

Levenson, J. C., Kay, D. B., & Buysse, D. J. (2015). The pathophysiology of insomnia. *CHEST Journal, 147*, 1179–1192.

Lichstein, K. L., & Riedel, B. W. (1994). Behavioral assessment and treatment of insomnia: A review with an emphasis on clinical application. *Behavior Therapy, 25*, 659–688.

Lichstein, K. L., Riedel, B. W., Wilson, N. M., Lester, K. W., & Aguillard, R. N. (2001). Relaxation and sleep compression for late-life insomnia: A placebo-controlled trial. *Journal of Consulting and Clinical Psychology, 69*, 227–239.

Liu, J., & Wang, L. N. (2012). Ramelteon in the treatment of chronic insomnia: Systematic review and meta-analysis. *International Journal of Clinical Practice, 66*, 867–873.

López-Muñoz, F., Ucha-Udabe, R., & Alamo, C. (2005). The history of barbiturates a century after their clinical introduction. *Neuropsychiatric Disease and Treatment, 1*, 329–343.

Loprinzi, P. D., & Cardinal, B. J. (2011). Association between objectively-measured physical activity and sleep, NHANES 2005–2006. *Mental Health and Physical Activity, 4*, 65–69.

McCall, C., & McCall, W. V. (2012). What is the role of sedating antidepressants, antipsychotics, and anticonvulsants in the management of insomnia? *Current Psychiatry Reports, 14*, 494–502.

Means, M. K., Lichstein, K. L., Epperson, M. T., & Johnson, C. T. (2000). Relaxation therapy for insomnia: Nighttime and day time effects. *Behaviour Research and Therapy, 38*, 665–678.

Michelson, D., Snyder, E., Paradis, E., Chengan-Liu, M., Snavely, D. B., Hutzelmann, J., . . . & Lines, C. (2014). Safety and efficacy of suvorexant during 1-year treatment of insomnia with subsequent abrupt treatment discontinuation: A phase 3 randomised, double-blind, placebo-controlled trial. *The Lancet Neurology, 13*, 461–471.

Monti, J. M., & Monti, D. (2000). Histamine H1 receptor antagonists in the treatment of insomnia. *CNS Drugs, 13*, 87–96.

Morin, C. M., & Benca, R. (2012). Chronic insomnia. *The Lancet, 379*(9821), 1129–1141.

Morin, C. M., Bootzin, R. R., Buysse, D. J., Edinger, J. D., Espie, C. A., & Lichstein, K. L. (2006). Psychological and behavioral treatment of insomnia: Update of the recent evidence (1998–2004). *Sleep, 29*, 1398–1414.

Morin, C. M., Colecchi, C., Stone, J., Sood, R., & Brink, D. (1999). Behavioral and pharmacological therapies for late-life insomnia: A randomized controlled trial. *JAMA, 281*, 991–999.

Morin, C. M., Vallières, A., Guay, B., Ivers, H., Savard, J., Mérette, C., . . . & Baillargeon, L. (2009). Cognitive behavioral therapy, singly and combined with medication, for persistent insomnia: A randomized controlled trial. *JAMA, 301*, 2005–2015.

Nicassio, P. M., Boylan, M. B., & McCabe, T. G. (1982). Progressive relaxation, EMG biofeedback and biofeedback placebo in the treatment of sleep-onset insomnia. *British Journal of Medical Psychology, 55*, 159–166.
Nicholson, A. N., Pascoe, P. A., & Stone, B. M. (1985). Histaminergic systems and sleep: Studies in man with HI and H2 antagonists. *Neuropharmacology, 24*, 245–250.
Okajima, I., Komada, Y., & Inoue, Y. (2011). A meta-analysis on the treatment effectiveness of cognitive behavioral therapy for primary insomnia. *Sleep and Biological Rhythms, 9*, 24–34.
Omvik, S., Sivertsen, B., Pallesen, S., Bjorvatn, B., Havik, O. E., & Nordhus, I. H. (2008). Daytime functioning in older patients suffering from chronic insomnia: Treatment outcome in a randomized controlled trial comparing CBT with zopiclone. *Behaviour Research and Therapy, 46*, 623–641.
Paterniti, S., Dufouil, C., & Alpérovitch, A. (2002). Long-term benzodiazepine use and cognitive decline in the elderly: The Epidemiology of Vascular Aging Study. *Journal of Clinical Psychopharmacology, 22*, 285–293.
Perlis, M. L., McCall, W. V., Krystal, A. D., & Walsh, J. K. (2004). Long-term, non-nightly administration of zolpidem in the treatment of patients with primary insomnia. *Journal of Clinical Psychiatry, 65*, 1–478.
Qaseem, A., Kansagara, D., Forciea, M., Cooke, M., & Denberg, T. (2016). Management of chronic insomnia disorder in adults. *Annuals of Internal Medicine, 165*, 125–133.
Rice, A. S. C., Maton, S., & Group1UK, P. N. S. (2001). Gabapentin in postherpetic neuralgia: A randomised, double blind, placebo controlled study. *Pain, 94*, 215–224.
Rickels, K., Case, W. G., Downing, R. W., & Winokur, A. (1983). Long-term diazepam therapy and clinical outcome. *JAMA, 250*, 767–771.
Risberg, A. M., Risberg, J., & Ingvar, D. H. (1975). Effects of promethazine on nocturnal sleep in normal man. *Psychopharmacologia, 43*, 279–284.
Roth, T. (2007). Insomnia: definition, prevalence, etiology, and consequences. *Journal of Clinical Sleep Medicine, 3*(5 Suppl), S7.
Roth, A. J., McCall, W. V., & Liguori, A. (2011). Cognitive, psychomotor and polysomnographic effects of trazodone in primary insomniacs. *Journal of Sleep Research, 20*, 552–558.
Ruigt, G. S. F., Kemp, B., Groenhout, C. M., & Kamphuisen, H. A. C. (1990). Effect of the antidepressant Org 3770 on human sleep. *European Journal of Clinical Pharmacology, 38*, 551–554.
Rush, A. J., Armitage, R., Gillin, J. C., Yonkers, K. A., Winokur, A., Moldofsky, H., . . . & Erman, M. K. (1998). Comparative effects of nefazodone and fluoxetine on sleep in outpatients with major depressive disorder. *Biological Psychiatry, 44*, 3–14.
Saletu, B., Grünberger, J., Krupka, M., & Schuster, P. (1987). Comparative double-blind, placebo-controlled sleep laboratory studies of a combination of lorazepam and diphenhydramine (SM-1014) and its single components. *Current Therapeutic Research, 42*, 1037–1058.
Sasseville, A., Paquet, N., Sévigny, J., & Hébert, M. (2006). Blue blocker glasses impede the capacity of bright light to suppress melatonin production. *Journal of Pineal Research, 41*, 73–78.
Scharf, M. B., Hirschowitz, J., Zemlan, F. P., Lichstein, M., & Woods, M. (1986). Comparative effects of limbitrol and amitriptyline on sleep efficiency and architecture. *Journal of Clinical Psychiatry, 47*, 587–591.
Seyffert, M., Lagisetty, P., Landgraf, J., Chopra, V., Pfeiffer, P. N., Conte, M. L., & Rogers, M. A. (2016). Internet-delivered cognitive behavioral therapy to treat insomnia: A systematic review and meta-analysis. *PloS One, 11*, 1–21.

Shahid, A., Chung, S. A., Phillipson, R., & Shapiro, C. M. (2012). An approach to long-term sedative-hypnotic use. *Nature and Science of Sleep, 4*, 53–61.

Shash, D., Kurth, T., Bertrand, M., Dufouil, C., Barberger-Gateau, P., Berr, C., . . . & Tzourio, C. (2015). Benzodiazepine, psychotropic medication, and dementia: A population-based cohort study. *Alzheimer's and Dementia, 12*, 604–613

Shipley, J. E., Kupfer, D. J., Griffin, S. J., Dealy, R. S., Coble, P. A., McEachran, A. B., . . . & Perel, J. M. (1985). Comparison of effects of desipramine and amitriptyline on EEG sleep of depressed patients. *Psychopharmacology, 85*, 14–22.

Singer, C. (2011). Placebo-controlled trial of quetiapine for sleep disturbance in AD. *Alzheimer's and Dementia, 7*, S773.

Sivertsen, B., Omvik, S., Pallesen, S., Bjorvatn, B., Havik, O. E., Kvale, G., . . . & Nordhus, I. H. (2006). Cognitive behavioral therapy vs zopiclone for treatment of chronic primary insomnia in older adults: A randomized controlled trial. *JAMA, 295*, 2851–2858.

Spielman, A. J. (1986). Assessment of insomnia. *Clinical Psychology Review, 6*, 11–25.

Sudak, D. M., Kloss, J., & Zamzow, J. (2014). Integration of cognitive-behavioral therapy and pharmacotherapy in the treatment of insomnia. *International Journal of Cognitive Therapy, 7*, 162–174.

Trauer, J. M., Qian, M. Y., Doyle, J. S., Rajaratnam, S. M., & Cunnington, D. (2015). Cognitive behavioral therapy for chronic insomnia: A systematic review and meta-analysis. *Annals of Internal Medicine, 163*, 191–204.

Vallières, A., Morin, C. M., & Guay, B. (2005). Sequential combinations of drug and cognitive behavioral therapy for chronic insomnia: An exploratory study. *Behaviour Research and Therapy, 43*, 1611–1630.

Vallières, A., Morin, C. M., Guay, B., Bastien, C. H., & LeBlanc, M. (2004). Sequential treatment for chronic insomnia: A pilot study. *Behavioral Sleep Medicine, 2*, 94–112.

Ware, J. C., Brown, F. W., Moorad, P. J., & Pittard, J. T. (1989). Effects on sleep: A double-blind study comparing trimipramine to imipramine in depressed insomniac patients. *Sleep: Journal of Sleep Research and Sleep Medicine, 12*, 537–549.

Winkler, A., Auer, C., Doering, B. K., & Rief, W. (2014). Drug treatment of primary insomnia: A meta-analysis of polysomnographic randomized controlled trials. *CNS Drugs, 28*, 799–816.

World Health Organization (1993). *The ICD-10 classification of mental and behavioural disorders: Diagnostic criteria for research*. Geneva: World Health Organization.

Wu, J. Q., Appleman, E. R., Salazar, R. D., & Ong, J. C. (2015). Cognitive behavioral therapy for insomnia comorbid with psychiatric and medical conditions: A meta-analysis. *JAMA Internal Medicine, 175*, 1461–1472.

Wu, R., Bao, J., Zhang, C., Deng, J., & Long, C. (2006). Comparison of sleep condition and sleep-related psychological activity after cognitive-behavior and pharmacological therapy for chronic insomnia. *Psychotherapy and Psychosomatics, 75*, 220–228.

Zachariae, R., Lyby, M. S., Ritterband, L. M., & O'Toole, M. S. (2016). Efficacy of internet-delivered cognitive-behavioral therapy for insomnia—A systematic review and meta-analysis of randomized controlled trials. *Sleep Medicine Reviews, 30*, 1–10.

9

Somatoform Disorders: Evidence-Based Integrated Biopsychosocial Treatment of Chronic, Persistent, Nonmalignant Pain

Douglas E. DeGood, Robert M. Julien, and Catherine A. DeGood

Current estimates suggest that more than 100 million Americans are currently suffering from pain (Califf, Woodcock, & Ostroff, 2016) and 9 million to 12 million of these have chronic or persistent pain. Indeed, 42% of US households report one or more persons with chronic pain, with about half of these individuals failing to achieve adequate pain relief. Over the past half-century, research and treatments have led to a significant increase in the incidence of pain, resulting in many books, research journals, and facilities dedicated to a better understanding of this problem. Yet, the problem of suffering from persistent pain continues.

It goes without saying that there really is no such thing as "benign" pain. To the person suffering from pain, no pain is "benign"; all pain is real, no matter the cause or origin. Nonetheless, benign pain refers to pain of either physical, noncancerous origin (e.g., arthritic diseases, musculoskeletal chronic back pain) or pain for which no clear organic cause can be elucidated, such as so called "psychogenic" pain or somatoform disorder. Successful treatment of most persistent pain can benefit from a multitiered approach that aims for integration of the pharmacological and nonpharmacological. Unfortunately, all too often medical personnel rely primarily on medication prescription, especially on prescription of opioid analgesics.[1] These range from relatively mild agents (e.g., tramadol), to potent, frequently addicting, agents (e.g., hydrocodone, oxycodone, morphine). Here, we will present evidence of the efficacy of narcotic and nonnarcotic pharmacological agents used in the treatment of benign pain, while highlighting issues of safety and pointing out their limitations. In this same vein, we will also present the efficacy and applicability of nonpharmacological psychosocial interventions in the treatment of this special patient population. It is assumed that even nonprescribers working in the field of pain management need to have some basic knowledge of pharmacological interventions, at least to the point where they can be integrated into a plan of comprehensive care, combining prescribed agents with nonpharmacological interventions. An example of such a need is found in the February 2016 initiative by the US Food and Drug Administration (FDA) to introduce sweeping new changes to opioid prescribing policies in an attempt to stem the tide of opioid use and opioid-related fatalities (Alford, 2016; Califf et al., 2016; Dart et al., 2015); such a proactive response to prescription abuse

Cognitive Behavioral Psychopharmacology: The Clinical Practice of Evidence-Based Biopsychosocial Integration, First Edition. Edited by Mark Dana Muse.

requires the awareness of all professionals involved in the treatment of chronic pain: prescriber and nonprescribing therapist. It also should be mentioned here that it is very difficult to evaluate the integration of medications and behavioral-based treatments for chronic pain, because the bulk of research comes from multidisciplinary pain centers where the treatments are seldom limited solely to medication or psychosocial interventions. Often patients in the pain clinic setting receive many other medical procedures as well as physical therapy and other supportive therapies, making it difficult to isolate the specific effects of individual components of the treatment package.

Acute versus Chronic Pain

Chronic pain, unlike acute pain, lasts beyond the usual time course for the normal healing process. Often the level of tissue pathology appears insufficient to explain the extent and/or presence of the ongoing pain. Seemingly, the pain has become the disease itself, requiring treatment as much as any underlying tissue pathology. It tends to persist over time and become increasingly resistant to medical treatment, and can ultimately cause dramatic and disruptive psychosocial consequences for the patient and family.

While chronic pain may be present without an identifiable cause, it may also accompany a known disease process such as degenerative spinal disc disease, rheumatoid arthritis, and many other myofascial and neuropathic syndromes. But when patients with such diagnoses are referred to tertiary pain centers, it is usually an indication of atypical difficulty with managing the associated pain.

The transition from acute to chronic pain appears to occur in three identifiable stages:

Stage 1 occurs when one becomes fearful that the pain will never end. The result may be the development of a state of anxiety and worry that is frequently treated with tranquilizing benzodiazepines and sleep agents. While short-term treatment with such drugs may be defensible, longer-term use almost invariably leads to dependency and other complications. For example, benzodiazepine prescriptions and abuse fatalities have increased considerably from 1996 through 2013 (Bachhuber, Hennessy, Cunningham, & Starrels, 2016). Drastically needed are new interventions to reduce benzodiazepine use or improve their safety. By the numbers, in 2013 an estimated 22,767 persons died of an overdose involving prescription drugs in the United States. Benzodiazepines were involved in approximately 31% of these fatal overdoses.

Stage 2 develops when poorly treated pain persists, and initial worry and frustration lead to learned helplessness (depression), preoccupation with symptoms and symptom magnification, often accompanied by sedative and opioid dependency. A corollary at this stage is the development of anger-generated distrust and feelings of entitlement.

Stage 3 enters into a true medical crisis that leads to the acceptance of a "sick" role that exempts the patient from normal responsibilities and obligations. Use of healthcare resources continues to increase during this final stage, and there is often a further escalation of maladaptive health behaviors such as increases in alcohol, opioid, and tobacco use, poor diet/weight concerns, and a lack of social and physical activities.

The Mind/Body Dilemma and Psychogenic Pain

All healthcare professionals working with chronic pain patients need to be sensitive to the potential for misunderstanding and misuse of a diagnostic label such as "psychogenic pain." With a psychogenic pain diagnosis the complex etiology of the pain sensation can be easily oversimplified and misconstrued (DeGood, 1983). Psychogenic pain is usually defined as physical pain that is caused, increased, or prolonged by mental, emotional, or behavioral factors. However, all too often after acquiring such a diagnostic label the patient is stigmatized as having pain that is "imaginary." This reaction represents a misleading dualistic separation of mind versus body. From a dualistic perspective, pain must either be somatic or psychic in origin, which quickly translates into artificial notions of "real" versus "not real" pain.

In short, the purpose of a psychosocial evaluation of the chronic pain patient is not concerned with determination of a mind versus bodily source of pain. Rather, the purpose of the evaluation is to identify as many factors as possible—physical, environmental, and psychological—which may be contributing to the persistent experience of pain.

The Biopsychosocial Model of Chronic Pain

The biopsychosocial approach to chronic pain (e.g., Gatchel, Howard, & Kishino, 2008) attempts to integrate the biological basis of pain with psychological (individual cognitions and emotions) and environmental social factors (e.g., family/friends, workplace, community). The model redefines nociceptive pain (acute tissue damage) as *disease* and chronic pain as an *illness*. Disease is considered an objective biological event involving body or organ system dysfunction, similar to the events associated with acute pain. Illness, in contrast, refers to a subjective experience or self-attribution that a disease is present. Illness also refers to how a sick person and his/her social support system live and respond to symptoms of pain and disability. Illness is characterized by the degree of suffering and intensity of observable pain-related behaviors. If one accepts this holistic biopsychosocial conceptualization of chronic pain, it becomes obvious that to manage chronic pain medical interventions must be integrated with psychosocial approaches.

Psychosocial Treatment for Pain

There is little mystery about what constitutes pharmacological treatment of pain, for analgesics have been used for this very purpose for millennia. On the other hand, what actually constitutes the psychosocial side of the integrated pain management equation is, perhaps, less obvious. A psychosocial intervention may involve addressing multiple personal and environmental factors tied to pain—educating the family about pain, encouraging modification in the work place, advice-giving in dealing with financial matters, teaching new behaviors for coping with pain, and, of course, addressing cognitive and mood disturbances that may accompany persistent pain. A psychosocial

Brief History of Multidisciplinary Biopsychosocial Management of Chronic Pain Treatment

Contemporary approaches to the treatment of chronic pain began in the mid-20th century at the University of Washington School of Medicine in Seattle. The key personalities were John Bonica, an anesthesiologist, John Loeser, a neurosurgeon, and Wilbert Fordyce, a clinical psychologist. The use of regional anesthetic injections for treatment of chronic pain, in so called "nerve block clinics," had become increasing commonplace after the end of World War II. But Dr. Bonica took pain management a step further. He initiated the study and treatment of pain as a multidisciplinary field (Bonica, 1953, 1990). He envisioned that a team approach, incorporating various specialties, would be the best way to move forward in pain management. The clinic he, Dr. Loeser, and Dr. Fordyce established at the University of Washington in the early 1970s is considered the first multidisciplinary pain center. Recognizing the psychosocial component of chronic pain, Fordyce (1976) conceptualized and elaborated the concept of "pain behaviors." He made the observation "that pain problems are signaled by the behavior of the patient" (Fordyce, 1984). One may be experiencing severe sensory nociceptive discomfort, but without visible or audible pain behaviors from the suffering person there is no communication of pain and thus no publically recognizable pain problem. He argued that these "operant pain behaviors" in turn are subject to the same factors that influence all operant behaviors. Thus, once a pain problem develops, and associated pain behaviors are emitted, it becomes inevitable that the behaviors will be further shaped by environmental contingencies. There may be direct positive benefits in the form of sympathy and financial compensation, or more subtle rewards in the form of reduction of responsibility, or avoidance of aversive working conditions. Of course, there may also be many aversive consequences, especially in the form of loss of income and general functioning. Continuing pursuit of pain relief through medical interventions may have mixed positive and negative consequences. Surgeries, injections, and pills may all provide the temporary reward of pain relief, but if long-term treatment benefits cannot be maintained, eventually greater suffering may result.

The Fordyce-led inpatient pain management program attempted to directly manipulate the contingency management of pain behaviors within the hospital environment. Active participation was required from the patient, rather than lying in bed waiting to be "cured" from pain. Attempts were made to apply behavioral contingency management principles to (1) appropriate analgesic medication use, (2) exercise and rest arrangements, and (3) attention and social feedback. Limited analgesic medication was delivered on a time contingent basis, rather than in response to complaints of pain, that is, pain behaviors. Reasonable exercise quotas were established for each patient, with rest contingent on achieving the quota rather than exercise to tolerance (i.e., pain tolerance). Quotas were gradually increased. As much as feasible, treatment staff members provided attention to performance of assigned treatment tasks, rather than to complaints of pain and suffering. Similarly, management of home behavioral contingency strategies was discussed with visiting family members.

The Fordyce behavioral contingency principles were adopted by many of the 1970s inpatient multidisciplinary programs. Although conceptualized as operant behavioral programs, they were, in fact, what today we would call a "cognitive-behavioral" therapy program. In addition to a direct effort to suppress exaggerated pain behavior and reward specific coping behaviors, there was a major cognitive educative component. Through individual and group discussions, faulty beliefs about pain and its treatment were addressed. Also, attention was given to addressing numerous other psychosocial factors at home and in the workplace that may be inadvertently supporting increased pain behavior.

intervention may consist largely of an attempt to educate the patient as to the nature of chronic pain and its treatment, or it may be much more specific to the unique problems faced by the individual. Formal individual or group counseling may consist of a range of psychotherapy strategies, but today most psychotherapeutic interventions are referred to as cognitive-behavioral therapy (CBT).

Clearly there is no single protocol or specific technique that defines CBT. One common CBT strategy applied to pain management is the teaching of behavioral self-generated relaxation skills via attention-focused meditation, slow-deep breath control, progressive muscle relaxation, and occasionally directed hypnosis. Such behavioral strategies can have both direct physiologic and psychic calming effects, which may result in a downturn in pain perception. Patients are encouraged to practice reliance on this type of "self-calming" in the face of stressors, including the stress of pain. Some therapist may conduct relaxation training sessions with the aid of biofeedback. Biofeedback involves electronic physiological monitoring of autonomic and central nervous system parameters such as muscle tension, skin conductance, heart rate, and brain waves. The purpose of the biofeedback monitoring is to provide direct physiological information (i.e., feedback) during the self-relaxation training. Biofeedback is not a medical treatment *per se* because it does not in itself do anything to the body; rather, it is a teaching aid to help the patient learn the self-regulation skills.

At a superficial level, the psychosocial side of pain treatment looks very much like any other counseling services. Patients participate individually and/or in groups with therapists, usually trained as clinical psychologists/counselors, social workers, or psychiatric nurses. As one might expect, much of the discussion centers on the patient's view of his or her pain problem and the resultant worries and fears that plague the patient and family. Reactions of frustration, anger, and depression are explored in detail. But there are distinct differences from the typical symptom-oriented counseling seen in mental health clinics, because in a pain clinic the presenting symptoms are seldom voiced directly in terms of cognitive or emotional concerns, but rather as physical pain concerns.

For psychotherapists working with this particular patient population, a certain amount of specialized knowledge is required to connect, and to be accepted as credible. Beyond standard mental health-focused information, effective CBT pain therapists should acquire additional knowledge about the medical aspects, both diagnostic and therapeutic, of pain. In their role as patient educators, they need to become familiar with the pros and cons of various surgical, injection, drug, and physical/exercise therapies. They need to be able to present not just the benefit/risk ratios of various treatments, but also the "whys" of these ratios, in terms that are understandable to the patient. For example, one should be able to discuss the neurochemical processes involved in how/why opioid tolerance and dependency develops. This includes how externally administered opioids suppress the production of natural endorphin analgesic substances, and trigger a down-regulation in the number of receptors to opioid-related molecules. Thus, one can explain drug rebound effects: when the relief from the most recent pill begins to wear off, the patient may feel worse pain than he or she did before treatment began. Also useful is an understanding of how workers' compensation, social security disability, and other forms of medical insurance operate. Patients need to understand fully how the medical insurance and disability insurance systems work because such financial concerns are common stressors for these individuals, and potentially lead to dysfunctional reinforcement contingencies.

The need for treatment staff members to address patients' maladaptive beliefs and expectations, as well as providing basic information about pain and its treatment, cannot be overemphasized. It is not uncommon, despite reporting multiple prior radiologic studies, invasive treatment failures, multiple medication trials, and lengthy periods of rest and inactivity, for patients to expect, and sometimes plaintively demand, more of the same failed efforts. Recommendations for conservative alternatives to surgery and medications will frequently be met with skepticism and disappointment, if not anger. In a similar vein, too often patients, sometimes with considerable justification, complain that no one had ever explained anything understandable to them about the cause of their pain problem. Thus, the patient, prior to entering the pain clinic, has felt compelled to persist in a desperate search for a doctor who "will just tell me what is wrong."

Frequently linked with a misplaced faith in medical (i.e., pharmacologic and surgical) interventions as the answer to all pain concerns is a passive acceptance of the "sick role" while waiting to be "cured." This passive attitude may include the belief that "staying off one's feet" or "bed rest" is essential, rather than active participation in physical therapy and exercise programs. Weight gain, further fitness deterioration, and depression (feelings of helplessness and hopelessness) are often the result. A fear that pain associated with activity is a sign of more damage can be pervasive, but can be modified by a discussion of "good vs. bad pain," and carefully supervised gradual increases in exercise to tolerance can be reframed in a positive, encouraging manner. Movement tolerance can also be facilitated by anticipating task requirements in advance and pacing oneself accordingly. Strategic use of stretching, rest–activity cycles, balance training, and limiting excessive bracing and guarding postures are just a few of the specific strategies that can further counter passivity and associated feelings of helplessness in the face of pain.

There is ample empirical evidence that maladaptive pain information and beliefs are predictive of moving from acute injury to chronic pain (Young Casey, Greenberg, Nicassio, Harpin, & Hubbard, 2008), and once chronicity has set in, the patients' level of physical disability and depression increase (Turner, Jensen, & Romano, 2000). Since such beliefs can directly impact how an individual behaviorally copes with pain, it is not surprising that maladaptive cognitions predict poor response to pain treatment (DeGood & Kiernan, 1997; Shutty, DeGood, & Hoekstra-Tuttle, 1990); alterations in such beliefs during treatment discriminate between good and poor outcomes (Jensen, Turner, & Romono, 2007). For example, the more an individual holds onto a belief that pain always signals physical harm and is necessarily uncontrollable and disabling, the poorer the treatment outcome (Roth & Geisser, 2002).

A cognitive research dimension closely related to addressing maladaptive beliefs has centered on the constructs of *catastrophizing* and *readiness to change.* Pain catastrophizing reflects an exaggerated helpless and hopeless response to the experience of pain. A heightened level of catastrophizing has been associated with many variables reflecting poor adjustment to pain, including psychological distress, poor response to treatment, more disability, and greater pain intensity (Keefe, Lefebvre, & Smith, 1999). Readiness to change, as measured by the Pain Stages of Change Questionnaire (Kerns, Rosenberg, Jamison, Caudill, & Haythornwaite, 1997), identifies patient cognitions that reflect how ready the patient is to work within a behavioral rehabilitation approach to pain management. In a study of 109 chronic pain patients participating in CBT treatment, the 50 patients who dropped out had significantly lower "Readiness" scores relative to patients who completed the treatment (Kerns & Rosenberg, 1999). Also pre-to-post increases in Readiness scores were associated with improved outcomes. Detailed descriptions and related research of numerous psychometric scales that have been developed for measuring these various dimensions of pain beliefs and coping strategies can be found in DeGood and Cook (2011).

Sleep is another concern that is often addressed in CBT therapy with chronic pain patients. Morin, Gibson, and Wade (1998) surveyed 105 consecutive patients referred to a multidisciplinary outpatient pain clinic about their quality of sleep. Two-thirds of the sample indicated significant difficulties initiating and maintaining sleep. There is a modest amount of clinical trial literature suggesting that the relationship between pain and poor sleep is reciprocal and that CBT intervention for pain or insomnia holds promise in reducing pain and improving sleep (Smith & Haythornthwaite, 2004), although the nature of pain-related sleep disturbance remains poorly defined (Bjurstrom & Irwin, 2016). Certainly inadequate sleep can confound coping with pain, and contribute to reductions in daytime cognitive alertness and behavioral functioning. Sedative/hypnotic sleep aids may be necessary during flare ups of pain, although the use of such sleep aids must be employed with caution given the risk of overdose, especially if the patient is already taking respiratory suppressing opioids and/or any other sedative/hypnotics. Therefore, before starting any pharmacological sleep aid it is critical that respiratory apnea be ruled out as a contributing factor to disturbed sleep. Finally, the inclusion of CBT-based instruction in understanding and improving sleep skills may be helpful. As with pain, presenting relevant information and instruction in self-controlled, cognitive-behavioral relaxation are commonly employed strategies in addressing insomnia. The person with chronic pain should understand how excess time spent in bed, or in otherwise prolonged inactivity, can disturb normal sleep cycles and lead to excessive sleep fragmentation. The patient must be dissuaded from the belief that the only good night of sleep is one that is free of awakenings. In fact, some individuals with chronic pain may do better with modifications of sleep schedules and sleep positions. For example, for those with severe low back pain, getting up every 2 or 3 h for a brief movement or stretching routine may actually improve their overall sleep experience.

In short, a patient's beliefs and expectations about pain and sleep and its treatment have a great deal to do with how people manage their pain and its consequences. In fact, the psychology of pain management is not primarily about reducing the sensory dimension of pain, but instead about trying to influence how people perceive and cope with their pain. If maladaptive beliefs directly influence coping, such beliefs should not be viewed simply as artifacts of the chronic pain experience that will disappear once a correct medical diagnosis and treatment is initiated. Rather, maladaptive cognitions and corresponding poor coping lie at the heart of the chronic pain problem.

Addressing the psychosocial dimensions of pain management is not just the task of psychotherapists in a chronic pain treatment facility. It must be a consistent message from all biopsychosocially oriented staff. This includes not only the professional staff, but also the office staff members who handle phone calls and schedule appointments. The message should never be presented in a dictatorial or punitive manner, but presented as information that is in the best interest of the patient.

Hypnotism, which clearly falls under the CBT rubric, deserves a brief mention here. Hypnosis for pain control has a strong foundation in the experimental literature, (e.g., Montgomery, DuHamel, & Redd, 2000; Patterson & Jensen, 2003), as well as numerous anecdotal reports. Hypnotically induced analgesia can be particularly dramatic following acute injury or during painful medical or dental procedures, where participants successfully hypnotized can experience a remarkable freedom from pain. Likewise, hypnosis can be used to create a highly relaxed cognitive-emotional state with focused attention that can help cope with chronic pain, especially for patients who can learn self-hypnosis. When successful with chronic pain, the key element is the ability of the patient to learn and then apply self-induced hypnotic analgesia as a behavioral coping skill in nearly any situation. However, the response to hypnotic analgesic suggestions can be quite unpredictable and for some individuals the term has a highly negative connotation. Furthermore, some patients report having bad experiences with hypnosis, particularly with exacerbation of anxiety and the triggering of unwanted or false memories. Granted that in the hands of a skilled hypnotist, knowledgeable about its use in pain management, hypnosis can be a useful tool in the teaching of pain coping, most pain management therapists prefer the less controversial route of teaching cognitive and physiologic relaxation via instruction in general muscle relaxation, breath control, positive imagery/visualization, and attention control (meditative) techniques, with or without the aid of biofeedback.

Evaluating Efficacy of Pain Treatments

Before we consider the evidence regarding the effectiveness of pharmacological and non-pharmacological treatments of chronic pain, there is a need to address the problem of gathering such empirical information. Many of the problems encountered in evaluating pain treatments are common to all treatment outcome research, but challenges are further multiplied when one looks at a phenomenon as amorphous as the experience of pain.

An immediate problem encountered in the evaluation of pain treatment outcomes is the fact that there is no truly objective way to measure pain. Pain is always a subjective individual perception and can only be quantified via self-report (usually a 10-point rating scale) or monitoring of behaviors that are indicative of pain.[2]

While self-reported pain relief is clearly an important outcome variable, it cannot stand as the sole criterion of treatment outcome. Of equal importance is the outcome variable of *functioning*—that is, is there indication of an improvement in functioning? Several dimensions of functioning should be monitored. Examples are *cognition* (e.g., attention and concentration, clarity of thinking), *emotions* and *emotional control* (e.g., anxiety, depression, anger), and specific *target behaviors* of interest, (i.e., self-care, return to work, social interaction, exercise, sleep). What conclusion do we draw if the patient reports subjective pain relief, but fails to demonstrate any meaningful improvement in functioning; or, contrariwise, how do we explain the case where function improves but without acknowledgement of pain relief? Despite frequent discrepancy between different outcome indicators, the need for multidimensional assessment remains critical in the clinical setting, and even more so in the clinical research setting.

Pharmacological Treatments for Chronic Pain

The evidence that opioid medications can reduce acute pain is overwhelming, and their importance in the management of acute pain generates little controversy. Undoubtedly, these medications can also reduce chronic pain, but often at the price of creating dependency and addiction with extended use. Some have argued (e.g., Portenoy & Foley, 1986) that with careful monitoring these problems can be adequately managed in many patients. No doubt some individuals can take well-regulated amounts of narcotic medications for extended periods of time, demonstrate minimal side effects, and continue to experience a useful degree of pain relief, without requiring increasing amounts of the drug. However, there is abundant evidence that, for many patients, the risks stemming from long-term use are very high, with little lasting improvement in functioning (Manchikanti, Fellows, Ailinani, & Pampati, 2010).

Jamison et al. (2010) tested whether the numbers of patients that can be safely managed on long-term opioids can be increased with a behavioral intervention. These research clinicians randomized high-risk patients to either a psychological intervention to improve compliance or to a no-intervention control group. The intervention group received structured education and worksheets on opioid risk and individual motivational counseling, all aimed to limit patterns of misuse. The results were encouraging in that the intervention group patients reduced their level of misuse down to the level of a low-risk comparison group while the high-risk controls remained unchanged in their abuse pattern. A follow up study (Wasan et al., 2012) produced similar positive results with a cognitive-behavioral intervention program geared at controlling the craving for medication in patients treated with opioids. Such studies are impressive examples of the power of psychosocial CBT strategies to reduce opioid misuse, but these are costly, time-consuming interventions that can be employed only with a highly trained staff.

Studies like those mentioned above do illustrate that where it is deemed necessary and appropriate to use opioid medication on a long-term basis, there are behavioral guidelines that may help control the risk. Nonmedical counselors can play an important role in screening, explaining, and enforcing these guidelines. The first step is to screen carefully for a personal and family history of substance abuse and addictions. If this screen does not raise a red flag, a *drug contract* should be explained to, and signed by, the patient. Typically the contract specifies the amount of medication that will be prescribed for a given period of time. Opioids must be used only as prescribed and requests for early refills are not responded to. Also early refill requests based on lost, stolen, or damaged medication are not honored. Any violation of the contract will result in termination of the agreement (e.g., Fishman & Kreis, 2002; Hariharan, Lamb, & Neuner, 2007). This contract presents an upfront behavior challenge to the patient to use opioids only in appropriate fashion and, in so doing, to participate responsibly in his or her pain management. The contract should also spell out the potential side effects, including the development of tolerance and dependency, and the likelihood of serious withdrawal effects if the medication is discontinued.

The patient may have to go through a medically supervised detoxification to regain the analgesic benefits of a lower dose. Another strategy is to take regular "drug holidays" to limit the build of tolerance/dependency. Patients may agree to take narcotic medication for 4 or 5 working days, allowing them to maintain a regular work schedule, but then discontinue, or greatly reduce the medication for 2 or 3 weekend days. Other patients accomplish the same goal by consciously limiting their use of the narcotic to only 3 or 4 "worse" pain days during the week, but never taking it every day. Some are able to get more pain relief with fewer narcotics with the use of an implanted drug pump that delivers the medication directly to the sight of pain. However, it should be noted that research to date has not entirely clarified the benefit/risk ratio of the intrathecal opioid drug pump.

How Do We Achieve "Opioid Sparing"?

Opioid sparing (Julien, Advokat, & Comaty, 2011) is the process of achieving pain relief without reliance on opioids. To properly approach opioid sparing it is important to note the co-morbidity of pain, anxiety, depression, and perhaps anger or frustration in most chronic pain patients. To treat these emotional states or reactions, opioids are largely ineffective while antidepressants and antiepileptic "mood stabilizers" are vital. Indeed, the value of antidepressants and mood stabilizers lies in two areas:

1) They possess analgesic actions.
2) They treat symptoms that trigger, exacerbate, or compound the effects of pain; notably depression, anxiety, sleep disturbances, anger, and other states of neural arousal/excitation.

On the other hand, benzodiazepine, nonbenzodiazepine sedatives, and "muscle relaxants" (e.g., cyclobenzaprine (Flexeril)) are not analgesic and impair psychomotor performance. These agents dull mentation and also impair driving abilities, even at blood concentrations considered to be therapeutic. Lacking fundamental analgesic qualities, these sedatives have little place in chronic pain management, although they are almost universally prescribed.

In addition to use of an analgesic-promoting antidepressant, especially the tricyclic antidepressants (Jain & Jain, 2011), and mood stabilizers (notably gabapentin and pregabalin), medical marijuana is emerging as a plausible pharmacological addition to pain therapy. At least two alkaloids found in marijuana tetrahydrocannabidiol (THC) and cannabidiol (CBD) possess potent analgesic and anxiolytic actions. One of these exhibits psychedelic action (THC) that may limit its use in chronic pain management, but the other alkaloid (CBD) is devoid of psychedelic action, retaining analgesic and anxiolytic actions. Indeed, CBD may provide yet another option in minimizing the use of potent opioid analgesics. Much remains, however, to be determined in the use of cannabis for pain management, including development of delivery system such as oral products (e.g., capsules) of near-pure CBD (Fine & Rosenfeld, 2013). Already marketed in several countries (but not the United States) is Sativex®, a mixture of equal parts of THC and CBD. Sativex® is used in the treatment of pain associated with multiple sclerosis as well as in the treatment of suffering in patients with advanced cancer disorders. Sativex®'s analgesia, sedation, and action in decreasing nausea and vomiting are impressive (Canadian Agency for Drugs and Technologies in Health, 2016).

In order to pharmacologically treat chronic pain with minimal use of opioids, we propose a tiered, multilayer approach for chronic pain medication:

1) Initiate therapy with a nonsteroidal anti-inflammatory drug (NSAID), such as aspirin, ibuprofen, naproxen, or a miscellaneous analgesic such as acetaminophen.
2) Should NSAIDs be insufficient, consider adding a mood stabilizer in the form of an anticonvulsant-analgesic (e.g., gabapentin or pregabalin).
3) Also consider adding an antidepressant with norepinephrine activity (e.g., a tricyclic antidepressant such as nortriptyline or amitriptyline; or, alternatively serotonin norepinephrine reuptake inhibitors (SNRIs) such as duloxetine or venlafaxine).
4) Omega-3-polyunsaturated fatty acid has mild analgesic actions and can be used as an add-on augmenting agent (Julien et al., 2011), while CBD extracted from marijuana possesses analgesic action in the absence of psychoactive effects.
5) Finally, if pain is so severe or persistent that the above regimen proves insufficient, then, and only then, should an opioid be prescribed.

Opioid Analgesics as a Last Resort

Should severe pain continue despite all other attempts at therapy, opioid analgesics have a limited role and should be used with great caution in chronic, benign pain. In 2008, 1.9 million persons in the United States were dependent upon or abusing prescription opioids. The United States makes up 4.8% of the world's population, yet uses 80% of the global supply of opioids and 99% of the global supply of hydrocodone. Deaths from prescription opioids now exceed auto accidents as cause of accidental deaths, and prescription opioids take more lives than heroin and cocaine combined.

Medications that bind to morphine receptors in the nervous system are of three types: *pure agonists*, *partial agonists*, and *pure antagonists.* Pure agonists include the powerful opioids, including morphine, hydrocodone, oxycodone, hydromorphone, oxymorphone, methadone, and fentanyl (and its derivatives). Partial agonists bind to morphine receptors, but exert less stimulant action on these receptors. They are thought to produce a somewhat lower level of pain relief and have less of a propensity to produce respiratory depression. Examples include buprenorphine, tapendolol, and the opioid-like synthetic analgesic tramadol. Finally, there is a series of pure antagonists that bind to opioid receptors, yield no analgesic effects, and block access of strong opioids to their receptors. Examples include: naloxone, naltrexone, and nalmefene. All of these antagonists are capable of reversing opioid-induced analgesia and respiratory depression.

In the product combination buprenorphine/naloxone, the partial agonist buprenorphine is combined with the pure antagonist naloxone. Here, if used as prescribed as an under-the-tongue film, the buprenorphine is absorbed while the naloxone is swallowed and not absorbed. However, if crushed or injected, the naloxone reaches the blood stream and precipitates withdrawal. In general, this pharmacologic agent has proven to be clinically successful in patients desiring to minimize their opioid dependency by careful manipulation of the biologic receptor system prominent in abuse.

There are other newer buphrenorphine formulations on the market that may decrease diversion/abuse risk. Probuphine is the first buprenorphine implant for the maintenance treatment of opioid dependence. Probuphine is designed to provide a constant, low-level dose of buprenorphine for 6 months in patients who are already stable on low-to-moderate doses of other forms of buprenorphine. However, due to both the cost of the product and the need for a surgical implantation procedure this is currently an impractical option for most patients and providers. More practical are some of the newer sublingual formulations of bupreneorphine; several are FDA approved for opioid use disorder only, but may be used off label for pain. Two low-dose buprennorphine products that have been recently FDA approved for pain include a sublingual tab (BELBUCA®) and a low-dose patch (BuTrans®). Although there can be challenges with getting insurance coverage for these expensive products, they remain a good option in the chronic pain patient with a history of an addictive disorder requiring ongoing opioid management.

Methadone and buprenorphine are both opioids that have analgesic properties but are thought to be of lower risk for abuse. Thus, they are frequently used as substitutes for higher-risk opioid formulations for patients who are already opioid dependent. Indeed, many persons feel that both drugs are opioid antagonists. This notion is wrong. Methadone is a pure agonist opioid, like morphine or oxycodone. Its claim to fame, and utility, is that it has a long half-life (about 24 h) and is well absorbed orally. As a result, it is taken orally and substitutes for other, shorter-acting opioids that are often used by injection. In methadone-maintenance programs, methadone is used as a transition from other, short-acting pure opioids to a longer-acting, orally administered one. Methadone is no "safer" than other pure agonist opioids. Buprenorphine as a partial agonist is used as a step-down drug in those patients desiring to eventually become opioid-free. Unfortunately, despite its alleged safety margin compared to other opioid-containing substances, the recent increase in prescriptions of buprenorphrine has been accompanied by increased reports (e.g., Sontag, 2013) of dependency and abuse. It is the authors' recommendation that this drug not be started solely for pain control, but that it be limited to those pain patients presenting with a concurrent addiction problem. These drugs and other opioid issues are discussed thoroughly in Julien's *Primer of Drug Action* (Advokat, Comaty, & Julien, 2014).

Efficacy of CBT for Chronic Pain

Efficacy reports of CBT treatment for chronic pain, based on randomized controlled trials (RCTs), come from both studies of specific pain problems and studies from pain centers combining many different types of pain problems.

The earliest reports regarding the use of variations of CBT for persistent pain involved patient education and biofeedback-aided relaxation training for headache management (Blanchard et al., 1985). The superiority of CBT supported by biofeedback over medication alone was particularly impressive at a 5-year follow up (Blanchard, Appelbaum, Guarnieri, Morrill, & Dentinger, 1987). Seemingly, the benefits of patient-learned, self-regulation skills continue to grow over time. In a later review of multiple studies (Andrasik, 2007), it was noted that CBT with biofeedback reliably produced a 30–60% reduction in headache activities, and these benefits are sustained many years after treatment. Meta-analysis of headache studies provides similar support for the value of CBT with biofeedback (or some other form of behavioral relaxation training) on improving both tension and migraine headaches, including the frequency and duration of headaches, when compared with a variety of control conditions (Nestoriuc & Martin, 2007; Nestoriuc, Rief, & Martin, 2008). CBT with biofeedback was generally found to be superior to therapeutic modalities without biofeedback for the treatment of migraine headaches, but equivalent with nonbiofeedback relaxation training for tension headaches.

The headache effects of CBT are more pronounced with tension headaches that are not concomitantly treated with drugs, and less effective with migraine (vascular) headaches when medication management/mismanagement forms a part of the treatment plan (Andrasik, Grazzi, Usai, Buse, & Bussone, 2009). Medication rebound, as part of the medication overuse syndrome, remains the most difficult headache pattern to treat, and can easily compromise an otherwise effective intervention. These patients may be better served in an inpatient setting that can directly monitor medication changes simultaneous with providing an educative CBT program. It seems reasonable to conclude that many of the outpatient effectiveness studies are based on moderately severe headaches with patients motivated to seek alternatives to drug treatments. Persistent drug-seeking individuals remain extremely challenging. However, this fact is true for all types of chronic pain, and not just with headache; for the patient who insists that medication is the only acceptable treatment, any approach that emphasizes the development of behavioral coping skills can be stymied.

Keefe et al. (1990) randomly assigned 100 older adults diagnosed as having osteoarthritis of the knee into one of three conditions: cognitive-behavioral pain coping skills training, education about arthritis, or continuation of standard treatment as usual (TAU). After 10 weeks, the patients receiving coping skills training had significantly lower levels of pain and reduced physical and psychological disability. Comprehensive meta-analyses of additional studies confirm the efficacy of CBT in reducing arthritis pain (Austin, Beckner, Soeken, Hochberg, & Berman, 2002; Knittle, Maes, & de Gucht, 2010). Meta-analyses of several studies also support the benefits of CBT for fibromyalgia pain (Glombiewski et al., 2010). In an early CBT study of back pain (Nicholas, Wilson, & Goyen, 1992) the relative efficacy of CBT combined with a physiotherapy back-education program was compared to a physiotherapy back-education and exercise program only. The combined-condition group displayed significantly greater improvement than the education/exercise-only condition, based on measures of other-rated functional impairment, use of active coping strategies, self-efficacy beliefs, and medication use. These differences were maintained at a 6-month follow up. Although, this was a small study of only 20 outpatients, it is important because it suggests that CBT adds something to chronic pain treatment effectiveness that goes beyond simple information sharing and increased compliance with exercise; the results hint at the possibility of a combination of treatments that interfaces psychosocial contributions with those of biological/medical treatments that go beyond simple pharmacotherapy.

Loisel et al. (1997) evaluated the components of a multidisciplinary return to work programs in patients with chronic back pain. The four comparison treatment groups were: (1) occupational medicine/ergonomic workplace intervention, (2) clinical functional restoration program—a CBT variation, (3) both interventions, or (4) TAU via the family physician. Group 3, receiving both interventions, had more than twice the return to work levels compared to those receiving care as usual. However, while group 3 alone reported a significant decrease in pain, only those combined with the workplace intervention also displayed an increased return to work. The results highlight the critical importance of involving the workplace in an intervention program if the primary goal is functional recovery with return to work.

The 1980s and 1990s saw the emergence of a variation of CBT in "back schools" for dealing with chronic back pain. Most back school programs consisted of some combination of group cognitive-behavioral education and intensive guided exercise. A systematic review by van Tulder, Koes, and Bouter (1997) assessed the effectiveness of 10 studies of varying experimental quality. Half of the 10 studies showed a positive reduction in back pain and improvement in functional status. Again, the most effective back schools were those with comprehensive programs that also involved integration with the work setting. Nonetheless, in another systematic review (Scheer, Watamabe, & Radack, 1997), it was reported that only two of six studies of back schools reported positive "vocationally-related outcomes." Similarly, Cohen, Goel, and Frank (1994), in a review of several similar studies, concluded that there is contradictory evidence that back schools are of benefit in the treatment of chronic low back pain.

Despite the back school dilemma, the overall value of CBT programs for back pain remains positive, with impressive superiority over usual community care (Cherkin et al., 2016). A meta-analysis of 22 RCTs for chronic back pain (Hoffman, Papas, Charkoff, & Kerns, 2007) suggested that CBT, contrasted with various control conditions, had significant positive effects on reducing pain, reducing pain-related interference with activities, increasing health-related quality of life, and reducing depression. In another Cochran Review of 30 RCTs of behavioral treatments for chronic back pain it was concluded that, immediately posttreatment, CBT was more effective than TAU for pain, but that there was no difference at intermediate to long-term follow up with regard to perceived pain or functional status (Henschke et al., 2010). This report highlights that group exercise instruction is an intimate component of most CBT programs, making it difficult to separate the specific effects of different components of the program. However, it should be noted that other studies have demonstrated that these components tend to be interactive, and that CBT, at a minimum, improves compliance with the exercise component.

A Cochran Review of CBT for chronic orofacial pain (Aggarwal et al., 2011) determined that CBT, often including biofeedback, resulted in long-term improvements in pain intensity, depression, and pain-related activity interference. The authors, however, note a lack of rigor in many of the studies covered by the review.

Finally, there are multiple pain syndromes other than headache, backache, and arthritic pain that have shown to be improved by adding a CBT component to their respective multimodal treatments, including temporomandibular joint pain (Stowell, Gatchel, & Wildenstein, 2007), chronic neuropathic pain following spinal cord injury(Heutink et al., 2012), complex regional pain syndrome (de Jong, Vlaeyer, Cuypers, den Hollander, & Ruijgrok, 2005), diabetic neuropathy (Otis et al., 2013), postherpetic neuralgia (Kanazi, Johnson, & Dworkin, 2000), irritable bowel syndrome (Blanchard & Schwarz, 1987), phantom limb pain (Jessup & Gaallegos, 1994), and postsurgery pain (Doering et al., 2016).

Noncondition-specific efficacy studies that are primarily generated in multidisciplinary pain centers where a wide spectrum of chronic pain problems are treated cover widely heterogeneous types of pain. In one of the first noncondition-specific meta-analytic reports, combining data from several prior studies, an effort was made to categorize and compare six classes of coping strategies with a no-treatment condition and a positive placebo/expectancy control condition (Fernandez & Turk, 1989). It was found that individual patients differ in which coping strategy is most effective for them, but overall the impact of the different individual strategies was not significantly different. However, all of the cognitive coping strategies were more effective in alleviating pain than were the two control conditions.

Ten years later, a much more comprehensive analysis of heterogeneous pain studies containing RCTs was completed, based on 33 previously published papers containing data suitable for meta-analysis (Morley, Eccleston & Williams, 1999). Effect sizes for CBT were compared with waiting list controls and several alternative treatment conditions. Compared with waiting list controls, CBT treatments were associated with significant positive effect sizes on all outcome measurement domains. Further comparisons with alternative treatments, including TAU, revealed that CBT produced significantly greater positive changes for the domains of pain experience, cognitive coping, and behavioral coping, and reduced behavioral expression of pain. There were no significant differences on measures of mood, catastrophizing, and social role functioning. TAU included a poorly defined category of "standard medical care," which presumably was primarily pharmacologic in nature. Other alternative treatment groups used in the meta-analysis included family support, education only, and biofeedback, all conditions that arguably could be considered partial forms of CBT. Despite these potential confounds, the authors concluded that a CBT based form of psychological treatment of chronic pain is effective. A later Cochrane Review of RCT studies, by the same British group (Willams, Eccleston, & Morley, 2012) again reached similar conclusions, noting this time that the superiority of CBT is much stronger in comparison with waiting list controls than with active treatment controls. Overall CBT effects were very modest in improving pain ratings, but stronger with improving mood and decreasing catastrophic thinking. Notably, positive results held up 6 months later.

CBT Applications to Special Populations with Pain

In their recent review, Ehde, Dillworth, and Turner (2014) describe several innovative application of CBT to special chronic pain populations that have been historically underserved such as children and adolescents, brain injured civilians and soldiers, older adults, and acute and subacute pain in primary care settings. A number of studies support the potential efficacy of behavioral treatments for these special populations, although in many cases definitive RCTs and high quality meta-analyses have yet to be done.

Children and Adolescents

Children and adolescents appear to benefit from CBT variants such as relaxation training, biofeedback, and parental guidance in the use of operant behavioral strategies. Most studies have targeted headaches (Trautmann, Lackschewitz, & Kroner-Herwig, 2006). Broader based meta-analyses including headaches as well as other types of pain (Eccleston, Morley, Williams, Yorke, & Mastroyannopoulou, 2002; Palermo, Eccleston, Lewandowski, Williams, & Morley, 2010) found that, relative to no-treatment controls, CBT-based therapies with children and adolescents resulted in a greater than 50% pain reduction, with improvement maintained for at least 3 months posttreatment.

Traumatic Brain Injury

Traumatic brain injury (TBI), often accompanied by chronic pain, is sustained by 1.4 million civilian Americans annually as well as numerous soldiers returning from the armed conflict (Gironda et al., 2009). In a review of 23 studies on chronic pain after TBI

(Nampiaparampil, 2008), a prevalence of 57.8% was found for chronic headaches. Other pain conditions often associated with TBI are pain due to spasticity, peripheral nerve injury, reflex sympathetic dystrophy, contracture, and heteropic ossification (Bell, Pepping, & Dikman, 2005). Several limited scope studies have reported positive results for CBT with pain from neurologic conditions such as spinal cord injury (Ehde & Jensen, 2004; Heutink et al., 2012; Perry, Nicholas, & Middleton, 2010) and multiple sclerosis (Ehde & Jensen, 2004; Jensen et al., 2011). Still other neurologic conditions receiving limited positive evidence include pain from stroke, HIV/Aids, and neuromuscular disease.

Elderly Population

Tthe prevalence of chronic pain tends to increase with age. In developed countries the reported rates are 47–63% for those over age 65 (Tsang et al., 2008). Medications for pain can be particularly risky for older adults, yet there is little research on alternatives. A recent study (Nicholas et al., 2013) found that an outpatient program combining CBT and exercise for elderly adults was superior to an exercise-only condition on posttreatment indicators of disability, pain-related distress, catastrophizing, and self-efficacy for managing pain. In an earlier meta-analysis of studies involving elderly patients, Lunde, Nordus, and Pallesen (2009) were able to identify only seven controlled studies. Nonetheless, this limited review indicated that CBT was efficacious for pain, with effect sizes comparable to those found with younger groups. However, this meta-analysis did not find significant reductions in medication use or depression after CBT treatment.

Subacute Pain in Primary Care

Those interested in the treatment of chronic pain have long recognized the desirability of preventing chronic pain by better management of pain before it has reached the 3 months or longer stage, which is typically used to define chronic pain. However, the vast majority of CBT studies have concerned established chronic pain. CBT is rarely involved during the acute (up to 7 weeks) and subacute stages (7 weeks to 3 months) of pain management. The Institute of Medicine's (2011) report on pain treatment urged providing patients with pain education about self-management and the role of biological and psychosocial factors early in the symptom development process before pain becomes chronic. There have been a few efforts to study the effect of CBT techniques for individuals with acute or subacute back or neck pain (e.g., Linton & Andersson, 2000; Slater et al., 2009; Sullivan, Adams, Rhondenizer, & Stanish, 2006), but these studies, although promising, offer insufficient evidence to conclude that psychosocial interventions at the early stage are effective in preventing the development of chronic pain (Nicholas et al., 2011). Pain is often inadequately managed in primary, secondary, and tertiary care settings, and psychosocial interventions in particular are underutilized in those contexts (Ehde et al., 2014; Keefe, Abernethy, & Campbell, 2005).

Summary

In summary, the available research evidence is strongly supportive of CBT as a useful treatment modality for pain, by itself and used in conjunction with other treatment approaches. CBT is endorsed as having significant empirical support for its treatment efficacy by the National Institutes of Health Consensus Program (1995) and the American Psychological Association Task Force on Treatment Efficacy (2005). According to Ehde et al. (2014, p. 153) "CBT is now a mainstream treatment, alone or in conjunction with medical or interdisciplinary rehabilitation treatments, for individuals with chronic pain problems of all types." A recent update by the British Pain Study group (Morley, Williams, & Eccleston, 2013) found CBT particularly effective in reducing negative mood, catastrophic thinking, and self-perceived disability, but only mildly so with self-rated pain. Curiously, Morley et al. conclude that after four decades of studies there is no further need for additional RCTs that simply report group means to demonstrate CBT's usefulness in the management of chronic pain. The report suggests a current need for more emphasis placed on clinical rather than mere statistical significance, and the need to identify which components of CBT work for what type of patients. Furthermore, future research should include direct comparisons of relative adverse outcomes associated with all treatments used in pain management. Such comparisons might be reasonably expected to be particularly favorable to CBT because of its minimal side effect risk when compared with medication treatments.

Best-Practice Recommendations

Table 9.1 presents a summary of our findings on evidence-based treatment of chronic, nonmalignant pain.

Apart from the indications found in Table 9.1, many of which are more applicable in the multidisciplinary pain clinic, we would like to make several points concerning best-practice recommendations in treating the chronic pain population within the primary care setting.

1) Treatment should begin with the six-tiered multilayered "opioid sparing" medication steps previously presented. A carefully tiered multilayered medication approach is the starting point for pain management. Avoiding opioid and sedative dependency is certainly preferable to having to treat it later.
2) With great care in medication prescribing, the primary care practitioner should attentively monitor and encourage exercise and weight control appropriate to the patient's condition or make a referral for services that can assist with maintaining physical functioning. A rapid loss of strength and flexibility following the onset of chronic pain only amplifies the downward spiral into chronicity and can greatly hamper future progress.
3) Throughout acute and subacute pain stages, the practitioner needs to be on the lookout for emotional and behavioral indicators of maladaptive beliefs about pain treatment and maladaptive personal coping that may be warning signs of emergence into a "sick role" pattern of behavior (Hill et al., 2011).
4) Care must be taken to encourage and help the patient to become informed about chronic pain, and CBT, where indicated, should be openly discussed with the patient in primary care and before referral for specialized tertiary care pain services.

Table 9.1 Integrative biopsychosocial intervention with chronic pain: Summary of best-practice recommendations by level of confidence derived from strength of evidence.

Chronic pain		
Level A	Recommended	• Integration of multidisciplinary approaches is essential to chronic pain management; this entails coordinating combination therapies of CBT with pharmacological and other medical approaches, as well as physical therapy, exercise, and nutrition • CBT is the first-line intervention once pain has become chronic, with pharmacological interventions forming an adjunctive role for many patients • Antidepressant medication, especially tricyclic medication, and mood stabilizers are considered first-line among pharmacological treatments of chronic pain
Level B	Suggested	• Combined with appropriate medication management, biofeedback-assisted relaxation training is indicated as a first-line intervention for chronic migraine headaches, while relaxation training, with or without biofeedback, is indicated for tension headaches • Management of arthritic pain is effectively assisted by CBT coping techniques, while low back pain treatment is enhanced by incorporating CBT into exercise and physical therapy regimens • There is limited but encouraging evidence that CBT can be effective with traumatic brain injury, children, and the elderly
Level C	May be considered	• Opioids are not a first-line treatment for chronic pain, but should be reserved as a tertiary approach, after other pharmacologic and psychosocial approaches have proved insufficient • If an opioid is essential, partial agonist therapy may present less risk for dependency and abuse, although the evidence remains limited • When prescribed, opioids require careful monitoring and should ideally be accompanied by psychosocial CBT strategies to reduce abuse, including the use of a drug contract

Notes

1 Because of serious problems associated with physical addiction and psychological dependency, the goal for treating chronic pain should be to try to ameliorate pain without major reliance on opioids. This can be defined as an "opioid sparing" treatment approach that minimizes or eliminates the need for these particularly potent drugs. In the mid-1980s, Portenoy and Foley (1986) raised a major challenge to the restriction against the use of opioid for nonmalignant pain. These pain doctors reported encountering few problems with 38 patients maintained on moderate levels of opioid therapy for 4–7 years. They concluded that opioid maintenance therapy can be carried out in a safe, low-risk manner, and that it is a more humane alternative than no treatment for those with intractable nonmalignant pain and no history of drug abuse. However, despite better pain control, they also noted there were no substantial gains in employment or social functioning following the institution of long-term opioid therapy. The floodgates for opioid prescriptions were suddenly opened based on this new, but minimal evidence. Sensing the potential for new profits, pharmaceutical companies were quick to move into this expanding market. In 1994 OxyContin (slow-release formulation of oxycodone)

appeared, promoted as a powerful slow-release opioid ideal for the treatment of moderate to severe pain for extended periods of time. With support from the FDA, doctors were informed that this new drug "would result in less abuse potential" since it was absorbed more slowly than other opioid products. Over the next 20 years the pharmaceutical industry released more than two dozen new extended-release opioids for the treatment of chronic pain. More recently, medical boards, acknowledging that overuse has led to thousands of deaths, have placed opioid prescribing under tighter control. "Zero pain" is no longer the goal of treatment (Lee, 2016). The dubious benefits of long-term opioid therapy in treating chronic, non-malignant pain must be weighed against their abuse and dependency issues.

2 See *Handbook of Pain Assessment* (Turk & Melzack, 2011) for a thorough presentation of pain measurement techniques and issues.

References

Advokat, C. D., Comaty, J. E. and Julien, R. M. (2014). *Julien's primer of drug action* (13th ed.). New York: Worth.

Aggarwal, V. R., Lovell, K., Peters, S., Javidi, H., Joughin, A., & Goldthorpe, J. (2011). Psychosocial interventions for the management of chronic orofacial pain. *Cochrane Database of Systematic Reviews*, Article No. CD008456.

Alford, D. P. (2016). Opioid prescribing for chronic pain – achieving the right balance through education. *The New England Journal of Medicine, 374*, 301–303.

American Psychological Association Task Force on Treatment Efficacy. (2005). *Evidence-based practice in psychology*. Washington DC: American Psychological Association.

Andrasik, F. (2007). What does the evidence show? Efficacy of behavioral treatments for recurrent headaches in adults. *Neurological Sciences, 28*(Suppl. 2), S70–S77.

Andrasik, F., Grazzi, L., Usai, S., Buse, D. C., & Bussone, G. (2009). Non-pharmacological approaches to treating chronic migraine with medication overuse. *Neurological Sciences, 30*(Suppl. 1), S89–S93.

Austin, J. A., Beckner, W., Soeken, K., Hochberg, M. C., & Berman, B. (2002). Psychological interventions for rheumatoid arthritis: A meta-analysis of randomized controlled trials. *Arthritis and Rheumatism, 47*, 291–302.

Bachhuber, M. A., Hennessy, S., Cunningham, C. O., & Starrels, J. I. (2016). Increasing benzodiazepine prescriptions and overdose mortality in the United States, 1996–2013. *American Journal of Public Health, 106*, 686–688.

Bell, K., Pepping, M., & Dikman, S. (2005). Rehabilitation after traumatic brain injury. In L. Robinson (Ed.), *Trauma rehabilitation* (pp. 91–114). Philadelphia, PA: Lippincott Williams & Wilkins.

Blanchard, E. B., Andrasik, F., Evans, D. D., Neff, D. F., Appelbaum, K. A., & Rodichok, L. D. (1985). Behavioral treatment of 250 chronic headache patients: A clinical replication series. *Behavioral Therapy, 16*, 308–327.

Blanchard, E. B., Appelbaum, K. A., Guarnieri, P., Morrill, B., & Dentinger, M. P. (1987). Five year prospective follow-up on the treatment of chronic headache with biofeedback and/or relaxation. *Headache, 27*, 580–583.

Blanchard, E. B., & Schwarz, S. P. (1987). Adaptation of a multi-component treatment program for irritable bowel syndrome to a small group format. *Biofeedback and Self-Regulation, 12*, 63–69.

Bjurstrom, M. F., & Irwin, M. R. (2016). Polysomnographic characteristics in nonmalignant chronic pain populations: A review of controlled studies. *Sleep Medicine Reviews, 26*, 74–86.

Bonica, J. (1953). *The management of pain.* New York: Lea & Febiger.

Bonica, J. (1990). *The management of pain* (2nd ed.). Philadelphia, PA: Lippincott Williams & Wilkins.

Califf, R. M., Woodcock, J., & Ostroff, S. (2016). A proactive response to prescription opioid abuse. *The New England Journal of Medicine, 374*, 1480–1485.

Canadian Agency for Drugs and Technologies in Health (2016). Cannabinoid buccal spray for non-cancer or neuropathic pain: A review of clinical effectiveness, safety, and guidelines. Ottawa, Canada. *Internet CADTH Rapid Response Reports* (available as a free online download).

Chapman, S. (1988). Chronic pain and the injured worker. In T. Lynch & S. Vasudevan (Eds.), *Persistant pain: Psychosocial assessment and intervention* (pp. 103–116). Boston, MA: Kluwer Academic Publishers.

Campbell, C. M., & Edwards, R. R. (2012). Ethnic differences in pain and pain management. *Pain Management, 2*, 219–230.

Carron, H., DeGood, D. E., & Tait, R. (1985). A comparison of low back pain patients in the United States and New Zealand: Psychosocial and economic factors affecting severity of disability. *Pain, 21*, 77–89.

Cherkin, D. C., Sherman, K. J., Balderson, B. H., Cook, A. J., Anderson, M. L., . . . & Turner, J. A. (2016). Effect of mindfulness-based stress reduction vs cognitive behavioral therapy or usual care on back pain and functional limitations in adults with chronic low back pain – a randomized clinical trial. *Journal of the American Medical Association, 315*, 1240–1249.

Cohen, J. E., Goel, V., & Frank, J. W. (1994). Group education interventions for people with low back pain: An overview of the literature. *Spine, 19*, 1214–1223.

Dart, R. C., Surratt, H. L., Cicero, T. J., Parrino, M. W., Severtson, G., Bucher-Bartelson, B., & Green, J. L. (2015). Trends in opioid analgesic abuse and mortality in the United States. *The New England Journal of Medicine, 372*, 241–248.

DeGood, D. E. (1983). Reducing medical patients' reluctance to participate in psychological therapies: The initial session. *Professional Psychology, 14*, 570–579.

DeGood, D. E., & Cook, A. J. (2011). Psychosocial assessment: Comprehensive measures and measures specific to pain beliefs and coping. In D. C. Turk, & R. Melzack (Eds.), *Handbook of pain assessment* (3rd ed.) (pp. 47–93). New York: Guilford.

DeGood, D. E., & Kierman, B. D. (1997). Pain related cognitions as predictors of pain treatment outcome. *Advances in Medical Psychotherapy, 9*, 73–90.

De Jong, J. R., Vlaeyer, P., Cuypers, C., den Hollander, M., & Ruijgrok, J. (2005). Reduction of pain-related fear in complex regional pain syndrome type I: The application of graded exposure in vivo. *Pain, 116*, 264–275.

Doering, L., McGuire, A., Eastwood, J., Chen, B., Bodan, R., Czer, L., & Irwin, M. (2016). Cognitive behavioral therapy for depression improves pain and perceived control in cardiac surgery patients. *European Journal of Cardiovascular Nursing, 15*, 417–424.

Eccleston, C., Morley, S., Williams, A., Yorke, L., & Mastroyannopoulou, K. (2002). Systematic review of randomized controlled trials of psychological therapy for chronic pain in children and adolescents, with a subset meta-analysis of pain relief. *Pain, 99*, 157–165.

Ehde, D. M., Dillworth, T. M., & Turner, J. A. (2014). Cognitive-behavioral therapy for individuals with chronic pain. *American Psychologist, 69*, 153–166.

Ehde, D. M., & Jensen, M. P. (2004). Feasibility of a cognitive restructuring intervention for treatment of chronic pain in persons with disabilities. *Rehabilitation Psychology, 49*, 216–224.

Fernandez, E., & Turk, D. C. (1989). The utility of cognitive coping strategies for altering pain perception: a meta-analytic review. *Pain, 49*, 221–230.

Fine, P. G., & Rosenfeld, M. J. (2013). "The endocannabinoid system, cannabinoids, and pain. *Ramban Maimonides Medical Journal, 4*, 1–19.

Fishman, S. M., & Kreis, P. G. (2002). The opioid contract. *Clinical Journal of Pain, 18*(4), S70–S75.

Fordyce, W. E. (1976). *Behavioral methods for chronic pain and illness. St.* Louis, MO: C. V. Mosby Co.

Fordyce, W. E. (1984). Behavioral science and chronic pain. *Postgraduate Medical Journal, 60*, 865–868.

Gatchel, R. J., Howard, K. J., & Kishino, N. D. (2008). The biopsychosocial approach. *Practical Pain Management, 8*(4), 1–6.

Gironda, R. J., Clark, M. E., Ruff, R. L., Chait, S., Craine, M., Walker, R., & Scholten, J. (2009). Traumatic brain injury, polytrauma, and pain: Challenges and treatment strategies for the polytrauma rehabilitation. *Rehabilitation Psychology, 54*, 247–258.

Glombiewski, J. A., Sawyer, A. T., Gutermann, J., Koenig, K., Rief, W., & Hoffmann, S. G. (2010). Psychological treatments for fibromyalgia: A meta-analysis. *Pain, 15*, 280–295.

Hariharan, J., Lamb, G. C., & Neuner, J. M. (2007). Long-term opioid contract use for chronic pain management in primary care practice: A five year experience. *Journal of General Internal Medicine, 22*, 485–490.

Henschke, N., Ostelo, R.W, van Tulder, M. W., Vlaeyen, J. W., Morley, S., Assendelft, W. J., & Main, C. J. (2010). Behavioural treatment for chronic low-back pain. *Cochrane Database of Systematic Reviews,* Article No. CD002014.

Heutink, M., Post, M. W., Bongers-Janssen, H. M., Dijkstra, C. A., Snoek, G. J., Spijkerman, D. C., & Linderman, E. (2012). The CONECSI trial: Results of a randomized controlled trial of a multidisciplinary cognitive-behavioral program for coping with chronic neuropathic pain after spinal cord injury. *Pain, 153*, 120–128.

Hill, J. C., Whitehurst, D. G., Lewis, M., Bryan, S., Dunn, K. M., Foster, N. E., . . . Hay, E. M. (2011). Comparison of stratified primary care management for low back pain with current best practice (STarT Back): A randomized controlled trial. *The Lancet, 378*, 1560–1571.

Hoffman, B. M., Papa, R. K., Chatkoff, D. K., & Kerns, R. D. (2007). Meta-analysis of psychological interventions for chronic low back pain. *Health Psychology, 26*, 1–9.

Institute of Medicine. (2011). *Relieving pain in America: A blueprint for transforming prevention, care, education, and research.* Washington, DC: National Academies Press.

Jain, R, & Jain, M. (2011). Antidepressants in the treatment of chronic pain. *Practical Pain Management, March*, 44–50.

Jamison, R. E. (1996). *Learning to master your chronic pain.* Sarasota, FL: Professional Resource Press.

Jamison, R. N., Ross, E. L., Michna, E., Chen, L. Q., Holcomb, C. & Wasan, A. D. (2010). Substance misuse treatment for high-risk chronic pain patients on opioid therapy: A randomized trial. *Pain, 150*, 390–400.

Jensen, M. P., Ehde, D. E., Gertz, K. J., Stoelb, B. L., Dillworth, T. M., Hirsh, A. T., . . . & Kraft, G. H. (2011). Effects of self-hypnosis training and cognitive restructuring on daily pain intensity and catastrophizing in individuals with multiple sclerosis and chronic pain. *Journal of Clinical and Experimental Hypnosis, 59*, 45–63.

Jensen, M. P., Turner, J. A., & Romano, J. M. (2007). Changes after multidisciplinary pain treatment in patient pain beliefs and coping are associated with concurrent changes in patient functioning. *Pain, 131*, 38–47.

Jessup, B. A., & Gallegos, X. (1994). Relaxation and biofeedback. In P. D. Wall & R. Melzack (Eds.), *Textbook of pain* (3rd ed.) (pp. 1321–1336). Edinburgh: Churchill Livingstone.

Johnson, R. E., Fudala, P. J., & Payne, R. (2005). Buphrenorphine: Considerations for pain management. *Journal of Pain and Symptom Management, 29*, 297–326.

Julien, R., Advokat, C., & Comaty, J. (2011). *A Primer of drug action*. Boston, MA: Worth Publishers.

Kanazi, G. E., Johnson, R. W., & Dworkin, R. H. (2000). Treatment of postherpic neuralgia: An empirical update. *Drugs 2000, May*, 1113–1126.

Keefe, F. J., Abernethy, A. P., & Campbell, C. (2005). Psychological approaches to understanding and treating disease-related pain. *Annual Review of Psychology, 56*, 601–630.

Keefe, F. J., Caldwell, D. S., Williams, D. A., Gill, K. M., Mitchell, D., Robertson, C., Marinez, S., & Helms, M. (1990). Pain coping skills training in the management of osteoarthritic knee pain: A comparative study. *Behavior Therapy, 21*, 49–62.

Keefe, F. J., Lefebvre, J. C., & Smith, S. J. (1999). Catastrophizing research: Avoiding conceptual errors and maintaining a balanced perspective. *Pain Forum, 8*, 176–180.

Kerns, R. D., & Rosenberg, R. (1999). Predicting responses to a self-management treatments for chronic pain: Application of the pain stages of change model. *Pain, 82*, 1–7.

Kerns, R. D., Rosenberg, R., Jamison, R. N., Caudill, M. A., & Haythornwaite, J. (1997). Readiness to adopt a self-management approach to chronic pain. The Pain Stages of Change Questionnaire (PSOCQ). *Pain, 72*, 227–234.

Knittle, K., Maes, S., & de Gucht, V. (2010). Psychological interventions for rheumatoid arthritis: Examing the role of self-regulation with a systematic review and meta-analysis of randomized controlled trials. *Arthritis Care and Research, 62*, 1460–1472.

Lee, T. H. (2016). Zero pain is not the goal. *Journal of the American Medical Association, 315*(15), 1575–1577.

Linton, S. J., & Andersson, T. (2000). Can chronic disability be prevented? A randomized trial of a cognitive-behavioral intervention and two forms of information for patients with spinal pain. *Spine, 25*, 2825–2831.

Loisel, P., Abenhaim, L., Durand, P., Esdaile, J. M., Suissa, S., Gosselin, L., . . . & Lemare, J. (1997). A population-based, randomized clinical trial on back pain management. *Spine, 22*, 2911–2918.

Lunde, L. H., Nordhus, I. H., & Pallesen, S. (2009). The effectiveness of cognitive and behavioral treatment of chronic pain in the elderly: A quantitative review. *Journal of Clinical Psychology in Medical Settings, 16*, 254–262.

Manchikanti, L., Fellows, B, Ailinani, H., & Pampati, V. (2010). Therapeutic use, abuse, and nonmedical use of opioids: A ten-year perspective. *Pain Physician, 13*, 401–435.

Melzach, R., & Wall, P. D. (1965). Pain mechanisms: A new theory. *Science, 150*, 971–979.

Montgomery, G. H., DuHamel, K. N., & Redd, W. H. (2000). A meta-analysis of hypnotically induced analgesia: How effective is hypnosis? *International Journal of Clinical and Experimental Hypnosis, 48*, 138–153.

Morin, C. M., Gibson, D, & Wade, J. (1998). Self-reported sleep and mood disturbance in chronic pain patients. *Clinical Journal of Pain, 14*, 311–314.

Morley, S., Eccleston, C., & Williams, A. (1999). Systematic review and meta-analysis of randomized controlled trials of cognitive behavior therapy for chronic pain in adults, excluding headache. *Pain, 80*, 1–13.

Morley, S., Williams, A., & Eccleston, C. (2013). Re-examining the evidence about psychological treatments for chronic pain: Time for a paradigm shift? *Pain, 154*, 1929–1931.

Nampiaparampil, D. E. (2008). Prevalence of chronic pain after traumatic brain injury: A systematic review. *JAMA, 300*, 711–719.

Nestoriuc, Y., & Martin, A. (2007). Efficacy of biofeedback for migraine: A meta-analysis. *Pain, 128*, 111–127.

Nestoriuc, Y. Rief, W., & Martin, A. (2008). Meta-analyis of biofeedback for tension-type headache: Efficacy, specificity, and treatment moderators. *Journal of Consulting and Clinical Psychology, 76*, 379–396.

National Institutes of Health, Technology Assessment Statement, October 1995. *Integration of behavioral and relaxation approaches into the treament of chronic pain and insomnia*, Washington, DC: National Institutes of Health, pp. 1–34.

Nicholas, M. K., Asghari, A., Blyth, F. M., Wood, B. M., Murray, R., McCabe, R., . . . & Overton, S. (2013). Self-management intervention for chronic pain in older adults: A randomized control trial. *Pain, 154*, 824–835.

Nicholas, M. K., Linton, S. J., Watson, P. J., Main, C. J., & "Decade of the Flags" Working Group. (2011). Early identification and management of psychological risk factors ("yellow flags") in patients with low back pain: A reappraisal. *Physical Therapy, 91*, 737–753.

Nicholas, M. K., Wilson, P. H., & Goyen, J. (1992). Comparison of cognitive-behavioral group treatment and an alternative non-psychological treatment for chronic low back pain. *Pain, 48*, 339–347.

Otis, J., Sanderson, K., Hardway, C., Pincus, M., Tun, C., & Soumekh, S. (2013). A randomized controlled pilot study of a cognitive-behavioral therapy approach for diabetic peripheral neuropathy. *Journal of Pain, 24*, 475–482.

Palermo,T. M., Eccleston, C., Lewandowski, A. S., Williams, A. D., & Morley, S. (2010). Randomized controlled trials of psychological therapies for management of chronic pain in children and adolescents: An updated meta-analytic review. *Pain, 14*, 387–397.

Patterson, D. R., & Jensen, M. P. (2003). Hypnosis and clinical pain. *Psychological Bulletin, 129*, 495–521.

Perry, K. N., Nicholas, M. K., & Middleton, J. W. (2010). Comparison of a pain management program with usual care in a pain management center for people with spinal cord injury related chronic pain. *Clinical Journal of Pain, 26*, 206–216.

Portenoy, R. K, & Foley, K. M. (1986). Chronic use of opioid analgesics in non-malignant pain: Report of 38 cases. *Pain, 25*, 171–186.

Roth, R. S., & Geisser, M. E. (2002). Educational achievement and chronic pain disability: Mediating role of pain-related cognitions. *Clinical Journal of Pain, 18*, 286–296.

Scheer, S. J., Watamabe, T. K., & Radack, K. L. (1997). Randomized controlled trials in industrial low back pain: III. Subacute/chronic pain interventions. *Archives of Physical Medicine and Rehabilitation, 78,* 414–423.

Shealy, C. N., Mortimer, J. T., & Hagfors, N. R. (1970). Dorsal column electroanalgesia. *Journal of Neurosurgery, 32,* 560–564.

Shutty, M. S., DeGood, D. E., & Hoekstra-Tuttle, D. H. (1990). Chronic pain patients' beliefs about their pain and treatment outcomes. *Archives of Physical Medicine and Rehabilitation, 71,* 128–132.

Slater, M. A., Weickgenant, A. L., Greenberg, M. A., Whalgren, D. R., Williams, R. A., Carter, C., & Atkinson, J. H. (2009). Preventing progression to chronicity in first onset, subacute low back pain: An exploratory study. *Archives of Physical Medicine and Rehabilitation, 90,* 545–552.

Smith, M. T., & Haythornthwaite, J. A. (2004). How do sleep disturbance and chronic pain inter-relate? Insights from the longitudinal and cognitive-behavioral clinical trials literature. *Sleep Medicine Reviews, 8,* 119–132.

Sontag, D. (2013). Addiction treatment with a dark side. *The New York Times,* November 16.

Stowell, A. W., Gatchel, R. J., & Wildenstein, L. (2007). Cost-effectiveness of treatments for temporomandibular disorders: Biopsychosocial intervention versus treatment as usual. *Journal of the American Dental Association, 138,* 202–208.

Sullivan, M. J., Adams, H., Rhodenizer, T., & Stanish, W. D. (2006). A psychosocial risk factor-targeted intervention for the prevention of chronic pain and disability following whiplash injury. *Physical Therapy, 86,* 8–18.

Trautmann, E., Lackschewitz, H., & Kroner-Herwig, B. (2006). Psychological treatment of recurrent headache in children and adolescents—a meta-analysis. *Cephalalgia, 26,* 1411–1426.

Tsang, A., Von Korff, M., Lee, S., Alonso, J., Karam, E., Angermeyer, M. C., & Watanabe, M. (2008). Common chronic pain conditions in developed and developing countries: Gender and age differences and comorbidity with depression-anxiety disorders. *Journal of Pain, 9,* 883–891.

Turk, D. C., & Melzack, R. (Eds.) (2011). *Handbook of pain assessment.* New York: Guilford.

Turner, J. A., Jensen, M. P., & Romano, J. M. (2000). Do beliefs, coping and catastrophizing independently predict functioning in patients with chronic pain? *Pain, 85,* 115–125.

Van Tulder, M. W., Koes, B. W., & Bouter, L. M. (1997). Conservative treatment of acute and chronic nonspecific low back pain. *Spine, 22,* 2128–2156.

Wasan, A. D., Ross, E. L., Michna, E., Chibnik, L., Greenfield, S. F., Weiss, R. D., & Jamison, R. N. (2012). Craving of prescription opioids in patients with chronic pain: A longitudinal outcome trial. *Journal of Pain, 13,* 146–154.

Williams, A. C., Eccleston, C., & Morley, S. (2012). Psychological therapies for the management of chronic pain (excluding headache) in adults. *Cochrane Database of Systematic Reviews, 2012*(11), CD007407.

Young Casey, C., Greenberg, M. A., Nicassio, P. M., Harpin, R. E., & Hubbard, D. (2008). Transition from acute to chronic pain and disability: A model including cognitive, affective, and trauma factors. *Pain, 134,* 69–79.

10

Eating Disorders: Evidence-Based Integrated Biopsychosocial Treatment of Anorexia Nervosa, Bulimia and Binge Eating Disorder

Marla Sanzone

While diagnostic categorization of eating disorders has expanded in number and detail with each revision of the Diagnostic and Statistical Manual of Mental Disorders (DSM), the current escalation in incidence of all eating disorders appears to be a function of increased prevalence among populations in which it was previously unusual to find eating disorders, including middle-aged adults, younger preadolescent children, and males. Epidemiologic studies have revealed significant increases in the incidence and prevalence of anorexia and bulimia among children under the age of 12, as well as among boys (Agency for Healthcare Research and Quality, 2009; Eddy et al., 2008; Field, Wren, Cooke, & Bloom, 1999; Hoek & van Hoeken , 2003; Rosen, 2003).

Dysregulations of the aminergic neurotransmitter systems are thought to be significant mediators in the maintenance of eating disorders through a complex interaction of genetic, biological, and behavioral factors. Anxiety as well as affective and substance abuse disorders appear to share with eating disorders a similar underlying serotonin, dopamine, and norepinephrine neurotransmission vulnerability (Akkerman, Paaver, Nordquist, Oreland, & Harro, 2008; Bosanac, Norman, Burrows, & Beumont, 2005; Bruce, Steiger, Ng Ying, & Kin, 2005; Bulik, Devlin, & Vacanu, 2003; Bulik, Hebebrand, & Keski-Rahkonen, 2007; Grice, Halmi, & Fichter, 2002; Kaye Gendall, & Strober, 1998; Rinaman, 2007; Wade, Bulik, & Neale, 2001). When serotonin levels are low and cortisol levels are elevated, biologic response mechanisms to stress and peripheral hunger/satiation signals are disrupted, increasing the propensity for eating disorder symptoms and symptoms of co-occurring conditions such as mood disorders and anxiety (Farooqi et al., 2007; Heal, Smith, Fisas, Codony, & Buschmann, 2008; Jimerson & Wolfe, 2004; Monteleone, Di Lieto, A., Castaldo, 2004). Eating disorders characteristically present with overt psychological as well as physical symptoms, often precipitating the initiation of some form of psychosocial, pharmacological, or combined progression of treatments aimed at ameliorating the eating disorder and its co-morbid mood and anxiety disorders (Halmi, 2005; Kaye & Strober, 1999; Keel & Brown, 2008; Keel & Haedt, 2008; Lewinsohn, Striegel-Moore, & Seeley, 2000; Mussell et al., 2000; NICE, 2004).

Empirical research demonstrates that adults with eating disorders of all types and subtypes most consistently respond to cognitive-behavioral therapy methods (CBT), particularly when combined with psychopharmacological therapies (American Psychiatric

Cognitive Behavioral Psychopharmacology: The Clinical Practice of Evidence-Based Biopsychosocial Integration, First Edition. Edited by Mark Dana Muse.

Association, 2006; Brambilla et al., 2009; Couturier, Kimber, & Szatmari, 2013; Darcy, Fitzpatrick, & Lock, 2015; Fairburn, 2008; Fairburn et al., 2015; Galsworthy-Francis, 2014; Halmi, 2013; Kaustav & Basu, 2010; Keel & Haedt, 2008; Mussell et al., 2000; NICE, 2004; Peterson, Becke, Treasure, Sharfran, & Brant-Waugh, 2016; Rosen, 2003; Schmidt, Lee, & Beecham, 2007; Schmidt, Wade, & Treasure, 2014; Turner, Marshall, Stopa, & Waller, 2015; Zipfel, Giel, Bulik, Hay, & Schmidt, 2015). Specific versions of CBT, alone and in combination with other forms of intervention, including medication, family, interpersonal, and group psychotherapies, have been found to be most suitable for particular patient populations by age and eating disorder subtype. For instance, children and adolescents under 16 with various eating disorders have exhibited best response and outcome to family-based treatments (Couturier et al., 2013; Dare & Eisler, 1997; Eisler, Simic, Russell, & Dare, 2007; Findlay, Pinzon, Taddeo, & Katzman, 2010; LeGrange & Eisler, 2009; Lilenfeld, Kaye, & Greeno, 1998; Lock, 2015; Lock, Couturier, & Agras, 2006; Lock, Le Grange, Agras, & Dare, 2001; Rosen, 2003; Russell, Szmukler, Dare, & Eisler, 1987; Schmidt et al., 2007), while adults with bulimia exhibit particularly robust positive outcomes to CBT and/or interpersonal therapy, combined with psychopharmacological interventions addressing co-morbid mood and compulsive symptomology (Agras, Walsh, Fairburn, Wilson, & Kraemer, 2000; American Psychiatric Association, 2006; Arcelus et al., 2009; Fairburn, 1992, 2008; Fairburn, Jones, Peveler, Hope, & O'Connor, 1993; Lock, 2015; NICE, 2004; Schmidt et al., 2014; Turner et al., 2015). Dialectical behavior therapy (DBT) is also yielding promising results for bulimics, particularly when chronicity and/or symptoms consistent with personality disorders are factors (Ben-Porath, Wisniewski, & Warren, 2009; Keel & Haedt, 2008; Mussell et al., 2000; NICE, 2004; Peterson et al., 2016; Safer, Telch, & Agras, 2001).

Standard of care protocols for inpatient hospital-based and residential-based treatment for anorexics and bulimics most often emphasize CBT in groups and behavioral nutrition therapies. Many programs also include a family therapy component. For instance, the Maudsley method (Le Grange & Eisler, 2009) and variations thereof are often introduced to parents of younger patients for the purposes of educating them about the least confrontational and most effective family meal implementation methods. Similarly, families and partners of older patients often need educating about the importance of posthospitalization family therapy, as systemic interactional problems are normative in this context and are common contributing causative factors to the chronic and more severe eating disorders (Crisp et al., 1991; Eisler et al., 2000a; Eisler et al., 2000b; Eisler et al., 2007; Robin, Siegel, & Moye, 1995; Russell et al., 1987). Family interaction patterns addressed might include triangulation, power struggles, boundary concerns, and identity/role confusion. When family therapy methods are integrated into treatment programs, relapse and rehospitalization rates have been lower (Boscolo, Cecchin, Hoffman, & Penn, 1987; Campbell, Draper, & Huffington, 1991; Findlay et al., 2010; Halmi, 2005; Hoffman, 1985; Howard, Evans, Quintero-Howard, Bowers, & Andersen, 1997; Kaplan & Olmstead 1997; LeGrange & Eisler, 2009; Lock, 2015; Lock et al., 2001; McIntosh, Jordan, & Carter, 2005; Rosen, 2003; Rosman, Minuchin, & Liebman, 1975; Russell et al., 1987; Schmidt et al., 2014; Vall & Wade, 2015; Zipfel, Reas, & Thornton, 2002; White & Boskind-White, 1984).

On the other hand, patients with binge eating disorder without symptoms of anorexia or bulimia are infrequently admitted to inpatient or residential programs unless they voluntarily admit themselves after failing to achieve the desired results in outpatient programs. Inpatient programs for binge eating disorder are often physically separate from units for anorexia and bulimia. Group therapies for binge eating tend to be behaviorally focused on learning new ways of eating, with emphases on nutrition education, healthy food preparation, and portion control, as well as body awareness training relevant to accurate physiological signal recognition and response. Except for bariatric surgery programs, inpatient and residential programs for binge eating are less common and are less likely to be covered by insurance unless inpatient medical necessity over outpatient treatment can be justified. In contrast, inpatient, partial and residential programs for anorexia and bulimia have become more common in the past decade as incidence and prevalence rates before and beyond puberty and adolescence have increased along with awareness about the importance of early treatment (Agency for Healthcare Research and Quality, 2009; Kaplan & Olmstead, 1997; Sigman, 1996; Zipfel et al., 2002).

Pharmacotherapy for Eating Disorders

Evidence supporting the use of medication as augmentation to psychosocial therapies for eating disorders has generally demonstrated superior results over psychotherapy alone or medication alone for most eating disorders (Brambilla et al., 2009; Halmi, 2005; Hilbert, 2015; Mitchell, Pyle, & Eckert, 1990; Peterson et al., 2016; Walsh et al., 1997; Wilson, Loeb, & Walsh, 1999). Response patterns to combination therapies, however, differ according to age, primary symptom manifestation, degree of emaciation, and co-morbidities. Given the preponderance of co-morbid mood and anxiety conditions in eating disorders, the data support the use of selective serotonin reuptake inhibitors (SSRIs) as first-order medication therapy, followed by serotonin–norepinephrine reuptake inhibitors (SNRIs) with most eating disordered types and subtypes, except for very young children or early adolescents, and with severely underweight anorexics of all ages whose systemic ability to respond to medication appears to interfere with its efficacy (Halmi, 2005; Peterson et al., 2016; Powers & Bruty, 2009; Reas & Grilo, 2015; Rossi et al., 2007; Walsh et al., 1997; Zhu & Walsh, 2002). For bulimia and binge eating disorder, SSRIs, SNRIs, and topiramate have demonstrated good to moderate levels of efficacy with regard to reducing the number of binge eating and binge eating/purging episodes among adult bulimics and binge eaters (Browne, 2002; McElroy, Guerdjikova, Mori, & O'Melia, 2012; McElroy & Arnold, 2003; Peterson et al., 2016; Powers & Bruty, 2009; Reas & Grilo, 2015; Steffen, Roerig, Mitchell, & Uppala, 2006; Walsh et al., 1997). Among more chronic and/or treatment resistant anorexics, off-label use of tricyclics and second-generation antipsychotics are occasionally employed for psychomotor and/or anxiety reduction, and for weight gain and sedating side effect. However, the efficacy results are mixed, and this may be in part due to the consistent idiopathic artifact that extremely low-weight anorexics tend not to respond to medication in general until weight restoration has been initiated (Biederman, Herzog, & Rivinus, 1985; Bruce et al., 2005; Halmi, Eckert, & LaDu, 1986; Bissada, Tasca, Barber, & Bradwejn, 2008; Lacey & Crisp, 1980; Powers & Bruty, 2009; Reas & Grilo, 2015; Steffen et al., 2006; Walsh et al., 1997). Not uncommonly, however, the body appears to begin responding to medication once body weight begins to increase, but the degree of weight gain required for a positive response to medications is not predictable (Black, Davis, & Kennedy, 1993; Kaye, Nagata, &Weltzin, 2001; Rossi et al., 2007). When weight begins to increase, the concomitant mood, anxiety, sleep, and cognitive disturbances also begin to exhibit responsiveness to other forms of therapy, including pharmacotherapy (Kaye, Frank, & McConah, 1999; Rosen, 2003; Rossi et al., 2007; Strober, 1992; Zipfel et al., 2015).

Pharmacotherapies for bulimia and binge eating disorders include antidepressants, anticonvulsants, atypical antipsychotics, psychostimulants (atomoxetine, lisdexamfetamine, methylphenidate), and antiobesity agents (orlistat, D-fenfluramine, locaserin) (Fidler et al., 20011; Hermanussen & Tresguerres, 2008; McElroy et al., 2012; Powers & Bruty, 2009). Medications are most effective when used to augment psychosocial therapies that address the maladaptive persistent behavior patterns associated with eating disorders, namely reducing the frequency of binge eating, weight reduction among binge eaters, reduced use of compensatory behaviors such as purging and obsessive exercise among bulimics, food restriction, mood-regulating and anxiety-reducing behaviors that are believed to emanate from, and contribute to, ongoing co-morbidities. Anticraving or antiaddiction drugs such as acamprosite and naloxone appear promising in the treatment of these eating disorders as a function of supporting the cognitive-behavioral efforts toward reducing urge intensity and impulsive reactivity, an inevitable component of conditioned responses to binge/purge urges (Goracci et al., 2015; McElroy & Arnold, 2003; McElroy et al., 2012; Reas & Grilo, 2014).

Second-generation antipsychotics such as risperdal, quetiapine, olanzapine, aripiprazole, lurasidone, and clomipramine are used in low doses with severely low-weight outpatient anorexics as well as hospitalized, highly co-morbid anorexics. They have moderate efficacy in the management of acute anxiety, excessive psychomotor activity, sleep disruption, and distorted, dichotomous thinking when these symptoms are treated concomitantly with psychosocial approaches. Second-generation antipsychotics moderately improve agitation and assist sleep, but do little to stimulate appetite among anorexics unless weight restoration has started (Bissada et al., 2008; Dold, Aigner, Klaubunde, Treasure, & Kasper, 2015; Kishi, Kafantaris, Sunday, Sheridan, & Correll, 2012; Lacey & Crisp, 1980; McKnight & Park, 2010; Powers et al., 2002; Rossi et al., 2007; Vandereycken & Pierloot, 1982).

In the early stages of both psychosocial and psychopharmacological treatment, anorexics are characteristically more resistant to treatment than are bulimics and binge eaters. SSRIs and SNRIs, separately or even in combination with small doses of antipsychotics, can at times render anorexics more available for psychosocial treatment by lowering levels of anxiety (Feld, Woodside, Kaplan, Olmsted, & Carter, 2001; Hepworth, Paxton, & Williams, 2007; Kaplan & Garfinkel, 1999; Kaustav & Basu, 2010; Vitousek, Watson, & Wilson, 1998). When antipsychotics are integrated as a component for treating anorexia, they are most often used in low doses with patients who exhibit extremely rigid cognitive distortions of a nearly delusional degree, such that physical health is compromised due to their demonstrated pattern of inability to ingest sufficient nutrition to sustain life. The diminished health, obsessive-compulsive weight and food focus, and concomitant behaviors that maintain the eating disorder, interfere with one's availability, cognitively and affectively, for productive engagement in psychotherapy (Halmi, 2005; Keel & Brown, 2010; Lewinsohn et al., 2000). Unless co-morbid mood and/or thought disorder symptomology justifies ongoing use of a neuroleptic, antipsychotic use with anorexics tends to be short term, specifically for the purposes of increasing their ability to constructively use cognitive-behavioral and/or other forms of psychosocial treatment, as well as to assist with treatment compliance toward nutritional improvement with less cognitive and emotional resistance (Aigner, Treasure, Kasper, & WFSBP Task Force on Eating Disorders, 2011; Dold et al., 2015).

Mood-regulating antidepressants such as SSRIs, SNRIs, tricyclic antidepressants (TCAs), and anticonvulsants have demonstrated reduced rates of relapse among eating disorder patients when integrated into a comprehensive treatment plan, as they work together to assist patients develop the ability to accurately integrate and regulate emotional and physical stimuli (Halmi et al., 1999; Lewinsohn et al., 2000; Walsh et al., 1997; Wilson et al., 1999). TCAs such as desipramine, imipramine, clomipramine, nortryptilline, and amytriptaline were among the early TCAs used to treat eating disordered patients before other antidepressant classes such as SSRIs were developed (Alger, Schwalberg, Bigaouette, Michalek, & Howard, 1991; Biederman et al., 1985; Bissada et al., 2008; Halmi, 1992; Lacey & Crisp, 1980, Pope, Hudson, Jonas & Yurgelun-Todd, 1983; Walsh, Hadigan, & Devlin, 1991). They were found to be moderately helpful toward reducing psychomotor restlessness, generalized anxiety, panic, and sleep disruption, and they have shown a slight tendency to increase appetite and weight gain.

SSRIs and SNRIs exhibit moderate efficacy with mood and anxiety improvement among anorexics, bulimics, and binge eaters when such patients also engage in CBT (Brambilla et al., 2009; Fichter, Leibl, Kruger, & Rief, 1997; Guerdjikova et al., 2008; Milano, Petrella & Sabatino, 2004; Wade et al., 2001; Walsh et al., 2000). They are better tolerated and have a safer suicidality profile than the TCAs. The TCAs are occasionally used in combination with the SSRIs or SNRIs to address symptoms consistent with double depression or a mix of dysthymia and major depression, or to assist regulation of sleep (Bissada et al., 2008; Kaye et al., 1999, 2001; Wade et al., 2001; Walsh et al., 1997; Zhu & Walsh, 2002).

Given the neurobiological interaction of eating disorders with co-morbid substance abuse, as well as affective and anxiety disorders, a treatment response in one of the co-occurring conditions is likely to positively influence responsiveness of the eating disorder to treatment. For example, changes in the dopaminergic, serotonergic, and opioid systems can serve to reinforce or diminish the behaviors associated with eating disordered behaviors, self-induced starvation, and bingeing/purging, as well as the associated cognitive rigidity/inflexibility and obsessive-compulsive thoughts and actions; and an improvement in mood or anxiety disturbances may translate to improvement in obsessive thinness pursuit thoughts and behaviors, as well as binge/purge and obsessive-compulsive food and weight-related symptoms (Bosanac et al., 2005; Halmi, 2005; Kaye et al., 2001; Peterson et al., 2016; Powers & Bruty, 2009; Reas & Grilo, 2015; Rossi et al., 2007; Wilson et al., 1999; Zhu & Walsh, 2002).

SSRIs are typically the first-line pharmacological agents used to treat the co-morbid symptoms of mood and anxiety seen with eating disorders, particularly with bulimics and binge eaters. Following an at least partial weight restoration, anorexics may exhibit responsiveness to this class of antidepressants (Aigner et al., 2011; Guerdjikova et al., 2008; Halmi, 2005; Jimerson & Wolfe, 2004; Kaye et al., 1999, 2001; Leombruni et al., 2008). The only SSRI currently Food and Drug Administration (FDA) approved for the treatment of bulimia is fluoxetine; however, sertraline, paroxetine, citalopram, escitalopram, as well as the newer agents such as vilazodone and vortioxetine, when prescribed off-label for eating disorders, demonstrate similar response rates (Browne, 2002; Hilbert, 2015; Kaye et al., 1998). All SSRIs tend to be efficacious in helping to improve mood, anxiety and appetite regulation among bulimics and binge eaters. These same agents appear to enhance weight restoration among anorexics. Nonetheless, trials of 60 mg/day fluoxetine were shown to have no benefit for inpatient underweight anorexics, but some evidence indicates that partial weight-restored anorexics on fluoxetine have lower relapse rates during the weight maintenance phase of treatment (Aigner et al., 2011; Halmi, 1992; Kaye et al., 1998; Jimerson & Wolfe, 2004).

While few double-blind placebo-controlled studies have been conducted on the clinical treatment of severe and complex anorexic conditions, paroxetine is an SSRI frequently preferred by prescribers for anorexics and low-weight bulimics due to its high propensity, relative to the other SSRIs, to induce weight gain. Demonstrated reductions in depression, general anxiety, and obsessionality, as well as improvement in sleep, have been shown with paroxetine and citalopram with anorexics previously intolerant of fluoxetine for reasons of elevated levels of irritability or activation on fluoxetine (Halmi, 2005; Kaye et al., 1999). While most SSRIs are generally well tolerated, sedation and weight gain are the most frequent causes cited by patients who discontinue them (Aigner et al., 2011; Browne, 2002; Bruce et al., 2005; Halmi, 2005; Kaye et al., 2001; Peterson et al., 2016; Rossi et al., 2007; Zhu & Walsh, 2002).

The SNRIs venlafaxine and duloxetine, or the newer desvenlafaxine or levomilnacipran, are generally not administered as first-line agents in the treatment of eating disorders. The SNRIs, however, may have particular benefit addressing mixed symptoms of anxiety and depression when dosed at higher levels that induce noradrenergic action, and after failed trials on SSRIs with patients with persistent levels of depression and anxiety (Rees & Grilo, 2015; Zipfel et al., 2015). Duloxetine has been shown to help improve response accuracy to appetite cues following reduced anxiety levels (Guerdjikova et al., 2012; Thase et al., 2007).

The atypical antidepressant buproprion has shown promise in the reduction of craving sensations and the associated obsessive food focus with appetite dysregulation seen among binge eaters and bulimics (McElroy et al., 2012; Powers & Bruty, 2009; Reas & Grilo, 2015). It is important to note, however, the contraindication of buproprion with active bulimic behavior, given the potential for a lower seizure threshold that increases vulnerability among this fragile population with possible electrolyte imbalance due to purging. Another effective utility of buproprion with a subset of binge eaters and bulimics is for those with attention deficit disorder. When attention deficit hyperactivity disorder (ADHD)-related conditions are treated with buproprion, eating disorder patients tend to exhibit improvements in mood, concentration, and impulsive decision-making, as well as with bulimia and binge eating (Ginawa, Al-Majed, & Al-Suwailem, 2005; Goracci et al., 2015; McElroy et al., 2012; Sokol, Gray, Goldstein, & Kaye, 1999; Weisler et al., 1994). The diagnostic co-occurrence and response to this agent among bulimics with ADHD and depressive symptomology lends support to the low dopamine hypothesis of eating/appetite, mood, attention, and energy dysregulation thought to be relevant to addictive and attentional disturbances (Goracci et al., 2015; Mond, Myers, Crosby, Hay, & Mitchell, 2008; Steffen et al., 2006).

Early studies looking at the use of atomoxetine with binge urges shows some promise toward reduced frequency of binge eating as well as reduction in ego-dystonic cognitive rumination about eating-related concerns relative to placebo controls (Hilbert, 2015; Reas & Grilo, 2015). Nevertheless, difficulty in tolerating side effects of increased dysphoric mood, constipation, and nervousness are not generally conducive to its use with binge eating and bulimia unless other options have not been well tolerated (McElroy et al., 2012; McElroy, & Arnold, 2003).

Several anticonvulsant medications have been effective in decreasing mood lability and impulsive reactivity to binge/purge urges. This class of medications may be particularly relevant with subpopulations of eating disordered individuals who exhibit co-morbid mood instability or bipolar disturbances that have been unresponsive to medications from other classes. Few controlled trials have been conducted, but several placebo-controlled double-blind trials with bulimics and binge eaters on relatively low doses of 100–200 mg of topiramate suggest considerable efficacy toward decreased uncontrolled eating, food, and body preoccupation, as well as frequency and intensity of urges to binge/purge (Hedges et al., 2003; Hoopes et al., 2003; McElroy & Arnold, 2003; Reas & Grilo, 2015). Preliminary studies of topiramate and zonisamide also report success when treating both affective and eating disorder symptoms, namely impulse control over eating and purging behavior (Rossi et al., 2007). Topiramate appears to demonstrate consistent positive appetite-regulating properties with bulimics and binge eaters who also describe decreased cognitive preoccupation with food (Field et al., 2008; Heal et al, 2008; McElroy & Arnold, 2003). Lamotrigine and zonisamide, in preliminary studies, have been reported to provide some assistance toward reduced binge eating frequency, but thus far improvements have not met significance levels in comparison with placebo response (Reas & Grilo, 2014).

Naltrexone is an opiate antagonist whose mechanism of action is thought to block the euphoric experience following the ingestion of a substance of choice. Reports of mild improvement in appropriate food intake by bulimics on 200–300 mg doses of the opiate antagonist suggests naltrexone may assist patients' ability to learn accurate interoception or physiological cue interpretation as well as to improve moderate regulation of hunger and satiation (Igoin-Apfelbaum & Apfelbaum, 1987; McElroy & Arnold, 2003; McElroy et al., 2012; Steffen et al., 2006).

Psychostimulants such as amphetamine, dextroamphetamine, lisdexamfetamine, and methylphenidate, indicated for the treatment of ADHD, have been shown to be therapeutic in improving appetite regulation and obsessive-cognitive foci when administered to eating disordered individuals (Sokol et al., 1999). With or without ADHD, binge eaters and bulimics who are prescribed stimulants have demonstrated improved ability to decrease food obsessions, reduce compulsive night eating behavior patterns, and to make more effective use of all forms of psychotherapy, particularly CBT. In 2015 lisdexamfetamine dimesylate was approved by the FDA for the treatment of binge eating disorder. Other psychostimulants, such as dextroamphetamine mixed salts, methylphenidate, methylphenidate extended release, and dexmethylphenidate, are used off-label adjunctively with psychotherapy to aid in appetite regulation (Goracci et al., 2015; Jimerson & Walsh, 2004; McElroy et al., 2012; Sokol et al., 1999; Sysko, Hildebrandt, Wilson, Wilfley, & Agras, 2010).

The antiemetic ondansetron is a $5HT_3$ antagonist, used to decrease nausea and vomiting in chemotherapy patients, and it appears to offer some efficacy toward reducing binge/purge behaviors in bulimics (Faris et al., 2000; Ginawa et al., 2005; Halmi, 2005). It has been hypothesized to moderate bulimia due to its ability to diminish afferent vagal activity (Faris et al., 2000; Halmi, 2005). Other seemingly unlikely agents in the repertoire of psychopharmacological treatments for eating disorders may be harbingers for future research. Early results suggest promise for compounds that antagonize glutamate-gated Ca^{2+} ion channels such as memantine (Hermanussen & Tresguerres, 2005). Selective 5-HT6 receptor ligands, sodium oxybate, baclofen, and locaserin, as well as other novel agents such as metabolism moderators and compounds that effect neurotransmission of corticotropin releasing factor, transporter system regulation, and complex endocrine interactions among such hormones as orexin, leptin, grehlin, and neuropeptide Y, may eventually clarify possible interactive metabolic, endocrine, immune, and neuropsychiatric system processes involved in eating disorders (Akkerman et al., 2008; Brambilla et al., 2009; Brennan et al., 2008; Broft, Spanos, & Corwin, 2007; Fidler, Sanchez, & Raether, 2011; Jimerson & Wolfe, 2004; Hermanussen & Tresguerres, 2005; McElroy et al., 2012; Reas & Grilo, 2014, 2015; Rinaman, 2007; Rossi et al., 2007; Steffen et al., 2006; Wilson et al., 1999; Zhu & Walsh, 2002).

Psychosocial Interventions in the Treatment of Eating Disorders

Because avoidance behavior serves to prevent encounters with aversive stimuli, eating disordered individuals can be particularly resistant to treatment. Cognitive restructuring of distortions and irrational thought processes with repeated adaptive rehearsal strategies has proved highly effective toward diminishing the degree of distress experienced when challenging the avoidant behavior patterns that have maintained them (Garner, 1988; Garner & Bemis, 1985). Helping a patient decondition behavioral avoidance patterns by preventing ongoing pairing of cognitive errors with associated eating disordered compensatory actions involves necessary exposure. In other words, the patient with the eating disorder must experience the exact circumstances that induce discomfort (e.g., eating foods they identify as "feared" or "bad" foods), allowing for weight gain, and experiencing the intrapsychic anguish that accompanies these normative behaviors. Fundamental aspects of CBT adapted for eating disorders include identifying and developing counters to idiosyncratic thoughts about eating particular foods, body image and function, irrational attitudes about the relationship between self-worth and weight/size, and distortions about relationships specific to the individual patient. By using strategies to increase appropriate self-monitoring, encourage conscious recognition and mindful awareness of distorted thoughts, confront conditioned meanings and emotions, and change aberrant behavior patterns, patients gradually develop the ability to accurately identify thinking and feeling states, to focus their attention, and consciously choose more appropriate and healthful emotional as well as behavioral responses to their thoughts and, in turn, to improve their ability to generate rational thoughts about the previously feared foods, based on relevant evidence that supports rational thoughts rather than conditioned emotional and behavioral reactivity.

Psychosocial therapy of eating disorder usually takes one of two forms: cognitive-behavioral approaches or systemic family approaches.

Cognitive-Behavioral Approaches

Similar to aspects of exposure therapy, with its underlying premise that aversive feelings dissipate after peaking when the compulsion to act or avoid has been resisted, CBT helps reinforce healthy cognitive control and affective tolerance as well as functional behaviors, while reinforcing resilience in the face of anxiety.

A CBT method that has demonstrated efficacy with cognitively inflexible and resistant patients and/or those with neurocognitive deficits from nutritional insufficiency is cognitive remediation therapy (CRT) (Lock et al., 2013). Lock and colleagues at Stanford University have demonstrated the utility of CRT-based exercises aimed at assisting eating disordered patients improve cognitive flexibility and other metacognition skills such as process versus outcome focusing, and set-shifting (Tchanturia, Davies, & Campbell, 2007; Tchanturia & Lock, 2011; Tchanturia, Lloyd, & Lang, 2013). CRT was developed during the latter decades of the 20th century in London to improve cognitive function deficits from traumatic brain injury (Tchanturia, Campbell, Morris, & Treasure, 2005). In the early 21st century, Tchanturia adapted CRT to improve treatment adherence and efficacy among anorexics who exhibited cognitive rigidity, hyperfocusing, perfectionism, perseveration, and related executive function challenges (Lock et al., 2013; Tchanturia et al., 2004, 2005, 2007, 2013; Tchanturia & Lock, 2011).

CRT has shown promise in early treatment with nutritionally and cognitively compromised patients. Anorexic patients unresponsive to pharmacotherapy due to severely low weight have been targeted by CRT for assistance in readiness and preparation for medication introduction (Tchanturia et al., 2004, 2005, 2007). CRT has been shown to minimize cognitive rigidity and overgeneralizations, which promote heightened anxiety and behavioral avoidance, and which interfere with medication compliance (Lock et al., 2013; Tchanturia et al., 2004, 2005, 2007).

Another form of CBT showing promise with this challenging population is enhanced CBT (CBT-E), a transdiagnostic reconceptualization of CBT. CBT-E is a derivation of cognitive-behavioral treatment, adapted to treat all eating disorder psychopathology, irrespective of the specific eating disorder diagnosis or subtype (Fairburn, Cooper, & Shafran, 2003; Fairburn et al., 2009, 2015). CBT-E applies evidence-based cognitive-behavioral treatment for bulimia, the eating disordered population upon whom most randomized controlled studies have been conducted, to all eating disorders regardless of type or subtype. The transdiagnostic view suggests that the processes that maintain psychopathology in individuals with eating disorders are essentially the same across all eating disorder manifestations (Fairburn et al., 2003; Hilbert et al., 2012; Wilson et al., 1999). Research comparing CBT-E to interpersonal psychotherapy (IPT) found that 65.5% of patients with any eating disorder met remission criteria following 20 weeks of CBT-E compared to 33% of those treated with IPT for 20 weeks (Fairburn et al., 2015). At 15 months posttreatment, 69.4% of the CBT-E group, compared to 49.0% of the IPT, no longer met criteria for an eating disorder. CBT-E is an effective outpatient treatment method for eating disorders that appears to continue to yield high rates of ongoing symptom improvement beyond 1 year posttreatment. Research to date comparing these approaches suggests that IPT is also effective across all eating disorder diagnoses, evidencing steady ongoing improvement after treatment completion. However, improvement with IPT appears to be more gradual than with CBT-E (Fairburn et al., 2009, 2015).

Systemic Family Therapy

Developed primarily as a maintenance treatment for unipolar depression in the 1970s, Yale researchers Gerald Klerman, Myrna Weissman, and Eugene Paykel developed IPT (Klerman, Weissman, & Paykel, 1974). Efficacy studies using IPT with other populations, including those with dysthymia, social phobia, and eating disorders, have been conducted with positive results (Browne, 2002; Fairburn et al., 1991; Frank, 1991; McIntosh et al., 2010; Wilfley, Frank, Welch, Spurrell, & Rounsaville, 1998). IPT was adapted for individual and group treatment of bulimia and binge eating disorder during the early and mid-1990s. Through the 1990s into the 2000s, IPT continued to be studied with the various subtypes of eating disorders, using Fairburn's three-stage IPT model in randomized controlled trials (Fairburn et al., 1991, 1995, 2003, 2015; Frank, 1991; Wilfley et al., 2000). Integrating IPT into CBT and family therapies for eating disordered adolescents, several eating disorder researchers demonstrated the efficacy of these combined therapies (Hilbert, 2015; LeGrange & Eisler, 2009; Lock, 2015; McIntosh, 2000; Rosen, 2003). Individuals presenting with eating disorder and social anxiety as well as other interpersonal deficits also exhibited consistent positive responses to combined IPT/CBT family therapy; and among adults the addition of medication, particularly to address mood and anxiety symptoms, yielded the best outcomes (Agras et al., 2000; Arcelus et al., 2009; Fairburn et al., 1991, 1992, 1993, 2015; Fairburn, Kirk, O'Connor, & Cooper, 1986; Garner, 1988; Garner & Bemis, 1985; Garner, Garfinkel, & Bemis, 1982; Guidano & Liotti, 1983; Liotti, 1993; McIntosh et al., 2005; Roth & Ross, 1988; Safran & Segal, 1990; Wilfley et al., 1993, 2003).

Family-based therapies have consistently shown good results for child and adolescent anorexics and bulimics (Halmi, 2005; Lock et al., 2006; Sargent, Liebman, & Silver, 1985; Selvini-Palazolli, 1978). Family therapy is not a single unified conceptual framework, but includes numerous models with considerable overlapping perspectives regarding specific change components. While many family therapy models have been applied to treating eating disorders, those with the most supporting research evidence are structural, strategic, and systemic family therapies (Brauhardt, de Zwaan, & Hilbert, 2014; Campbell et al., 1991; Couturier et al., 2013; Dare & Eisler, 1997; Eisler et al., 2007; Halmi, 2005; Russell et al., 1987; Selvini-Palazolli, 1978). The relatively recent strong emergence of the Maudsley model (Schmidt et al., 2014) is one example of family therapy applied to the eating disorder population. In the Maudsley model, parents are involved in the treatment procedures at home, with specific emphasis on eating behaviors and mealtime communication processes. This pragmatic approach is particularly relevant given the characteristic current-day short inpatient hospitalization durations of 1–3 weeks relative to the 1970s when family therapies were initially demonstrated to be highly effective with this population and a typical inpatient hospitalization for an adolescent anorexic would last several months (Agency for Healthcare Research and Quality, 2009; Boscolo et al., 1987; Campbell et al., 1991; Crisp et al., 1991; Dare & Eisler, 1997).

Combined Therapy for Eating Disorders

CBT with psychopharmacological intervention has been demonstrated to be the most well-researched individual treatment combination for all types of adult eating disorders, particularly when no or minimal personality disturbance is evident (American Psychiatric Association, 2006; Fairburn, 2008; Halmi, 2005). For children with anorexia nervosa, family psychotherapy with behavioral interventions, but without pharmacotherapy, appears to be the exception with regard to integrated, evidence-based treatment (Boscolo, 1987; Couturier et al., 2013; Eisler et al., 2007; Findlay et al., 2010; LeGrange & Eisler, 2009; Lock, 2015; NICE, 2004; Rosen, 2003; Schmidt et al., 2014). All other age groups and eating disorder types/subtypes appear most responsive to CBT as the primary modality of individual psychotherapy, with variations in specific CBT presentation according to co-morbidities, age, and receptivity at time of treatment (Agras et al., 2000; American Psychiatric Association, 2006; Couturier et al., 2013; Eisler et al., 2007; Fairburn et al., 2009, 2015; Halmi, 2005; Keel & Haedt, 2008; Mussell et al., 2000; NICE, 2004; Tchanturia et al., 2013).

When concomitant personality disorder is evident, particularly borderline personality, eating disorder symptoms are most effectively resolved with a combination of therapies, including psychopharmacological treatment for mood disturbances and anxiety, while CBT/IPT address specific eating behaviors and associated distorted cognitions, as well as relevant family dynamics (Agras et al., 2000; American Psychiatric Association, 2006; Arcelus et al., 2009; Brauhardt et al., 2014; Bruce et al., 2005; Crosby et al., 2009; Halmi, 2005; NICE, 2004).

Psychotherapy that integrates scaled, individually tailored components of cognitive-behavioral, DBT-informed, and interpersonal therapeutic modalities with relevant psychopharmacologic management of co-morbid mood/affective and anxiety symptoms, usually with SSRIs, SNRIs, anticonvulsants, and/or low-dose atypical antipsychotics, consistently appears the most effective, both in the short and the long term. Adjusting treatment modalities, intensities, and combinations according to acute and chronic symptom management is required. As eating disorder symptoms resolve and co-morbid mood, anxiety, and developmental issues surface, coping abilities, identity reorganization, and relationship dynamics shift and require therapeutic attention. Therapeutic revisions carefully attuned to address such evolutions are central to long-term stabilization and relapse prevention of eating disorders and related symptom management (American Psychiatric Association, 2006; Brambilla et al., 2009; Bruce et al, 2005; Darcy et al., 2015; Fairburn et al., 2015; Halmi, 2005; Zhu & Walsh, 2002).

In summary, the treatment of eating disorders is one area where combining medical/pharmacotherapy with psychosocial interventions is unapologetically preferred to monotherapeutic approaches. In fact, eating disorders require a multimodal approach that integrates medical interventions, including nutrition and pharmacology, with psychosocial interventions, including personal psychotherapy as well as social and family components, to address the whole person, and not just the symptom.

Table 10.1 presents the treatment recommendations derived from our review of evidence-based research in the area of eating disorders.

Table 10.1 Integrative biopsychosocial intervention with eating disorders: Summary of best-practice recommendations by level of confidence derived from strength of evidence.

Anorexia nervosa (AN)		
Level A	Recommended	• Cognitive-behavioral therapy (CBT) is demonstrated to be the most efficacious first-line treatment for adults with AN • Family psychotherapy is indicated as first-line for children under 16 with AN, with the inclusion of CBT when the patient is cognitively and developmentally capable of using these methods • Nutritional education and behavioral intervention are recommended when patients with AN are insufficiently nourished/significantly malnourished such that they are cognitively compromised and unable to make use of psychotherapy
Level B	Suggested	• Switching to another individual psychosocial approach such as psychodynamic, interpersonal, or supportive therapy and group therapy may be considered when CBT proves ineffective, and when a patient exhibits the cognitive and developmental capacity to process forms of therapy other than behavioral • Low-dose atypical antipsychotics may be considered to improve sleep and decrease agitation or anxiety. Olanzapine and quetiapine also induce increased appetite/weight gain, though they are often not well tolerated in this population • Psychopharmacology may be best considered as adjunctive to psychosocial interventions; however, it is important to keep in mind that the use of pharmacological intervention may be compromised when body weight is extremely low
Level C	May be considered	• Selective serotonin reuptake inhibitors (SSRIs) are usually recommended as the first choice once weight restoration is underway provided there is no indication of bipolar disorder. Paroxetine is a frequent choice with AN as it may be more likely to induce weight gain than the other SSRIs • Switching out of the SSRIs to a serotonin–norepinephrine reuptake inhibitor (SNRI) may be considered if the patient fails to respond to one or more SSRIs, or if anxiety is insufficiently managed with SSRIs and psychosocial interventions
Bulimia nervosa (BN)		
Level A	Recommended	• CBT and interpersonal psychotherapy are considered first-line treatment for bulimia nervosa • DBT appears indicated when the eating disorder presents with borderline personality disorder • Fluoxetine or another SSRI, in combination with psychotherapy, is indicated when depressive and/or anxiety co-morbid exist • Family psychotherapy is indicated as first-line for children under 16 with BN
Level B	Suggested	• If response to SSRI is insufficient, augmentation with SNRIs, atypical antipsychotics, or anticonvulsants may help manage symptoms of affective, anxiety, and/or personality disorder(s) • Topiramate, often in combination with an SSRI or SNRI and psychosocial treatment, helps decrease frequency and intensity of binge urges • The appetite suppressant effects of psychostimulants can augment SSRI or other antidepressant and psychosocial therapy

Table 10.1 (Continued)

Level C	May be considered	• Group therapy can be a useful augment to individual and pharmacotherapies to address the interpersonal challenges frequently accompanying bulimia nervosa
Binge eating disorder (BED)		
Level A	Recommended	• CBT plus SSRI is the preferred treatment combination • If response to CBT and SSRI is insufficient, consider shift to SNRI or buproprion • Psychostimulant to improve appetite management in combination with antidepressant and CBT or other psychosocial therapy
Level B	Suggested	• Buproprion without SSRI/SNRI if no concomitant mood or anxiety disorder, provided patient is not bulimic • Nutrition counseling/support • Antiobesity drugs
Level C	May be considered	• Group psychotherapy • Self-help programs face-to-face • Self-help programs via internet

Case Example

A 20-year-old single, Caucasian female, Camille presents to outpatient psychotherapy for the first time after her mother calls to make an appointment for her while Camille is home for the summer having completed her junior year at a prestigious east coast college. Camille is sitting rigidly in the waiting room, appearing both eager and anxious.

Camille describes "struggling with eating and weight" issues for "about 3–4 years," since 11th grade when she started a "normal diet" after her then boyfriend, Matt, told her she probably only made the JV instead of varsity lacrosse team, because she had "gotten a little chunkier." Camille said she was "devastated" by his comment and shocked that he had "acted like he loved me for almost 2 years and all this time thought I was a fat pig." She wanted to believe the team captain who told her she didn't make the team because of a recurrent ankle injury, but no matter how much she tried to make herself believe that, she couldn't get Matt's words out of her head. Anytime she was around boys after that, even those she used to think were her friends, she felt "stupid and fat" and thought she "had been a fool." Despite her boyfriend's repeated apologies, Camille ended their 2-year relationship a week later with the explanation that she didn't deserve him as her boyfriend anymore. She said she felt like a "loser" and wouldn't let herself even think of having another boyfriend until she lost at least 10 pounds.

In her initial session, Camille explained that she didn't believe she had an eating disorder until the day she finished her final exams and was walking back to her dorm and fainted. Her mom had come to campus to help her move her stuff back home for the summer, and told Camille she "almost didn't recognize [her]." She admitted having lost about 10 pounds over the past month, but that she needed to because she was "getting too close" to the weight she was in 11th grade when Matt told her she was chunky.

At 5′5″, Camille weighed 111 pounds. Of a small frame, she explained she was a normal weight because the weight charts that say a normal weight between 115 and 140 for her

(Continued)

height and age were intended for medium-framed women. In 11th grade, when she started dieting, she weighed 128 pounds. She started dieting in the fall of 11th grade by cutting out lunch and all snacks, but after the first month she was disappointed that she had only lost 8 pounds. She felt disgusted with herself, calling herself "weak-willed and lazy" and she decided to cut out as much dinner as she could stand to. She continued to cut back the size of her meals until breakfast was only a hard-boiled egg and dinner was a salad with vinegar and maybe a few bites of tuna fish. If she ran more than 5 miles in a given day, she might allow herself a yogurt after dinner. By the end of her senior year of high school she weighed only 100 pounds, having lost nearly 30 pounds. She had stopped menstruating, her hair had become thin and dull, she felt cold all the time, and no longer wanted to hang out with friends, saying "they were immature and didn't have anything in common anymore." When her mother told her she thought she was anorexic and that if she didn't gain 10 pounds she wasn't going to let her move in the fall to start college, Camille became furious and insisted she wasn't anorexic, but was just trying to be healthy. She yelled at her mother saying she couldn't tell her how to live her life anymore.

Angry, but also terrified by her mother's ultimatum, Camille cut her running down to 3 miles per day, 5 days per week instead of 5–8 miles 6 or 7 days per week, and she forced herself to eat three meals so her mother would see her eating and no longer accuse her of having anorexia. By mid-August, nearly time to move to college, Camille had gained 14 pounds. Her mother never mentioned her weight being a problem again, and together they excitedly moved her to campus as though there had never been a concern.

Once in college, Camille was determined to get straight As to prove to herself that she could keep up with the other students she thought must be smarter than she, because three of her five suitemates had scholarships and she didn't. She began staying up late and getting up early, getting only 4–5 h of sleep per night so she could fit in a run and still have time to double check her homework assignments and read ahead to the next day's assignments. Some nights she described feeling like she had a "pit" in her stomach. She couldn't tell if the feeling was hunger or fear, but she figured she must be hungry because she couldn't identify anything that should be scaring her. The first time she felt this way was before a biology mid-term. The feeling in her stomach was so persistent she couldn't fall asleep, so she decided to get up and eat a bowl of ice cream. She immediately felt better and fell asleep easily. The next morning she was a little nervous about the mid-term, but she knew that she was ready. She aced the exam and felt better than she'd felt in months. Excited she'd done so well, she invited her suitemates out that night to celebrate.

After a night of drinking and eating greasy appetizers at the local bar, she felt bloated and guilty about having "been such a glutton." Her suitemate she'd become close friends with told her that when she felt that way she just stuck her fingers down her throat and "all the guilt went away." Initially thinking her friend was gross, she later thought, "Why not? That way I can eat and not have to gain the weight. Besides, with all my homework, I don't have time like I used to to run all of the time."

That night, and most nights thereafter, Camille engaged in the routine of eating dinner with her friends, provoking vomiting, studying until 10, eating ice cream, vomiting again, drinking a beer or smoking a joint to "help get calm to fall asleep fast," then getting up early the next morning to make sure she remembered what she studied last night and was ready for class. Some nights she was too tired to go out to get the ice cream so instead she'd order in a pizza to be delivered and eat the whole thing. Pizza was harder to throw up than ice cream so the mornings after eating and throwing up pizza, she would skip her extra study time and instead go for a run "to make up for the extra calories."

When asked why the fainting episode was the signal to her that she had a problem and not the daily binge eating and purging, she said, "It became pretty clear that most of my suitemates, and probably just about any other girl on campus who was smaller than a size 6, was doing it, so it couldn't be too abnormal. I heard about people having really bad eating disorders and having to be hospitalized and stuff like that, but I figured if it was really a problem I wouldn't be able to get straight As, and I wouldn't be able to stop doing it; but, I can stop it if I want to."

When asked what alerted her that she might need help, Camille answered that the week before exams she had eaten one small meal each day of no more than 400 calories. She tried repeatedly to stop herself from throwing up these small meals, but she could not, and when she fainted she realized she couldn't lie to herself anymore; that, indeed, she was not able to stop vomiting.

Camille agreed to complete several questionnaires assessing her levels of depression, anxiety, obsessive-compulsive thought processes, eating patterns and related attitudes, and a personality inventory. The scores from these suggested a highly anxious, moderately depressed, interpersonally sensitive, accommodating, risk averse, perfectionistic individual with a high need for approval and strong desire to please those she cares about. She is achievement-oriented, determined, goal-oriented, and tends toward sensation-seeking activities, particularly when stressed. She also agreed to keep track of her eating and exercising, as well as of purging behavior and associated moods over the next several days before her next appointment.

At her next appointment, Camille was pleased to bring in a new file folder with several forms, including some of the checklists from the last session, color-coded lists of her food and behavior tracking progress, complete with graphs and spreadsheets.

Labs were drawn, including a complete blood count (CBC), high sensitivity thyroid screen, vitamin B and D levels, and a follow-up appointment for a bone density evaluation was scheduled. The lab results appeared largely within normal limits with low normal levels of vitamin D, low normal potassium, high normal thyroid stimulating hormone (TSH) levels, high normal levels of T4 free, and low normal levels of T3 free. Also of note was a slightly elevated triglyceride level relative to Camille's age, weight, and otherwise normal lipid panel. Elevated triglyercides are sometimes found among bulimic and binge eating individuals whose food intake consists of high levels of high sugar, high fat baked goods, desserts, and processed carbohydrates. The low normal potassium, vitamin D, and T3 free, and high normal TSH values are consistent with thyroid function vulnerabilities, fatigue, and/or depression (Aigner et al., 2011; Halmi, 1992).

Camille was receptive to considering medication for anxiety and depression "as long as it doesn't change my personality or make me fat," and she also readily signed on for cognitive-behavioral strategies that built upon her previous efforts at charting of food, mood, behavior, feelings, thoughts, activities, and interaction patterns among these. The charting proved instrumental in helping Camille understand what factors contributed to her feelings and beliefs about food, eating, weight, her body, relationships, responsibilities, maturation, and control. In addition to twice-weekly individual cognitive-behavioral psychotherapy, and a

(Continued)

process group for bulimia and anorexia that met twice monthly, Camille also began a trial of 10 mg escitalopram to help decrease her pervasive level of general anxiety, the obsessive-compulsive rumination about her body and what others thought about her. She was scheduled for weigh-in every 3 months and intermittent repeat labs.

Over the next 6 months, Camille participated actively in individual therapy, always showing up early with "homework" completed in great detail. She made considerable progress identifying and challenging cognitive errors, particularly those associated with negative self-appraisals that often triggered a decline in mood and/or increased anxiety, anxious avoidance of anything that threatened to show her to be less than perfect, especially new experiences or things she hadn't tried before. She recognized how dichotomous, all-or-nothing, overpersonalized, and catastrophic thinking about how she presumed others were viewing her contributed to food choices and interfered with eating in public for fear she'd be perceived as gluttonous. Through her homework, Camille began to see patterns in her thought processes and how they interfered with engaging with others, feeling confident, and not constantly self-conscious, as well as how the cascade of negative thoughts and feelings disrupted making healthy reasonable choices of food.

The patient's mood and anxiety gradually improved, but she was still anxious most of the time, and had trouble falling asleep or staying asleep at times. She also continued to feel "that pit in my stomach a lot, especially if I'm going to be with friends I haven't seen in a while or if my weight is a little higher." We discussed possible medication changes and the escitalopram was subsequently increased to 20 mg.

Over the next 3 months, Camille continued to improve on mood regulation, sleep continuity, eating regularity, decreased purging, excessive exercise, and she gradually increased weight, with slight improvements in tolerance of higher weight than she'd been in 2 years. She acknowledged considerable cognitive dissonance between her logical awareness of her near-normal weight, and struggling to "feel okay" with it. Visualization and relaxation exercises that accompanied DBT and CBT constructs around mindfulness and conscious awareness development of "willfulness" and "deliberateness" were particularly helpful exercises for Camille. By reminding herself of the facts about her body as demonstrated by the scale, clothing size, improvements in lab results, and physical wellbeing, she was able to consciously focus on positive emotions and wellbeing, and to further attend to the feelings that emanate from her body, mind, and mood from that awareness.

Ten months after Camille started 10 mg escitalopram, it was discontinued and a trial of 75 mg of venlafaxine was started. Venlafaxine was eventually titrated to 150 mg because general anxiety and internal physiological sense of uneasiness persisted. Three months later, Camille was maintaining 119–123 pounds and had not binged or purged in 2 months.

Camille has completed her undergraduate degree in biology with a 3.9 average, which she is pleased with. She admits that a year ago she would have been very angry with herself for not having a 4.0, but she considers 3.9 proof of "learning to live realistically." She still struggles with occasional urges to binge when a big project is due at work. She decreased venlafaxine to 75 mg a few months after graduating and, while she hopes to one day try taking no medication, she finds it is particularly helpful premenstrually and during significantly stressful times. She continues in twice-monthly individual psychotherapy, and recently decided to consider joining the process group as she recognized that since graduating from college she has a tendency to socially isolate more than she thinks is healthy; the isolation increases internal cognitive rumination, whereas social involvement helps her challenge her cognitive appraisals and catch irrational, self-critical, all-or-nothing or perfectionistic thoughts or associations.

Camille recently indicated that, since developing a healthier relationship with her body and realizing her feelings about herself and the world around her are at least in part determined by how she thinks and what she believes about them, she now feels ready to change her relationship with her parents, whereas before she felt powerless to effect any such change. She has developed an internal locus of control and is therefore now more capable of recognizing her feelings and relating to her physical, emotional and social needs with proactive awareness and redirection instead of as a passive recipient. She said she feels less bothered by her father's seeming lack of interest in much of a relationship with her, and is less irritated with her mother's intrusive, controlling tendencies. She states, "they are who they are and I'm not going to change that by trying to be perfect or by hating myself because I didn't get the kind of love I always hoped for from them. They act how they act because of who they are, not because of me or because I'm thin or fat, smart or dumb. That sounds so obvious now."

References

Agency for Healthcare Research and Quality (2009). *Eating disorders sending more Americans to the hospital. AHRQ News and Numbers.* Retrieved from www.ahrq.gov/news/nn/nn040109.htm

Agras, W., Walsh, B., Fairburn, C., Wilson, G., & Kraemer, H. (2000). A multicenter comparison of cognitive-behavioural therapy and interpersonal psychotherapy for bulimia nervosa, *Archives of General Psychiatry, 57,* 459–466.

Aigner, M., Treasure, J., Kasper, S., & WFSBP Task Force on Eating Disorders (2011). World Federation of Societies of Biological Psychiatry (WFSBP) guidelines for the pharmacological treatment of eating disorders. *World Journal of Biological Psychiatry, 12,* 400–443.

Akkermann, K., Paaver, M., Nordquist, N., Oreland, L., & Harro, J. (2008). Association of 5-HTT gene polymorphism, platelet MAO activity, and drive for thinness in a population-based sample of adolescent girls. *International Journal of Eating Disorders, 41,* 399–204.

Alger, S., Schwalberg, M., Bigaouette, J., Michalek, A., & Howard, L. (1991). Effects of a tricyclic antidepressant and opiate antagonist on binge-eating behavior in normoweight bulimic and obese, binge-eating subjects. *American Journal of Clinical Nutrition, 53,* 865–871.

American Psychiatric Association (2006). Practice guideline for the treatment of patients with eating disorders (revision). *American Journal of Psychiatry, 163*(Suppl. 1), 1–54.

Arcelus, J., Whight, D., Langham, C., Baggott, J., McGrain, L., Meadows, L., & Meyer, C. (2009). A case series evaluation of a modified version of interpersonal psychotherapy (IPT) for the treatment of bulimic eating disorders: A pilot study. *European Eating Disorders Review, 17,* 260–268.

Ben-Porath, D., Wisniewski, L., & Warren, M. (2009). Differential treatment response for eating disordered patients with and without a comorbid borderline personality diagnosis using a dialectical behavior therapy (DBT)-informed approach. *Eating Disorders, 17,* 225–241.

Biederman, J., Herzog, D., & Rivinus, T. (1985). Amitriptyline in the treatment of anorexia nervosa: a double-blind, placebo-controlled study. *Journal of Clinical Psychopharmacology, 5*, 10–16.

Bissada, H., Tasca, G., Barber, A., & Bradwejn, J. (2008). Olanzapine in the treatment of low body weight and obsessive thinking in women with anorexia nervosa: A randomized double-blind placebo-controlled trial. *American Journal of Psychiatry, 165*, 1281–1288.

Black, R., Davis, C., & Kennedy, S. (1993). Alterations in metabolism and energy expenditure in eating disorders. In A. Kaplan, &P. Garfinkel, P. (Eds.), *Medical issues and the eating disorders: The interface* (pp. 144–164). New York: Brunner/Mazel.

Bosanac, P., Norman, T., Burrows, G., & Beumont, P. (2005). Serotonergic and dopaminergic systems in anorexia nervosa: A role for atypical antipsychotics? *Australia and New Zealand Journal of Psychiatry, 39*, 146–153.

Boscolo, L., Cecchin, G., Hoffman, L., & Penn, P. (1987). *Milan systemic family therapy.* New York: Basic Books.

Brambilla, F., Samek, L., Company, M., Lovo, F., Cioni, L., & Mellado, C. (2009). Multivariate therapeutic approach to binge-eating disorder: Combined nutritional, psychological and pharmacological treatment. *International Journal of Clinical Psychopharmacology, 24*, 312–317.

Brauhardt, A., de Zwaan, M., & Hilbert, A. (2014). The therapeutic process in psychological treatments for eating disorders: A systematic review. *International Journal of Eating Disorders, 46*, 565–584.

Brennan, B., Roberts, J., Fogarty, K., Reynolds, K., Jonas, J., & Hudson, J. (2008). Memantine in the treatment of binge eating disorder: An open-label, prospective trial. *International Journal of Eating Disorders, 41*, 520–526.

Broft, A., Spanos, A., & Corwin, R. (2007). Baclofen for binge eating: An open-label trial. *International Journal of Eating Disorders, 40*, 687–691.

Browne, G. (2002). Sertraline and interpersonal psychotherapy, alone and combined, in the treatment of patients with dysthymic disorder in primary care: A 2 year comparison of effectiveness and cost. *Journal of Affective Disorders, 68*, 317–330.

Bruce, K., Steiger, H., Ng Ying, N., & Kin, M. (2005). Reduced platelet [3H] paroxetine binding in anorexia nervosa: Relationship to eating symptoms and personality pathology. *Psychiatry Research, 142*, 225–232.

Bulik, C., Devlin, B., & Vacanu, S. (2003). Significant linkage on chromosome 10p in families with bulimia nervosa. *American Journal of Human Genetics, 72*, 200–207.

Bulik, C., Hebebrand, J., & Keski-Rahkonen, A. (2007). Genetic epidemiology, endophenotypes, and eating disorder classification. *International Journal of Eating Disorders, 40*, S52–S60.

Campbell, D., Draper, R., & Huffington, C. (1991). *Second thoughts on the theory and practice of the Milan approach to family therapy.* London: Draper Campbell.

Couturier, J., Kimber, M., & Szatmari, P. (2013). Efficacy of family-based treatment for adolescents with eating disorders: A systematic review and meta-analysis. *International Journal of Eating Disorders, 46*, 1, 3–11.

Crisp, A., Norton, K., Gowers, S., Halek, C., Bowyer, C., & Yeldham, D. (1991). A controlled study of the effect of therapies aimed at adolescent and family psychopathology in anorexia nervosa. *British Journal of Psychiatry, 159*, 325–333.

Crosby, R., Wonderlich, S., Engel, S., Simonich, H., Smyth, J., & Mitchell, J. (2009). Daily mood patterns and bulimic behaviors in the natural environment. *Behaviour Research and Therapy, 47*, 181–188.

Dare, C., & Eisler, I. (1997). Family therapy for anorexia nervosa. In D. Garner, & P. Garfinkel (Eds.), *Handbook of treatment for eating disorders* (2nd ed.) (pp. 307–324). New York: Guilford Press.

Darcy, A., Fitzpatrick, K., & Lock, J. (2015). Cognitive remediation therapy and cognitive behavior therapy for anorexia nervosa. In H. Thompson-Brenner (Ed.), *Casebook of evidence-based therapy for eating disorders* (pp. 102–128). New York: Guilford Press.

Dold, M. Aigner, M., Klaubunde, M., Treasure, J., & Kasper, S. (2015). Second-generation antipsychotic drugs in anorexia nervosa: A meta-analysis of randomized controlled trials. *Psychotherapy and Psychosomatics, 84,* 110–116.

Eddy, K., Dorer, D., Franko, D., Tahilani, K., Thompson-Brenner, H., & Herzog, D. (2008). Diagnostic crossover in anorexia nervosa and bulimia nervosa: Implications for DSM-V. *American Journal of Psychiatry, 165,* 245–250.

Eisler I., Dare, C., Hodes, M., Russell, G., Dodge, E., & LeGrange, D. (2000a). Family therapy for adolescent anorexia nervosa: The results of a controlled comparison of two family interventions. *Journal of Child Psychiatry, 41,* 727–736.

Eisler I., Dare, C., Russell, G., Szmukler, G., LeGrange, D., & Dodge, E. (2000b). Family and individual therapy in anorexia nervosa: A 5-year follow-up. *Archives of General Psychiatry, 54,* 1025–1030.

Eisler, I., Simic, M., Russell, G., & Dare, C. (2007). A randomized controlled treatment trial of two forms of family therapy in adolescent anorexia nervosa: A five year follow-up. *Journal of Child Psychology and Psychiatry, 48,* 552–560.

Fairburn, C. (2008). *Cognitive behavior therapy and eating disorders.* New York: Guilford Press.

Fairburn, C. (1992). Interpersonal psychotherapy for bulimia nervosa. In G. L. Klerman, & M. W. Weissman (Eds.), *New applications of interpersonal psychotherapy* (pp. 353–378). Washington, DC: American Psychiatric Press.

Fairburn, C., Bailey-Straebler, S., Basden, S., Doll, H., Jones, R., Murphy, R., . . . & Cooper, Z. (2015). Transdiagnostic comparison of enhanced cognitive behaviour therapy (CBT-E) and interpersonal psychotherapy in the treatment of eating disorders. *Behaviour Research and Therapy, 70,* 64–71.

Fairburn C., Cooper, Z., Doll, H., O'Connor, M., Bohn, K., Hawker, D., . . . & Palmer, R. (2009). Transdiagnostic cognitive behavioral therapy for patients with eating disorders: A two-site trial with 60-week follow-up. *American Journal of Psychiatry, 166,* 311–319.

Fairburn, C., Cooper, Z., & Shafran, R. (2003). Cognitive behaviour therapy for eating disorders: A "transdiagnostic" theory and treatment. *Behaviour Research and Therapy, 41,* 509–528.

Fairburn, C, Jones, R., Peveler, R., Carr, S., Solomon, R., O'Connor, M., . . . & Hope, R. A. (1991). Three psychological treatments for bulimia nervosa: A comparative trial. *Archives of General Psychiatry, 48,* 463–469.

Fairburn, C., Jones, R., Peveler, R., Hope, R., & O'Connor, M. (1993). Psychotherapy and bulimia nervosa: The longer-term effects of interpersonal psychotherapy, behaviour therapy and cognitive behaviour therapy. *Archives of General Psychiatry, 50,* 419–428.

Fairburn, C., Kirk, J., O'Connor, M., & Cooper, P. (1986). A comparison of two psychological treatments for bulimia nervosa. *Behaviour Research Therapy, 24,* 629–643.

Fairburn, C., Norman, P., Welch, S., O'Connor, M., Doll, H., & Peveler, R. (1995). A prospective study of outcome in bulimia nervosa and the long-term effects of three psychological treatments. *Archives of General Psychiatry, 52,* 304–312.

Faris, P., Kim, S., Meller, W., Goodale, R., Oakman, S., & Hofbauer, R. (2000). Effect of decreasing afferent vagal activity with ondansetron on symptoms of bulimia nervosa: A randomized, double-blind trial. *Lancet, 355*, 792–979.

Farooqi, I., Bullmore, E., Keogh, J., Gillard, J., O'Rahilly, S., & Fletcher, P. (2007). Leptin regulates striatal regions and human eating behavior. *Science, on-line.* doi:10.1126/science.1144599

Feld, B., Woodside, D., Kaplan, A., Olmsted, M., & Carter, J. (2001). Pretreatment motivational enhancement therapy for eating disorders: A pilot study. *International Journal of Eating Disorders, 29*, 393–400.

Fichter, M., Leibl, C., Kruger, R., & Rief, W. (1997). Effects of fluvoxamine on depression, anxiety, and other areas of general psychopathology in bulimia nervosa. *Pharmacopsychiatry, 30*, 85–92.

Fidler, M., Sanchez, M., & Raether, B. (2011). A one-year randomized trial of lorcaserin for weight loss in obese and overweight adults: The BLOSSOM trial. *Journal of Clinical Endocrinology and Metabolism, 96*, 3067–3077.

Field, B., Wren, A., Cooke, D., & Bloom, S. (2008). Gut hormones as potential new targets for appetite regulation and the treatment of obesity. *Drugs, 68*, 147–163.

Findlay, S., Pinzon, J., Taddeo, D., & Katzman D. (2010). Canadian Paediatric Society, Adolescent Health Committee. Family-based treatment of children and adolescents with anorexia nervosa: guidelines for the community physician. *Paediatric Child Health, 15*, 31.

Frank, E. (1991). Interpersonal psychotherapy as a maintenance treatment for patients with recurrent depression. *Psychotherapy and Psychosomatics, 28*, 259–266.

Galsworthy-Francis, L. (2014). Cognitive-behavioural therapy for anorexia nervosa: A systematic review. *Clinical Psychology Review, 34*, 54–72.

Garner, D. (1988). Anorexia nervosa. In M. Hersen, & C. Last (Eds.), *Child behavior therapy casebook* (pp. 263–276). New York: Plenum Press.

Garner, D., & Bemis, K. (1985). Cognitive therapy for anorexia nervosa. In D. Garner, & P. Garfinkel (Eds.), *Handbook of psychotherapy for anorexia nervosa and bulimia* (pp. 107–146). New York: Guilford Press.

Garner, D., Garfinkel, P., & Bemis, K. (1982). A multidimensional psychotherapy for anorexia nervosa. *International Journal of Eating Disorders, 1*, 3–46.

Ginawa, O., Al-Majed, A., & Al-Suwailem, A. (2005). Ondansetron, a 5-HT3 antagonist, antagonizes methamphetamine-induced anorexia in mice. *Pharmacological Research, 51*, 255–259.

Goracci, A., diVolo, S., Casamassima, F., Bolognesi, S., Benbow, J., & Fagiolini, A. (2015). Pharmacotherapy of binge-eating disorder: A review. *Journal of Addictions Medicine, 9*, 1–19.

Grice, D., Halmi, K., & Fichter, M. (2002). Evidence for a susceptibility gene for anorexia nervosa on chromosome 1. *American Journal of Human Genetics, 70*, 787–792.

Guidano, V., & Liotti, G. (1983). *Cognitive processes and emotional disorders: A structural approach to psychotherapy.* New York: Guilford Press.

Guerdjikova, A., McElroy, S., Kotwal, R., Welge, J., Nelson, E., & Lake, K. (2008). High-dose escitalopram in the treatment of binge-eating disorder with obesity: A placebo-controlled monotherapy trail. *Human Psychopharmacology, 23*, 1–11.

Halmi, K. (1992). Psychobiology and treatment of anorexia nervosa and bulimia nervosa. In K. Halmi (Ed.), *Psychobiology and treatment of anorexia nervosa and bulimia nervosa* (pp. 79–90). Washington DC: American Psychiatric Association Press.
Halmi, K. (2005). The multimodal treatment of eating disorders. *World Psychiatry, 4*(2), 69–73.
Halmi, K., Eckert, E., & LaDu, T. (1986). Anorexia nervosa: Treatment efficacy of cyproheptadine and amitriptyline. *Archives of General Psychiatry, 43*, 177–181.
Heal, D., Smith, S., Fisas, A., Codony, X., & Buschmann, H. (2008). Selective 5-HT6 receptor ligands: progress in the development of a novel pharmacological approach to the treatment of obesity and related metabolic disorders. *Pharmacological Therapeutics, 117*, 207–231.
Hedges, D., Reimherr, F., Hoopes, S., Rosenthal, N., Kamin, M., & Kamin, R. (2003). Treatment of bulimia nervosa with topiramate in a randomized, double-blind, placebo-controlled trial, part 2: Improvement in psychiatric measures. *Journal of Clinical Psychiatry, 64*, 1449–1454.
Hoopes, S., Reimherr, F., Hedges, D., Rosenthal, N., Kamin, M., & Kamin, R. (2003). Treatment of bulimia nervosa with topiramate in a randomized, double-blind, placebo-controlled trial, part 1: Improvement in binge and purge measure. *Journal of Clinical Psychiatry, 64*, 1335–1341.
Hepworth, N., Paxton, J., & Williams, B. (2007). Predictors of attitudes towards treatments for bulimia nervosa. *Australia and New Zealand Journal of Psychiatry, 41*, 247–256.
Hermanussen, M., & Tresguerres, J. (2005). A new anti-obesity drug treatment: First clinical evidence that antagonising glutamate-gated Ca2+ ion channels with memantine normalises binge-eating disorders. *Economics and Human Biolology, 3*, 329–337.
Hilbert, A. (2015). Advances in the treatment of eating disorders. *Psychotherapie, Psychosomatik, Medizinische, Psychologie, 65*, 28–29.
Hoek, H., & van Hoeken, D. (2003). Review of the prevalence and incidence of eating disorders. *International Journal Eating Disorders, 34*, 383–396.
Hoffman, L. (1985). Beyond power and control: Toward a "second order" family systems therapy. *Family Systems Medicine, 3*, 381–396.
Howard, W., Evans, K., Quintero-Howard, C., Bowers, W., & Andersen, A. (1997). Predictors of success or failure of transition to day hospital treatment for inpatients with anorexia nervosa. *American Journal of Psychiatry, 156*, 1697–1702.
Igoin-Apfelbaum, L., & Apfelbaum, L. (1987). Naltrexone and bulimic symptoms. *Lancet, 2*, 1087–1088.
Jimerson, D., & Wolfe, B. (2004). Neuropeptides in eating disorders. *CNS Spectrums, 9*, 516–522.
Kaplan A., & Garfinkel, P. (1999). Difficulties in treating patients with eating disorders: A review of patient and clinician variables. *Canadian Journal of Psychiatry, 44*, 665–670.
Kaplan A., & Olmstead, M. (1997). Partial hospitalization. In D. Garner, & P. Garfinkel (Eds.), *Handbook of treatment for eating disorders* (2nd ed.) (pp. 354–360). New York: Guilford Press.
Kaustav, C., & Basu, D. (2010). Management of anorexia and bulimia nervosa: An evidence-based review. *Indian Journal of Psychiatry, 52*, 174–186.
Kaye, W., Frank, G., & McConah, A. (1999). Altered dopamine activity after recovery from restricting-type anorexia nervosa. *Neuropsychopharmacology, 21*, 503–506.

Kaye, W., Gendall, K., & Strober, M. (1998). Serotonin neuronal function and selective serotonin reuptake inhibitor treatment in anorexia and bulimia nervosa. *Biological Psychiatry, 44*(9), 825–838.

Kaye, W., Nagata, T., &Weltzin, T. (2001). Double-blind placebo-controlled administration of fluoxetine in restricting and restricting-purging type anorexia nervosa. *Biological Psychiatry, 49*, 644–652.

Kaye, W., & Strober, M. (1999). Neurobiology of eating disorders. In D. Charney, E. Nestler, & B. Bunny (Eds), *Neurobiological foundations of mental illness* (pp. 891–906). New York: Oxford University Press.

Keel, P., & Brown, T. (2010). Update on Course and outcome in eating disorders. *International Disorders of Eating Disorders, 43*, 195–204.

Keel, P., & Haedt, A. (2008). Evidence-based psychosocial treatment for eating problems and eating disorders. *Journal of Clinical Child and Adolescent Psychology, 37*, 39–61.

Kishi, T., Kafantaris, V., Sunday, S., Sheridan, E., & Correll, C. (2012). Are antipsychotics effective for the treatment of anorexia nervosa? Results from a systematic review and meta-analysis. *Journal of Clinical Psychiatry, 73*, e757–e766.

Klerman, G., Weissman, M., & Paykel, E. (1974). Treatment of depression by drugs and psychotherapy. *American Journal of Psychiatry, 131*, 186–191.

Lacey, J., & Crisp, A. (1980). Hunger, food intake and weight: The impact of clomipramine on a refeeding anorexia nervosa population. *Postgraduate Medical Journal, 56*, 79–85.

LeGrange, D., & Eisler, I. (2009). Family interventions in adolescent anorexia nervosa. *Child Adolescent Psychiatric Clinics of North America, 18*, 159–173.

Leombruni, P., Piero, A., Lavagnino, L., Burstolin, A., Campisi, S., & Fassino, S. (2008). A randomized, double-blind trial comparing sertraline and fluoxetine 6-month treatment in obese patients with binge eating disorder. *Progress in Neuropsychopharmacology and Biological Psychiatry, 32*, 1599–1605.

Lewinsohn, P., Striegel-Moore, R., & Seeley, J. (2000). Epidemiology and natural course of eating disorders in young women from adolescence to young adulthood. *Journal of the American Academy of Child and Adolescent Psychiatry, 39*, 1284–1292.

Lilenfeld, R., Kaye, W., & Greeno, C. (1998). A controlled family study of anorexia nervosa and bulimia nervosa: Psychiatric disorders in first degree relatives and effects of proband comorbidity. *Archives of General Psychiatry, 55*, 603–610.

Liotti, G. (1993). Disorganized attachment and dissociative experiences: An illustration of the developmental-ethological approach to cognitive therapy. In K. Kuehlwein, & H. Rosen (Eds.), *Cognitive therapies in action: Evolving innovative practice* (pp. 213–239). San Francisco, CA: Jossey-Bass.

Lock, J. (2015). An update on evidence-based psychosocial treatments for eating disorders in children and adolescents. *Journal of Clinical Child and Adolescent Psychology, 44*, 707–721.

Lock, J., Agras, W., Fitzpatrick, K., Bryson, S., Jo, B., & Tchanturia, K. (2013). Is outpatient cognitive remediation therapy feasible to use in randomized clinical trials for anorexia nervosa? *International Journal of Eating Disorders, 46*, 567–575.

Lock, J., Couturier, J., & Agras, W. (2006). Comparison of long-term outcomes in adolescents with anorexia nervosa treated with family therapy. *Journal of the American Academy of Child and Adolescent Psychiatry, 45*, 666–672.

Lock, J., Le Grange, D., Agras, W., & Dare, C. (2001). *Treatment manual for anorexia nervosa: A family-based approach*. New York: Guildford Publications, Inc.

McElroy, S., & Arnold, M. (2003). Topiramate in the treatment of binge eating disorder associated with obesity: a randomized, placebo-controlled trial. *American Journal of Psychiatry, 160*, 255–261.
McElroy, S., Guerdjikova, A., Mori, N., & O'Melia, A. (2012). Pharmacological management of binge eating disorder: current and emerging treatment options. *Therapeutics and Clinical Risk Management, 8*, 219–241.
McIntosh, V. (2000). Interpersonal psychotherapy for anorexia nervosa. *International Journal of Eating Disorders, 27*, 125–139.
McIntosh, V., Jordan, J., & Carter, F. (2005). Three psychotherapies for anorexia nervosa: A randomized, controlled trial. *American Journal of Psychiatry, 162*, 741–747.
McKnight, R., & Park, R. (2010). Atypical antipsychotics and anorexia nervosa: A review. *European Eating Disorders Review, 18*, 10–21.
Milano, W., Petrella, C., & Sabatino, C. (2004). Treatment of bulimia nervosa with sertraline: A randomized controlled trial. *Advanced Therapeutics, 21*, 232–237.
Mitchell, L., Pyle, R., & Eckert, D. (1990). A comparison study of antidepressants and structured group therapy in patients in the treatment for bulimia nervosa. *Archives of General Psychiatry, 47*, 149–160.
Mitchell, L., Pyle, R., & Hatsukami, D. (1989). A 2 to 5 year follow-up study of patients treated for bulimia. *International Journal of Eating Disorders, 8*, 157–165.
Mond, J., Myers, T., Crosby, R., Hay, P., & Mitchell, J. (2008). Excessive exercise and eating-disordered behavior in young adult women: Further evidence from a primary care sample. *European Eating Disorders Review, 16*, 215–221.
Monteleone, P., Di Lieto, A., & Castaldo, E. (2004). Leptin functioning in eating disorders. *CNS Spectrums, 9*, 523–529.
Mussell, M., Crosby, R., Crow, S., Knopke, A., Peterson, C., Wonderlich, S., & Mitchell, J. (2000). Utilization of empirically supported psychotherapy treatments for individuals with eating disorders: A survey of psychologists. *International Journal of Eating Disorders, 27*, 230–237.
National Institute for Clinical Excellence (NICE) (2004). *Eating disorders: Core interventions in the treatment and management of anorexia nervosa, bulimia nervosa, and related eating disorders*. London: National Institute for Clinical Excellence.
Peterson, C., Becke, C., Treasure, J., Sharfran, R., & Brant-Waugh, R. (2016). The three-legged stool of evidence-based practice in eating disorder treatment: Research, clinical and patient perspectives. *BMC Medicine, 14*, 69.
Pope, H., Hudson, J., Jonas, J., & Yurgelun-Todd, D. (1983). Bulimia treated with imipramine: A placebo controlled, double blind study. *American Journal of Psychiatry, 140*, 554–558.
Powers, P., & Bruty, H. (2009). Pharmacotherapy for eating disorders and obesity. *Child Adolescent Psychiatric Clinics of North America, 18*, 175–187.
Powers, P., Santana, C., & Bannon, Y. (2002). Olanzapine in the treatment of anorexia nervosa: An open label trial. *International Journal of Eating Disorders, 32*, 146 151.
Reas, D., & Grilo, C. (2015). Pharmacological treatment of binge eating disorder: Update review and synthesis. *Expert Opinion Pharmacotherapy, 16*, 1463–1478.
Reas, D., & Grilo, C. (2014). Current and emerging treatments for binge eating disorder. *Expert Opinion Emerging Drugs, 19*, 99–142.
Rinaman, L. (2007). Visceral sensory inputs to the endocrine hypothalamus. *Frontiers in Neuroendocrinology, 28*, 50–60.

Robin, A., Siegel, P., & Moye, A. (1995). Family versus individual therapy for anorexia: Impact on family conflict. *International Journal of Eating Disorders, 17*, 313–322.
Rosen, D. (2003). Eating disorders in children and young adolescents: Etiology, classification, clinical features, and treatment. *Adolescent Medicine, 14*, 49–59.
Rosman, B., Minuchin, S., & Liebman, R. (1975). Family lunch session: An introduction to family therapy in anorexia nervosa. *American Journal of Orthopsychiatry, 45*, 846–853.
Rossi, G., Balottin, U., Rossi, M., Chiappedi, M., Fazzi, E., & Lanzi, G. (2007). Pharmacological treatment of anorexia nervosa: A retrospective study in preadolescents and adolescents. *Clinical Pediatrics, 46*, 806–811.
Roth, D., & Ross, D. (1988). Long-term cognitive-interpersonal group therapy for eating disorders. *International Journal of Group Psychotherapy, 38*, 4591–4510.
Russell, G., Szmukler, G., Dare, C., & Eisler, I. (1987). An evaluation of family therapy in anorexia nervosa and bulimia nervosa. *Archives of General Psychiatry, 44*, 1047–1056.
Safran, J., & Segal, Z. (1990). *Interpersonal process in cognitive therapy*. New York: Basic Books.
Safer, D., Telch, C., & Agras, W. (2001). Dialectical behavior therapy for bulimia nervosa. *American Journal of Psychiatry, 158*, 632–634.
Schmidt, U., Lee, S., & Beecham, J. (2007). A randomized controlled trial of family therapy and cognitive behavior therapy guided self-care for adolescents with bulimia nervosa and related disorders. *American Journal of Psychiatry, 164*, 591–598.
Schmidt, U., Wade, T., & Treasure, J. (2014). The Maudsley model of anorexia nervosa treatment for adults (MANTRA): Development, key features, and preliminary evidence. *Journal of Cognitive Psychotherapy, 2*, 48–71.
Selvini-Palazolli, M. (1978). Self-starvation: From individual to family therapy. In *the treatment of anorexia nervosa*. New York: Jason Aronson.
Sigman, G. (1996). How has the care of eating disorder patients been altered and upset by payment and insurance issues? Let me count the ways. *Journal of Adolescent Health, 19*, 317–318.
Sokol, M., Gray, N., Goldstein, A., & Kaye, W. (1999). Methylphenidate treatment for bulimia nervosa associated with cluster B personality disorder. *International Journal of Eating Disorders, 25*, 233–237.
Steffen, K., Roerig, J., Mitchell, J., & Uppala S. (2006). Emerging drugs for eating disorder treatment. *Expert Opinion on Emerging Drugs, 11*, 315–336.
Strober, M. (1992). Family genetics studies. In K. Halmi (Ed.), *Psychobiology and treatment of anorexia nervosa and bulimia nervosa* (pp. 61–76). Washington DC: American Psychiatric Association Press.
Sysko, R., Hildebrandt, T., Wilson, G., Wilfley, D., & Agras, W. (2010). Heterogeneity moderates treatment response among patients with binge eating disorder. *Journal of Consulting and Clinical Psychology, 78*, 681–690.
Tchanturia, K., Campbell, I., Morris, R., & Treasure, J. (2005). Neuropsychological studies in AN [Special issue: Anorexia nervosa]. *International Journal of Eating Disorders, 37*, 572–576.
Tchanturia, K., Davies, H., & Campbell, I. (2007). Cognitive remediation therapy for patients with anorexia nervosa: Preliminary findings. *Annals of General Psychiatry, 6*, 14.

Tchanturia, K., Lloyd, S., & Lang, K. (2013). Cognitive remediation therapy for anorexia nervosa: Current findings and future directions. *International Journal of Eating Disorders, 46*, 492–495.
Tchanturia, K., & Lock, J. (2011). Cognitive remediation therapy for eating disorders: Development, refinement and future directions. *Current Topics in Behavioral Neuroscience, 6*, 269–287.
Tchanturia, K., Morris, R., Anderluh, M., Collier, D., Nikolaou, V., & Treasure, J. (2004). Can cognitive exercises help treat anorexia nervosa? *Eating and Weight Disorders, 11*, e112–e116.
Thase, M., Pritchett, Y., Ossanna, M., Swindle, R., Xu, J., & Detke, M. (2007). Efficacy of duloxetine and selective serotonin reuptake inhibitors: Comparisons as assessed by remission rates in patients with major depressive disorder. *Journal of Clinical Psychopharmacology, 6*, 672–676.
Turner, H., Marshall, E., Stopa, L., & Waller, G. (2015). Cognitive-behavioural therapy for outpatients with eating disorders: Effectiveness for a transdiagnostic group in a routine clinical setting. *Behaviour Research and Therapy, 68*, 70–75.
Vall, E., & Wade, T. (2015). Predictors of treatment outcome in individuals with eating disorders: A systematic review and meta-analysis. *International Journal of Eating Disorders, 48*, 946–971.
Vandereycken, W., & Pierloot, R. (1982). Pimozide combined with behavior therapy in the short term treatment of anorexia nervosa. *Acto Psychiatry Scandinavia, 66*, 445–450.
Vitousek, K., Watson, S., & Wilson, G. (1998). Enhancing motivation for change in treatment-resistant eating disorders. *Clinical Psychology Review, 18*, 391–420.
Wade, T., Bulik, C., & Neale, M. (2001). Anorexia nervosa and major depression: Shared genetic and environmental risk factors. *American Journal of Psychiatry, 157*, 469–471.
Walsh, B., Agras, W., Devlin, M., Fairburn, C., Wilson, G., & Kahn, C. (2000). Fluoxetine for bulimia nervosa following poor response to psychotherapy. *American Journal of Psychiatry, 157*, 1332–1334.
Walsh, B., Hadigan, C., & Devlin, M. (1991). Long-term outcome of antidepressant treatment for bulimia nervosa. *American Journal of Psychiatry, 148*, 1206–1212.
Walsh, B., Wilson, G., Loeb, K., Devlin, M., Pike, K., Roose, S., . . . & Waternaux, C. (1997). Medication and psychotherapy in the treatment of bulimia nervosa. *American Journal of Psychiatry, 154*, 523–531.
Weisler, R., Johnston, J., Lineberry, C., Samara, B., Branconnier, R., & Billow, A. (1994). Comparison of bupropion and trazodone for the treatment of major depression. *Journal of Clinical Psycopharmacology, 14*, 170–179.
White, W., & Boskind-White, M. (1984). An experimental behavioral treatment program for bulimarexic women. In W. Hawkins, W. Fremouw, & P. Clement (Eds.), *Binge-eating: Theory, rresearch and treatment* (pp. 77–103). New York: Springer.
Wilfley, D., Agras, W., Telch, C., Rossiter, E., Schneider, J., Cole, A., . . . & Raeburn, S. D. (1993). Group cognitive-behavioural therapy and group interpersonal psychotherapy for the non-purging bulimic individual: A controlled comparison. *Journal of Consulting and Clinical Psychology, 61*, 296–305.

Wilfley, D., Frank, M., Welch, R., Spurrell, E., & Rounsaville, B. (1998). Adapting interpersonal psychotherapy to a group format (IPT-G) for binge eating disorder: Toward a model for adapting empirically supported treatments. *Psychotherapy Research, 8*, 379–391.

Wilfley, D., Mackenzie, K., Welch, R., Ayres, V., & Weissman, M. (2000). *Interpersonal psychotherapy for group*. New York: Basic Books.

Wilson, G., Loeb, K., & Walsh, B. (1999). Psychological versus pharmacological treatment of bulimia nervosa: Predictors and processors of change. *Journal of Consulting and Clinical Psychology, 67*, 451–459.

Zipfel, S., Giel, K., Bulik, C., Hay, P., & Schmidt, U. (2015). Anorexia nervosa: Aetiology, assessment, and treatment. *Lancet, 2*, 1099–1011.

Zipfel, S., Reas, D., & Thornton, C. (2002). Day hospitalization programs for eating disorders: A systematic review of the literature. *International Journal of Eating Disorders, 31*, 105–117.

Zhu, A., & Walsh, B. (2002). Pharmacologic treatment of eating disorders. *Canadian Journal of Psychiatry, 47*, 227–234.

11

Childhood and Adolescent Disorders: Evidence-Based Integrated Biopsychosocial Treatment of ADHD and Disruptive Disorders

George Kapalka, Ronald T. Brown, David F. Curtis,[1] Tony C. Wu, and Mario Marquez

The term, "disruptive" is a descriptor that has recently entered the diagnostic nomenclature. The Diagnostic Statistical Manual of Mental Disorders (DSM) system, in its current revision, includes a section on disruptive, impulse-control, and conduct disorders (DSM-5; American Psychiatric Association, 2013). This chapter conceptualizes disruptive behaviors as those which emanate from internal urges that most individuals would be able to suppress in a given situation, while individuals who behave disruptively seemingly cannot. Thus, impulsivity and limited self-control are thought herein to underlie disruptive behaviors.

Disruptive features and behaviors are core symptoms that are listed in the diagnostic criteria for many behavioral disorders. Impulsivity and self-control problems (sometimes including aggression) are thought to be the central aspects of disruptive disorders seen in childhood and adolescence. While attention deficit hyperactivity disorder (ADHD) is not classified as a disruptive disorder *per se* in the DSM-5, it shares many of the common features of disruptive behavior disorders (DBDs). This chapter focuses on three childhood disorders: ADHD, and the disruptive disorders of oppositional defiant disorder (ODD) and conduct disorder (CD).

Attention Deficit Hyperactivity Disorder

ADHD is "a persistent pattern of inattention and/or hyperactivity-impulsivity that interferes with functioning or development" (American Psychiatric Association, 2013, p. 61). The disorder is estimated to affect between 3% and 10% of school aged children and 2–6% of adolescents (Raishevich-Cunningham & Jensen, 2011).

Treatment Considerations

ADHD is a chronic neurodevelopmental disorder in which it is estimated that 80% will continue to retain some of the ADHD symptoms well into adulthood (Barkley, Murphy, & Fischer, 2008; Wolraich et al., 2011). There now exist several evidence-based

Cognitive Behavioral Psychopharmacology: The Clinical Practice of Evidence-Based Biopsychosocial Integration, First Edition. Edited by Mark Dana Muse.

therapies for the management of ADHD that include pharmacological therapies, psychosocial treatments, and their combination. Because the associated symptoms of the disorder are quite heterogeneous, it is likely that various treatment modalities are appropriate for different children with the disorder. Frequently, successful treatment is contingent on the child's developmental level (e.g., preschool, elementary school, adolescence). Behavioral therapy is apt to prove to be an efficacious therapy for preschoolers with ADHD (Wolraich et al., 2011), while family therapy might prove to be a successful therapy for adolescents with the disorder (Robbins & Barkley, 2000). Regardless of the developmental level of the child, when selecting an intervention it is important to specify those specific target behaviors to address.

Pharmacotherapy for ADHD

Stimulants

For the management of ADHD in school-aged children and adolescents the most commonly prescribed medications are in the class of agents known as stimulants (Zuvekas & Vitiello, 2012). The prescribing of stimulants has increased dramatically over the past three decades, and prescriptions for stimulants from 2007 to 2010 have increased more than five-fold relative to 1988 through 1994 (Visser et al., 2014). Although stimulants have been the most extensively investigated psychotropic medications in the field of child and adolescent psychiatry (for a review, see Brown & Daly, 2009), public debate continues with considerable controversy regarding the long-term use of stimulant medication in the management of ADHD, and whether the stimulants are overly prescribed for ADHD (LeFever, Arcona, & Antonuccio, 2013).

A number of explanations have been posited to explain the increase in stimulant prescribing, including better identification of the disorder, less stigma than in previous years attached to medication as a treatment option, the recognition that there are specific subgroups of the disorder, and finally the fact that there is poor access to alternative mental health services, particularly among those less affluent individuals who do not have health insurance. A consensus of the literature suggests that stimulants are not generally overprescribed to children and adolescents in the United States (Connor, 2011), although epidemiological studies do suggest that stimulants are inappropriately or overly prescribed in some regions of the country (Angold, Erkanli, Egger, & Costello, 2000).

Stimulants are believed to exert their effects through modulating neurotransmitters, particularly dopamine and norepinephrine, although epinephrine and serotonin also have been implicated (Nigg & Barkley, 2014). The increase in neurotransmitter availability at the synapses leads to the enhancement of extracellular dopamine and norepinephrine activity in the central nervous system, particularly in the prefrontal cortex and basal ganglia regions of the brain (for a review, see Brown & Daly, 2009). Stimulant medication increases neurotransmitter activity and inhibits problematic behavior associated with impulsivity, as well as enhancing attention, concentration, self-regulation, and executive functioning (Nigg & Barkley, 2014).

The literature is clear that stimulants enhance attention and concentration, but, while stimulants exert some moderating effect on hyperactivity and impulsivity, the actual effects of the stimulants in these two areas are poorly understood. Further, the effects of stimulants on social skills are generally equivocal, with very little evidence to suggest that children with ADHD are actually more likeable or rated as more socially desirable while receiving these medications.

Stimulants have been demonstrated to improve some of the specific core symptoms associated with ADHD in the short term, including attention and concentration, while at the same time reducing hyperactivity and impulsivity among children with ADHD (Barbaresi, Katusic, Colligan, Weaver, & Jaconsen, 2007; Pliszka & AACAP Work Group on Quality Issues, 2007). There is compelling evidence that children treated with stimulant medication make fewer errors on vigilance tasks, are less disruptive in the classroom setting, increase their academic productivity on-task behavior, and attain improved teacher ratings (for a review, see Nigg & Barkley, 2014).

Nonetheless, the limitations of stimulants are evident in the observation that children who demonstrate a positive response on some measures of ADHD rarely experience total normalization of behavior (Nigg & Barkley, 2014). Stimulants also have limited impact on domains of functional secondary impairment associated with ADHD, including social behavior and academic performance (Nigg & Barkley, 2014). Although stimulant medication has been shown to enhance certain social functioning to a statistically significant level in research trials, these improvements do not always translate to clinically improved functioning (Tannock & Brown, 2000). The final limitations of stimulants involve their dubious long-term efficacy as well as their potential for abuse.

Despite the fact that the US Food and Drug Administration (FDA) has not endorsed the use of stimulants for children who are less than 6 years of age due to limited safety and efficacy data, there has been a substantial increase in the number of off-label prescriptions of stimulants for preschoolers (Zito et al., 2007), and several studies have attempted to determine benefits and risks among this young population. In a large multisite clinical trial sponsored by the National Institute of Mental Health (NIMH), which examined the safety and efficacy of immediate-release methylphenidate for preschool children ranging from 3 to 5 years of age, findings indicated that methylphenidate may be both safe and efficacious for preschool children with ADHD. Based on the NIMH findings, Greenhill et al. (2006) nonetheless recommend initiating treatment with lower doses of stimulants since preschoolers metabolize stimulants at a slower rate relative to school-age children. Greenhill et al. also caution that preschoolers experience greater adverse side effects when treated with high doses of stimulant medication relative to their school-aged counterparts. Despite the Greenhill et al. findings, recommendations based on clinical research data to date generally suggest that stimulant medication for preschoolers be employed only as a second-line option and only for children with moderate to severe ADHD, when behavior therapy has not proven to be effective and when the symptoms of the disorder have persisted for at least 9 months (Wolraich et al., 2011).

There appears to be no evidence to suggest that the use of stimulant medication during childhood increases the chance of an older child or adolescent developing problems with substance use or dependence. In fact, research evidence has generally indicated that the use of stimulant medication during childhood reduces the risk for substance abuse in adulthood (Barkley, Fischer, Smallish, & Fletcher, 2003; Biederman, Wilens, Mick, Spencer, & Faraone, 1999; Wilens et al., 2008). Nonetheless, a recent meta-analysis has revealed that stimulant medication employed to manage ADHD in childhood did not either increase or decrease the risk of later developing substance use disorder (Humphreys, Eng, & Lee, 2013).

Adverse side effects of stimulant medication may include decreased appetite, stomach ache, insomnia, and headache (Barbaresi et al., 2006). Less common side effects include motor tics, headaches, nausea, fatigue, irritability, and increases in heart rate and blood pressure (Pliszka & AACAP Work Group on Quality Issues, 2007). Many of the adverse side effects associated with the stimulants typically abate after a short period of time or may even disappear depending on the dosage or timing of administration (Shier, Reichenbacher, Ghuman, & Ghuman, 2013).

Nonstimulant Medications Used to Manage ADHD

While a consensus of the data clearly attests to the efficacy of stimulant medication in the management of ADHD, for those children and adolescents who do not evidence any response to the stimulants, or where they experience too many adverse effects associated with the stimulants, the prescriber may turn to other nonstimulant medications. There are several nonstimulant medications that have been approved by the FDA for the management of ADHD in children and adolescents, and one of these is atomoxetine, a nonstimulant medication that affects the neurotransmitter norepinephrine. Atomoxetine is believed to inhibit presynaptic norepinephrine reuptake, thereby increasing extracellular norepinephrine; atomoxetine exerts little effect on serotonin and neurotransmitters other than norepinephrine. Unlike the stimulants, the increase in dopamine in the prefrontal cortex is believed to be more indirect (Nigg & Barkley, 2014; Wilens, 2006). The therapeutic effect of atomoxetine is believed to occur through its influence on the posterior attentional systems (Wilens, 2006). Wietech et al. (2009, 2013) found evidence of atomoxetine's effectiveness in treating ADHD symptoms in children, but the comparison was only against placebo. There are few clinical trials in which atomoxetine is compared head-to-head with stimulants in the child and adolescent population (Garnock-Jones & Keating, 2009), but where such studies have been done it has been found to be less effective than methyphenidate and amphetamine. Ni et al. (2013), however, found evidence that its effectiveness was similar to methylphenidate in improving executive functioning in adults, and somewhat superior for spatial planning.

Clonidine and guanfacine are alpha-adrenergic agents that have been approved by the FDA for the treatment of ADHD in the long-acting 24-h release form. Clonidine has been demonstrated to be most efficacious in the reduction of hyperactivity and aggression, and less support has been shown for problems with focusing and sustaining attention (Ming, Mulvey, Mohanty, & Patel, 2011). Guanfacine XR (extended release) also is an antihypertensive and has a very different mechanism of action whereby the medication "fine-tunes" the alpha-2 receptors on nerve cells in the prefrontal cortex thereby producing enhanced signal strength and conductivity (Nigg & Barkley, 2014). The therapeutic effects of the alpha-adrenergics are posited to exert their positive benefits in the prefrontal cortex, resulting in enhanced neuropsychological functioning among children and adolescents with ADHD (Wilens, 2006). The research evidence on the effectiveness of guanfacine in comparison with the stimulants is equivocal, at best (Bilder, Loo, McGough, & McCracken, 2016).

Psychosocial Therapies for ADHD

While the evidence for pharmacotherapy and particularly stimulant medication for the management of ADHD has been compelling, parents of ADHD children and other caregivers often rate the option of medication lower in acceptability relative to nonpharmacotherapies (Fiks et al., 2012). Fortunately, a number of psychosocial treatments, mostly behavioral or family-oriented (Barkley, 2006), have demonstrated efficacy for symptoms associated with ADHD as well as other co-occurring symptoms such as depression, aggression, and low self-esteem.

Behavioral therapies are well supported by research in their employment for children and adolescents with ADHD (for a review, see Reiff & Tippins, 2004). Based on the principles of social learning and contingency management, behavior therapy for ADHD typically includes interventions that are taught to both caregivers and teachers. Changes in parenting practice are conceptualized as the mechanism of action by which parent training influences the behavior of children and adolescents with ADHD (Weersing & Weisz, 2002). Findings have typically demonstrated that children and adolescents demonstrate the greatest degree of behavior change when they receive consistent responses for their behaviors and actions. Techniques that reinforce positive behavior, applied in the classroom or at home, have been demonstrated to be quite effective in the management of ADHD. Methods of behavior therapy typically include management skills for caregivers and teachers, contingency management approaches (e.g., time-outs, positive reinforcement), self-management strategies for the child (e.g., self-monitoring and self-reinforcement), and training that targets social skills and problem-solving.

With follow up periods of up to 5 years, studies have generally demonstrated that behavioral interventions in the home and at school are effective and are associated with reductions of ADHD symptoms as well as functional impairments associated with the disorder (Evans, Owens, & Bunford, 2014). Research in this area has generally yielded moderate effect sizes, although Pelham and Waschbusch (1999) have provided data to indicate that tightly controlled behavior management programs are equivalent to low to moderate doses of stimulant medication. Studies of behavioral therapies have focused on the functional impairments associated with ADHD, and the effects of behavioral therapies appear to improve long-term outcomes associated with the disorder, including parenting practices, peer relationships, and school functioning (for a review, see Brown et al., 2008a, 2008b).

Those behavioral therapies that have provided well-established evidence for the management of symptoms associated with ADHD include behavioral parent training, behavioral peer interventions, behavioral classroom management, and organizational skills training (Evans et al., 2014). Contingency management approaches employed in behavioral parent training emphasize behavior modification, cue and consequences, reward systems, and discipline (Chronis, Chacko, Fabiano, Wymbs, & Pelham, 2004). Behavioral peer intervention is designed to promote cooperation, communication, and participation in peer social situations among children with ADHD.

Children with ADHD frequently are described as annoying, immature, intrusive, and overbearing (Pelham et al., 2005). While there has been some evidence that a focus on social skills deficits may improve social functioning and peer relationships among children with ADHD (Gol & Jarus, 2005), the positive effects from this type of therapy have been demonstrated to be beneficial only when it is part of a more intensive multimodal behavioral treatment package that is delivered within the child's social milieu (Pelham et al., 2005).

Children with ADHD often pose a challenging management problem for teachers, and there is evidence attesting to the efficacy of behavioral therapies in the classroom setting (Daly, Creed, Xanthopoulos, & Brown, 2007). One intervention that has shown strong empirical support is the Daily Report Card (DRC; Fabiano et al., 2010), an approach that entails collaboration among the child, caregivers, and the teacher in the selection of two to three clearly defined behavioral goals (e.g., completion of assigned seat work, obeying classroom rules, on-task behavior, getting along with other classmates).

Combined Treatments for ADHD

The "gold standard" in the management of ADHD is medication in combination with behavioral interventions with children and their caregivers. The data from research have been clear that multimodal treatment is moderately superior to pharmacotherapy or nonpharmacologic interventions employed alone (Sibley, Kuriyan, Evans, Waxmonsky, & Smith, 2014). The largest and most comprehensive clinical trial of ADHD treatment outcomes to date is the NIMH Multimodal Treatment Study of Children with ADHD (MTA Cooperative Group, 1999). Participants in this multisite study included 579 children between the ages of 7 and 10 years who were assigned randomly to one of four treatment groups: state-of-the-art medication management, intensive behavioral intervention, medication and behavioral interventions combined, and a community treatment control group that received routine standard care (usually medication). Findings revealed that while all four treatment groups improved over time, the medication management and combined intervention groups demonstrated significantly greater improvement in core ADHD symptoms relative to the behavioral treatment alone and the community care group. Importantly, the children in the combined group exhibited better outcomes than those in the community care group across a number of important functioning domains (e.g., disruptive behavior, parent–child relationships, social skills, academic achievement). Moreover, the results for the combined treatment group were found to be superior to those in the medication alone group with co-morbid conditions (e.g., anxiety). Children who received integrated multimodal treatment required lower stimulant doses than those treated with medication alone. Of interest was the finding that caregivers reported most satisfaction with the behavioral and combined treatment approaches over medication as a stand-alone.

An MTA follow up investigation of the participants who ranged in age from 6 to 8 years old did not find support for the durability of the therapies (Molina et al., 2009); the original four groups did not differ on variables such as school grades, arrests, and psychiatric hospitalizations, the data on which were obtained at the follow up assessment. Thus, while the use of medication and behavioral therapies initially produce significant reductions of symptoms and functional impairments, these differential effects dissipate upon the discontinuation of treatment. A further comparison of children participating in the MTA group with a group of children without ADHD revealed that, while children in the MTA study sustained functional improvements relative to their baseline functioning at pretreatment, they demonstrated poorer outcomes posttreatment than their peers without ADHD on the majority of dependent measures originally assessed at baseline, including higher ratings of overactivity and impulsivity as well as lower standardized test scores of academic functioning. Children in the MTA group also had a greater frequency of grade retention, delinquency, arrest records, and psychiatric hospitalizations in comparison to non-ADHD counterparts who did not receive the MTA protocol (Molina et al., 2009).

In a recent investigation, Helseth et al. (2015) compared the unique and combined effects of evidence-based treatments on ADHD that include stimulant medication and behavior modification on children's rates of reinforcement for deviant peer behavior. Participants included over 200 elementary school-age children receiving various combinations of behavior modification and various doses of stimulant medication in a highly structured summer camp program. Findings revealed that children with ADHD encouraged (reinforced) the deviant behavior of their peers at a higher rate than control children. The difference, however, dissipated in the presence of both behavior management and stimulant drug therapy. Specifically, both low- and high-intensity behavior modification, as well as medium and high doses of stimulant medication, significantly reduced the rate of ADHD children's reinforcement for deviant peer behavior to levels similar to the control group. The data were interpreted to suggest that evidence-based interventions can substantially decrease the presence of reinforcement for deviant behavior, thereby diminishing the potential disruptive behavior of ADHD children's peers.

Important questions remain with regard to the appropriate duration of treatments, and the intensity as well as the sequencing of treatments. The preponderance of evidence suggests that medication should be implemented as a first-line treatment for children, particularly for those children with less severe symptoms and impairments, while multimodal treatments may be more appropriate for those ADHD children with a more guarded prognosis (e.g., co-morbid conditions, more severe symptoms, and associated functional impairments). Nonetheless, there is evidence that stand-alone medication is not as equally effective as behaviorally reinforced medication regimens, and combination treatment might well be considered the treatment of choice when access to both medication and therapy exist. With regard to stand-alone psychotherapies, behavior modification is the only nonmedication therapy that has a compelling evidence base for the management of ADHD. In fact, the MTA trials have suggested that the use of behavior management therapy may reduce the amount of stimulant medication needed to manage behaviors associated with ADHD.

ADHD and Co-Morbid Disorders

There have been few studies that have compared the efficacy of various interventions for ADHD children with and without co-morbid conditions, and results of these studies have been mixed. With regard to the internalizing disorders, various pharmacological and behavioral therapies have been demonstrated to be efficacious for the co-morbidity of anxiety disorders and ADHD (Antshel et al., 2011). Co-morbidity of anxiety disorders has not been found to impact the efficacy of stimulant drug therapy (Garcia et al., 2009) and there is evidence to indicate that children treated with stimulant medication are less likely to develop other psychiatric co-morbidities at adolescence (Biederman, Monuteaux, Spencer, Wilens, & Farone, 2009). In fact, the data from the MTA study demonstrated that children with co-morbidity of ADHD and anxiety disorders responded similarly to both behavioral and medication interventions relative to those with ADHD without co-morbidity. Geller et al. (2007) provided further data that indicate that children with various types of anxiety disorders, including co-morbid generalized anxiety disorder, separation anxiety disorder, and social phobia, demonstrated significant reductions in both symptoms of ADHD and anxiety following a 3-month trial of atomoxetine relative to placebo.

Several pharmacotherapies may be beneficial for ADHD with co-morbidity of depression. Atomoxetine, a drug that is similar in mechanism of action to many antidepressants, has been found to be effective in the management of ADHD symptoms, but it has been found to have less direct impact on depressive symptoms among children with co-morbidity of ADHD and depression (Kratochvil et al., 2005). On the other hand, youth with ADHD and co-morbid depression were managed with fluoxetine or placebo for 2 months, followed by the addition of atomoxetine for 5 weeks; findings revealed that both groups demonstrated similar responses in their symptoms of ADHD, although children who received a combination of atomoxetine and fluoxetine demonstrated the greatest improvement in depressive symptoms. Further, there has been some preliminary evidence from small open-label trials to suggest that bupropion as well as the combination of fluoxetine and methylphenidate may be effective in the management of the co-morbidity of ADHD and depressive symptoms (Bond et al., 2012). Although there is some evidence suggesting efficacy of a combination of medications in the management of co-morbid conditions, several experts have recommended that single medication should be employed for the purpose of targeting the more severe disorder prior to implementing polypharmacy (Pliszka et al., 2006; Texas Children's Medication Algorithm Project, AACAP Work Group on Quality Issues, 2006).

With regard to the externalizing disorders, data from the MTA study indicate that children with ADHD and co-morbidity of ODD or CD responded best to the combined intervention of pharmacotherapy and behavior management (MTA Cooperative Group, 1999). Furthermore, it has been found that children with ADHD and co-morbid aggression may benefit from methylphenidate employed either alone or in combination with flueoxetine (Patel & Barzman, 2013). Few studies have actually examined the efficacy of pharmacotherapies on children with co-morbidity of ADHD and aggression, although there is preliminary evidence for the efficacy of clonidine, guanfacine, risperidone, lithium, and valproic acid for aggression specifically (Patel & Barzman, 2013). However, much more research is necessary prior to endorsing the efficacy of these agents in combination with the stimulants.

For children and adolescents with co-morbidity of ADHD and learning disabilities, combined treatment including both medication and psychoeducational interventions has been demonstrated to be the treatment of choice (DuPaul, Gormley, & Laracy, 2013). Pharmacotherapy for ADHD and co-morbid learning disabilities has been demonstrated to enhance academic productivity (Williamson, Murray, Damaraju, Asher, & Starr, 2014), although DuPaul et al. (2013) have cautioned that medication alone is simply not a sufficient treatment for youth with co-morbidity of ADHD and learning disabilities. Typically, children with co-morbid ADHD and learning disabilities perform best with those psychosocial interventions that demonstrate efficacy in improving academic functioning, organizational skills, and peer tutoring.

With regard to children and adolescents with co-morbidity of ADHD and tics, there has been ongoing concern that the stimulants exacerbate tic disorders, and for this reason providers were warned against prescribing the stimulants for youth with such co-morbidities. However, many of these recommendations were based on uncontrolled case reports and retrospective chart reviews. Recent prospective controlled clinical trials have provided some encouraging data to suggest that the stimulants are not likely to evoke or exacerbate tics (Tourette's Syndrome Study Group, 2002). In one randomized controlled clinical trial, children with co-morbid ADHD and chronic tic disorders evidenced marked improvement in ADHD symptoms when managed with methylphenidate or clonidine, or their combination. More importantly, for those receiving methylphenidate, no exacerbation of tics was found relative to the placebo group. While these data are clearly encouraging, more controlled clinical trials are needed prior to endorsing the safety and efficacy of the stimulants for youth with co-morbidity of ADHD and tic disorders.

Oppositional Defiant Disorder

ODD is a disorder, predominantly occurring in children and adolescents, that is characterized by patterns of negative reactions to authority, willful noncompliance, irritable mood, and negative attention-seeking behaviors. The DSM-5 reports that ODD affects approximately 3.3% of all children and adolescents with a lifetime prevalence of 12.6% (American Psychiatric Association, 2013).

The developmental course of ODD symptoms often reveals a consistent increase in severity over time that frequently progresses to diagnoses of CD, depression or other major mental health concerns. Thus, when ODD is manifest, early intervention may prevent exacerbation of symptoms and progression into more severe disorders. Behavior therapy, especially including parent training, has been a mainstay treatment for decades, and continues to exhibit robust support in clinical investigations. More severe cases, however, may exhibit severely compromised development of self-control, and in those instances intervening with behavior therapy alone may not produce sufficient improvement in a reasonable time frame. In addition, when co-morbid disorders are present, a single treatment modality may not be sufficient.

Pharmacotherapy for ODD

Pharmacological research dedicated exclusively to the treatment of ODD is very limited. These interventions are difficult to study due to core symptoms often being conflated with those of CD (Loeber, Burke, & Pardini, 2009). Consequently, many pharmacological studies examine aggression and emotional dysregulation, collapsing the ODD and CD diagnoses to focus upon specific symptoms. In addition, as discussed below, ODD is highly co-morbid with other conditions (e.g., ADHD, anxiety, and mood disorders). Although many of the medications used to treat these co-morbid disorders may also reduce symptoms of ODD, the evidence and the biological mechanisms for improving oppositional behaviors remain unclear.

Studies of pharmacological treatment of children with ODD have examined divalproex sodium, lithium, and atypical antipsychotics such as risperidone. One randomized clinical trial and two open-label studies of divalproex sodium revealed significant improvement in "hostility" in children with ODD (Donovan et al., 1997, 2000; Saxena et al., 2010). Lithium salts have been used extensively in the treatment of aggression over the past 35 years; however, they have primarily been intended for pediatric onset bipolar disorder. Only a handful of controlled trials have examined the efficacy of lithium salts for child and adolescent conduct problems and aggression (Campbell et al., 1995; Malone, Delaney, Luebbert, Cater, & Campbell, 2000; Rifkin et al., 1997), with none specifically for ODD. Atypical antipsychotics, on the other hand, have received greater empirical support for treating ODD than has lithium, particularly for aggressive symptoms. Risperidone has been the most studied of these atypicals

(Pappadopulos et al., 2006), although most investigations of "pure" ODD (i.e., without co-morbidity) have been limited to children with below-average intelligence (Aman, De Smedt, Derivan, Lyons, & Findling, 2002; Snyder et al., 2002). Though providing some support for improving conduct, these studies also report significant confounds (e.g. low IQ, short treatment duration, questionable follow up phases, use of combined medication treatments) and a high rate of adverse events (98%) (Aman et al., 2002; Snyder et al., 2002).

Because of limited research support for pharmacological treatments for ODD, pharmacotherapy should not be considered a first-line intervention for ODD. It may be considered as a secondary treatment option in more complex cases, only when evidence-based psychosocial interventions have been insufficient or when co-morbid conditions require stabilization. Practice parameters recommended by the American Academy of Child and Adolescent Psychiatry (AACAP) suggest that, "medications for youth with ODD are mostly considered to be adjunctive, palliative, and noncurative" and "should not be the sole intervention in ODD" (ACTION, 2007, p. 137). Similarly, international consensus on the management of ODD recommends that pharmacological treatment be limited to patients who have not first benefited from psychosocial interventions, or exhibit extreme levels of aggression or destructive behaviors (Kutcher et al., 2004). The evidence to date suggests that risperidone may offer the most potential benefits for ameliorating aggression, but with few benefits for improving primary symptoms of noncompliance or other conduct issues. However, studies of risperidone have been limited to children with intellectual disabilities, and frequent negative side effects such as somnolence, extrapyramidal effects, and weight gain suggest the need for extreme caution.

Psychosocial Therapies for ODD

Evidence-based psychosocial interventions are recommended as the gold standard treatment approach for children with ODD. The interventions in this section have all been supported by well-conducted randomized controlled trials (RCTs) and found superior to no treatment or wait list control conditions. In addition to demonstrating robust positive treatment outcomes, these programs have demonstrated longitudinal and generalized effects, proving to be both effective and durable interventions (McNeil, Eyberg, Eisenstadt, Newcomb, & Funderburk, 1991). Parent training programs, especially those targeting younger children, are among the most extensively studied treatments for children with behavioral problems such as ODD, and they are recommended as the first-line approach (Eyberg, Nelson, & Boggs, 2008). Interventions for youth in middle-childhood and adolescence generally focus on individual or group sessions with the child. Children in these stages of development present a greater capacity to benefit from cognitive-behavioral approaches in which they are primary agents of change. However, given that maladaptive parenting behaviors, family conflict, and family instability are associated with the development and maintenance of disruptive behaviors in children (Frick et al., 1992; Patterson, 1982), child-focused interventions often include a parent training component. Below is an overview of the evidence-based, manualized interventions that have received the greatest research support for treating ODD, as well as additional programs that emphasize the same evidence-based practice principles.

Behavioral Parent Training (BPT) Programs

Parent–child interaction therapy (PCIT) is a BPT program for children of ages 2–7 (McNeil & Hembree-Kigin, 2010). The typical PCIT structure consists of weekly, 60-min therapy sessions in which the therapist, usually behind a one-way mirror, coaches parents on their use of skills with their child. There are two stages in PCIT: child-directed interaction (CDI) and parent-directed interaction (PDI). CDI sessions focus on coaching parents' positive attending and active ignoring skills when interacting with their child. During PDI, limit setting and discipline techniques are emphasized to help parents follow through with behavioral strategies in a consistent and predictable manner. Parents learn to balance their warmth and responsiveness with their demands and discipline. PCIT therapists code parent–child interactions to measure parents' skill progression and to determine mastery of skills. "Graduation" from PCIT depends on parents' mastery of the specific skills taught, their self-reported confidence in handling child behaviors, and their ratings of disruptive behavior on the Eyberg Child Behavior Inventory (ECBI) falling within normal limits (Eyberg & Pincus, 1999).

Helping the Noncompliant Child (HNC) is a program for children aged 3–8 (McMahon & Forehand, 2003). The parent and child are seen together for sessions of 60–90 min, held once or twice weekly over the course of approximately 10 weeks. HNC skills are achieved through therapist modeling, parent–therapist role-play, and live practice with the child in the clinic and at home. Therapist coaching occurs within the therapy room or from behind a one-way mirror. Similar to PCIT, the HNC program consists of two treatment phases. During the first phase (differential attention), parents learn skills to increase the child's prosocial behaviors (using positive verbal and physical attention) and to reduce minor misbehaviors (utilizing attending, positive reinforcement, and ignoring strategies). The second phase (compliance training) focuses on teaching parents to give clear instructions and follow through consistently with effective consequences (e.g., time out or loss of privileges) for noncompliance.

The Incredible Years (IY) training series is a set of three training programs: the child program (IY CT, ages 3–8), the parent program (IY-PT, ages 2–10), and the teacher program for children up to age 12 (Webster-Stratton & Reid, 2003). Each IY program is delivered by a trained facilitator and carried out in a group format. Parent and child programs are typically delivered in conjunction with one another over a course of 12–22 weeks, with sessions lasting 2–3 h. Sessions incorporate videotaped vignettes tailored to the specific target audience (e.g., parent, teacher, or child groups). Vignettes include common challenging situations followed by group discussions comparing ineffective and effective ways of dealing with the problem situations.

Triple P-Positive Parenting Program is a treatment designed for children from birth to age 12, with extensions for ages 13 to 16, and focuses on enhancing parenting confidence and skills (Sanders, 1999). Triple P can be delivered in individual, group, self-directed, or in a combination of these formats. Triple P is multileveled (Levels 1 through 5) and families participate in a specific level depending on the severity of child behavioral problems. Level 4 (Standard Triple P) and Level 5 (Enhanced Triple P) have received the most empirical support (Eyberg et al., 2008). Standard Triple P involves 10 individual, or eight group parent sessions on topics such as differential attention, effective commands, logical consequences, quiet time, and time out. Level 5 is an enhanced version that incorporates home visits and three to five additional sessions designed to address family stressors (e.g., parental depression, marital conflict) (Sanders, Murphy-Brennan, & McAuliffe, 2003).

Parent Management Training Oregon Model (PMTO) is supported for use with the widest age range of children: 3–12 years of age (Patterson, Reid, Jones, & Conger, 1975). PMTO can be provided in group or individual formats. Individual family sessions are 60 min and are held weekly for approximately 25–30 weeks. Group sessions are 90 min and are held weekly for 14 weeks. Treatment also includes midweek calls from the therapist to encourage successful implementation of home procedures and skill generalization. The therapist teaches parents via role-play and modeling of skills across five content areas: skill encouragement (e.g., incentive chart and rewards for positive behaviors), limit setting, monitoring, problem-solving, and positive involvement. The order of skill content and time allocated to each skill varies, based upon the family's presenting needs and level of child participation in sessions. Parent mastery of skill encouragement is a prerequisite to learning discipline strategies such as giving effective directions, and consistent and calm use of consequences (e.g., time out, privilege removal) for noncompliance.

Child-Focused Individual and Group Interventions

Problem-solving skills training (PSST) uses cognitive restructuring and problem-solving skills (e.g., identifying the problem, generating solutions, evaluating solutions, and perspective-taking) to help youth with ODD cope with interpersonal difficulties (Kazdin, 2010). Treatment is designed for children aged 7–13 and consists of 12 weeks of individual child therapy sessions that last 30–50 min. The therapist employs interactive exercises, games, modeling, and role-play of different scenarios often encountered by the child. A token economy system with response cost is used by the therapist. Initial sessions focus on child participation, but parents are more actively included in later sessions in order to practice challenging daily scenarios and to assist the child in generalizing skills to use at home (Kazdin, 2010).

Anger Control Skills Training (ACST) is a school-based, group intervention that targets negative, defiant, and hostile behavior toward school authority figures (Larson & Lochman, 2002). Eighteen (60–90-min) weekly sessions for children aged 8–12 focus on cognitive coping strategies, awareness of physiological cues, perspective-taking, and problem-solving skills. Following skill-building sessions, participants watch videos of other children experiencing interpersonal difficulties, and then discuss alternative, appropriate social responses. Children participate in role-play rehearsal of alternative skill choices, using strategies introduced through the program. Final sessions provide children with opportunities to act out real-life situations and apply new skills instead of reacting with defiance or aggression. Similarly, Coping Power is a clinic-based program that was developed as an extension of ACT. Coping Power offers individual sessions for children as well as a BPT component (Lochman, Boxmeyer, Powell, Barry, & Pardini, 2010).

Programs Emphasizing Evidence-Based Practice Principles

While the aforementioned programs have received the greatest empirical support, there are also many interventions that are based exclusively upon the evidence-based principles that define these programs (e.g. Barkley's (2013) *Defiant Children*; Kapalka's (2007) *Parenting Your Out of Control Child*; Kazdin's (2009) *The Kazdin Method for Parenting the Defiant Child*; and Greene's (2010) *The Explosive Child*). Each program emphasizes use of positive reinforcement to promote appropriate behaviors, increasing the effectiveness of commands, consistent limit setting, and use of nonphysical/nonpunitive discipline techniques. However, each program also adds strategies that may be a focus of a particular family's treatment. For example, Barkley's (2013) 10-session program provides both proactive and reactive strategies for addressing negative behavior (e.g., contingency management, time out, problem prediction, and school collaboration), while Kazdin's (2009) BPT incorporates behavioral shaping in-session, teaching parents to create clear definitions of behavioral goals and reinforcing successive approximations toward desired outcomes. In addition to managing argumentative and defiant behaviors, Kapalka (2007) emphasizes strategies for managing emotional dysregulation and "out of control" behaviors, specifically for common problem situations such as transitions between activities, during homework, and while in public places. Similarly, Greene's (2010) Explosive Child program highlights difficulties related to emotion regulation as well as cognitive inflexibility among children who become explosive. Greene's approach teaches parents to recognize the warning signs of a meltdown, remove parent behaviors that may be fueling a meltdown, and gradually to "downshift" to allow the child to consider options when they are frustrated.

Intervening early with an evidence-based psychosocial intervention for ODD proves not only cost effective, but also potent as the best clinical practice. Positive treatment outcomes have been demonstrated for these interventions in RCTs, providing a strong evidence base for their use in the treatment of ODD (e.g., Webster-Stratton, Reid, & Hammond, 2004). In follow up studies, these interventions also demonstrate maintenance of treatment gains for years after treatment has ended (e.g., Forgatch, Patterson, DeGarmo, & Beldavs, 2009). Given the posttreatment durability of positive therapeutic effects, psychosocial interventions are considered the gold standard for children with ODD, and an especially attractive option for families, communities, and prescribing therapist alike, as first-line intervention (Edidin, Karnik, Hunter, & Steiner, 2012).

Psychosocial interventions for ODD focus on the child and authority figure(s) learning techniques that will create new, healthy patterns of interacting, and interrupt the negative coercive cycle that results in defiant behavior (Patterson, 1982). The skills learned in treatment can then be applied whenever necessary after treatment has ended, with follow up care done on an as-needed basis. By comparison, maintenance of a psychotropic medication regimen requires careful monitoring and consistent maintenance over time for the duration of medication use. In addition, medications obviously do not teach skills to change child or caregiver patterns of interactions, and are therefore not viable long-term solutions. In addition, medications produce highly variable outcomes for children with DBD depending on their age and co-morbidities.

Combined Treatments for ODD

There is a dearth of research related to combined psychosocial and pharmacological interventions in the treatment of ODD. This largely stems from the fact that psychosocial approaches are preferred as front-line interventions; whereas, medications are often used as adjuncts to treat co-morbidities or to help manage aggression (ACTION, 2007; Turgay, 2009). Despite the lack of research for pharmacotherapy in the management of ODD, clinical practice parameters set by the AACAP still suggest that a multimodal treatment is often needed to successfully treat ODD. Further, AACAP recommends that clinicians develop individualized treatment plans for children and adolescents, as any given modality of treatment may vary in effectiveness from patient to patient (ACTION, 2007).

At present, existing data regarding the combined treatment of ODD must be extrapolated from studies primarily focused on other DBDs, namely ADHD (MTA Cooperative Group, 1999; Swanson et al., 2001). The Multimodal Treatment of Attention-Deficit Hyperactivity Disorder study compared the efficacy of various treatment modalities for ADHD (MTA Cooperative Group, 1999). A subset of this study's sample was identified as having co-morbid ODD, and secondary analyses found that medication combined with behavioral treatment is significantly more effective than medication alone, although the effect was small (Swanson et al., 2001), and the effect of psychosocial intervention may be partially attributable to variability in treatment fidelity and effectiveness across sites. Some sites found moderate to large positive effects for psychosocial treatment, while others found small to large negative effects (p. 177). Given the absence of evidence to support pharmacological intervention and the strong body of evidence for parenting interventions and child-focused skill-building interventions, psychosocial interventions are clearly the most effective treatments for ODD. Since very few pharmacological studies to date have even attempted to specifically treat ODD, more research is needed to explore the efficacy of adding pharmacological support to first-line psychosocial intervention.

Current practice parameters may suggest the addition of stimulants, α2-agonists, or even atypical antipsychotics to psychosocial therapies to address child behaviors that are significantly aggressive, destructive, or nonresponsive to evidence-based behavior therapy. However, guidelines for the use of these pharmacological agents in the treatment of ODD are based upon clinical expert consensus rather than empirical data based upon RCTs or even open-label trials. Pharmacological treatments should, therefore, be considered with caution when addressing symptoms of "pure" ODD, given the unanswered questions about their long-term effectiveness and safety with this population. Adverse events related to the use of medications (e.g., fatigue, nausea, tics, weight gain, and overdose potential) may outweigh benefits for many children, and, in the interest of informed consent, practitioners should discuss these issues with families carefully. Indeed, from a practical standpoint, titration needs may also present significant challenges given the relative lack of research or published medication algorithms for this population. Finally, the use of these medications for ODD is considered off-label, with FDA approval only granted for co-morbid conditions such as ADHD, thus further prompting the need for caution (Charach et al., 2011).

ODD and Co-Morbid Disorders

ODD is frequently complicated by co-morbidity with other conditions. In fact, this appears to be the rule rather than the exception with nearly 50% of all ODD cases presenting co-occurring ADHD (Martel, Nikolas, Jernigan, Friderici, & Nigg, 2012; Willcutt et al., 2012), 40% reporting significant anxiety symptoms (Drabick, Ollendick, & Bubier, 2010; Greene et al., 2002), and 12% being diagnosed with depression (Stoep et al., 2012). When depression later follows childhood onset of ODD, it is best predicted by the prominence of ODD-related negative affect. Likewise, children presenting more dominant symptoms of defiance and antagonistic behaviors frequently progress from ODD to later display symptoms more representative of CD. There is an estimated .81 correlation between the symptoms of ODD and CD, which ultimately reflects an extremely high degree of symptom co-morbidity (Boden, Fergusson, & Horwood, 2010; Loeber et al., 2009). Despite the strong evidence supporting ODD as a predictor of future behavioral and emotional problems, it still remains unclear if its role is causal, prodromal, or simply a precursor to future concerns (Burke & Loeber, 2010).

Psychostimulant medication, considered the first-line treatment for ADHD, also presents potential benefits for treating co-morbid externalizing symptoms of ODD (Swanson et al., 2001). Methylphenidate has been particularly well supported in both open-label (e.g., Serra-Pinheiro, Mattos, Souza, Pastura, & Gomes, 2004) and controlled studies (e.g., Kolko, Bukstein, & Barron, 1999; Pliszka, Browne, Olvera, & Wynne, 2000) for reducing disruptive behaviors and aggression in addition to improving core symptoms of ADHD. More recent studies also suggest that atomoxetine, a SNRI, may be effective for ODD symptoms when co-morbid with ADHD (Bangs et al., 2008; Dell'Agnello et al., 2009; Dittmann et al., 2011). A major advantage of atomoxetine treatment compared to stimulant therapy is the longer duration of effects, thus potentially addressing symptoms occurring during early morning and evening periods when stimulant effects have typically subsided. After methylphenidate and atomoxetine, alpha-2 adrenergic receptor agonists such as clonidine and guanfacine may be considered second-line medications for treating co-morbid symptoms of ODD and ADHD. Clinical trials of clonidine or guanfacine alone or in combination with stimulant treatments have been shown to reduce oppositionality in children with co-morbid ADHD (e.g., Connor et al., 2010; Palumbo et al., 2008); however, significant caution is also warranted due to serious overdose potential (Hazell, 2010). Nonetheless, international treatment guidelines currently support the clinical use of α2-agonists for children with ADHD and co-morbid CD, severe ODD, or tic disorder, as well as those with co-morbid ADHD and ODD who fail to respond favorably to either stimulant or atomoxetine treatment (Turgay, 2009).

Pharmacological treatments for ODD with co-morbid anxiety and mood disorders (AMD) have also been examined, though to a lesser extent. Two recent studies suggest promising support for selective serotonin reuptake inhibitor (SSRI) treatment among youth with ODD and co-morbid AMD (Jacobs et al., 2010; Kodish, Rockhill, & Varley, 2011). However, current AACAP clinical practice parameters for ODD indicate that there is insufficient evidence at this time to support the use of SSRIs for treating ODD symptoms alone (ACTION, 2007). With the introduction of the new diagnostic category of disruptive mood dysregulation disorder (DMDD), now used to reflect these kinds of presenting problems, SSRI prescriptions are more likely to be directed toward the DMDD population rather than to a subset of children with co-morbid ODD and AMD (Leibenluft, 2011).

When co-morbid with ADHD, the strongest empirical evidence supports the combined use of stimulants and atomoxetine for treating ODD. Methylphenidate is the most supported for use with potentially substantial benefits for reducing noncompliance and reactive aggression associated with ADHD. Atomoxetine should be limited to those considered to be minimal responders to stimulants or for those experiencing negative side effects. Alpha-2-agonists such as clonidine and guanfacine currently have the least support for treating co-morbid ADHD and ODD. When co-morbid with anxiety and mood-related problems, pharmacological treatment data for ODD suggest benefits for judicious use of SSRIs.

Challenges to Treatment Interventions

ODD is a high base rate condition that causes significant behavioral, emotional, and interpersonal difficulties for the individual diagnosed as well as for family, teachers, and friends (Olfson, Blanco, Wang, Laje, & Correll, 2014). Without treatment, ODD symptoms tend to persist and worsen over time (Shaw, Lacourse, & Nagin, 2005), often evolving from childhood disruptive behavior to an adolescence and adulthood marked by emotional problems and/or antisocial behaviors such as crime and violence. Fortunately, children and adolescents with ODD have been shown to respond very positively to intervention, both during treatment and in long-term follow up studies. More encouraging is the notion that psychosocial treatments are evidenced to be most effective for ODD, thus not requiring pharmacotherapy. In fact, pharmacological intervention studies to date are so few and unclear in their findings that medication is not even recommended as an option for combined treatment of ODD unless risks or co-morbid symptoms suggest the need for additional support (ACTION, 2007). There are many behavior therapies available for first-line intervention comprising either parent training or child-focused psychotherapies delivered in individual and group formats.

On the other hand, psychosocial and behavioral therapies require adherence to regularly scheduled sessions, which may be a challenge for families dealing with a variety of stressors. Access to care, availability of insurance coverage, and transportation to regularly scheduled sessions may be difficult for families with impoverished resources. The treatment strategies covered herein also require therapist familiarity with these techniques, the underlying behavioral principles to be applied, and the nature of the disorder, since psychotherapy conceptualized more generally as "treatment as usual" (TAU) does not utilize these techniques and is much less likely to be effective. As with ADHD, treatment adherence is also a challenge, especially when family members are not in agreement with regard to treatment plans or when there are relationship problems between caregivers and youth.

Conduct Disorder

Individuals with CD display consistent aggressive or rule-breaking behaviors toward others, including bullying, threatening, fighting, using weapons, forcing others into sexual activity, and other socially inappropriate behaviors (American Psychiatric Association, 2013). Children with CD have poor prognoses in later years: they are more likely to have criminal histories, histories of domestic violence, mental and medical problems, financial difficulties, lower cognitive abilities, poor temperaments, and lower socioeconomic status (SES), and are likely to abuse alcohol and drugs. Depending on the samples and methods used in the studies, the prevalence of CD has been estimated to be between 2 and 16% (Wu, 2011).

Treatment Considerations

In preschool children, prodromal symptoms include irritable temperament and inattentiveness, and some theoreticians hypothesize these may result from poor maternal–child attachment (Sanders & Schaechter, 2007). As they age, children with CD in elementary school come to demonstrate quick, angry temperaments and poor social skills, and tend to blame the victim in scenarios involving physical aggression. In middle and high school, children with CD commonly break rules, overreact emotionally, and often do not take responsibility for their actions. Research has shown that people with childhood-onset CD, known as "early starters," are likely to exhibit antisocial personality disorder (APD) as adults (Kimonis & Frick, 2010). According to Hinshaw, Lahey, and Hart (1993), childhood-onset CD often begins with ODD. In fact, 80% of boys with childhood-onset CD had been previously diagnosed with ODD (Lahey & Loeber, 1994). As adults, early starters tended to have more criminal convictions, incarcerations, and other legal involvements than their adolescent-onset counterparts. In fact, between a third and a half of these children were diagnosed with disorders characterized by antisocial behaviors (Loeber, Burke, & Lahey, 2002).

Compared to early starters, individuals with adolescent-onset CD tend to be less aggressive and violent. This population has fewer cognitive, neuropsychological, and behavioral deficits than early starters. Furthermore, individuals with adolescent-onset CD are more likely to have stable family units that use effective parenting strategies more often than those with early-onset CD. However, later-onset individuals are at a greater risk for continued substance abuse problems (Odgers et al., 2007).

Since the developmental course of ODD symptoms often reveals a consistent increase in severity over time, a parallel may be drawn with CD, suggesting that when early symptoms are present prompt intervention may prevent exacerbation of symptoms and progression into more severe disorders. Behavior therapy, especially including parent training, has been a mainstay treatment for decades, and continues to exhibit robust support in clinical investigations. More severe cases, however, may exhibit severely compromised development of self-control, and in those instances intervening with behavior therapy alone may not produce sufficient improvement in a reasonable time frame. In addition, when co-morbid disorders are present, a single treatment modality may not be sufficient, and combined treatment may become the intervention of choice.

Pharmacotherapy for CD

Pharmacological interventions for CD have been used for decades; nonetheless, they are mostly used in conjunction with psychotherapy. Studies on pharmacological interventions for CD are often further complicated by the presence of co-morbid disorders such as ADHD, anxiety, major depression, substance use, and other related impulse-control problems. Overall, there are five classes of medications commonly prescribed to children and adolescents with CD: antipsychotics, mood stabilizers, antidepressants, stimulants, and adrenergic agents (Tcheremissine & Lieving, 2006).

Antipsychotics

Historically, antipsychotics have been the medications most commonly prescribed to adolescents with CD (Kaplan, 1994). RCTs of conventional antipsychotic medications for CD reveal a decrease in behavioral symptoms. For example, in a double-blind study of 31 hospitalized children with aggressive behavior between the ages of 6 and 11, the effects of molindone and thioridazine were examined over an 8-week period (Greenhill, 1985). The results on standardized rating scales indicated a decrease in aggressive behaviors, but a placebo control group was not used, so these conclusions are not definitive. In addition, these medications often cause significant adverse effects, including extrapyramidal symptoms (EPSs) caused by dopamine blockade or depletion in the basal ganglia (Blair, 1992). Side effects of typical antipsychotics include acute dyskinesia and dystonic reactions, tardive dyskinesia, Parkinsonism, akinesia, akathisia, and a risk of neuroleptic malignant syndrome.

Atypical antipsychotics, including risperidone, aripiprazole, quetiapine, and olanzapine, may offer the benefits of decreased behavioral aggression with reduced risk of EPSs. Generally, these medications block dopamine and serotonin receptors, and may decrease aggressive behavior. For example, risperdone was effective in children with CD, as demonstrated in a 10-week trial on 20 outpatient children of ages 5 to 15. A decrease in aggressive behavior was noted, and no EPSs were reported during the study. These results were replicated in two additional double-blind, placebo-controlled studies with small sample sizes: one with children with borderline intellectual functioning (Van Bellinghem, 2001) and the other with children with borderline intellectual functioning or mild mental retardation (Buitelaar, 2001). Similarly, aripiprazole has been found to be effective and well tolerated in adolescents (Findling, 2009). Safety, dosage, and effectiveness were evaluated in 23 children and adolescents with CD, between the ages of 6 and 17. The participants showed improvements in symptoms, but during the study the dose had to be reduced due to vomiting and sedation. After dosage adjustments, however, aripiprazole was generally well tolerated and improvements in aggressive behavior were noted.

Quetiapine was similarly assessed as a treatment for CD in a 7-week randomized, double-blind, placebo-controlled pilot study (Connor, 2008) with 19 children. The study demonstrated that quetiapine was superior to placebo on all clinician-assessed measures and on a parent-assessed quality-of-life rating scale. One patient on quetiapine developed akathisia, but no other EPS was observed. However, weight gain and metabolic disturbances are significant risks with this medication. Finally, in a retrospective study of 23 adolescents diagnosed with CD, participants responded well to olanzapine treatment (Masi, 2006). Nevertheless, as with quetiapine, risk of significant weight gain and Type II diabetes are major concerns with this medication and may limit its utility.

Mood Stabilizers

Lithium's effectiveness in treating CD has been evaluated in three RCTs, and once in a retrospective study. Campbell (1995) conducted a double-blind, placebo-controlled clinical trial with 50 children diagnosed with CD. The results indicated that lithium is superior to placebo in decreasing aggression, but only a modest effect was noted on some of the measures. A second double-blind RCT, conducted by Rifkin (1997), evaluated 33 adolescents in an inpatient setting. Subjects were randomly assigned after 1 week of placebo, and 26 subjects completed the study. After 2 weeks of treatment, it was concluded that lithium did not improve symptoms of aggression. Since lithium poses significant risks of weight gain and thyroid disturbances, its limited efficacy may not outweigh concerns over serious adverse effects.

The effectiveness of anticonvulsant mood stabilizers in treating CD has also been investigated. Donovan (1997) evaluated the use of divalproex sodium in a two-part investigation. Initially, in an open-label treatment, 10 adolescents with DBD exhibited significant improvement. A double-blind placebo-controlled study was then performed to replicate these findings with 20 children and adolescents, aged 10 to 18, with CD or ODD and mood lability. The results confirmed clinically significant improvements after

6 weeks. Another study by Steiner (2003), evaluated the efficacy of divalproex sodium in 71 youth with CD. All subjects were adolescent males with at least one criminal conviction. A 7-week RCT was carried out in which participants were randomized to high- and low-dose groups. Participants in the low-dose group were administered a dose of 125 mg/day, and those in the high-dose group a dose of 1,000 mg/day. The results indicated that divalproex sodium produced significant, dose-dependent improvements in the impulse control and self-restraint measures completed by the clinicians and subjects. A more recent study utilized the same sample to examine weekly slopes of emotions and cognitions of varying degrees of complexity (Khanzode, 2006). By measuring more basic states such as anger, depression, happiness, and anxiety, as well as complex states such as impulse control, consideration of others, responsibility, and self-esteem, the researchers attempted to evaluate varying levels of psychopathology for youth with CD. The outcome of this study was mixed, however, and no definitive conclusions could be drawn from it other than a need for further studies.

Another mood stabilizer, carbamazepine, has also been used as a treatment for aggressive behavior in children. Kafantaris (1992) completed a pilot study of carbamazepine in 10 hospitalized aggressive and explosive children diagnosed with CD. This study showed that the use of carbamazepine is associated with clinically and statistically significant reductions in the target symptoms of aggressiveness and explosiveness. These results were promising and suggested that a critical assessment of the efficacy and safety of carbamazepine was warranted under double-blind and placebo-controlled conditions in this population. The common side effects of anticonvulsant mood stabilizers often include nausea, vomiting, diarrhea, weight gain, drowsiness, hives, rashes, confusion, cognitive blunting, slurred speech, and in rare cases Stevens–Johnson syndrome and liver damage. These risks must carefully be weighed against any potential clinical benefits.

Antidepressants

Aggressive and impulsive symptoms of CD are often targeted with serotonin-based antidepressants (Armenteros, 2002). For example, trazodone, a serotonin agonist and reuptake inhibitor, was evaluated by Zubieta and Alessi (1992) for efficacy in children with DBDs. Their sample consisted of 22 inpatient children between the ages of 5 and 12. After treatment, 13 of the children demonstrated a decrease in aggressive behavior, and follow up interviews with parents showed continued positive effects. Fluoxetine was also evaluated in an RCT of 126 adolescents with CD, major depressive disorder, and substance use disorder. The outcomes were promising in that the medication improved the participants' symptoms (Riggs et al., 2007). Citalopram, another SSRI, was evaluated in an open-label study by Armenteros (2002). Twelve subjects of ages 7 to 15 with impulsive aggression were administered citalopram for 6 weeks. In the study, impulsive aggression was defined as a pattern of aggressive behavior over the preceding 6 months, including at least three acts of aggression within 1 week of the study screening. Eleven subjects completed the study; one subject withdrew due to hyperactivity, which required additional pharmacotherapy. The results indicated that citalopram pro duces a clinically significant decrease in impulsive aggression on all outcome measures. No significant adverse effects of the medication were reported. Researchers concluded that this medication was effective and well tolerated in this sample of children and adolescents.

Psychostimulants

Stimulant medications have historically been used to address hyperactive and impulsive behavior; however, early research has shown benefits with aggressive behavior as well. Eisenberg (1963) examined the efficacy of dextroamphetamine in a double-blind, placebo-controlled study of 28 institutionalized boys with delinquent behavior. The results demonstrated improvement in symptoms according to teachers, observers, and peers. Decades later, beginning in 1990, studies of the stimulant methylphenidate have demonstrated similar decreases in aggressive behavior. In a 7-week crossover study with nine adolescents (ages 13–16) with ADHD and CD, Kaplan (1990) found a significant decrease in aggressive behavior during methylphenidate treatment when compared with placebo. Similarly, Klein (1997) examined the efficacy of methylphenidate in an RCT of 83 children with CD. Children aged 6–15 were assigned to the methylphenidate or the placebo group for 5 weeks, and over this period their behavior was rated by parents, teachers, and clinicians, and through direct classroom observations. The results indicated that the children's behaviors that were specific to CD decreased significantly with methylphenidate treatment. The researchers concluded that the effects of methylphenidate on symptoms of CD were not a function of the severity of ADHD symptoms because the positive medication effects remained after researchers statistically controlled for the severity of ADHD. Although stimulants may be effective (especially with co-morbid ADHD), side effects may include headache, upset stomach, increased blood pressure, decreased appetite, weight loss, nervousness, sleep problems, and emotional instability.

Antihypertensives

This class of medications (especially α-adrenergic agonists) has also been used to treat aggressive behaviors arising from CD. Kemph (1993) investigated the effectiveness of clonidine in treating aggressive behavior in a pilot study with 17 children and adolescents (ages 5–15). After a mean of 5.2 months, 88% of the participants had significantly improved in their emotions and behavior. A more recent study by Hazell (2003) evaluated the effects of clonidine when added to psychostimulant therapy in children diagnosed with ADHD as well as CD or ODD. This randomized, placebo-controlled study involved 60 children between the ages of 6 and 14. The outcome measure, on Conners' Rating Scales, demonstrated a greater reduction in symptoms in the clonidine group. Adverse effects including, drowsiness and dizziness, were reported in the clonidine group but these were noted to be transient. Common side effects may also include dry mouth, bowel-movement difficulties, drowsiness, dizziness, and low energy levels; and subjects may feel weak, especially upon the onset of treatment or after a dose increase.

To summarize, medication can be an effective treatment modality for CD. Psychotropic medications used to treat individuals with CD have included antipsychotics, antidepressants, mood stabilizers, stimulants, and antihypertensive agents. However, prescribers and patients need to fully understand the reasons for using a medication, as well as its therapeutic benefits and potential adverse effects. Usually, a comprehensive psychological and medical evaluation is warranted to minimize risks. It is also critical that prescribers and patients discuss the initial use as well as the criteria for continuation or termination of any of the psychotropic medications discussed above, with full informed consent forming an essential element in such agents' implementation.

Psychosocial Therapies for CD

As suggested by Pardini and Frick (2013), it may be beneficial to individualize treatments for children with CD based on the different developmental pathways of their problem behaviors. For instance, treatment that emphasizes anger management and works to decrease harsh parenting might be helpful for children with anger problems and emotional dysregulation issues (Lochman & Wells, 2004). On the other hand, interventions based on enhancing the parent–child relationship might help children with CD and callous-unemotional traits (Thomas & Zimmer-Gembeck, 2007). Kolko and Pardini (2010) further noted that empirically based interventions are generally helpful in assisting children with CD (Somech & Elizur, 2012).

Problem-Solving Skills Training

Psychosocial treatments for CD may focus on the individual youth, the parents, the family system, and the community. Some treatments focus on only one of these aspects, while others include a more comprehensive set of modalities. For example, cognitive therapy has been used especially to teach adolescents with CD better problem-solving skills that help reduce aggressive behaviors. In other cases, adolescents with CD may fail to recognize alternative interpretations of social situations, and may often make negative attributions regarding the motivations of others. They may also have difficulty understanding how others view them and understanding the consequences of their own actions (Kazdin, 2002). PSST (Kazdin, 2003) addresses this by teaching interpersonal problem-solving skills, and adolescents are encouraged to take a step-by-step approach to social situations, and to focus on all aspects of a situation before deciding how to respond. Therapists use in-session modeling of prosocial behavior, role-playing, corrective feedback, and social reinforcement. Several meta-analytic reviews of the effectiveness of PSST have supported its usefulness. One review of 36 studies using participants between the ages of 4 and 17 found that the effectiveness of self-statement modification, modeling, and problem-solving training exceeded that of the placebo and attention-control groups (Baer & Nietzel, 1991). Research using randomized clinical trials also suggested particular benefit to children aged 11 and older (Durlak, Fuhrman, & Lampman, 1991). Overall, these studies showed reduced aggressive and antisocial behavior at home, at school, and in the community at the end of treatment and at a 1-year follow up (Kazdin, 2002).

Parent Management Training

Parent management training (PMT) has also been noted to be an effective and empirically supported treatment for CD (Kazdin, 2005a). In PMT, parents are taught to modify their adolescents' behavior in the home using social learning principles. They are taught basic principles regarding reinforcement and consequences, and they learn alternative strategies for using these to manage their adolescents' behavior. Adolescents are also brought into the therapy for behavioral contracting. Basic characteristics of PMT include having parents identify, define, and observe problem behavior, target specific behaviors for change, implement social learning principles, and provide contingent consequences (Kazdin, 2005a).

PMT is considered one of the most empirically validated treatments for CD. For instance, Brestan and Eyberg (1998) examined 82 studies and suggested that 20 interventions had a significant probability of meeting criteria for efficacious treatment for youth identified as conduct-disordered. The results of these studies showed that adolescents with parents who had participated in PMT showed marked improvement in behavior as reported by parents and teachers and in school and police reports. Many of the behavioral improvements could be directly connected to parental behavior and practices. These treatment gains were maintained for up to 14 years (Long, Forehand, Wierson, & Morgan, 1994). A more recent meta-analysis of parent training effectiveness was conducted by McCart, Priester, Dacies, and Azen (2006). Their results suggested that PMT was effective in reducing aggressive behavior, and also significantly reduced the parents' own psychosocial distress.

Parent–Child Interaction Therapy (PCIT)

As mentioned earlier in the chapter, PCIT is an evidence-based intervention approach for young children with emotional and behavioral disorders that works on improving the quality of the parent–child relationship and dyadic patterns. In fact, many parent training programs based on PCIT and Webster-Stratton's parent training program (1990) have been repeatedly shown to have empirical support in comparison to control groups, although these studies have generally only looked at children under the age of 10. Research has suggested that adolescents appear to respond less well to parent management techniques than children do (Dishion & Patterson, 1992), which has motivated a search for programs that are more effective with adolescents. In 2008, Eyberg and colleagues conducted a study to examine well-established and efficacious treatments for CD in this population group, and their review identified two evidence-based multicomponent treatment approaches for adolescents with significant delinquent behavior, both of which included both parent- and child-training components. These were Multisystemic Therapy (MST) and Multidimensional Treatment Foster Care (MTFC).

Multisystemic Therapy

MST (Henggeler & Bordiun, 1990) is a family-systems-based approach that considers adolescent delinquent behavior as it is embedded within the family, school, community, and peer system. Therefore MST interventions combine cognitive-behavioral approaches, behavior therapies, parent training, and pragmatic family therapies. Strong evidence in support of MST has come from multiple randomized, controlled clinical trials involving youth with disruptive behaviors. In one such study, male adolescents who had committed criminal offenses or were on probation showed significant treatment gains and lower recidivism under MST than members of the control groups (Henggeler, Schoenwald, Borduin, Rowland, & Cunningham, 2009). In addition, efficacy trials for MST among violent and chronic juvenile offenders have shown improved family relations, decreased youth behavior problems, and decreased recidivism when compared to individual counseling after a 4-year follow up (Borduin et al., 1995). Similar results have been found with juvenile sex offenders. When compared to those in individual counseling, adolescent sex offenders participating in MST demonstrated a 93% lower rate of sexual reoffending and 72% lower rate of other criminal offending (Borduin, Henggeler, Blaske, & Stein, 1990).

When compared to TAU sex offender services, MST has also shown decreased out-of-home placements, decreased delinquency, and improved family relations for juvenile sex offenders (Borduin, Schaeffer, & Heiblum, 2009).

Multidimensional Treatment Foster Care

MTFC is a community-based program, originally developed as an alternative to institutionalization for youth with severe and chronic delinquent behavior (Chamberlain & Smith, 2003). During treatment, youths are placed in a foster home for 6–9 months and undergo intensive support and treatment in the foster home setting. In addition, the foster parents receive a 20-h PMT course where they learn to implement basic social learning principles. After their training, the foster parents implement a daily token-reinforcement system in which the youth receives points for engaging in appropriate and positive behaviors and loses points for negative behaviors. In addition to the parent management component, each youth participating in MTFC meets weekly with an individual therapist who provides support and works with them on problem-solving skills, anger management, social skills, and educational or vocational planning. The adolescent also meets weekly with a behavior support specialist trained in applied behavior analysis, who focuses on teaching prosocial behaviors through one-on-one interactions within the community setting. Positive outcomes for this approach have been demonstrated (Rhoades, Chamberlain, Roberts, & Leve, 2011). Rhoades, Chamberlain, Roberts, and Leve (2013), for example, found that adolescent girls showed significant decreases in delinquent behaviors after participating in this type of intervention.

Functional Family Therapy

Research on family-based treatments of CD and delinquency in adolescents has also focused on two other interventions: Functional Family Therapy (FFT) and Brief Strategic Family Therapy (BSFT). FFT (Alexander et al., 1994) integrates systems, behavioral, and cognitive approaches to therapy. Overall, FFT focuses on the functions that various behaviors serve, and requires that a functional analysis be conducted prior to intervention. FFT considers how the behavior of each family member functions within the family system. The therapy's treatment goals are to increase reciprocity and positive reinforcement among family members. Early research using randomized trials showed that FFT was more effective than three other comparison conditions at improving family interactions and decreasing recidivism for statutory offenses, but not for criminal offenses (Alexander & Parsons, 1973). More recent research using a randomized efficacy study with substance-abusing youth did not find FFT to be more effective than the comparison groups (Waldron, Slesnick, Brody, Turner, & Peterson, 2001). Overall, though, research indicated that adolescents participating in FFT had better results than those participating in client-centered family groups or psychodynamically oriented family therapy, and those receiving no treatment (Alexander et al., 1994).

Brief Strategic Family Therapy

BSFT (Henggeler & Sheidow, 2012; Szapocznik, Hervis, & Schwartz, 2003), initially developed for use with Hispanic youth in the Miami, Florida area, is another emerging approach for treating adolescent conduct problems. As with most treatments discussed herein, BSFT also views adolescent behavior problems in terms of family dysfunction, and is therefore problem-focused and attempts to alter the interaction patterns among family members (Kazdin, 2002). Therapy is generally delivered in a weekly format, either at a clinic or in the family's home, for a duration of 8–24 sessions, depending on family needs. Two randomized trials with adolescents referred for treatment showed more posttreatment reduction in conduct symptoms among youth who completed BSFT than among youths in the control group (Coatsworth, Santisteban, McBride, & Szapocznik, 2001). Youth completing BSFT also had greater improvement in behavior problems posttreatment than those in a participatory-learning condition (Santisteban et al., 2003).

Overall, a number of psychosocial treatments for CD have shown promise in research trials. Since the etiology of CD may include psychological and sociological aspects such as disordered cognitions, deviant peer groups, and dysfunctional family systems, these treatments may work because they address precipitating and maintenance factors directly. According to Kazdin (2002), familial criminal behavior, family relational difficulties, both harsh punishment and permissive parenting, and low levels of affection, emotional support, acceptance, and attachment all contribute to conduct problems. Interventions that focus on parent, youth, and family characteristics that contribute to or maintain the child's conduct problems may in turn directly focus on causal factors of the disorder.

Notwithstanding their proven effectiveness, there are limitations associated with using psychosocial treatment methods. For example, treatments with a parent training component tend to have high dropout rates. In addition, these treatments require that families learn and implement social learning principles, which may be difficult in many family circumstances. When the adolescent's problems are more severe, their parents may also find it more difficult to implement these strategies. Many of the treatment programs are also intensive; MST, for example, requires cognitive treatment for the adolescent, PMT, intervention with the school, community interventions when necessary, and therapists who are readily available.

Combined Treatment of Conduct Disorder

CD is considered difficult to treat, with decades of research making only small steps in identifying successful interventions (Burke, Loeber, & Birmaher, 2004). Within the past two decades, cognitive and behavioral therapies have been the most researched for children and adolescents with CD, while pharmacological therapies continue to be among those least studied (Mpofu, 2002). Even among psychosocial treatments for CD youth, many have proven to be ineffective due to their failures to incorporate factors linked to the development of CD (Frick, 2001). Despite their allure, integrated approaches for treating youth with CD have not been well researched, and very few studies have evaluated the effects of combined psychosocial and pharmacological treatment protocols for this patient population (Brown et al., 2008b). When considering treatment options, it is important to target the processes that have been demonstrated by research to contribute to the development and maintenance of CD. These include biological factors (predispositions), functional factors (child temperament, academic performance, impulsivity, social cognition, etc.), and psychosocial factors (parenting methods, child abuse, peer effects, socioeconomic stresses, trauma, life stressors, ability to cope, etc.) (Burke et al., 2004).

The identification of effective treatments for children and adolescents with CD should ideally address the two-factor reality that CD not only consists of the individual's conduct, but also that individual's systemic context. At an individual level, many youths with CD show significant psychosocial impairments, including low educational achievement, poor social relationships, conflict with parents and teachers, involvement with the legal system, and high emotional distress (Frick, 2001). Clinical data and outcomes from longitudinal studies have demonstrated that the prognosis for CD youths is relatively poor and that uninformed and ill-conceived treatments for youth CD can do more harm than good. According to Frick (2001), intervention programs for children with CD need to be implemented with caution, as some approaches might be harmful to children. Given this poor prognosis and the detrimental effects of subpar treatments for CD youth, it is crucial to identify treatments that have strong empirical support for effectiveness and positive outcomes.

At a systemic level, it is important for schools and communities to identify effective treatments of CD youth as part of a comprehensive approach to decreasing violence in schools and in the community. School violence continues to occur and to threaten the physical, psychological, and emotional well-being of students and school staff (National Association of School Psychologists, 2006). Given the aggressive nature of students with CD, targeting this population for intervention may be an important step in the effort to reduce violence.

There are several exceptions to the general paucity of research on combined treatment of CD. As early as 1974, Maletzky evaluated dextroamphetamine in a double-blind, placebo-controlled study of 28 teenagers with antisocial behavior (Maletzky, 1974). When dextroamphetamine was added to ongoing therapy, there was a significant reduction in antisocial behavior in these teenagers. Additionally, when adolescents between the ages of 15 and 19 were placed for 16 weeks into either a fluoxetine group with cognitive-behavioral therapy (CBT), a CBT-only group, or a placebo group, the fluoxetine-and-CBT group had greater efficacy and gains than did either the placebo group or the CBT-only group on one of two depression measures, and was not associated with greater decline in self-reported substance use or CD symptoms These results suggested that combined treatment was superior to the other two groups (Riggs et al., 2007).

Brown et al. (2008a, 2008b), reviewed a randomized placebo-controlled study that examined separate and incremental effects of methylphenidate and behavior modification in 16 children with ADHD and ODD. The results revealed that both treatment modalities showed positive effects when the treatment was a stand-alone rather than a combined approach. The authors also discussed the Multimodal Treatment of Attention-Deficit Hyperactivity Disorder (MTA) study, which included 579 children randomly assigned either to routine community care (CC) or to one of three study-delivered treatments, each lasting 14 months. The three MTA treatments consisted of monthly medication management (usually methylphenidate), intensive behavioral treatment, and the combination. According to Brown et al., the MTA study found that children with ADHD and ODD/CD responded well to stimulant medication alone, while children with ADHD and other disorders responded well to a combined treatment of medication and psychosocial interventions.

Apart from little evidence-based research to support multimodal treatment over stand-alone treatments, there are potential benefits of using a combined pharmacological and psychotherapeutic approach when treating children and adolescents with CD. These may include having a more comprehensive and individualized approach that is wider in scope and one that may be more likely to target the wide array of risk factors linked to the development and maintenance of CD symptoms for each individual child. However, the few studies that reviewed combined pharmacological and psychological treatments for youth with CD revealed inconsistent results, and the studies have many limitations. As previously discussed, there are very few studies on the efficacy of combined interventions for youth with CD, so further research is warranted. To assist in this effort, research for combined approaches may begin with interventions, both psychological and pharmacological, that possess empirical data supporting their effectiveness as unimodal treatment approaches; and, in the case of psychological treatments, interventions that target factors that have been linked to the development and maintenance of CD. Data detailing and comparing the cost effectiveness of combined and unimodal treatment approaches might also be worth exploring.

CD and Co-morbid Disorders

Co-morbid diagnoses are commonly observed in children with CD. In general, children with CD are also more likely to have co-occurring ADHD, depression, anxiety, learning disabilities, impulse-control problems, and addictions. Adolescents with both CD and alcohol abuse problems have a much greater risk of displaying antisocial behaviors (Howard, Fin, Jose, & Gallagher, 2012). When CD and other disorders are present, both must be addressed in treatment.

Aggressive behavior is often targeted in treatment alongside ADHD. Two antidepressant medications, buproprion and reboxetine (currently not available in the US, although atomoxetine, available in the US, is a similar substance), have been evaluated for their efficacy in addressing aggression, impulsivity, and hyperactivity. Buproprion was evaluated in an open-label pilot study (Riggs, 1998). Thirteen boys with CD and ADHD diagnoses in a residential treatment program were administered buproprion for 5 weeks. Outcome measures included Conners' Hyperactivity Index and Daydream Attention scores. The data showed a decrease in symptoms, suggesting buproprion may be useful in adolescents with CD and co-morbid ADHD. Likewise, reboxetine was evaluated by Mozes (2005) for efficacy in treating aggression in CD and hyperactivity. An open-label trial was conducted with 15 children (ages 5 to 14) in inpatient treatment. Twelve patients completed the 12-week trial. This study showed significant reduction in symptoms by week 8. While reboxetine was well tolerated, adverse effects such as drowsiness, decreased appetite, bed-wetting, and hair loss were reported among the participants.

Challenges to Integrated Treatment Interventions with CD

With a myriad of factors contributing to CD, it is logical to assume that targeting many of these factors may require more than one intervention, as any single modality will not generally suffice to treat these multidimensional problems (Burke et al., 2004). In addition to a multimodal approach, there is evidence showing that interventions must be individualized and tailored to the unique needs of each child and adolescent with CD (Frick, 2001). These needs vary depending upon the specific mechanisms underlying each subject's cognitive, emotional, and behavioral disturbances. Given the complexity and multidimensional nature of CD, combined approaches may hold real promise for treating children and adolescents with this disorder. By combined, one should not limit thinking in the sense of pharmacology combined with psychotherapy; rather, combined could be any combination of interventions with evidence-based efficacy in treating any component of the CD syndrome.

Combined treatments may involve integrating various psychosocial treatments, such as MST and FFT, both of which focus on the interaction of systems, environments, and cognitive and behavioral interventions (Kazdin, 1997). Combined approaches may also involve a combination of pharmacological and psychotherapeutic modalities. For instance, medications may be used to treat maladaptive, impulsive, or dangerous symptoms, as part of a comprehensive treatment plan, while cognitive or behavioral interventions are incorporated to enhance effective coping mechanisms. One benefit of adding pharmacological interventions to psychosocial interventions is that the pharmacological intervention may enhance the child or adolescent's responsiveness to the psychological interventions. For example, stimulant medication has been shown to reduce conduct problems in children with ADHD and co-morbid CD. It has also been shown to decrease the rate of disruptive classroom behaviors, including verbal and physical aggression, teasing, destruction of property, and cheating (Frick, 2001).

If a child with CD is able to reduce his or her aggression through the use of medication, then he or she may be better able to take active part in interventions aimed at building and practicing social skills. A child with CD taking stimulant medication may also be better able to reduce his or her verbal aggression toward adults, and consequently may be more receptive to and capable of engaging in psychotherapy aimed at developing coping skills to deal with anger. As disruptive behaviors decrease and the child develops a repertoire of alternative socially acceptable behaviors, he or she may begin to experience success in interactions with others and consequently experience a more rewarding quality of life.

Recommendations for the Treatment of ADHD and Disruptive Disorders

Co-morbidity among ADHD types and the various disruptive disorders is striking, and many of the treatments applied to one disorder are transferable to the other disorders. Yet, each disorder has its individual etiology, and its peculiarities of dynamics and presentation, and so it is essential to identify what specific intervention works for each of the disorders, although they may share many characteristics in common. There is an obvious need for much greater research with disruptive disorders to further explicate the nuances among them. We present our treatment recommendations in Table 11.1, based on the evidence to date.

Table 11.1 Integrative biopsychosocial intervention with ADHD, ODD, and CD: Summary of best-practice recommendations by level of confidence derived from strength of evidence.

Attention deficit hyperactivity disorder (ADHD)		
Level A	Recommended	• Medication management is considered first-line in the treatment for ADHD • Behavioral therapy is considered first-line treatment for ADHD • There is compelling evidence that combined treatments, consisting of stimulant medication and behavioral management methods, are especially efficacious in the management of ADHD
Level B	Suggested	• There is emerging evidence to suggest that nonstimulant medications (serotonin–norepinephrine reuptake inhibitors (SNRIs) and alpha-2 adrenergic receptor agonists) may also help as a second-line intervention for ADHD, particularly when children are refractory to stimulant medication or when they evidence unsatisfactory adverse effects to stimulants
Level C	May be considered	• Cognitive-behavioral skills-based intervention has some promise for late adolescents and adults when it is combined with stimulant medication
Oppositional defiant disorder (ODD)		
Level A	Recommended	• Psychosocial interventions should be first-line treatments for ODD, with evidence of large treatment effects that are also generalizable across settings and are long lasting • Behavioral parent training (BPT) has demonstrated the greatest benefits and is recommended across all age groups • Problem-solving skills training (PSST) and anger control skills training (ACST) are also well-established interventions, but they typically complement BPT for ages 7 and up • Pharmacological treatments are not recommended as solitary or even combined treatments for uncomplicated ODD due to an inability to reduce core symptoms and risk of negative side effects
Level B	Suggested	• Child-focused skills training therapies (i.e., PSST and ACST) without direct parent involvement is suggested when behavioral parent training is not available • Psychosocial interventions combined with either an alpha-2 adrenergic agonist or an atypical antipsychotic is suggested for reducing ODD-related symptoms of aggression and/or emotional dysregulation • Combined psychosocial and psychostimulant treatment is suggested when ODD is co-morbid with ADHD, but not for ODD alone
Level C	May be considered	• Combined psychosocial treatment with selective serotonin reuptake inhibitors (SSRIs) may be considered for ODD to address co-morbid anxiety and/or depression, but not for ODD alone • Adding any pharmacotherapy to an existing psychosocial intervention may be considered as adjunctive, palliative, and noncurative for "associated symptoms" or highly impairing co-morbidities only, and not used for pure ODD

Table 11.1 (Continued)

Conduct disorder (CD)		
Level A	Recommended	• Although pharmacotherapy has been shown to be effective in the treatment of CD, evidence does not show it to be more effective that psychosocial treatments, and its side effect profile is concerning when used with a population that is still developing • The first-line treatment for CD should be psychosocial, with a parent management component particularly indicated
Level B	Suggested	• Cognitive-behavioral therapy (CBT) or behavioral therapy have been shown to be effective, but traditional individual therapy does not appear to be as effective as psychosocial treatment that incorporates multisystemic approaches involving patient, parents, and family dynamics
Level C	May be considered	• Psychotropic medication may be tried when psychosocial interventions are insufficient. Start with SSRIs, such as fluoxetine and citalopram. Switching to atypical antipsychotics, such as risperidone, may be indicated if one or more SSRI trials do not work effectively

Illustrative Case Study in the Clinical Practice of Biopsychosocial Integration with ADHD

Tonya is a third grade student who was recently diagnosed with ADHD and co-morbid learning disabilities. At school her teachers describe her as having significant difficulty attending to tasks at hand, which poses particular difficulties in academic areas including reading and mathematics. At home, Tonya is being raised by a single mother who frequently has difficulty negotiating childcare and work responsibilities. Tonya has two other younger male siblings who evidence formidable management difficulties. Tonya and her siblings visit with her father and his wife on weekends, and Tonya's mother has noted that she has considerable difficulty in "settling down" on Sunday evening and getting ready for the school week. Because she is frequently off-task at school, and this has resulted in significant academic difficulties, Tonya's teacher has recommended that Tonya be placed on stimulant medication for the purpose of managing her off-task behavior during the school day. While Tonya's mother is willing to consider a trial of stimulant medication, her father is vehemently opposed to any type of medication for the purpose of managing Tonya's behavior.

Tonya's mother consulted with a specialized university-affiliated clinic that has particular expertise in the management of ADHD and other externalizing disorders. Tonya was carefully evaluated and also received psychoeducational testing for the purpose of assessing any possible learning disabilities that may be contributing to her academic difficulties. With the consent of Tonya's mother, who has custody of Tonya, the developmental pediatrician discussed the results of the assessment with both Tonya's mother and her father during separate visits. Because of Tonya's father's objection to the use of medication, it was suggested that Tonya and her parents participate in a behavior management program during the school year for the purpose of working on transitions and rewarding on-task behavior at home and at school. A DRC was employed whereby Tonya's teacher would assess Tonya's on-task behavior on a daily basis and report this information to Tonya's parents. If Tonya received four good reports

(Continued)

throughout the week, she was permitted by her father to engage in a special activity on the weekend. During the week, for each day that Tonya's on-task behavior was reported to be satisfactory, Tonya's mother would provide a special treat at the end of the day.

Psychoeducational testing revealed that Tonya suffered from a specific learning disability in the areas of reading and mathematics, which in part accounted for her difficulties in these subject areas. As a result, Tonya received special education services in these two subject areas.

Tonya's behavior at home improved significantly, particularly with regard to transitions on the weekend. Tonya's mother reported that she encountered fewer difficulties in managing Tonya's behavior as well as that of her siblings. Teacher reports of Tonya's behavior at school were only slightly improved as a result of the behavior therapy and, again, stimulant medication was recommended. After some family therapy, Tonya's father was able to accept the possibility of conducting a trial of stimulant medication over the course of a month to determine whether Tonya would actually benefit from such therapy and whether this would result in enhanced on-task behavior at school.

The results of the stimulant medication trial was overwhelmingly positive, with Tonya evidencing much greater on-task behavior at school and concomitant increases in academic productivity and performance. This enhanced academic performance was attributed to the special education services that Tonya was receiving at school coupled with the stimulant medication. When Tonya returned home from school each afternoon, Tonya's mother noticed that she was encountering particular difficulties with focusing on homework and that she was now encountering difficulty with bedtime routines. This was attributed to the rebound effect of the stimulant medication, and Tonya's mother focused on the behavior therapy for the purpose of directing more goal-oriented behavior at home, particularly during the rebound period of the medication.

After 5 months of stimulant medication, behavior therapy, and special education services at school, Tonya evidenced marked improvement, and her on-task behavior at school increased by 75%. During the summer months, she was enrolled in a summer camp program for ADHD children that employed ongoing behavior therapy throughout the course of the day. She was able to have a drug-free holiday during the summer months and both of Tonya's parents were quite pleased with the outcome.

Note

1 Dr. Curtis wishes to acknowledge Sara R. Elkins, Samantha Miller, Margaret J. Areizaga, Elizabeth Brestan-Knight, and Timothy Thornberry for their contributions to the section on oppositional defiant disorder.

References

ACTION, A. O. (2007). Practice parameter for the assessment and treatment of children and adolescents with oppositional defiant disorder. *Journal of the American Academy of Child and Adolescent Psychiatry, 46*. doi:10.1097/01.chi.0000246060.62706.af

Alexander, J. F., Holtzworth-Munroe, A., & Jameson, P. (1994). The process and outcome of marital and family therapy research: Review and evaluation. In A. E. Bergin, & S. L. Garfield (Eds.), *Handbook of behavior therapy and behavior change* (4th ed.) (pp. 595–630). New York: Wiley.

Alexander, J. F., & Parsons, B. V. (1973). Short-term behavioral intervention with delinquent families: Impact on family process and recidivism. *Journal of Abnormal Psychology, 81*, 219–255.

Aman, M. G., De Smedt, G., Derivan, A., Lyons, B., & Findling, R. L. (2002). Double-blind, placebo-controlled study of risperidone for the treatment of disruptive behaviors in children with subaverage intelligence. *American Journal of Psychiatry, 159*, 1337–1346.

American Psychiatric Association. (2013). *Diagnostic and statistical manual of mental disorders* (5th ed.). Washington, DC: American Psychiatric Association.

Angold, A., Erkanli, A., Egger, H. L., & Costello, E. J. (2000). Stimulant treatment for children: A community perspective. *Journal of the American Academy of Child and Adolescent Psychiatry, 39*, 975–984. Discussion, 984–994.

Antshel, K. M., Hargrace, T. M., Simonescu, M., Kaul, P., Hendricks, K., & Farone, S. V. (2011). Advances in understanding and treating ADHD. *BMC Medicine, 9*, 72–83.

Armenteros, J. L. (2002). Citalopram treatment for impulsive aggression in children and adolescents: An open pilot study. *Journal of the American Academy of Child and Adolescent Psychiatry, 41*, 522–529.

Bangs, M. E., Hazell, P., Danckaerts, M., Hoare, P., Coghill, D. R., Wehmeier, P. M., . . . & Levine, L. (2008). Atomoxetine for the treatment of attention-deficit/hyperactivity disorder and oppositional defiant disorder. *Pediatrics, 121*, e314–e320.

Baer, R. A., & Nietzel, M. T. (1991). Cognitive and behavioral treatment of impulsivity in children: A meta-analytic review of the outcome literature. *Journal of Clinical Child Psychology, 20*, 400–412.

Barbaresi, W. J., Katusic, S. K., Colligan, R. C., Weaver, A. L., Leibson, C. L., & Jacobsen, S. J. (2006). Long-term stimulant medication treatment of attention-deficit/hyperactivity disorder: Results from a population-based study. *Journal of Developmental and Behavioral Pediatrics, 27*, 1–10. http://doi.org/10.1097/00004701-200602000-00001

Barbaresi, W. J., Katusic, S. K.,Colligan, R. C., Weaver, A. L., & Jacobsen, S. J. (2007). Modifers of long-term school outcomes for children with attention-deficit/hyperactivity disorder: Does treatment with stimulant medication make a difference? Results from a population-based study. *Journal of Developmental and Behavioral Pediatrics, 28*, 274–287. http://doi.org/10.1097/DBP.0b013e3180cabc28

Barkley, R. A. (2006). *Attention-deficit hyperactivity: A handbook for diagnosis and treatment* (3rd ed.). New York: Guilford Press.

Barkley, R. A. (2013). *Defiant children. A clinician's manual for assessment and parent training* (3rd ed.). New York: Guilford Press.

Barkley, R. A., Fischer, M., Smallish, L., & Fletcher, K. (2003). Does the treatment of attention-deficit/hyperactivity disorder with stimulants contribute to drug use/abuse? A 13-year prospective study. *Pediatrics, 111*, 97–109. http://doi.org/10.1542/peds.111.1.97

Barkley, R. A., Murphy, K. R., & Fischer, M. (2008). *ADHD in adults: What the science says.* New York: Guilford Press.

Biederman, J., Swanson, J. M., Wigal, S. B., Kratochvil, C. J., Boellner, S. W., Earl, C. W., & Greenhill, L. (2005). Efficacy and safety of modafinil film-coated tablets in children and adolescents with attention-deficit/hyperactivity disorder: Results of a randomized, double-blind, placebo-controlled, flexible-dose study. *Pediatrics, 116*, e777–e784. http://doi.org/10.1542/peds.2005–0617

Biederman, J., Monuteaux, M. C., Spencer, T., Wilens, T. E., & Farone, S. V. (2009). Do stimulants protect against psychiatric disorders in youth with ADHD? A 10-year follow-up study. *Pediatrics, 124*, 71–78. http://doi.org/10.1542/peds.2008–3347

Biederman, J., Wilens, T., Mick, E., Spencer, T., & Farone, S. V. (1999). Pharmacotherapy of attention-deficit/hyperactivity disorder reduces risk for substance use disorder. *Pediatrics, 104*, e20–e24. http://doi.org/10.1542/peds.104.2.e20

Bilder, R., Loo, S., McGough, J., & McCracken, J. (2016). Cognitive effects of stimulant, guanfacine, and combined treatment in child and adolescent attention-deficit/hyperactivity disorder. *Journal of the American Academy of Child and Adolescent Psychiatry, 55*, 667–673.

Blair, D. D. (1992). Extrapyramidal symptoms are serious side-effects of antipsychotic and other drugs. *The Nurse Practitioner, 17*, 62–64.

Boden, J. M., Fergusson, D. M., & Horwood, L. J. (2010). Risk factors for conduct disorder and oppositional/defiant disorder: Evidence from a New Zealand birth cohort. *Journal of the American Academy of Child and Adolescent Psychiatry, 49*, 1125–1133.

Bond, D. J., Hadjipavlou, G., Lam, R. W., McIntyre, R. S., Neaulieu, S., Schaffer, A., & Weiss, M. (2012). The Canadian Network for Mood and Anxiety Treatments (CANMAT) task force recommendations for the management of patients with mood disorders and comorbid attention-deficit/hyperactivity disorder. *Annals of Clinical Psychiatry, 24*, 23–37.

Borduin, C. M., Henggeler, S., Blaske, D. & Stein, R. (1990). Multisystemic treatment of adolescent sexual offenders. *International Journal of Offender Therapy and Comparative Criminology, 35*, 105–114.

Borduin, C. M., Mann, B., Cone, L., Henggeler, S., Fucci, B., . . . & Williams, R. (1995). Multisystemic treatment of serious juvenile offenders: Long-term prevention of criminality and violence. *Journal of Consulting and Clinical Psychology, 63*, 569–578.

Borduin, C. M., Schaeffer, C. & Heiblum, N. (2009). A randomized clinical trial of multisystemic therapy with juvenile sexual offenders: Effect on youth social ecology and criminal activity. *Journal of Consulting and Clinical Psychology, 77*, 26–37.

Brestan, E. V., & Eyberg, S. M. (1998). Effective psychosocial treatments of conduct-disordered children and adolescents: 29 years, 82 studies, and 5,272 kids. *Journal of Clinical Child Psychology, 27*, 180–189.

Brown, R. T., Antonuccio, D., DuPaul, G., Fristad, M., King, C., . . . & Vitiello, B. (2008). *Oppositional defiant and conduct disorders. Childhood mental health disorders: Evidence base and contextual factors for psychosocial, psychopharmacological, and combined interventions.* Washington, DC: American Psychological Association. doi:10.1037/11638-003

Brown, R. T., Antonuccio, D., DuPaul, G. J., Fristad, M., King, C. A., Leslie, L. K., . . . & McCormick, G. (2008). *Psychopharmacological, psychosocial, and combined interventions for childhood disorders: Evidence base, contextual factors, and future directions.* Washington, DC: American Psychological Association.

Brown, R. T., & Daly, B. P. (2009). Neuropsychological effects of stimulant medication on children's learning and behavior. In C. R. Reynolds & E. Fletcher-Janzen (Eds.), *Handbook of clinical child neuropsychology* (3rd ed.) (pp. 529–580). New York: Plenum.

Buitelaar, J. V. K. (2001). A randomized controlled trial of risperidone in the treatment of aggression in hospitalized adolescents with subaverage cognitive abilities. *Journal of Clinical Psychiatry, 62*, 239–248.

Burke, J., & Loeber, R. (2010). Oppositional defiant disorder and the explanation of the comorbidity between behavioral disorders and depression. *Clinical Psychology: Science and Practice, 17*, 319–326.

Burke, J. D., Loeber, R., & Birmaher, B. (2004). Oppositional defiant disorder and conduct disorder: A review of the past 10 years, part II. *Focus: The Journal of Lifelong Learning in Psychiatry, 11*, 558–576.

Campbell, M. A. (1995). Lithium in hospitalized aggressive children with conduct disorder: A double-blind and placebo-controlled study. *Journal of the American Academy of Child & Adolescent Psychiatry, 34*, 445–453.

Campbell, M., Adams, P. B., Small, A. M., Kafantaris, V., Silva, R. R., Shell, J., . . . & Overall, J. E. (1995). Lithium in hospitalized aggressive children with conduct disorder: A double-blind and placebo-controlled study. *Journal of the American Academy of Child and Adolescent Psychiatry, 34*, 445–453.

Chamberlain, P., & Smith, D. K. (2003). Antisocial behavior in children and adolescents: The Oregon Multidimensional Treatment Foster Care Model. In A. E. Kazdin & J. R. Weisz (Eds.), *Evidenced-based psychotherapies for children and adolescents*. New York: Guilford.

Charach, A., Dashti, B., Carson, P., Booker, L., Lim, C., Lillie, E., . . . & Schachar, R. (2011). Attention deficit hyperactivity disorder: Effectiveness of treatment in at-risk preschoolers; long-term effectiveness in all ages; and variability in prevalence, diagnosis, and treatment. *Comparative Effectiveness Review No. 44*. AHRQ Publication No. 12-EHC003-EF. Rockville, *MD:* Agency for Healthcare Research and Quality. Retrieved from www.effectivehealthcare.ahrq.gov/reports/final.cfm

Chronis, A. M., Chacko, A., Fabiano, G. A., Wymbs, B. T., & Pelham, W. E., Jr. (2004). Enhancements to the behavioral parent training paradigm for families of children with ADHD: Review and future directions. *Clinical Child and Family Psychology Review, 7*, 1–27. http://doi.org/10.1023/B:CCFP.0000020190.60808.a4

Coatsworth, J. D., Santisteban, D. A., McBride, C. K., & Szapocznik, J. (2001). Brief strategic family therapy versus community control: Engagement, retention, and an exploration of the moderating role of adolescent symptom severity. *Family, Process, 40*, 313–332.

Connor, D. F. (2008). Randomized controlled pilot study of Quetiapine in the treatment of adolescent conduct disorder. *Journal of Child and Adolescent Psychopharmacology, 18*, 140–156.

Connor, D. F. (2011, August 11). Problems of overdiagnosis and overprescribing in ADHD. *Psychiatric Times,* Retrieved from http://www/psychiatrictimes.com/adhd/problems-overdiagnosis-and-overprescribing-adhd/page/0/1

Connor, D. F., Findling, R. L., Kollins, S. H., Sallee, F., López, F. A., Lyne, A., & Tremblay, G. (2010). Effects of guanfacine extended release on oppositional symptoms in children aged 6–12 years with attention-deficit hyperactivity disorder and oppositional symptoms. *CNS Drugs, 24*, 755–768.

Daly, B. P., Creed, T., Xanthopoulos, M., & Brown, R. T. (2007). Psychosocial treatments for children with attention deficit/hyperactivity disorder. *Neuropsychology Review, 17*, 73–89. http://doi.org/10.1007/s11065-006-9018-2

Dell'Agnello, G., Maschietto, D., Bravaccio, C., Calamoneri, F., Masi, G., Curatolo, P., . . . & Zuddas, A. (2009). Atomoxetine hydrochloride in the treatment of children and adolescents with attention-deficit/hyperactivity disorder and comorbid oppositional defiant disorder: A placebo-controlled Italian study. *European Neuropsychopharmacology, 19*, 822–834.

Dishion, T. J., & Patterson, G. R. (1992). Age effects in parent training outcomes. *Behavior Therapy, 23*, 719–723.

Dittmann, R., Schacht, A., Helsberg, K., Schneider-Fresenius, C., Lehmann, M., Lehmkuhl, G., & Wehmeier, P. (2011). Atomexetine versus placebo in children and adolescents with attention-deficit/hyperactivity disorder and comorbid oppositional defiant disorder: A double-blind, randomized, multicenter trial in Germany. *Journal of Child and Adolescent Psychopharmacology, 21*, 97–110.

Donovan, S. J., Stewart, J. W., Nunes, E. V., Quitkin, F. M., Parides, M., Daniel, W., . . . & Klein, D. F. (2000). Divalproex treatment for youth with explosive temper and mood lability: A double-blind, placebo-controlled crossover design. *American Journal of Psychiatry, 157*, 818–820.

Donovan, S. J., Susser, E. S., Nunes, E. V., Stewart, J. W., Quitkin, F. M., & Klein, D. F. (1997). Divalproex treatment of disruptive adolescents: A report of 10 cases. *Journal of Clinical Psychiatry, 58*, 12–15.

Donovan, S. S. (1997). Divalproex treatment of disruptive adolescents: A report of 10 cases. *Journal of Clinical Psychiatry, 58*, 12–15.

DuPaul, G. J., Gormley, M. J., & Laracy, S. D. (2013). Comorbidity of LD and ADHD: Implications of DSM-5 for assessment and treatment. *Journal of Learning Disabilities, 46*, 43–51.

Drabick, D. A. G., Ollendick, T. H. & Bubier, J. L. (2010). Co-occurrence of ODD and anxiety: Shared risk processes and evidence for a dual-pathway model. *Clinical Psychology: Science and Practice, 17*, 307–318.

Durlak, J. A., Fuhrman, T. & Lampman, C. (1991). Effectiveness of cognitive-behavioral therapy for maladaptive children: A meta-analysis. *Psychological Bulletin, 110*, 204–214.

Edidin, J. P., Karnik, N. S., Hunter, S. J., & Steiner, H. (2012). Disruptive behavior disorders. In W. M. Klykylo, & J. Kay (Eds.) *Clinical child psychiatry* (3rd ed.). Chichester: John Wiley & Sons, Ltd.

Eisenberg, L. L. (1963). A psychopharmacologic experiment in a training school for delinquent boys. *American Journal of Orthopsychiatry, 33*, 431–437.

Evans, S. W., Owens, J. S., & Bunford, N. (2014). Evidence-based psychosocial treatments for children and adolescents with attention-deficit/hyperactivity disorder. *Journal of Clinical Child and Adolescent Psychology, 43*, 527–551. http://doi.org/10.1080/15374416.2013.850700

Eyberg, S. M., Nelson, M., & Boggs, S. (2008). Evidence-based psychosocial treatments for children and adolescents with disruptive behavior. *Journal of Clinical Child and Adolescent Psychology, 37*, 215–237.

Eyberg, S. & Pincus, D. (1999). *Eyberg Child Behavior Inventory and Sutter-Eyberg student behavior inventory—revised: professional manual.* Odessa, FL: Psychological Assessment Resources.

Fabiano, G. A., Vujnovic, R. K., Pelham, W. E., Waschnusch, D. A., Massetti, G. M., Pariseau, M. E., & Volker, M. (2010). Enhancing the effectiveness of special education programming for children with Attention Deficit Hyperactivity Disorder using a daily report card. *School Psychology Review, 39*, 219–239.

Fiks, A. G., Mayne, S., Highes, C. C., Debartolo, E., Behrens, C., Guevara, J. P., & Power, T. (2012). Development of an instrument to measure parents' preferences and goals for the treatment of attention deficit-hyperactivity disorder. *Academic Pediatrics, 12*, 445–455. http://doi.org/10.1016/j.acap.2012.04.009

Findling, R. K. T. (2009). An open-label study of aripiprazole: Pharmacokinetics, tolerability, and effectiveness in children and adolescents with conduct disorder. *Journal of Child and Adolescent Psychopharmacology, 19*, 431–439.

Frick, P. (2001). Effective interventions for children and adolescents with conduct disorder. *Canadian Journal of Psychiatry, 46*, 597–608.
Frick, P. J. (2012). Developmental pathways to conduct disorder: Implications for future directions in research, assessment, and treatment. *Journal of Clinical Child and Adolescent Psychology, 41*, 378–389.
Frick, P. J., Lahey, B. B., Loeber, R., Stouthamer-Loeber, M., Christ, M. A. G., & Hanson, K. (1992). Familial risk factors to oppositional defiant disorder and conduct disorder: Parental psychopathology and maternal parenting. *Journal of Consulting and Clinical Psychology, 60*, 49–55.
Forgatch, M. S., Patterson, G. R., DeGarmo, D. S., & Beldavs, Z. G. (2009). Testing the Oregon delinquency model with 9-year follow-up of the Oregon divorce study. *Development and Psychopathology, 21*, 637–660.
Garcia, S. P., Guimaraes, J., Zampieri, J., Martinez, A. L., Polanczyk, G., & Rohde, L. A. (2009). Response to methylphenidate in children and adolescents with ADHD: Does comorbid anxiety disorders matters? *Journal of Neural Transmission, 116*, 631–636.
Garnock-Jones, K., & Keating, G. (2009). Atomoxetine: A review of its use in attention-deficit hyperactivity disorder in children and adolescents. *Paediatric Drugs, 11*, 203–226.
Geller, D., Donnelly, C., Lopez, F., Rubin, R., Newcorn, J., Sutton, V., . . . & Sumner, C. (2007). Atomoxetine treatment for pediatric patients with attention-deficit/hyperactivity disorder with comorbid anxiety disorder. *Journal of the American Academy of Child and Adolescent Psychiatry, 46*, 1119–1127. http://doi.org/10.1097/chi.0b013e3180ca8385
Gol, D., & Jarus, T. (2005). Effect of a social skills training group on everyday activities of children with attention-deficit-hyperactivity disorder. *Developmental Medicine and Child Neurology, 47*, 539–545. http://doi.org/10.1111/j.1469–8749.2005.tb01188x
Greene, R. W. (2010). *The explosive child: A new approach for understanding and parenting easily frustrated, "chronically inflexible" children* (4th ed.). New York: Harper Collins.
Greene, R. W., Biederman, J., Zerwas, S., Monuteaux, M., Goring, J. C., & Faraone, S. V. (2002). Psychiatric comorbidity, family dysfunction, and social impairment in referred youth with oppositional defiant disorder. *American Journal of Psychiatry, 159*, 1214–1224.
Greenhill, L. S. (1985). Molindone hydrochloride treatment of hospitalized children with conduct disorder. *Journal of Clinical Psychiatry, 46*, 20–25.
Greenhill, L., Kollins, S., Abikoff, H., McCracken, J., Riddle, M., Swanson, J., & Cooper, T. (2006). Efficacy and safety of immediate-release methylphenidate treatment for preschoolers with ADHD. *Journal of the American Academy of Child and Adolescent Psychiatry, 45*, 1284–1293. http://doi.org/10.1097/01.chi.0000235077.32661.61
Hazell, P. S. (2003). A randomized controlled trial of clonidine added to psychostimulant medication for hyperactive and aggressive children. *Journal of the American Academy of Child and Adolescent Psychiatry, 42*, 886–894.
Hazell, P. (2010). Review of attention-deficit/hyperactivity disorder comorbid with oppositional defiant disorder. *Australasian Psychiatry, 18*, 556–559.
Ni, H. C., Shang, C. Y., Gau, S. S., Lin, Y. J., Huang, H. C., & Yang, L. K. (2013). A head-to-head randomized clinical trial of methylphenidate and atomoxetine treatment for executive function in adults with attention-deficit hyperactivity disorder. *International Journal of Neuropsychopharmacology, 16*, 1959–1973.
Helseth, S. A., Waschbusch, D. A., Gnagy, E. M., Onyango, A. N., Burrows, A., MacLean, L., . . . & Pelham, W. E. (2015). Effects of behavioral and pharmacological therapies on peer reinforcement of deviancy in children with ADHD-only, ADHD and

conduct problems, and controls. *Journal of Consulting and Clinical Psychology, 83*, 280–292.
Henggeler, S. W., & Borduin, C. M. (1990). *Family therapy and beyond: A multisystemic approach to teaching the behavior problems of children and adolescents.* Pacific Grove, CA: Brooks/Cole.
Henggeler, S. W., & Sheidow, A. J. (2012). Empirically supported family-based treatments for conduct disorder and delinquency in adolescents. *Journal of Marital and Family Therapy, 38*, 30–58.
Henggeler, S. W., Schoenwald, S., Borduin, C., Rowland, M., & Cunningham, P. (2009). *Multisystemic therapy for antisocial behavior in children and adolescents* (2nd ed.). New York: Guilford Press.
Hinshaw, S. P., Lahey, B., & Hart, E. (1993). Issues of taxonomy and comorbidity in the development of conduct disorder. *Developmental Psychology, 20*, 1120–1134.
Howard, R., Fin, P., Jose, P., & Gallagher, J. (2012). Adolescent-onset alcohol abuse exacerbates the influence of childhood conduct disorder on late adolescent and early adult antisocial behavior. *Journal of Forensic Psychiatry and Psychology, 23*, 7–22.
Humphreys, K. L., Eng, T., & Lee, S. S. (2013). Stimulant medication and substance use outcomes: A meta-analysis. *JAMA Psychiatry, 70*, 740–749. http://doi.org/10.1001/jamapsychiatry.2013.1273
Jacobs, R. H., Becker-Weidman, E. G., Reinecke, M. A., Jordan, N., Silva, S. G., Rohde, P., & March, J. S. (2010). Treating depression and oppositional behavior in adolescents. *Journal of Clinical Child and Adolescent Psychology, 39*, 559–567.
Kafantaris, V. C. G. (1992). Carbamazepine in hospitalized aggressive conduct disorder children: An open pilot study. *Psychopharmacology Bulletin, 28*, 220.
Kapalka, G. (2007). *Parenting your out of control child.* Oakland, CA: New Harbinger Publications.
Kaplan, S. B. (1990). Effects of methylphenidate on adolescents with aggressive conduct disorder and ADHD: A preliminary report. *Journal of the American Academy of Child and Adolescent Psychiatry, 29*, 719–723.
Kaplan, S. S. (1994). Prescribing practices of outpatient child psychiatrists. *Journal of the American Academy of Child and Adolescent Psychiatry, 33*, 35–44.
Kazdin, A. E. (1997). Practitioner review: Psychosocial treatments for conduct disorder in children. *Journal of Child Psychology and Psychiatry, 38*, 161–178.
Kazdin, A. E. (2002). Psychosocial treatments for conduct disorder in children and adolescents. In P. E. Nathan & J. M. Gorman (Eds.), *A guide to treatments that work* (2nd ed.). New York: Oxford University Press.
Kazdin, A. E. (2003). Problem-solving skills training and parent management training for conduct disorder. In A. E. Kazdin & J. R. Weisz (Eds.), *Evidence-based psychotherapies for children and adolescents.* New York: Guilford.
Kazdin, A. E. (2005a). *Parent management training: Treatment for oppositional, aggressive, and antisocial behavior in children and adolescents.* New York: Oxford University Press.
Kazdin, A. E. (2005b). Child, parent, and family based treatment of aggressive and anti-social child behavior. In E. D. Hibbs & P. S. Jensen (Eds.), *Psychosocial Treatments For Child And Adolescent Disorders: Empirically Based Strategies For Clinical Practice* (2nd ed.). Washington, DC: American Psychological Association.

Kemph, J. D. (1993). Treatment of aggressive children with clonidine: Results of an open pilot study. *Journal of the Academy of Child and Adolescent Psychiatry, 32,* 577–581.
Khanzode, L. S. (2006). Efficacy profiles of psychopharmacology: Divalproex sodium in conduct disorder. *Child Psychiatry and Human Development, 37,* 55–64.
Kimonis, E. R., & Frick, P. J. (2010). Oppositional defiant disorder and conduct disorder grown up. *Journal of Developmental and Behavioral Pediatrics, 31,* 244–254.
Klein, R. A. (1997). Clinical efficacy of methylphenidate in conduct disorder with and without attention deficit hyperactivity disorder. *Archives of General Psychiatry, 54,* 1073–1080.
Kodish, I., Rockhill, C., & Varley, C. (2011). Pharmacotherapy for anxiety disorders in children and adolescents. *Dialogues in Clinical Neuroscience, 13,* 439.
Kolko, D. J., Bukstein, O. G., & Barron, J. (1999). Methylphenidate and behavior modification in children with ADHD and comorbid ODD or CD: Main and incremental effects across settings. *Journal of the American Academy of Child and Adolescent Psychiatry, 38,* 578–586.
Kolko D. J., Pardini, D. A. (2010). ODD dimensions, ADHD, and callous-unemotional traits as predictors of treatment response in children with disruptive behavioral disorders. *Journal of Abnormal Psychology, 119,* 713-725.
Kollins, S. H. (2008). ADHD, substance use disorders, and psychostimulant treatment: Current literature and treatment guidelines. *Journal of Attention Disorders, 12,* 115–125. http://doi.org/10.1177/1087054707311654
Kratochvil, C. J., Newcorn, J. H., Arnold, L. E., Duesenberg, D., Emslie, G. L., Quintanna, H., & Biederman, J. (2005). Atomoxetine alone or combined with fluoxetine for treating ADHD with comorbid depressive or anxiety symptoms. *Journal of the American Academy of Child and Adolescent Psychiatry, 44,* 915–924. http://doi.org/10.1097/01
Kutcher, S., Aman, M., Brooks, S. J., Buitelaar, J., van Daalen, E., Fegert, J., . . . & Tyano, S. (2004). International consensus statement on attention-deficit/hyperactivity disorder (ADHD) and disruptive behaviour disorders (DBDs): Clinical implications and treatment practice suggestions. *European Neuropsychopharmacology, 14,* 11–28.
Lahey, B. B., & Loeber, R. (1994). Framework for a developmental model of oppositional defiant disorder and conduct disorder. In: Routh D. K., (ed.), *Disruptive behavior disorders in childhood.* New York: Plenum.
Larson, J., & Lochman, J. E. (2002). *Helping school children cope with anger: A cognitive-behavioral intervention.* New York: Guildford Press.
LeFever, G. B., Arcona, A. P., & Antonuccio, D. O. (2003). ADHD among American school-children: Evidence of overdiagnosis and overuse of medication. *Scientific Review of Mental Health Practice, 2,* 49–60.
Leibenluft, E. (2011). Severe mood dysregulation, irritability, and the diagnostic boundaries of bipolar disorder in youths. *American Journal of Psychiatry, 168,* 129–142.
Lochman, J. E., Boxmeyer, C. L., Powell, N. P., Barry, T. D., & Pardini, D. A. (2010). Anger control training for aggressive youths. In A. E. Kazdin & J. R. Weisz, (Eds.), *Evidence-based psychotherapies for children and adolescents* (2nd ed.). New York: Guilford Press.
Lochman, J. E., & Wells, K. C. (2004). The Coping Power Program for preadolescent aggressive boys and their parents: Outcome effects at the 1-year follow-up. *Journal of Consulting and Clinical Psychology, 72,* 571–578.

Loeber, R., Burke, J. D., & Lahey, B. (2002). What are adolescent antecedents to antisocial personality disorder? *Criminal Behaviour and Mental Health, 12*, 24–36.

Loeber, R., Burke, J. D., & Pardini, D. A. (2009). Development and etiology of disruptive and delinquent behavior. *Annual Review of Clinical Psychology, 5*, 291–310.

Long, P., Forehand, R., Wierson, M., & Morgan, A. (1994). Does parent training with young noncompliant children have long-term effects? *Behaviour Research and Therapy, 32*, 101–107.

Maletzky, B. (1974). d-Amphetamine and delinquency: Hyperkinesis persisting. *Diseases of the Nervous System, 35*, 543–547.

Malone, R. P., Delaney, M. A., Luebbert, J. F., Cater, J., & Campbell, M. (2000). A double-blind placebo-controlled study of lithium in hospitalized aggressive children and adolescents with conduct disorder. *Archives of General Psychiatry, 57*, 649.

Martel, M. M., Nikolas, M., Jernigan, K., Friderici, K., & Nigg, J. T. (2012). Diversity in pathways to common childhood disruptive behavior disorders. *Journal of Abnormal Child Psychology, 40*, 1223–1236.

Masi, G. M. (2006). Olanzapine treatment in adolescents with severe conduct disorder. *European Psychiatry , 21*, 51–57.

McCart, M. R., Priester, P., Dacies, W., & Azen, R. (2006). Differential effectiveness of behavioral parent-training and cognitive-behavioral therapy for antisocial youth: A meta-analysis. *Journal of Abnormal Child Psychology, 34*, 527–573.

McMahon, R. J., & Forehand, R. (2003). *Helping the noncompliant child: Family-based treatment for oppositional behavior* (2nd ed.). New York: Guilford.

McNeil, C. B., Eyberg, S., Eisenstadt, T. H., Newcomb, K., & Funderburk, B. (1991). Parent-child interaction therapy with behavior problem children: Generalization of treatment effects to the school setting. *Journal of Clinical Child Psychology, 20*, 140–151.

McNeil, C. B., & Hembree-Kigin, T. L. (2010). *Parent-child interaction therapy* (2nd ed.). New York: Springer.

Ming, X., Mulvey, M., Mohanty, S., & Patel, V. (2011). Safety and efficacy of clonidine and clonidine extended-release in the treatment of children and adolescents with attention deficit and hyperactivity disorders. *Adolescent Health, Medicine, and Therapeutics, 2*, 105–112. http://doi.org/10/2147/AHMT.S15672

Molina, B. S. G., Hinshaw, S. P., Swanson, J. M., Arnold, L. E., Vitiello, B., Jensen, P. S., & Houck, P. R. (2009). The MTA at 8 years: Prospective follow-up of children treated for combined-type ADHD in a multisite study. *Journal of the American Academy of Child and Adolescent Psychiatry, 48*, 484–500. http://doi.org/10.1097/CHI.0b013e31819c23d0

Mozes, T. M.-A. (2005). Reboxetine as an optional treatment for hyperkinetic conduct disorder: A prospective open-label trial. *Journal of Child and Adolescent Psychopharmacology, 15*, 259–269.

Mpofu, E. (2002). Psychopharmacology in the treatment of conduct disorder children and adolescents: Rationale, prospects, and ethics. *South African Journal of Psychology, 32*, 9–21.

MTA Cooperative Group (1999). The Multimodal Treatment Study of Children with ADHD: A 14-month randomized clinical trial of treatment strategies for attention-deficit/hyperactivity disorder. *Archives of General Psychiatry, 56*, 1073–1086. http://doi.org/10/1001/archpsyc.56.12.1073

National Association of School Psychologists (2006). *School violence* (Position Statement). Bethesda, MD: National Association of School Psychologists.

Nigg, J. T., & Barkley, R. A. (2014). Attention-deficit/hyperactivity disorder. In E. J. Mash, & R. A. Barkley (Eds.), *Child psychopathology* (3rd ed.). New York: Guilford Press.

Odgers, C. L., Caspi, A., Broadbent, J., Dickson, N., Hancox, R. . . . , & Moffitt, T. (2007). Prediction of differential adult health burden by conduct problem subtypes in males. *Archives of General Psychiatry, 64*, 476–484.

Olfson, M., Blanco, C., Wang, S., Laje, G., & Correll, C. U. (2014). National trends in the mental health care of children, adolescents, and adults by office-based physicians. *JAMA Psychiatry, 71*, 81–90.

Palumbo, D. R., Sallee, F. R., Pelham, W. E., Bukstein, O. G., Daviss, W. B., & McDermott, M. P. (2008). Clonidine for attention-deficit/hyperactivity disorder: I. Efficacy and tolerability outcomes. *Journal of the American Academy of Child and Adolescent Psychiatry, 47*, 180–188.

Pappadopulos, E., Woolston, S., Chait, A., Perkins, M., Connor, D. F., & Jensen, P. S. (2006). Pharmacotherapy of aggression in children and adolescents: Efficacy and effect size. *Journal of the Canadian Academy of Child and Adolescent Psychiatry, 15*, 27–39.

Pardini, D., & Frick, P. J. (2013). Multiple developmental pathways to conduct disorder: Current conceptualizations and clinical implications. *Journal of the Canadian Academy of Child and Adolescent Psychiatry, 22*, 20–25.

Patel, B. D., & Barzman, D. H. (2013). Pharmacology and pharmacogenetics of pediatric ADHD with associated aggression: A review. *Psychiatric Quarterly, 84*, 407–415. http://doi.org/10.1007/s11126-013-9253-7

Patterson, G. R. (1982). *Coercive family process*. Eugene, OR: Castalia.

Patterson, G. R., Reid, J. B., Jones, R. R., & Conger, R. E. (1975). *A social learning approach to family intervention: Families with aggressive children (volume 1)*. Eugene, OR: Castalia.

Pelham, W. E., Fabiano, G. A., Gnagy, E. M., Greiner, A. R., Hoza, B., & Manos, M. J. (2005). The role of summer treatment programs in the context of comprehensive treatment for ADHD. In E. D. Hibbs & P. S. Jensen (Eds.), *psychosocial treatments for child and adolescent disorders: Empirically based strategies for clinical practice* (2nd ed.). Washington, DC: APA Press.

Pelham, W. E., & Waschbusch, D. A. (1999). Behavioral interventions in attention deficit/hyperactivity disorder. In H. Quay & A. Hogan (Eds.), *Handbook of disruptive behavior disorders*. New York: Kluwer Academic

Pliszka, S. R., & AACAP Work Group on Quality Issues (2007). Practice parameter for the assessment and treatment of children and adolescents with attention-deficit/hyperactivity disorder. *Journal of the American Academy of Child and Adolescent Psychiatry, 46*, 894–921. http://doi.org/10.1097/chi.0b013e318054e724

Pliszka, S. R., Browne, R. G., Olvera, R. L., & Wynne, S. K. (2000). A double-blind, placebo-controlled study of Adderall and methylphenidate in the treatment of attention-deficit/hyperactivity disorder. *Journal of the American Academy of Child and Adolescent Psychiatry, 39*, 619–626.

Pliszka, S. R., Crismon, M. L., Hughes, C. W., Conners, C. K., Emslie, G. J., Jensen, P. S., & AACAP Work Group on Quality Issues (2006). Texas Consensus Conference on Pharmacotherapy of Childhood Attention Deficit-Hyperactivity Disorder: The Texas Children's Medication Algorithm Project: Revision of the algorithm for pharmacotherapy of attention-deficit/hyperactivity disorder. *Journal of the American Academy of Child and Adolescent Psychiatry, 45*, 642–657. http://doi.org/10.1097/01.chi.0000215326.51175eb

Raishevich-Cunningham, N., & Jensen, P. (2011). Attention-deficit/hyperactivity disorder. In R. M. Kliegman, B. M. D. Stanton, J. St. Geme, N. F., Schor, & R. E., Behrman (Eds.), *Nelson textbook of pediatrics* (19th ed.). Philadelphia, PA: Saunders.

Reiff, M. I., & Tippins, S. (2004). *ADHD: A complete and authoritative guide.* Oak Grove Village, IL: American Association of Pediatrics.

Rhoades, K. A., Chamberlain, P., Roberts, R., & Leve, L. (2013). MTFC for high-risk adolescent girls: A comparison of outcomes in England and the United States. *Journal of Child and Adolescent Substance Abuse, 22,* 435–449.

Rifkin, A. K. (1997). Lithium treatment of conduct disorders in adolescents. *American Journal of Psychiatry, 154,* 554–555.

Rifkin, A., Karajgi, B., Dicker, R., Perl, E., Boppana, V., Hasan, N., & Pollack, S. (1997). Lithium treatment of conduct disorders in adolescents. *American Journal of Psychiatry, 154,* 554–555.

Riggs, P. L. (1998). An open trial of bupropion for ADHD in adolescents with substance use disorders and conduct disorder. *Journal of American Academy of Child and Adolescent Psychiatry, 37,* 1271–1278.

Riggs, P., Mikulich-Gilbertson, S, K., Davies, R. D., Lohman, M., Klein, C., & Stover, S. K. (2007). A randomized controlled trial of fluoxetine and cognitive behavioral therapy in adolescents with major depression, behavior problems, and substance use disorders. *Archives of Pediatric Adolescent Medicine , 161*(11), 1026–1034.

Sanders, L. M., & Schaechter, J. (2007). Conduct disorder. *Pediatrics in Review, 28,* 433–343.

Sanders, M. R. (1999). Triple P-positive parenting program: Towards an empirically validated multilevel parenting and family support strategy for the prevention of behavior and emotional problems in children. *Clinical Child and Family Psychology Review, 2,* 71–90.

Sanders, M. R., Murphy-Brennan, M., & McAuliffe, C. (2003). The development, evaluation and dissemination of a training program for general practitioners in evidence-based parent consultation skills. *International Journal of Mental Health Promotion, 5,* 13–20.

Santisteban, D. A., Perez-Vidal, A., Coatsworth, J., Kurtines, W. M., Schwartz, S. J., LaPerriere, A., & Szapocznik, J. (2003). Efficacy of brief strategic family therapy in modifying Hispanic adolescent behavior problems and substance use. *Journal of Family Psychology, 17,* 121–133.

Saxena, K., Mora, L., Torres, E., Hall, R., Delizonna, L., Torres, A., & Steiner, H. (2010). Divalproex sodium-ER in outpatients with disruptive behavior disorders: A three month open label study. *Child Psychiatry and Human Development, 41,* 274–284.

Serra-Pinheiro, M. A., Mattos, P., Souza, I., Pastura, G., & Gomes, F. (2004). The effect of methylphenidate on oppositional defiant disorder comorbid with attention deficit/ hyperactivity disorder. *Archives of Neuropsychiatry, 62,* 399–402.

Shaw, D. S., Lacourse, E., & Nagin, D. S. (2005). Developmental trajectories of conduct problems and hyperactivity from ages 2 to 10. *Journal of Child Psychology and Psychiatry, 46,* 931–942.

Shier, A. C., Reichenbacher, T., Ghuman, H. S., & Ghuman, J. K. (2013). Pharmacological treatment of attention deficit hyperactivity disorder in children and adolescents: Clinical strategies. *Journal of Central Nervous System Disease, 5,* 1–17.

Sibley, M. H., Kuriyan, A. B., Evans, S. W., Waxmonsky, J. G., & Smith, B. H. (2014). Pharmacological and psychosocial treatments for adolescents with ADHD: An updated systematic review of the literature. *Clinical Psychology Review, 34*, 218–232. http://doi.org/10.1016/j.cpr.2014.02.001

Snyder, R., Turgay, A., Aman, M., Binder, C., Fisman, S., & Carroll, A. (2002). Effects of risperidone on conduct and disruptive behavior disorders in children with subaverage IQs. *Journal of the American Academy of Child and Adolescent Psychiatry, 41*, 1026–1036.

Somech, L. Y., & Elizur, Y. (2012). Promoting self-regulation and cooperation in pre-kindergarten children with conduct problems: A randomized controlled trial. *Journal of the American Academy of Child and Adolescent Psychiatry, 51*, 412–422.

Steiner, H. P. (2003). Divalproex sodium for the treatment of conduct disorder: A randomized controlled clinical trial. *Journal of Clinical Psychiatry, 64*, 1183–1191.

Stoep, A. V., Adrian, M. C., Rhew, I. C., McCauley, E., Herting, J. R., & Kraemer, H. C. (2012). Identifying comorbid depression and disruptive behavior disorders: Comparison of two approaches used in adolescent studies. *Journal of Psychiatric Research, 46*, 873–881.

Swanson, J., Kraemer, H., Hinshaw, S., Arnold, L., Conners, C., Abikoff, H., . . . & Wu, M. (2001). Clinical relevance of the primary findings of the MTA: Success rates based on severity of ADHD and ODD symptoms at the end of treatment. *Journal of the American Academy of Child and Adolescent Psychiatry, 40*, 168–179.

Szapocznik, J., Hervis, U., & Schwartz, S. (2003). *Brief strategic family therapy for adolescent drug abuse* (NIH Publication No. 03-4751). Bethesda, MD: National Institute on Drug Abuse.

Tannock, R., & Brown, T. E. (2000). Attention-deficit disorders with learning disorder in children and adolescents. In T. E. Brown (Ed.), *Attention-deficit disorders and comorbidities in children, adolescents, and adults*. Washington, DC: American Psychiatric Press.

Tcheremissine, O. L., & Lieving, L. M. (2006). Pharmacological aspects of the treatment of conduct disorder in children and adolescents. *CNS Drugs, 20*, 549–565.

Thomas, R., & Zimmer-Gembeck, M. J. (2007). Behavioral outcomes of Parent Child Interaction Therapy and Triple P-Positive Parenting Program: A review and meta-analysis. *Journal of Abnormal Child Psychology, 35*, 475–495.

Tourette's Syndrome Study Group (2002). Treatment of ADHD in children with tics: A randomized controlled trial. *Neurology, 58*, 527–536.

Turgay, A. (2009). Psychopharmacological treatment of oppositional defiant disorder. *CNS Drugs, 23*, 1–17.

Van Bellinghem, M. D. (2001). Risperidone in the treatment of behavioral disturbances in children and adolescents with borderline intellectual functioning: A double-blind, placebo-controlled pilot trial. *Journal of Child and Adolescent Psychopharmacology, 11*, 5–13.

Visser, S. N., Danielson, M. L., Bitsko, M. L., Holbrook, J. R., Kogan, M. D., Ghandour, R. M., & Blumberg, S. J. (2014). Trends in the parent-report of health care provider diagnosed and medicated attention-deficit/hyperactivity disorder: United States, 2003–2011. *Journal of the American Academy of Child and Adolescent Psychiatry, 53*, 34–46. http://doi.org/10.1016/j.jaac.2013.009.001

Waldron, H. B., Slesnick, N., Brody, J., Turner, C., & Peterson, T. (2001). Treatment outcomes for adolescent substance abuse at 4 and 7 month assessments. *Journal of Consulting and Clinical Psychology, 69*, 802–813.

Webster-Stratton, C. H., & Reid, M. J. (2003). The incredible years parents, teachers, and children training series: A multifaceted treatment approach for young children with conduct disorders. In A. E. Kazdin, & J. R. Weisz, (Eds.), *Evidence-based psychotherapies for children and adolescents.* New York: Guilford Press.

Webster-Stratton, C., Reid, M. J., & Hammond, M. (2004). Treating children with early-onset conduct problems: Intervention outcomes for parent, child, and teacher training. *Journal of Clinical Child and Adolescent Psychology, 33,* 105–124.

Weersing, V. R., & Weisz, J. R. (2002). Mechanisms of action in youth psychotherapy. *Journal of Child Psychology and Psychiatry, 43,* 3–29. http://doi.org/10.1111/1469-7610.00002

Wilens, T. E. (2006). Attention deficit hyperactivity disorder and substance use disorders. *American Journal of Psychiatry, 163,* 2059–2063. http://doi.org/10.1176/appi.ajp.163.12.2059

Wilens, T. E., Adamson, J., Monuteaux, M. C., Farone, S. V., Schillinger, M., Westerberg, D., & Biederman, J. (2008). Effect of prior stimulant treatment for attention-deficit/hyperactivity disorder on subsequent risk for cigarette smoking and alcohol and drug use disorders in adolescents. *Archives of Pediatric and Adolescent Medicine, 162,* 916–921. http://doi.org/10/1001/archpedi.162.10.916

Willcutt, E. G., Nigg, J. T., Pennington, B. F., Solanto, M V. Rohde, L. A., Tannock, R., . . . & Lahey, B. B. (2012). Validity of DSM-IV attention-deficit/hyperactivity disorder symptom dimensions and subtypes. *Journal of Abnormal Psychology, 121,* 991–1010.

Williamson, D., Murray, D. W., Damaaju, C. V., Ascher, S., & Starr, H. L. (2014). Methylphenidate in children with ADHD with or without learning disability. *Journal of Attention Disorders, 18,* 95–104. http://doi.org/10.1177/1087054712443411

Wolraich, M. L., Brown, L., Brown, R. T., DuPaul, G. J., Earls, M., Feldman, H. M., & Visser, S. (2011). Clinical practice guideline for the diagnosis, evaluation, and treatment of attention-deficit/hyperactivity disorder in children and adolescents. *Pediatrics, 128,* 1007–1022. http://doi.org/10.1542/peds.2011-2654

Wu, T. (2011). Conduct disorder. In S. Goldstein & J. Naglieri (Eds.), *The encyclopedia of child behavior and development.* Berlin: Springer.

Zito, J. M., Safer, D. J., Valluri, S., Gardner, J. F., Korelitz, J. J., & Mattison, D. R. (2007). Psychotherapeutic medication prevalence in Medicaid-insured preschoolers. *Journal of Child and Adolescent Psychopharmacology, 17,* 195–203. http://doi.org/10.1089/cap.2007.0006

Zubieta, J. K., & Alessi, N. E. (1992). Acute and chronic administration of trazadone in the treatment of disruptive behavior disorders. *Journal of Clinical Psychopharmacology, 12,* 346–351.

Zuvekas, S. H., & Vitiello, B. (2012). Stimulant medication use in children: A 12-year perspective. *American Journal of Psychiatry, 169,* 160–166. http://doi.org/10/1176/appi.ajp.2011.11030387

12

Geriatric Disorders: Evidence-Based Integrated Biopsychosocial Treatment of Depression, Dementia, and Dementia-Related Disorders in the Elderly

Robert E. McCue and Mary Kelleher

In 2030, 20% of the US population will be 65 years of age or older; the number of people 85 years and older will more than have doubled to 8.9 million. The relatively small number of subspecialists in geriatric care will be unable to treat this large number of older adults, and mental health general practitioners who treat adults will increasingly service a sizable number of elderly patients. Recognizing and treating their problems will be essential.

The most pressing mental health conditions encountered in the elderly population include: (1) late-life depression, (2) dementia, and (3) co-morbid disorders associated with dementia, including depression, psychotic symptoms, and behavioral disturbances.

Late-Life Depression

A 2006 review (Djernes, 2006) of prevalence studies of depression in elderly Caucasians (65 and older) found rates of major depressive disorder (MDD) ranging from 0.9% to 9.4% for those living at home, and from 14% to 42% for those living in institutions. In 2012, the Institute of Medicine (Institute of Medicine, 2012) reported the following 12-month prevalence rates for community-dwelling adults, 65 years or older:

MDD = 3.0–4.3%
dysthymic disorder = 0.6–1.6%
depressive symptoms =1.1–11.1%.

Late-life depression (LLD) is frequently associated with cognitive impairment and structural changes in the brain affecting the orbital-frontal region of the frontal lobes, the hippocampus, amygdala, and basal ganglia. Additionally, white matter hyperintensities on magnetic resonance imaging (MRI) scans of many older adults are believed to indicate vascular injury to white matter tracts. In some cases, these vascular lesions lead to a depressive syndrome called "vascular depression" (Krishnan, Hays, & Blazer, 1997) or to a depressive-executive dysfunction syndrome (Alexopoulos, 2005) from frontostriatal dysfunction that is characterized by psychomotor retardation, loss of interest,

Cognitive Behavioral Psychopharmacology: The Clinical Practice of Evidence-Based Biopsychosocial Integration, First Edition. Edited by Mark Dana Muse.

limited insight, with fewer depressive vegetative signs and poor response to antidepressants. Earlier LLD treatment studies may not have recognized these subclasses, and results should be interpreted accordingly.

Pharmacotherapy with Late-Life Depression

Over the past 50 years, there have been many studies of antidepressant treatment of LLD completed using a wide variety of methodologies. Systematic reviews of LLD antidepressant trials from 1964–1986 (Gerson, Plotkin, & Jarvik, 1988), 1987–1995 (Anstey & Brodaty, 1995), and 1996–2001 (Salzman, Wong, & Wright, 2002) all found that antidepressants improved depression with no differences among medication classes (tricyclic antidepressants (TCAs), selective serotonin reuptake inhibitors (SSRIs), monoamine oxidase inhibitors (MAOI)) in efficacy and side effects. A 2010 update to an original 2001 Cochrane Review (Wilson, Mottram, Sivanranthan, & Nightingale, 2001) found in a meta-analysis of 17 studies comparing antidepressants in depressed older adults (age range 55–90 years) that all classes of antidepressants had equally modest effects compared with placebo. It should be noted that this meta-analysis included diagnoses other than MDD.

Multiple meta-analyses lead one to conclude that antidepressant versus placebo response rates in LLD have ranged from a broad 63.1% vs. 27.2% (Mittmann et al., 1997) to a narrow 44.4% vs. 34.7% (Nelson, Delucchi, & Schneider, 2008). Katona and Livingston (2002) performed a number needed to treat (NNT) analysis of antidepressant trials between 1966 and 1999 and found different antidepressant classes to be similar, with an NNT for treatment response of 2–4. Nonetheless, a 2004 systematic review of 18 placebo-controlled antidepressant trials (Taylor & Doraiswamy, 2004) calculated an NNT of 7–8 for antidepressant response with no significant difference in response between TCAs and SSRIs; a high placebo response rate was noted. Sneed and colleagues' (2008) meta-analysis of 16 antidepressant trials from 1985–2008 found the antidepressant response rates in comparator trials to be significantly larger (60%) than in placebo-controlled trials (46%). A plausible explanation for this difference attributed the results to subjects knowing that they would be getting an active treatment in comparator studies, thereby reinforcing the importance of the placebo effect in LLD.

In a 2008 meta-analysis of 10 second-generation antidepressant trials (Nelson et al., 2008), the estimated NNT for antidepressant response was 13, and 20 for remission. Many of the studies were noted to have high dropout rates in the antidepressant groups. Longer studies, of 10–12 weeks, seemed to yield better antidepressant response. A further analysis (Nelson, Delucchi, & Schneider, 2013) found a strong drug–placebo difference only in those adults who had a moderately severe depression or duration-of-episode over 10 years. The authors concluded that antidepressants were not effective in short-duration LLD. Kok and colleagues' systematic review of 51 studies (Kok, Nolen, & Heeren, 2012) included other depressive categories, but the meta-analyses were limited to those with MDD. Overall antidepressant response rate for MDD was 48.0% vs. 38.6% for placebo, with an NNT of 6.7. The antidepressant remission rate was 33.7% vs. 27.2% for placebo, with an NNT of 14.4. There were no differences in efficacy and effectiveness among antidepressant classes. Only in aggregate were antidepressants significantly better than placebo. When each class of antidepressant was compared separately against placebo, the advantage disappeared.

A meta-analysis and meta-regression in 2011 (Tedeschini et al., 2011) looked at 15 studies between 1980 and 2010 with a variety of antidepressants. Significant heterogeneity of the studies was noted. Antidepressant-treated subjects had significantly better response rates than placebo *only* in the age group 55–65 years. There was no drug–placebo difference in those subjects of 65–75 years old. Only six studies had subjects in the older age range, though. Possible reasons for the lack of efficacy were cerebral damage with neuropsychiatric consequences, inadequate trial length, inadequate dosing, and the small number of subjects in that age group.

Considering that antidepressants alone do not produce high response rates in LLD, what about other pharmacological treatments? A randomized, placebo-controlled 8-day trial of methylphenidate in 16 older (mean age = 72.3 years) patients with MDD and a medical illness (Wallace, Kofoed, & West, 1995) found that methylphenidate produced significant improvement. Similarly, lithium augmentation has been reported to be helpful in treatment-resistant cases (Cooper et al., 2011). However, no Class I studies have substantiated the above treatments in LLD. In a randomized, placebo-controlled study (Reynolds III et al., 2011) with a 2-year follow up in 130 nondemented patients with MDD (mean age = 73 years), augmentation with donepezil decreased the progression of mild cognitive impairment, when present, but also increased the recurrence of depression. For those with no cognitive impairment, donepezil provided no benefit. The best-substantiated pharmacological approach to treatment-resistant depression in older adults comes from a 2015 study by Lenze et al. (2015). Subjects with MDD who had failed a trial of venlafaxine of at least 12 weeks were randomized to augmentation with either aripiprazole or placebo for another 12 weeks. The aripiprazole group had a significantly greater remission rate (44%) than the placebo group (26%) with an NNT of 6.6. A subsequent analysis (Kaneriya et al., 2016) of this study showed that baseline executive dysfunction, as demonstrated by a low score on the Trail Making Test, predicted poor response to aripiprazole augmentation.

Most studies have looked at MDD; far fewer have examined the pharmacological treatment of milder forms of depression, such as dysthymia, minor depression, or subsyndromal depressive symptoms in older adults. A 2003 systematic review (Bartels et al., 2003) suggested antidepressants may be better than placebo for dysthymia and minor depression, but evidence was not Class I. A 2013 meta-regression by Calati et al. (2013) looked at 34 randomized, double-blind, controlled trials for older adults with MDD, minor depression, or dysthymia. Among the significant findings were that a *lower* antidepressant response rate was associated with a lower baseline severity of symptoms (such as present in minor depression) and a longer duration of illness (such as with dysthymia). Locher et al. (2015) performed a meta-analysis of 19 randomized, placebo-controlled studies of older adults with MDD, minor depression, or dysthymia. The average age in the studies ranged from 59–79 years. Both antidepressants and placebo had significant response rates, but the only clinically meaningful difference between antidepressant and placebo were for those with the most severe depression.

Although the inclusion criteria for most of the antidepressant trials has been 55 or 60 years of age or older, with the mean age running in the 60s or low 70s, the fastest growing group of seniors is the "old-old" (75 years and above). In a review of three studies treating older depressed adults with either nortriptyline or paroxetine, Gildengers et al.

(2002) found that patients aged 76–99 years improved as much as did patients aged 59–75. Response rates after 10 weeks of treatment were 67–75%. On the other hand, a randomized, placebo-controlled, 8-week study with 175 patients 75 years and older (Roose & Schatzberg, 2005) found no overall significant difference with remission rates between citalopram (35%) and placebo (31%). The subgroup of patients with the most severe depression did significantly better on citalopram. A follow up analysis (Culang et al., 2009) showed that those patients who had not responded to citalopram developed worsening cognition (verbal learning and psychomotor speed) if they remained on it. Nonresponders to placebo had no similar deterioration.

There is a growing understanding that some older patients may have executive dysfunction and that this will affect response to antidepressant treatment. Alexopoulos et al. (2000) followed 58 older adults with MDD and varying degrees of cognitive impairment who had improved with nortriptyline. During a 2-year maintenance period, those with executive dysfunction, particularly with abnormal initiation and perseveration, had a significantly worse outcome with more relapses and recurrences. Memory impairment did not have this effect. Sneed et al. (2010) used data from the study of patients 75 years and older (Roose & Schatzberg, 2005) that was mentioned above. Those who had deficient response inhibition based on the Stroop Color Word Test had a worse response to citalopram than to placebo. A review (Pimontel, Culang-Reinlieb, Morimoto, & Sneed, 2012) of the topic concluded that executive dysfunction, notably verbal fluency and response inhibition, negatively affect antidepressant response rates in LLD, and are likely manifestations of a disruption in the frontostriatal limbic circuit, particularly the anterior cingulate and dorsolateral prefrontal cortex.

Psychosocial Therapy with Late-Life Depression

As we have seen, many studies examining the efficacy of antidepressants in LLD were remarkable for high placebo response rates. The regular meetings with study personnel, who at the very least inquired about symptoms and side effects, clearly had a therapeutic effect for many in placebo groups. Disengagement from the social environment is strongly linked to LLD (Fiske, Wetherell, & Gatz, 2009); therefore, the supportive personal nature of psychotherapy is likely to be beneficial for depression.

Five types of psychotherapy have been most studied in the treatment of LLD. They are the following:

1) Cognitive-behavioral therapy (CBT): teaches how to identify distorted cognitions that lead to distress and to increase behaviors that improve mood.
2) Interpersonal therapy (IPT): focuses on problems in current relationships that may be related to depression.
3) Problem-solving therapy (PST): teaches how to methodically analyze problems and decide on solutions that will reduce distress if implemented.
4) Reminiscence and life review therapy: reviews and re-evaluates past events and puts them in perspective.
5) Brief psychodynamic therapy (BPD): explores emotions and events in the past in order to gain insight into the unconscious meaning of symptoms and behavior.

We will review controlled trials evaluating the efficacy of these forms of psychotherapy in treating MDD in older adults. Thompson, Gallagher, and Breckenridge (1987) compared 6-week trials of behavioral therapy, cognitive therapy, and BPD with wait list controls in 91 older (average age = 66 years) patients with MDD. All active therapies had significant improvement as compared to the control group. There was no difference in outcomes among the types of therapy.

Areán et al. (1993) randomized 75 older (average age = 66 years) adults with MDD to weekly group treatment for 12 weeks with either PST or reminiscence therapy, or to a wait list control. Both therapies had significantly more improvement than the control group. PST was superior to reminiscence therapy in reducing depressive symptoms. A later study (Areán, Hegel, Vannoy, Fan, & Unützer, 2008) compared PST adapted for primary care sites (PST-PC) with community-based psychotherapy in 433 older (average age = 70 years) primary care patients. Those who had been randomly assigned to PST-PC had significantly improved depression over the control, up to 24 months.

Thompson, Coon, Gallagher-Thompson, Sommer, and Koin (2001) randomly assigned 102 older (average age = 66.8 years) patients with MDD to treatment with CBT, desipramine, or the combination. All treatments resulted in substantial improvement, with the CBT (alone) and the combination groups having similar results, which were better than the drug treatment by itself. Strachowski et al. (2008) randomized 48 older (average age = 62 years) patients with MDD and an elevated risk for cardiovascular disease to either 16 weeks of CBT or wait list control. After treatment, 57% of the CBT group were in remission compared to 4% of the control group. In their randomized study, Laidlaw et al. (2008) compared CBT with treatment-as-usual (TAU) in 44 older primary care patients with MDD (average age = 74 years). There were significant reductions in depressive symptoms in both groups, but 74% of the CBT were in remission at the end of treatment, compared to 42% of the control group. This difference persisted at 3 months. Serfaty et al. (2009) randomized 204 older (mean age = 74 years) primary care patients with MDD into three groups for 4 months: CBT, TAU with a talking control, and TAU. CBT produced significantly more improvement than the other two groups.

Van Schaik et al. (2006) looked at 143 depressed primary care patients (average age = 68 years) who were randomized to treatment with either IPT for 10 sessions or TAU. IPT was significantly more effective in moderately to severely depressed patients, but not in mildly depressed ones.

Bartels and colleagues' (2003) systematic review of psychosocial treatments for LLD concluded that CBT, cognitive, and behavioral therapies had well-substantiated evidence as effective treatments for MDD. There was insufficient evidence regarding dysthymia and minor depression. Another evidence-based review in 2005 (Scogin, Welsh, Hanson, Stump, & Coates, 2005) of psychotherapies in older adults with a wide variety of depressive syndromes found behavioral therapy, CBT, PST, BPD, reminiscence therapy, and cognitive bibliotherapy to be significantly efficacious. In their systematic review of psychotherapeutic interventions for LLD in 17 randomized controlled trials (RCTs), Francis and Kumar (2013) found that CBT, PST, IPT, reminiscence therapy, and BPD were all equally efficacious.

A meta-analysis (Cuijpers, van Straten, & Smit, 2006) of 25 randomized studies of CBT, IPT, PST, behavioral therapy, and reminiscence therapy in older adults with clinically relevant depressive symptoms provided further evidence of the effectiveness of psychosocial approaches with LLD. Seventeen of the studies had controls, and there was low heterogeneity. Psychological treatments produced significant improvement with an overall effect size of 0.72. For those patients with MDD, the effect size was 0.84.

There was no difference in efficacy among the treatments and no difference between those treatments administered individually or in groups. Another meta-analysis (Pinquart, Duberstein, & Lyness, 2007) looked at 57 controlled studies with older adults with MDD, minor depression, and dysthymia. The largest effect sizes were for CBT (1.06) and reminiscence therapy (1.00). Wilson, Motram, and Vassilas 2008) conducted a meta-analysis of seven RCTs of older adults with MDD who received CBT, BPD, IPT, or supportive therapy. CBT was more effective than control, and BPD was similarly effective to CBT. A recent meta-analysis and systematic review (Huang, Delucchi, Dunn, & Nelson, 2015) included 27 RCTs of formal psychotherapy in the acute phase treatment of LLD. Psychotherapy was shown to be an effective treatment, but the effect size varied with the type of control group. The effect size was large with wait list controls, but smaller when compared to supportive therapy and TAU. Types of psychotherapy were not identified in their study.

There are few studies looking at psychotherapy for milder forms of depression in older adults. Williams et al. (2000) randomized 415 older (mean age = 71 years) primary care patients with dysthymic disorder or minor depression to three treatments: paroxetine plus supportive monitoring, PST-PC, or placebo plus supportive monitoring. After 11 weeks, the benefit of PST-PC was small and not different from placebo. However, its outcome varied among sites. Ciechanowski et al. (2004) randomized 1,387 older (average age = 73 years) adults with minor depression or dysthymia to home-based treatment with PST or TAU. After 12 months, 43% of the treatment group responded vs. 15% of the control group; additionally, 36% were in remission compared to 12% of controls.

As noted previously, older patients with MDD and executive dysfunction do not appear to respond well to antidepressants. Areán et al. (2010) looked at 221 older (mean age = 73 years) patients with MDD and executive dysfunction who were randomized to treatment with either PST or supportive therapy (control). After 12 weeks, 56.7% of the patients who received PST had responded and 45.6% were in remission. In the control group, the rates were 34.0% and 27.8%, respectively. NNT for PST was 4.4–5.6. These results tend to argue in favor of psychosocial approaches, and in particular PST, over pharmacotherapy for older patients with executive dysfunction who suffer from MDD.

Pharmacotherapy and Psychosocial Therapy as Monotherapies and in Combination in Late-Life Depression

Both pharmacotherapy and psychotherapy are efficacious treatments for LLD, but how do they compare with each other? Gerson, Belin, Kaufman, Mintz, and Jarvik (1999) conducted a meta-analysis of RCTs between 1974 and 1998 of LLD treated with either antidepressants or psychotherapy. More studies were available for medication treatment, and those showed a significantly greater reduction in depressive symptoms than placebo, while fewer psychotherapy studies found response rates equivalent to those of TCAs and SSRIs. CBT and BPD were significantly better than placebo. Zeiss and Breckenridge (Zeiss, 2003) compared results of meta-analyses looking at the efficacies of pharmacotherapy and psychotherapy and concluded that psychotherapy was at least as efficacious as pharmacotherapy for LLD. In the study that was discussed above of primary care patients with minor depression or dysthymia (Williams et al., 2000), paroxetine had a stronger positive effect than did PST. When Thompson et al. (2001) compared CBT, desipramine, and the combination in older outpatients with MDD, CBT was at least as efficacious as desipramine alone. In a 2007 meta-analysis (Pinquart et al., 2007), antidepressants and psychotherapy had similar effect sizes in older adults with MDD and other depressive disorders. In a recent 2013 review of treatment for LLD (Kok, 2013), Kok concluded that there was no definitive guide as to whom would best be treated with antidepressants or psychotherapy. He suggested that antidepressants are preferable for more severe cases.

There are few studies looking at the combination of pharmacotherapy and psychotherapy versus either treatment alone in LLD. Maintenance treatment of LLD with the combination of nortriptyline and IPT has been shown to be superior to either treatment alone by Reynolds et al. (2006). However, in the trial by Thompson et al. (2001) mentioned above, CBT plus desipramine was *not* more efficacious than CBT alone.

Practice Guidelines for the Treatment of Late-Life Depression

We conclude from our findings that, for older adults who do not have executive dysfunction and who are on the young end of the range (60s–early 70s), antidepressants are an effective treatment for MDD. The response rate is 45–60% with an NNT of 6–13. The remission rate is 30–40% with an NNT of 15–20. No single class of antidepressant is superior. Potential for side effects will govern the choice of agent; many, but not all, studies find side effect burden less with SSRIs than with TCAs. An adequate antidepressant trial is 8–12 weeks. Nonresponders would best be treated with aripiprazole augmentation.

There is insufficient evidence whether medication provides a significant benefit above placebo for depressive conditions outside of MDD. Likewise, adults in the old-old range have not been adequately studied to provide definitive treatment recommendations. Antidepressants are worth a try if the depression is severe and there are no signs of executive dysfunction. If there is executive dysfunction, particularly deficient response inhibition, antidepressants may make the patient worse.

Psychotherapy is an efficacious treatment for MDD in late life. As with antidepressants, most trials have involved patients in the young-old range. A variety of psychotherapies have been studied: CBT, IPT, PST, BPD, reminiscence therapy, and engage therapy. The types of therapy with the strongest support against controls are CBT, PST, and BPD. However, there is insufficient evidence that any type of psychotherapy is superior to another in LLD. Most treatments were administered individually for periods of 6–52 weeks.

For LLD, the evidence shows that antidepressants and psychotherapy are equally efficacious. The conventional wisdom is that most severe MDD should be treated with antidepressants, but there is no conclusive evidence for this. In cases of LLD with executive dysfunction, psychotherapy, particularly PST, is the treatment of choice. Otherwise, treatment selection should be based on patient preference and clinician competency. While studies have shown the combination of antidepressants and psychotherapy is efficacious for LLD, it is not clear that it is better than either treatment alone.

Cognitive Deficits Associated with Dementia

As our population ages, an increasing number of older adults will develop dementia, a condition whose primary risk factor is age. Dementia is a major neurocognitive disorder with impairment of both cognitive functioning and the ability to perform everyday activities, as per the Diagnostic and Statistical Manual of Mental Disorders,

Fifth Edition (DSM-5) (American Psychiatric Association, 2013). A 2007 population study (Plassman et al., 2007) estimated that 14% of people in the US over the age of 70 have dementia. Results from the Einstein Aging Study (Katz et al., 2012) that looked at 1944 community-dwelling urban adults over the age of 70 found the prevalence of dementia to be 6.5%. A 2013 systematic review and meta-analysis (Prince et al., 2013) arrived at a 5–7% global prevalence of dementia in people aged 60 and above. As a result of improvement in mid-life cardiovascular health, the prevalence of dementia in the US and UK appears to be declining. However, this reduction will be offset by the increased number of the oldest-old (75 years and above) who are most vulnerable for dementia.

The most common form of dementia is Alzheimer's disease (AD), making up 60–70% of the cases. It is a progressive disorder whose typical early manifestation is a difficulty in learning new information. Its prevalence increases with age: 3.0% in adults 65–74, 17.6% for ages 75–84, and 32.3% in 85 and older (Hebert, Weuve, Scherr, & Evans, 2013). The vast majority (81%) of people with AD are 75 years and older (Alzheimer's Association, 2016).

Vascular dementia (VaD) is the next most prevalent type, estimated to be 20% of dementia cases. However, this is a heterogeneous disorder with a variety of pathologies: microbleeds, infarcts, cortical laminar necrosis, hippocampal sclerosis, and white matter lesions from chronic hypoxemia. The varying pathologies and diagnostic criteria make a precise estimate of VaD's prevalence difficult. Many cases of AD also have evidence of vascular pathology, and this mixed form of dementia is now believed to be the most prevalent type (Schneider, Arvanitakis, Bang, & Bennett, 2007).

Dementia with Lewy bodies (DLB) constitutes 4.2% of dementia cases in the community and 7.5% in secondary care settings (Vann Jones & O'Brien, 2014). Many cases may be undiagnosed. Visuospatial, executive, and attention deficits are prominent. Aside from cognitive impairment, DLB is notable for greater functional impairment, greater risk of falls, fluctuations in alertness, extrapyramidal symptoms (including extreme sensitivity to neuroleptics), autonomic dysfunction, rapid eye movement (REM) sleep disorders, and visual hallucinations. Psychotic symptoms are more frequent in the earlier stages of the disease than in AD. The mean age of onset is 75 years. The classic pathology is the Lewy body, an intraneuronal aggregate of the protein α-synuclein, which is also found in Parkinson's disease. Pathologically, the hippocampus and medial temporal structures are less affected than in AD; functional neuroimaging has shown DLB (occipital hypoperfusion) can be reliably distinguished from AD (parietotemporal hypoperfusion).

Frontotemporal dementia is another type of dementia. However, as its onset is typically in middle age, we will not include it in this discussion.

Pharmacotherapy to Remediate Cognitive Deficits of Dementia

Alzheimer's Disease

The loss of acetylcholine neurons in AD was an early focus of medication development. The US Food and Drug Administration (FDA) has approved three acetylcholinesterase inhibitors (AChEIs) for AD to increase levels of acetylcholine in the brain: donepezil, galanatamine, and rivastigmine. These medications slow the progression of AD, rather than cure it; most studies establishing their efficacy have been industry-sponsored with durations of 6 months.

A meta-analysis by Birks and Harvey (2006) included 15 RCTs of donepezil in the treatment of AD for periods ranging from 12–52 weeks. They concluded that donepezil (5 mg and 10 mg) produced improvement in cognition, behavior, and activities of daily living (ADLs) in patients with mild, moderate, and severe stages of AD. The higher dose produced marginally better results. In the United States, donepezil was initially only approved for the treatment of mild-to-moderate AD; the manufacturer sought approval for a 23-mg tablet for moderate-to-severe AD. An RCT by Farlow et al. (2010) showed that the increase of donepezil from 10 mg daily to 23 mg improved one outcome measure but not another. Nonetheless, in 2010 the 23-mg tablet was approved for the treatment of moderate-to-severe AD. A subsequent RCT (Doody et al., 2012) comparing the 10-mg versus 23-mg dose in moderate-to-severe AD, found inconsistent evidence that the higher dose was more efficacious, but it did produce more side effects.

Galantamine is approved for treatment of mild-to-moderate AD. A meta-analysis (Loy & Schneider, 2006) of eight RCTs of galantamine in mild-to-moderate AD found improved cognition and global ratings after 3–6 months of treatment. An RCT (Burns et al., 2009) looking at galantamine in patients with severe AD found improvement in cognition after 6 months, but not in ADLs. Hwang, Ahn, Kim, and Kim (2016) performed a prospective, 52-week, open label trial of galantamine in patients with mild-to-moderate AD who had failed treatment with donepezil. Patients treated with galantamine after failing donepezil did as well as those patients in the control group treated with galantamine who had never been given an AChEI. This suggests that failure of one AChEI does not mean failure of AChEIs as a class. If there is an insufficient response with an AChEI, another should be tried.

The third AChEI, rivastigmine, has the distinction of being available in a transdermal patch. Unlike the other two AChEIs, it is considered a "pseudo-irreversible" inhibitor of AChE, with an effect that may outlast its half-life. A 2015 meta-analysis (Birks, Chong, & Grimley Evans, 2015) of seven RCTs examining the efficacy of rivastigmine in mild-to-moderate AD for periods of 12–52 weeks found that there were small positive effects on cognition, ADLs, and global assessment, but not on behavior or caregiver impact. The authors noted the high number of dropouts, particularly from the rivastigmine group. A 24-week RCT by Farlow, Grossberg, Sadowsky, Meng, and Somogyi (2013) looked at rivastigmine patch in severe AD. They found that the high-dose patch (13.3.mg) produced benefit in both cognition and ADLs over the lower-dose patch (4.6 mg) without increased side effects. However, only 64% of the patients were able to complete the study. Although the transdermal patch is easier to administer, particularly in those with severe AD, it has increased risk. A review of pharmacovigilance databases from both the United States and Canada (Ali, Schleret, Reilly, Chen, & Abagyan, 2015) found disproportionate fatal outcomes with the use of the rivastigmine patch. Many of these were overdoses from the inadvertent application of multiple patches.

A fourth drug to treat AD is memantine, an N-methyl-D-aspartate glutamate (NDMA) receptor antagonist. It is approved for use in moderate-to-severe AD. McShane, Areosa Sastre, and Minakaran (2006) reviewed the efficacy of memantine in AD: three RCTs for 6 months in patients with mild-to-moderate AD showed marginal benefit on cognition and no benefit on ADLs and behavior; three RCTs for 6 months in patients with moderate-to-severe AD showed a small positive effect on cognition, ADLs, and behavior. Current practice is to combine memantine with an AChEI in patients with moderate-to-severe AD. One RCT (Grossberg et al., 2013) found giving memantine to patients with moderate-to-severe AD who were already taking an AChEI improved cognition, behavior, and global assessment, but not ADLs; however, two other RCTs (Doody et al., 2012; Howard et al., 2012) did not find that adding memantine to donepezil in patients with moderate-to-severe AD produced any additional benefit. Atri et al. (2015) conducted an area-under-the-curve analysis of four RCTs of memantine or memantine + donepezil in patients with moderate-to-severe AD. After 6 months, there was superior efficacy from the combination of memantine and donepezil that was additive and 50% greater than with either drug alone. They concluded that previous analyses had underestimated this effect.

The approved drugs for AD were generally studied for periods of 1 year or less. As AD deteriorates over many years, is there long-term efficacy of these drugs? An open-label study (Rogers, Doody, Pratt, & Ieni, 2000) followed 133 patients with mild-to-moderate AD who had completed an RCT with donepezil for up to 5 years. Improvement on donepezil was maintained for 6–9 months, after which there was deterioration. An RCT (Courtney et al., 2004) looked at 565 patients with mild-to-moderate AD who had been treated with donepezil. After 2 years, patients maintained on donepezil had sustained a small improvement in cognition and ADLs, but there was no difference compared to the placebo group in institutionalization, progression of disability, or behavioral disturbances. A recent large-scale observational study in Japan of the long-term use of donepezil in AD (Arai et al., 2016) found continued improvement through 18 months, with deterioration at 24 months. In an RCT (Scarpini et al., 2011) looking at whether there was additional benefit of continuing galantamine after 12 months of treatment in mild-to-moderate AD found that after 24 months patients who were switched to placebo were significantly more likely to drop out (including from lack of efficacy), yet the cognitive scores of those who remained were not significantly different between groups. Hogan's (2014) systematic review of the long-term use of AChEIs concluded that current evidence is mixed and is limited by methodological problems.

Vascular Dementia

The diagnosis of VaD is evolving and, as many cases of AD are believed to have signs of vascular injury, looking for a treatment specific for VaD presents theoretical and methodological challenges. A meta-analysis (Malouf & Birks, 2004) identified only two RCTs and found that for subjects with mild-to-moderate VaD, 6 months of treatment with donepezil showed benefit in cognition, ADLs, and global assessment. Another meta-analysis (Birks & Craig, 2013) found two acceptable RCTs of galantamine on VaD and VaD + AD. There was evidence of improvement in cognition and global assessment, but also a high dropout rate due to side effects. The authors concluded that there was no consistent evidence of galantamine's benefit. Rivastigmine for VaD has also been studied. Birks, McGuinness, and Craig (2013) found three RCTs but could not use them for a meta-analysis. One of the studies showed improvement in cognition with rivastigmine after 24 weeks, but a significant proportion of patients on the drug dropped out due to side effects. A recent meta-analysis by Chen, Zhang, Wang, Yuan, and Hu (2016) on the efficacy of AChEIs in VaD identified 12 studies. Five studies looked at donepezil and another five looked at galantamine; both drugs showed improvement on one cognitive measure, but not another. No conclusion could be drawn from the two studies examining rivastigmine. The authors concluded that both donepezil and galantamine offer modest benefit for VaD, but side effects were a major reason for discontinuing treatment. In a meta-analysis (McShane et al., 2006), two identified RCTs of memantine in VaD showed some benefit in cognition and behavior, but these were not apparent in global clinical assessments.

Along a different line of inquiry, huperzine A is derived from a Chinese herb and is believed to have neuroprotective properties. A 2011 review (Hao, Liu, Liu, & Lu, 2009) found no high-quality evidence to support its use in VaD. However, a later RCT (Xu et al., 2012) of huperzine A in 78 patients with mild-to-moderate VaD found that there was significant improvement in cognition after 12 weeks. Although aspirin is routinely prescribed for patients with VaD, an updated review in 2012 by Rands and Orrell (2000) found no evidence that aspirin is useful in patients with VaD. A randomized, controlled, open-label trial of the antidepressant fluoxetine in 50 nondepressed patients with VaD (Liu et al., 2014) found that 12 weeks of treatment produced significant increases in cognition and brain-derived neurotrophic factor compared to those who did not take fluoxetine.

Dementia with Lewy Bodies

Rolinski, Fox, Maidment, and McShane (2012) reviewed and meta-analyzed the efficacy of treating DLB and Parkinson's disease dementia with AChEIs. Six trials met their criteria, but only one (McKeith et al., 2000) included patients with DLB. In it, rivastigmine produced no benefit over placebo. The meta-analysis did show benefit of AChEIs in Parkinson's disease dementia, and the authors suggested that since this condition is similar to DLB, subsequent trials may prove the efficacy of AChEIs with the latter. Ikeda, Mori, Matsuo, Nakagawa, and Kosaka (2015) performed an RCT of donepezil in 142 patients with DLB. After 12 weeks, there was improvement in cognition in those patients taking donepezil 10 mg daily compared to donepezil 5 mg or placebo. An open-label extension of that trial (Mori et al., 2015) found that 110 of the patients with DLB had sustained improvement on donepezil 10 mg for up to 52 weeks. Side effects were easily managed.

Psychosocial Therapy to Remediate Cognitive Deficits of Dementia

A variety of psychotherapeutic techniques have been reported as effective with demented patients (Douglas, James, & Ballard, 2004), but few of these studies used a sufficiently rigorous methodology. The most significant studies and strongest evidence for efficacy are for cognitive interventions. The three major categories of cognitive interventions are cognitive training (teaching strategies and skills to optimize specific cognitive functions), cognitive rehabilitation (developing strategies to address specific goals with the aim of improving performance in everyday life), and cognitive stimulation (engagement in activities to enhance cognitive and social functioning in a nonspecific manner).

Reality-orientation therapy has been developed to assist older, confused people. It can be integrated into nursing care or administered in a group; the focus is on memory and orientation. A 2000 systematic review (Spector, Davies, Woods, & Orrell, 2000) of the efficacy of reality-orientation therapy in patients with dementia included eight RCTs lasting 4–21 weeks. There was evidence of its efficacy in improving cognition and behavior, equivalent to raising the Mini-Mental State Exam (MMSE) (Folstein, Folstein, & McHugh, 1975) by 2.1 points. Long-term efficacy was not addressed.

Spector et al. (2003) conducted an RCT with 115 people with mild-to-moderate dementia. They received either a combination of reality-oriented therapy and cognitive stimulation twice a week for 7 weeks or "usual activities" as a control. The intervention group had significant improvement in objective cognitive measures. The authors conclude that this intervention was as efficacious as available medication with a NNT = 4.

Olazarán et al. (2004) randomly assigned 72 patients with mild-to-moderate AD on AChEIs to treatment with cognitive-motor stimulation (cognitive exercises, social and psychomotor activities) or an active control of psychosocial support. At 6 months, the control group had deteriorated cognitively, but the intervention group had not. At 12 months, both groups had deteriorated cognitively, but the intervention group deteriorated to a lesser degree and also had a persistent improvement in mood. A 2012 systematic review (Woods, Aguirre, Spector, & Orrell, 2012) of the efficacy of cognitive stimulation in mild-to-moderate dementia included 15 RCTs with 718 participants. Variable trial quality was noted. However, the authors concluded that cognitive stimulation produced benefits in cognition above that of medication, and also appeared to improve the quality of life for people in the earlier stages of dementia.

Requena, Maestú, Campo, Fernández, and Ortiz (2006) randomized patients with mild AD to one of four groups: cognitive training + AChEI, AChEI alone, cognitive training alone, and no treatment. The cognitive training program consisted of small-group sessions of 45 min, 5 days a week, for 2 years. Other participants watched television as a control condition. At the end of the first year, subjects in both the cognitive training + AChEI and the cognitive training alone groups had significant improvement in cognitive functioning; the other two groups gradually deteriorated. At 2 years, all groups had deteriorated but less so with the group who had cognitive training. Another RCT (Tárraga et al., 2006) had 46 subjects with mild AD on AChEIs receive a 24-week program of cognitive training + psychostimulation, psychostimulation (as active control), or medication only. The cognitive training + psychostimulation group had significant improvement at both 12 and 24 weeks, equivalent to two points on the MMSE. The psychostimulation alone group had early improvement that was not sustained. A meta-analysis of cognitive training in AD by Sitzer, Twamley, and Jeste (2006) included 19 studies (14 RCTs). Although, the quality of the studies was variable, the authors found evidence that cognitive training was able to improve cognitive and functional ability in AD, and that the effect can be maintained for 4–5 months.

Loewenstein, Acevedo, Czaja, and Duara (2004) studied the efficacy of a program of cognitive rehabilitation with mild AD by randomly assigning 44 subjects to an individualized program of cognitive rehabilitation over 12–16 weeks versus an active control of nonspecific mental stimulation. At the end of treatment and at a 3-month follow up, the actively treated group was significantly better at a variety of cognitive and functional tasks than the control group, whose performance deteriorated. Clare et al. (2010) studied 69 subjects with mild AD on AChEIs who were randomized to eight weekly sessions of cognitive rehabilitation, relaxation therapy (active control), or no treatment. The group that received cognitive rehabilitation had significant improvements in cognitive performance and satisfaction; the other groups were unchanged. At a 6-month follow up, subjects who had received cognitive rehabilitation sustained their improvements.

In a systematic review (Alves et al., 2013) of cognitive interventions in AD, four RCTs were identified (three used cognitive training and another used cognitive stimulation). These interventions appeared to benefit global cognitive function, but not other specific cognitive and functional domains. Another systematic review in 2013 (Bahar-Fuchs, Clare, & Woods, 2013) looked at cognitive training and cognitive rehabilitation in mild-to-moderate AD or VaD. Eleven RCTs were included, 10 of which involved cognitive training. The cognitive training studies were judged to be of variable quality and showed no consistent effects. The one cognitive rehabilitation study was of high quality and showed a beneficial effect.

Practice Guidelines to Remediate Cognitive Deficits of Dementia

There is evidence that a number of pharmacological and psychotherapeutic interventions are beneficial for people with dementia. However, the efficacy of these treatments does not appear to be sustained after 2 years.

All AChEIs have shown significant, if not clinically substantial, efficacy for mild-to-moderate AD. There is evidence that these drugs also are efficacious in severe AD. The benefit of adding memantine to an AChEI in moderate-to-severe stages of AD has also been shown. Donepezil and galantamine have been found to be efficacious in mild-to-moderate VaD, the former also in DLB.

Reality-orientation therapy, which has multiple iterations, is efficacious in improving memory and behavior in dementia. Cognitive stimulation, cognitive training, and cognitive rehabilitation have all been shown to be efficacious in early stages of dementia. However, the intensity, content, and duration of these treatments can vary, and the optimal method of administering them remains to be established.

Co-morbid Conditions Associated with Dementia

Depression Concomitant with Dementia

Although people with dementia may frequently complain of being depressed and, at times, appear depressed, it is not easy to determine whether they have a clinically significant mood disorder. There are many confounding factors. The prevalence of depressive symptoms will vary widely depending on whether information is obtained by a direct examination of the patient or through a family member or caregiver. Additionally, there is overlap between the clinical features of MDD and dementia; anxiety, sleep, and appetite disturbances, decrease in activities, and cognitive dysfunction are common in both. Since psychiatric diagnoses rely on descriptive criteria, there is no unequivocal way to resolve this. As a screening tool, Alexopoulos, Abrams, Young, and Shamoian (1988) developed a rating scale to measure the severity of depression in demented patients that relies on information from both the caregiver and patient. The National Institute of Mental Health organized a workshop of experts who proposed standardized criteria for MDD in AD (Olin et al., 2002) that were intentionally inclusive to minimize the risk of missing cases of clinical importance. However, the inclusiveness increases the rate of false-positives, which will stymie efforts to identify effective treatments. Whatever their theoretical merits, these criteria have not been used consistently in studies.

Steinberg et al. (2008) calculated the 5 year prevalence of depression in dementia to be 77%. There appears to be no relationship between the severity of cognitive impairment and having depression. It may be more prevalent in early-onset dementia, before 65 years (Rosness, Barca, & Engedal, 2010). Studies have found depression with VaD, as compared to AD, is characterized by complaints of weakness and tiredness, psychomotor retardation, and emotional withdrawal.

Pharmacotherapy of Depression Concomitant with Dementia

Reifler et al. (1989) treated 28 demented outpatients with MDD for 8 weeks with either imipramine or placebo. There was no difference between groups' improvement, and the imipramine group had worsening of cognition. In a 6-week study (Roth, Mountjoy, & Amrein, 1996), moclobemide, a reversible monoamine oxidase inhibitor, was significantly better than placebo in 511 patients with dementia and MDD. A 12-week trial (Lyketsos et al., 2000) comparing sertraline and placebo in 22 patients with AD and MDD had equivocal results: sertraline was better than placebo by some, but not all, clinical ratings. The same protocol with an enlarged sample of 44 patients with AD (Lyketsos et al., 2003) found sertraline to be significantly better than placebo. In this study, 84% of the sertraline-treated patients were either full or partial responders, compared to 35% of the placebo group.

Demented subjects have been studied who have more broadly defined depressive syndromes, including minor depression or dysthymia as well as MDD, or have "depression in dementia" from criteria similar to those proposed by Olin et al. (2002). Nyth et al. (1992) compared citalopram with placebo in 29 patients with dementia and moderate-to-high depression ratings; after 6 weeks, the citalopram group improved more than the placebo group in both mood and cognitive function. Petracca, Tesón, Chemerinski, Leiguarda, and Starkstein (1995) treated 21 depressed AD patients with either clomipramine or placebo, and found that the drug produced more improvement in mood, but worsening of cognition. Other studies found no differences between sertraline and placebo (Magai, Kennedy, Cohen, & Gomberg, 2001), fluoxetine and placebo (Petracca, Chemerinski, & Starkstein, 2001), and venlafaxine and placebo (de Vasconcelos Cunha et al., 2007) in patients with both depression and dementia. In a multicenter trial (Rosenberg et al., 2010) comparing sertraline and placebo in AD patients with the "depression of dementia," after 12 weeks there were no differences in response, ratings, and remission between the sertraline and placebo groups. As in other studies, the drug-treated group had more side effects. Continuing the treatment for an additional 12 weeks did not change the results (Weintraub et al., 2010).

Head-to-head comparisons have been rare. Taragano, Lyketsos, Mangone, Allegri, and Comesaña-Diaz (1997) compared fluoxetine and amitriptyline in 37 patients with AD and MDD. After 45 days, both groups showed similar improvement in mood, but more than 50% of the amitriptyline group had dropped out. Katona, Hunter, and Bray (1998) treated 198 patients with dementia and depression (MDD and minor depression) for 8 weeks with either paroxetine or imipramine. Both had similar efficacy. Lastly, Banerjee et al. (2011) studied 218 depressed patients with AD who were treated for 13 weeks either with sertraline, mirtazapine, or placebo. All groups showed improvement at 13 weeks with, curiously, the greatest improvement in the placebo group. This group also had the *fewest* adverse events. At a 39-week follow up, the results were unchanged.

Two meta-analyses, which included some of the above trials, had opposite conclusions. One (Thompson, Herrmann, Rapoport, & Lanctôt, 2007) included five RCTs of patients with AD, and concluded that antidepressants were efficacious and effective, with NNTs = 5. Interestingly, of the five studies, only two had shown improvement over placebo and both required MDD for inclusion. The second (Nelson & Devanand, 2011) included seven RCTs in the meta-analysis. The authors noted the studies used a variety of methods, were probably underpowered, and could not confirm the efficacy of antidepressants in depression and dementia.

Psychosocial Therapy of Depression Concomitant with Dementia

Very few studies have examined the efficacy of psychotherapy as a treatment for a formally diagnosed depressive syndrome in people with dementia. Teri, Logsdon, Uomoto, and McCurry (1997) conducted an RCT of two forms of behavioral treatment (pleasant events focused for patients, or problem-solving for caregivers) versus two control groups (TAU or wait list). The subjects were 72 patients with probable AD and either MDD (75%) or minor depression (25%). After 9 weeks, 52–68% of the behavioral groups had shown significant clinical improvement (no longer meeting criteria for baseline depressive disorder) compared to 20% of the control groups. At a 6-month follow up, 69% of the treatment responders had maintained improvement.

A 2015 systematic review and meta-analysis looked at psychological treatments for depression in demented patients (Orgeta, Qazi, Spector, & Orrell, 2015). Treatments were considered for the study if they were designed to treat depression, were based on a psychological theory, and had a structured intervention. The six RCTs included in the meta-analysis used variations of CBT, interpersonal therapy, and counseling. Baseline depressive diagnoses were not specified. The authors concluded that there was evidence of moderate quality that these psychological treatments were efficacious in treating depression in patients with dementia. However, there was variability in the duration and intensity of treatments among the studies.

The mood of patients with dementia is very dependent on their living arrangements, the people around them, and the institutional rules and restrictions. Additionally, with progressive dementia, more traditional forms of psychotherapy may be less feasible. As a result, alternative psychosocial interventions have been developed to improve the mood of these patients. Teri, McKenzie, and LaFazia (2005) systematically reviewed the efficacy of psychosocial interventions in patients with "depression in dementia." The review included 11 RCTs. In seven studies, interventions produced significant improvement in depression as compared to controls. These successful interventions included teaching behavioral approaches to the staff and enhancing social engagement of the patients. Six of the studies showed sustained effects of these interventions.

Some studies have looked at the effect of psychosocial interventions on the mood of demented patients who have not been formally diagnosed with a depressive disorder. Since the criteria for a depressive disorder in someone with dementia are far from being firmly established, these interventions are relevant. A systematic review (O'Connor, Ames, Gardner, & King, 2009) looked at psychosocial treatments of the psychological symptoms of dementia (including depressed mood or negative affect). Twelve RCTs were identified of sufficient quality and six had positive results. Three of the six studies had strong quality ratings. One of these, a study of behavioral interventions by Teri et al. (1997), was described above. In a second study (Beck et al., 2002), demented nursing home residents were randomly assigned to one of three treatments (activity of daily living intervention, psychosocial enhancement, or both) or to one of two controls (non specific attention or TAU) for 12 weeks. The treatment groups had significantly more positive affect on a number of rating scales as compared to the controls. A third trial (Williams & Tappen, 2007) compared an exercise program, a supervised walking group, and a social conversation group in patients with AD. After 10 weeks, the exercise group showed significantly more positive affect than the other two groups. Two of the remaining positive studies in the systematic review had ratings of moderate quality. These studies found improvements in mood by personalized recreational activities

(Kolanowski, Litaker, & Buettner, 2005) and validation group therapy (Toseland et al., 1997). The latter is a form of psychotherapy designed to stimulate communication and empathically validate those communications, both verbal and nonverbal, of patients with dementia.

Psychosocial interventions that have *not* been shown by RCTs to have a positive effect on mood are the following: caregiver training in emotionally sensitive care, using a rocking chair, multisensory stimulation, muscle relaxation training, simulated presence using a family audiotape, and music during mealtimes.

Practice Guidelines for Depression Concomitant with Dementia

For antidepressants, there is moderately strong evidence that they are effective in demented patients, particularly those with AD, if a diagnosis of MDD is made by conventional criteria. The lack of head-to-head studies does not allow for recommending a specific class of antidepressant.

For the broader category of "depression in dementia," the efficacy of antidepressants has not been proved. However, for these patients, there is moderate evidence for the efficacy for interventions that teach behavioral approaches to the staff, and enhance the patients' social engagement. Other psychosocial interventions that may improve mood in demented patients with depression include focusing on enhancing ADLs, exercise programs, personalized recreational activities, and group validation therapy.

Psychotic symptoms Concomitant with Dementia

Delusions and hallucinations are common in dementia and are classified among the neuropsychiatric symptoms (NPS) or behavioral and psychological symptoms of dementia (BPSD). About 60% of patients with dementia in the community and over 80% in nursing homes have BPSD, which presents a challenge to caregivers, clinicians, and patients. They are associated with agitation, aggression, higher rates of institutionalization, greater functional impairment, faster cognitive decline, and earlier death.

Psychotic symptoms often are seen in the moderate-to-severe stages of dementia. Psychosis has a 40–50% prevalence rate in AD, the most common type of dementia. The most common psychotic symptoms in AD are delusions, with a median prevalence of 36%; about 18% of AD patients experience hallucinations, and 13% have both delusions and hallucinations (Paulsen et al., 2000; Ropacki & Jeste, 2005). About 50% of patients with DLB develop psychosis with visual hallucinations as a core symptom (Borroni, Agosti, & Padovani, 2008). In VaD, patients are more likely to develop depression and anxiety rather than frank psychosis.

In patients with AD and psychosis, the frontal and parietotemporal neocortical regions show metabolic and perfusion abnormalities, with poor perfusion of the anterior cingulate cortex. Delusions are associated with decreased gray matter density in the left frontal lobe, right frontoparietal cortex, and left claustrum. Frontal lobe deficits in attention and fluency are the cognitive functions most strongly associated with delusions and hallucinations in AD, supporting the frontal lobe hypoperfusion hypothesis.

Visual hallucinations are associated with occipital atrophy and vision loss. In a study of 30 demented patients with visual hallucinations compared with 30 demented patients without this symptom, 50% of those with hallucinations had poor vision versus 27% of those without (Murgatroyd & Prettyman, 2001). McKeith et al. (2005) found that DLB patients with visual hallucinations have profound visuoperceptual dysfunction compared to those without visual hallucinations.

Abnormal levels of the neurotransmitters dopamine, acetylcholine, serotonin, and norepinephrine have all been linked to dementia-related psychosis. These neurotransmitter deficits lend support to the use of AChEIs and SSRIs to treat BPSD.

Pharmacotherapy of Psychotic Symptoms Concomitant with Dementia

The FDA has not approved any medication to treat BPSD, making all medication use off-label. Atypical antipsychotics, particularly risperidone, aripiprazole, and olanzapine, can be effective but the side effects often outweigh benefits. In a meta-analysis of four RCTs of patients with AD and psychosis, risperidone led to significant improvement in psychosis as compared to placebo (Katz et al., 2007). Another meta-analysis of 23 RCTs by Tan et al. (2015) found that aripiprazole and risperidone reduced psychotic symptoms at 12 weeks. In the multicenter Clinical Antipsychotic Trial of Intervention Effectiveness—Alzheimer's Disease (CATIE-AD) study (Schneider et al., 2006b), 421 outpatients with AD and psychosis, agitation, or aggression were randomized to risperidone, olanzapine, quetiapine, or placebo for up to 36 weeks. The primary outcome of the study was time to discontinuation from either lack of effect or side effects. In this regard, risperidone (mean dose 1 mg) and olanzapine (mean dose 5.5 mg) were superior to quetiapine and placebo.

The efficacy of atypical antipsychotics in dementia is limited by the high rates of adverse events, including strokes and death. Atypical antipsychotics increase the mortality rate in dementia-related psychosis by a factor of 1.6 (Schneider, Dagerman, & Insel, 2005). As a result, in 2005 the FDA issued a black box warning on the use of atypical antipsychotics to treat dementia-related psychosis; in 2008 this warning was expanded to include typical antipsychotics. However, other long-term studies have not found the same increased mortality rate, but these latter studies may have had methodological flaws (Kales, Gitlin, & Lyketsos, 2015; Lopez et al., 2013; Raivio, Laurila, Strandberg, Tilvis, & Pitkälä, 2007).

Atypical antipsychotics also cause a statistically and clinically significant decline in cognition in patients with dementia (Vigen et al., 2011). Other side effects include drowsiness, urinary tract infections, extrapyramidal symptoms (EPSs), and gait abnormalities. As for typical antipsychotics, there is no evidence for their efficacy in treating NPS; adverse effects such as death, somnolence, and EPSs outweigh any benefits (Lonergan, Luxenberg, Colford, & Birks, 2002; Sink, Holden, & Yaffe, 2005). In general, antipsychotics also do not improve function or quality of life in patients with dementia (Ravona-Springer & Davidson, 2014).

AChEIs may help with psychosis in both AD and DLB. In an open-label study (Paleacu, Mazeh, Mirecki, Even, & Barak, 2002) of 28 patients with AD, 6 months of donepezil significantly improved BPSD, including delusions and hallucinations. A multicenter open-label study (Carrasco, Agüera, Gil, Moríñigo, & Leon, 2011) of 529 patients with AD had similar positive findings from donepezil after 18–20 weeks of treatment. An RCT by Mori, Ikeda, and Kosaka (2012) that treated 140 patients with DLB with either donepezil or placebo for 12 weeks found that the active group had fewer delusions and hallucinations. In an RCT (McKeith et al., 2000) of 120 patients with DLB who were given either rivastigmine or placebo, those treated with rivastigmine had significant improvement in hallucinations and delusions after 20 weeks.

SSRIs have also shown benefit. In the CitAD study (Leonpacher et al., 2016), 186 patients with AD were randomized to a 9-week trial of either citalopram or placebo. Citalopram at a dose of 30 mg reduced the frequency of delusions and the severity of hallucinations. However, further studies are needed at lower doses, as the FDA has imposed a dosage limit of 20 mg citalopram for patients over age 60 because of concerns about cardiac side effects.

Psychosocial Therapy of Psychotic Symptoms Concomitant with Dementia

Psychotherapeutic interventions have not been widely studied for dementia-related psychosis. There are more data when BPSD treatment is considered as a whole. But while current studies may lack rigor and power, the broader category of nonpharmacological interventions, including psychotherapy, are nonetheless considered first-line treatments for BPSD due to their lack of adverse effects.

An important question for a patient with dementia and psychosis is whether any treatment is needed. The frequency and severity of symptoms, including the patient's level of distress and the risk of harm to the patient or caregiver need to be assessed. Certain delusions, for example that a deceased person is alive, might comfort a patient and should be tolerated. In general, hallucinations and delusions that do not distress the patient or pose a threat to the patient or caregiver can be ignored or diverted.

The broader strategy in a psychotherapeutic approach to delusions in dementia is to try to understand the etiology of the delusional belief and then address symptom-related problems with the patient and environment of care, including caregivers. Some symptoms may involve a misinterpretation of reality or result from sensory problems like vision loss rather than represent actual psychosis. If a patient claims that a caregiver he has forgotten is an imposter, then caregivers should be introduced at each visit and be educated about how a person with dementia may perceive them. Delusions of theft can be from forgetfulness and can be alleviated by buying multiple copies of items. Similarly, nursing home placement may make patients feel abandoned and this may lead to delusions of spousal infidelity. To help resolve this, family visits and phone calls can re-establish trust.

Specific types of psychotherapy have been used to address psychosis in dementia. While some studies have found simulated presence therapy, which entails playing audiotaped memories from earlier life, to be beneficial for agitation arising from abandonment beliefs (Camberg et al., 1999), a 2011 systematic review (O'Neil et al., 2011) found that quality evidence for this type of therapy is lacking and might even worsen behavior in dementia. Validation therapy accepts a patient's reality and validates the expression of emotion, but there is insufficient evidence of its efficacy (O'Neil et al., 2011). Reality-orientation therapy targets orientation information like the date and use of names. A systematic review of its efficacy in treating NPS (Livingston, Johnston, Katona, Paton, & Lyketsos, 2005) identified 11 studies (one RCT) and concluded that there was insufficient evidence of its benefit.

Practice Guidelines for Psychotic Symptoms Concomitant with Dementia

There are no psychotherapeutic interventions with clear evidence of efficacy for dementia-related psychosis. However, nonpharmacological methods tailored to the patient and caregiver should be tried first since psychotic symptoms are classified as BPSD, and most expert guidelines recommend such interventions as the first-line treatment for BPSD given the lack of side effects.

Next, patients should be prescribed AChEIs, particularly donepezil, which can reduce psychosis in AD and also slow cognitive decline. Most patients would be on these medications already to preserve memory. After AChEIs, clinicians should try citalopram, which has shown promise for treating delusions in AD dementia, though the optimal dose needs further study given FDA warnings against using more than 20 mg in people older than 60 years.

Atypical antipsychotics should be prescribed as a last resort if nonpharmacological methods and the above medications fail. They should be used only on a short-term or emergency basis given their side effects, and if the psychosis is dangerous to the patient or others. If use is justified, risperidone or aripiprazole are preferred, followed by olanzapine. Risks and benefits must be carefully discussed. Typical antipsychotics, quetiapine, anticonvulsants and benzodiazepines should not be used for dementia-related psychosis since they lack efficacy and cause harmful side effects.

Behavioral Disturbances Concomitant with Dementia

Behavioral symptoms in dementia include repetitive questioning, sleep disturbances, wandering, agitation, aggression, pacing, irritability, hoarding, and purposeless movements. They are highly prevalent: almost all patients with dementia develop behavioral problems and most manifest more than one symptom. About 60–90% of AD patients develop NPS (Cummings et al., 2016), and a major part of these symptoms have behavioral components that correspond to BPSD. Agitation is defined as excess motor activity and may manifest as physical or verbal aggression, signifying emotional distress. It occurs in 20–45% of dementia patients and increases with the severity of dementia. Depression and apathy are common in VaD and AD, while DLB patients have marked visual hallucinations and REM sleep disorders. Sleep disturbances occur in up to 35% of community-dwelling demented patients (Bombois, Derambure, Pasquier, & Monaca, 2010) and up to 55% of patients with DLB (Borroni et al., 2008).

Behavioral symptoms are associated with early nursing home placement, more rapid deterioration, increased mortality, psychiatric admissions, and caregiver stress and depression. Greater cognitive impairment, lower premorbid agreeableness, psychosis, and depression are risk factors for agitation and aggression in dementia. More severe medical co-morbidity also increases the risk of agitation, irritability, and aberrant motor behavior.

Neurofibrillary tangles and amyloid plaques are associated with NPS in AD, and tau pathology has been implicated in agitation. Agitation in dementia has been associated with functional deficits and volume loss in the frontal and anterior cingulate cortices, the posterior cingulate, the amygdala, and the hippocampus (Rosenberg, Nowrangi, & Lyketsos, 2015).

Imbalances in acetylcholine, serotonin, and dopamine are thought to be involved. Theories of cholinergic deficits in the limbic system and frontal lobes support the use of AChEIs to treat the NPS of AD. Reduced 5-HT_{1A} receptor binding in the temporal cortex has been correlated with aggression in AD (Lai et al., 2003).

Pain, increased caregiver burden, and undiagnosed medical illness increase the risk of agitation. As verbal skills fail, behavioral symptoms can express unmet needs from physical discomfort, boredom, loneliness, or recognizing the losses from dementia. Dull, noisy, or unstructured environments can trigger BPSD. Pre-existing psychiatric illness and personality disorders can also manifest as BPSD.

Pharmacotherapy of Behavioral Disturbances Concomitant with Dementia

Atypical antipsychotics can reduce NPS but have serious side effects. A meta-analysis of 15 RCTs (Schneider, Dagerman, & Insel, 2006a) looked at their efficacy and adverse effects in treating BPSD. Aripiprazole and risperidone had small effect sizes, while the efficacy of olanzapine and quetiapine was unconfirmed. Dropout rates and adverse effects limited medication efficacy. Patients still had significant behavioral symptoms despite antipsychotic treatment. In a systematic review by Ballard and Howard (2006) of three RCTs, they concluded that olanzapine (5–10 mg) was efficacious for agitation and aggression but not psychosis. In the CATIE-AD study (Schneider et al., 2006b) mentioned above, risperidone and olanzapine were superior to placebo for efficacy but not side effects. Side effects like EPSs and sedation made the authors recommend against atypical antipsychotics for aggression and agitation in AD. Another analysis of CATIE-AD data indicated olanzapine and risperidone could be effective for anger, aggression, and paranoia, but did not improve quality of life and overall functioning (Sultzer et al., 2008).

Lonergan et al. (2002) reviewed five RCTs that examined the efficacy of haloperidol, a typical antipsychotic, in treating agitation in dementia. Haloperidol was efficacious in controlling aggression in patients with agitated dementia. However, there was no overall reduction in agitation as compared to placebo. The authors concluded that there was little evidence to support a benefit of haloperidol on manifestations of agitation other than aggression, and that haloperidol should not be used routinely to treat patients with agitated dementia. A systematic review (Sink et al., 2005) included two RCTs and two meta-analyses looking at typical antipsychotics in dementia. They acknowledged the slight benefit of haloperidol with aggression, but suggested that the side effects of EPSs and sedation may outweigh the benefit. In general, they found insufficient evidence that typical antipsychotics were efficacious in the treatment of BPSD.

Antipsychotics have an elevated risk of stroke and death in dementia patients because of a 1.6–1.7 increased risk of mortality that led the FDA to issue a black box warning against the use of all antipsychotics in elderly patients with dementia-related psychosis. Canada, which had approved risperidone for severe dementia, restricted its use in 2015 to short-term control of aggression and psychosis only in severe AD due to a higher risk of cerebrovascular events in patients with mixed or vascular dementia. Fatigue, urinary tract infections, incontinence, worsening cognitive test scores, and increased stroke risk are among the other deleterious side effects of atypical antipsychotics in dementia. The stroke risk may be even higher with atypical antipsychotics than with typical ones (Ballard & Howard, 2006; Schneider et al., 2006a). Risperidone and olanzapine are associated with abnormal gait and EPSs. EPSs are particularly problematic in patients with DLB.

SSRIs have fewer side effects and can improve agitation, likely because there is disturbed serotonin metabolism in dementia. Sertraline and citalopram have been shown to reduce agitation in dementia, though more safety and efficacy studies are needed (Seitz et al., 2011). A 16-week multicenter double-blind + open study (Nyth & Gottfries, 1990) of 98 patients with various types of dementia looked at the efficacy of citalopram in the "emotional disorders" of dementia. For patients with AD, citalopram at 20–30 mg improved confusion, irritability, emotional bluntness, depressed mood, and restlessness with few and mild side effects. However, there was no benefit for those with VaD. Porsteinsson et al. (2014) reported on the efficacy of citalopram on agitation from the CitAD study. Patients randomized to citalopram (target dose = 30 mg) had reduced agitation and caregiver distress, though they also had worsening cognition and QTc prolongation. In a 6-week RCT of 40 patients with AD (Barak, Plopski, Tadger, & Paleacu, 2011), escitalopram had similar efficacy to risperidone in reducing agitation. Although SSRIs are better tolerated than antipsychotics, they also have side effects that may include hyponatremia, headaches, sleep changes, and gastrointestinal bleeding.

AChEIs improve behavioral symptoms in AD, and their use is supported by theories linking cholinergic deficits to behavioral problems. In a 2003 meta-analysis (Trinh, Hoblyn, Mohanty, & Yaffe, 2003) of 29 RCTs, AChEIs showed modest benefit for neuropsychiatric and functional outcomes in AD after at least 1 month of treatment. In a more recent meta-analysis (Campbell et al., 2008) that included nine RCTs, after 3–12 months of treatment AChEIs showed a statistically significant benefit in reducing NPS in AD. Not all the evidence has been positive. In a 12-week RCT of 272 patients (Howard et al., 2007), donepezil was not more effective than placebo for agitation in AD. In another multiyear RCT of 565 patients with mild-to-moderate AD (Courtney et al., 2004), donepezil was no better than placebo in behavioral or psychological outcomes after 48 weeks of treatment. However, an RCT (Mori et al., 2012) found that donepezil did improve BPSD and lessen delusions and hallucinations in DLB.

Memantine may have a small beneficial effect on behavior in moderate-to-severe AD, though not in mild-to-moderate AD, and has shown a small but clinically undetectable benefit on behavior in mild-to-moderate VaD (McShane et al., 2006). In an analysis of two RCTs (Gauthier, Wirth, & Möbius, 2005), memantine improved behavioral symptoms, particularly agitation and aggression, in moderate-to-severe AD.

Some have postulated the antiagitation benefits of antipsychotics and citalopram come from antagonism of the alpha-1 adrenoreceptor (Raskind & Wang, 2014). In an RCT of 22 patients with AD and agitation or aggression (Wang et al., 2009), prazosin, an alpha-1 blocker, was well tolerated and improved aggression and agitation over placebo after 8 weeks of treatment.

For stereotypies or repetitive behaviors, small studies have reported benefit from fluvoxamine, buspirone, trazodone, donepezil, and galantamine. However, a 2013 review (Cipriani, Vedovello, Ulivi, Nuti, & Lucetti, 2013) found that there had been no systematic studies about this phenomenon. For example, no medications have been found to be efficacious for wandering in dementia (Cipriani, Lucetti, Nuti, & Danti, 2014).

In a 2008 meta-analysis (Konovalov, Muralee, & Tampi, 2008) of the efficacy of anticonvulsants in BPSD, five RCTs showed no benefit of valproic acid. Carbamazepine showed modest benefit for agitation but only in two small studies of short duration and suboptimal methodologies. Benzodiazepines have not shown benefit in controlling dementia-related behaviors, and should be avoided except in REM sleep behavior disorders (Hugo & Ganguli, 2014).

Psychosocial Therapy of Behavioral Disturbances Concomitant with Dementia

Most guidelines recommend the use of nonpharmacological interventions, including psychotherapeutic strategies, as the treatment of choice for BPSD, except in emergencies. These interventions cause less harm, provide more attention and care to patients, and curb the use of psychotropic medications. Unfortunately, data about the efficacy of psychotherapeutic interventions are inconclusive due to lack of RCTs, underpowered studies, and studies that focus only on people with severe dementia in nursing homes. Given the heterogeneity of behaviors, there is no standard psychotherapeutic approach to managing behavioral problems in dementia. Lack of training and familiarity, as well as reimbursement and time limitations, are also obstacles to the use of nonpharmacological methods, despite guidelines recommending them.

Psychotherapeutic interventions should stem from an assessment of behavioral problems, including triggers, and the characterization of the behavior with its repercussions on the patient and caregiver. Treatments should be patient-centered and individualized, and address unmet needs like boredom, loneliness, and physical discomfort that often underlie agitated behavior. The needs of most patients with dementia are psychosocial: being respected, having social contact, and coping with their illness.

Caregivers, often stressed, tired and depressed, can provoke agitation by yelling, being confrontational, or underestimating patients' impairments. A systematic review by Livingston et al. (2005) included nine studies (seven RCTs) looking at psychoeducation of caregivers to change their interactions with patients with dementia. The authors concluded that there is compelling evidence for this type of intervention, and that the positive effects can be sustained over several months. Another systematic review using three high-quality RCTs (Olazarán et al., 2010) confirmed this finding: interventions work best when individualized.

In the systematic review noted above (Livingston et al., 2005), there was good evidence that behavioral management strategies focusing on individual behaviors can reduce BPSD. Examples of such efficacious strategies include manualized-guided treatments focused on pleasant events, progressive muscle relaxation, social skills training, and a functional analysis of patient-centered bathing. Educating staff on nonpharmacological management of BPSD is also important in reducing the unnecessary use of antipsychotic medication in nursing homes.

Cognitive stimulation uses information processing rather than factual knowledge to address problems in functioning in patients with dementia. Livingston et al. (2005) looked at four RCTs using cognitive stimulation to treat BPSD. Three showed positive results, although there was variability in how they were implemented and assessed. Olazarán et al. (2010) reviewed three RCTs examining the efficacy of group cognitive stimulation sessions over 4–11 weeks in improving behavior in demented patients and found evidence to support its use.

Some analyses have found short-term benefit from music and Snoezelen therapy, which use relaxation techniques and sensory stimuli such as light and sound to create a pleasant nonverbal environment for patients with more severe dementia (Cohen-Mansfield, 2001; Kverno, Black, Nolan, & Rabins, 2009; O'Neil et al., 2011). A meta-analysis of 21 nonpharmacological therapies (Kverno et al., 2009) found some evidence for aromatherapy with lavender and lemon balm oils. Hand massage and touch might be options for short-term agitation and eating problems, though more RCTs are needed (Viggo Hansen, Jørgensen, & Ørtenblad, 2006). Systematic reviews have found insufficient data of good quality for any of these nonpharmacological treatments including Snoezelen rooms (Chung, Lai, Chung, & French, 2002), aromatherapy (Forrester et al., 2014), and music (Vink, Bruinsma, & Scholten, 2004). There is also insufficient evidence to recommend the use of reminiscence therapy, validation therapy, simulated presence therapy, therapeutic activity programs, reality-orientation therapy, enforced social interaction, and family counseling to treat BPSD (Livingston et al., 2005).

Practice Guidelines for Behavioral Disturbances Concomitant with Dementia

Nonpharmacological interventions should be the first treatment tried for BPSD. These approaches should be directed toward patients, the environment, or caregivers. Sensory modalities like music and massage, as well as interventions targeted at family caregivers, have the most evidence, and should be attempted before medication is used.

If nonpharmacological interventions fail, AChEIs, especially donepezil, and the SSRI citalopram should be used next. These medications have fewer side effects than antipsychotics and can reduce agitation. Of note, the FDA issued a warning that citalopram should not be dosed at more than 20 mg in patients over age 60 due to cardiac conduction risks. For moderate-to-severe AD, memantine should be prescribed next as it might prevent NPS and protects memory.

Atypical antipsychotics, while somewhat effective for agitation, should be avoided except as a last option due to their risk of stroke and death. These medications should be prescribed on a short-term and emergency basis for dangerous agitation. If used, risperidone, aripiprazole, and olanzapine are recommended; there is no reason to use quetiapine in AD.

Typical antipsychotics and anticonvulsant medications should not be used as there is no evidence of their general efficacy and they have potentially harmful side effects. Benzodiazepines should be avoided in elderly patients with dementia, given the risk of falls and cognitive impairment.

Conclusions

Treating mental disorders in older adults can be a challenge. Problems are often multifactorial and syndromes can result from overlapping diagnoses. As a result, clinical trials have led to a large number of possible treatments to consider. However, the evidence substantiating the efficacy of these treatments is variable. We have examined the treatments currently available, and have rated them based on the strength of the evidence. Our findings are presented in Table 12.1.

Table 12.1 Integrative biopsychosocial intervention with depression, dementia, and dementia-related disorders in the elderly: Summary of best-practice recommendations by level of confidence derived from strength of evidence.

Late-life depression		
Level A	Recommended	• Antidepressant for major depressive disorder (MDD) if ≤ 75 years and no executive dysfunction; 8–12 weeks of treatment • Augmentation with aripiprazole • Cognitive-behavioral therapy (CBT), problem-solving therapy (PST), or brief psychodynamic therapy (BPD)
Level B	Suggested	• Antidepressant for severe MDD > 75 years if no executive dysfunction • PST if MDD and executive dysfunction • Interpersonal therapy (IPT) or reminiscence therapy
Level C	May be considered	• Methylphenidate • Augmentation with lithium • PST for dysthymia or minor depression
Cognitive deficits of dementia		
Level A	Recommended	• Acetylcholinesterase inhibitors (AChEIs) for Alzheimer's disease (AD), up to 2 years • Memantine + AChEI for moderate-to-severe AD • Reality-oriented therapy
Level B	Suggested	• AChEIs for AD, past 2 years • Donepezil or galantamine for vascular dementia (VaD) • Donepezil for dementia with Lewy bodies (DLB) • Memantine + AChEI for VaD • Pioglitazone (if diabetic) • Cognitive stimulation or rehabilitation for early stages
Level C	May be considered	• Cognitive training for early stages
Depression concomitant with dementia		
Level A	Recommended	• Antidepressants if MDD criteria • Behavioral therapy groups • Teaching behavioral approaches to staff • Enhancing social engagement of patients
Level B	Suggested	• Antidepressants if depressive symptoms • CBT, IPT, or counseling
Level C	May be considered	• Personalized recreational activities • Activities of daily living (ADL) interventions • Validation group therapy
Psychotic symptoms concomitant with dementia		
Level A	Recommended	• No interventions meet this level of evidence
Level B	Suggested	• AChEIs • Citalopram
Level C	May be considered	• Atypical antipsychotics

Table 12.1 (Continued)

Behavioral symptoms concomitant with dementia		
Level A	Recommended	• Caregiver training and psychoeducation
Level B	Suggested	• Behavioral management strategies • Cognitive stimulation groups • Music therapy • Snoezelen therapy • AChEIs • Memantine • Citalopram
Level C	May be considered	• Aromatherapy • Hand massage • Atypical antipsychotics

Illustrative Case Study of the Clinical Practice of Biopsychosocial Integration with Late-life Depressive and Cognitive Symptoms

Ms. P is a 69-year-old woman who was referred for psychiatric consultation by her internist for worsening of depression. Ms. P is college-educated and had retired 7 years previously from her administrative job in municipal government. She lives with her husband of 46 years, who is also retired. They have two grown children. Since retirement, Ms. P has been volunteering at a local cat rescue and adoption group. She has always loved animals; at home, they have three cats and a dog.

Ms. P has no history of psychiatric problems. Her medical problems include hypertension and hypercholesterolemia, both being treated. She is overweight, but not obese. She has not smoked cigarettes for 30 years, has no significant use of illicit drugs, and uses alcohol moderately.

Ms. P's problems started 8 months previously. One of her duties as a volunteer was to deliver a cat to the home of the person who had been approved to adopt it. On this occasion, in the process of delivering a cat, she found herself lost. Even though she had been in the area many times, she was unable to determine the direction to the address. She was overwhelmed and confused. She called for assistance and another volunteer came to complete the delivery. Subsequently, she refrained from making deliveries. The leaders of the group, concerned about Ms. P's safety, told her that she needed to take a "break" from the group.

Ms. P became saddened by the loss of her volunteer responsibilities. Her husband noticed her low mood and the growing difficulty which she had doing some routine household chores. At his insistence, she visited her internist. Her medical condition was stable. As Ms. P was coherent and able to recount her history, the internist assessed Ms. P as being cognitively intact. He acknowledged her low mood and prescribed duloxetine for depression. Ms. P took three doses of the duloxetine, but was unable to tolerate it because of side effects of jitteriness and sweating. The internist discontinued the duloxetine and started escitalopram. Ms. P was able to tolerate the medication, but its effect on her mood was minor.

In the succeeding months, Ms. P did household chores and socialized with her husband and their friends. Her husband noticed that she would repeat the same questions and would often

(Continued)

claim to have lost items that invariably resurfaced later. Two weeks before psychiatric consultation, Ms. P and her husband were preparing to attend a dinner party. On the day before the party, Ms. P called the hostess and asked her that since they were to be there at 7:30 pm, how could she determine whether it was am or pm? The hostess became concerned and contacted Ms. P's husband. He contacted the internist who referred her for psychiatric consultation.

During the assessment by the psychiatrist, Ms. P was a polite, well-dressed woman who was easy to engage in conversation. She reported no significant difficulties with her husband or their children. Her speech was normal and her thoughts were logical and coherent. There was no evidence of psychosis. She was clearly distressed at the events that had been happening to her, but described her mood as "okay." She acknowledged becoming anxious and overwhelmed at times, but could not provide further insight into these episodes. She retained a desire for social activities and wished to resume volunteering. She admitted to occasionally forgetting things, but did not see this as that much of a problem. There were no problems with her sleep and appetite. There was no hopelessness or thoughts of suicide.

Her husband reported that he became annoyed with her at times because of her repeating herself. He had always handled the finances, but reported that, to his knowledge, Ms. P had no problems buying things at local stores. However, he felt that Ms. P was "different": more passive and more easily overwhelmed.

GDS (15-item) was 3; MMSE was 23 with major difficulties in short-term recall. The provisional diagnosis was that this was an early stage of dementia, probably AD. There was insufficient evidence to diagnose MDD or a clinically significant depressive syndrome. Laboratory tests were unremarkable, and an MRI of the brain showed moderate atrophy of the medial temporal and parietal lobes. These findings ruled out a reversible cause of dementia and are typical findings in AD.

The findings were discussed with Ms. P and her husband. The psychiatrist offered to continue to see Ms. P regularly to help her through this difficult time. Ms. P wished to continue taking the escitalopram, but did not want to take an AChEI. The plan of therapy included two approaches: PST and cognitive rehabilitation. The psychiatrist planned weekly sessions of PST and a referral to a neuropsychologist for cognitive rehabilitation. Ms. P refused the latter. She was then offered a referral to the local Alzheimer's Association, which had a free cognitive training program for early-stage dementia. Ms. P also refused this.

Ms. P did participate in the PST sessions. A major goal of these sessions was to help Ms. P recognize her cognitive strengths and weaknesses—taking advantage of the former to compensate for the latter. After 2 months, Ms. P acknowledged, and was proud of, her cognitive strengths (intelligence, persistence in effort, using categories to organize information). She agreed to see the neuropsychologist as a way of building on her strengths. She continued to refuse AChEIs and a referral to the Alzheimer's Association. Her husband reported that she seemed more confident and was "losing" things less often. Future treatment goals in therapy will be directed toward helping her decide if she would be able to volunteer again and, if so, under what circumstances, exploring her refusal to accept evidence-based treatments (i.e., AChEI, cognitive training), and helping her and her husband plan for a possible deterioration in her functioning.

References

Alexopoulos, G. S. (2005). Depression in the elderly. *Lancet, 365*, 1961–1970. doi:10.1016/S0140-6736(05)66665-2

Alexopoulos, G. S., Abrams, R. C., Young, R. C., & Shamoian, C. A. (1988). Cornell Scale for depression in dementia. *Biological Psychiatry, 23*, 271–284. doi:10.1016/0006-3223(88)90038-8

Alexopoulos, G. S., Meyers, B. S., Young, R. C., Kalayam, B., Kakuma, T., Gabrielle, M., . . . & Hull, J. (2000). Executive dysfunction and long-term outcomes of geriatric depression. *Archives of General Psychiatry, 57*, 285–290. doi:10.1001/archpsyc.57.3.285

Ali, T. B., Schleret, T. R., Reilly, B. M., Chen, W. Y., & Abagyan, R. (2015). Adverse effects of cholinesterase inhibitors in dementia, according to the pharmacovigilance databases of the United States and Canada. *PLoS One, 10*, e0144337. doi:10.1371/journal.pone.0144337

Alves, J., Magalhães, R., Thomas, R. E., Gonçalves, Ó. F., Petrosyan, A., & Sampaio, A. (2013). Is there evidence for cognitive intervention in Alzheimer disease? A systematic review of efficacy, feasibility, and cost-effectiveness. *Alzheimer Disease and Associated Disorders, 27*, 195–203. doi:10.1097/WAD.0b013e31827bda55

Alzheimer's Association. (2016). 2016 Alzheimer's disease facts and figures. *Alzheimer's and Dementia, 12*, 459–509. doi:10.1016/j.jalz.2016.03.001

American Psychiatric Association. (2013). *Diagnostic and statistical manual of mental disorders* (5th ed.). Arlington, VA: American Psychiatric Publishing.

Anstey, K., & Brodaty, H. (1995). Antidepressants and the elderly: Double-blind trials 1987–1992. *International Journal of Geriatric Psychiatry, 10*, 265–279. doi:10.1002/gps.930100403/abstract

Arai, H., Sumitomo, K., Sakata, Y., Daidoji, K., Takase, T., & Toyoda, T. (2016). Disease state changes and safety of long-term donepezil hydrochloride administration in patients with Alzheimer's disease: Interim results from the long-term, large-scale J-GOLD study in Japan. *Psychogeriatrics, 16*, 107–115. doi:10.1111/psyg.12130

Areán, P. A., Hegel, M., Vannoy, S., Fan, M. Y., & Unützer, J. (2008). Effectiveness of problem-solving therapy for older, primary care patients with depression: Results from the IMPACT project. *The Gerontologist, 48*, 311–323. doi:10.1093/geront/48.3.311

Areán, P. A., Perri, M. G., Nezu, A. M., Schein, R. L., Christopher, F., & Joseph, T. X. (1993). Comparative effectiveness of social problem-solving therapy and reminiscence therapy as treatments for depression in older adults. *Journal of Consulting and Clinical Psychology, 61*, 1003–1010. doi:10.1037/0022-006X.61.6.1003

Areán, P. A., Raue, P., Mackin, R. S., Kanellopoulos, D., McCulloch, C., & Alexopoulos, G. S. (2010). Problem-solving therapy and supportive therapy in older adults with major depression and executive dysfunction. *American Journal of Psychiatry, 167*, 1391–1398. doi:10.1176/appi.ajp.2010.09091327

Atri, A., Hendrix, S. B., Pejović, V., Hofbauer, R. K., Edwards, J., Molinuevo, J. L., & Graham, S. M. (2015). Cumulative, additive benefits of memantine-donepezil combination over component monotherapies in moderate to severe Alzheimer's dementia: A pooled area under the curve analysis. *Alzheimer's Research and Therapy, 7*, 28. doi:10.1186/s13195-015-0109-2

Bahar-Fuchs, A., Clare, L., & Woods, B. (2013). Cognitive training and cognitive rehabilitation for mild to moderate Alzheimer's disease and vascular dementia. *Cochrane Database Systematic Review*, CD003260. doi:10.1002/14651858.CD003260.pub2

Ballard, C., & Howard, R. (2006). Neuroleptic drugs in dementia: Benefits and harm. *Nature Review Neuroscience, 7*, 492–500. doi:10.1038/nrn1926

Banerjee, S., Hellier, J., Dewey, M., Romeo, R., Ballard, C., Baldwin, R., . . . & Katona, C. (2011). Sertraline or mirtazapine for depression in dementia (HTA-SADD): A randomised, multicentre, double-blind, placebo-controlled trial. *Lancet, 378*, 403–411. doi:10.1016/S0140-6736(11)60830-1

Barak, Y., Plopski, I., Tadger, S., & Paleacu, D. (2011). Escitalopram versus risperidone for the treatment of behavioral and psychotic symptoms associated with Alzheimer's disease: A randomized double-blind pilot study. *International Psychogeriatrics, 23*, 1515–1519. doi:10.1017/S1041610211000743

Bartels, S. J., Dums, A. R., Oxman, T. E., Schneider, L. S., Areán, P. A., Alexopoulos, G. S., & Jeste, D. V. (2003). Evidence-based practices in geriatric mental health care: An overview of systematic reviews and meta-analyses. *Psychiatric Clinics of North America, 26*, 971–990. doi:10.1016/S0193-953X(03)00072-8

Beck, C. K., Vogelpohl, T. S., Rasin, J. H., Uriri, J. T., O'Sullivan, P., Walls, R., . . . & Baldwin, B. (2002). Effects of behavioral interventions on disruptive behavior and affect in demented nursing home residents. *Nursing Research, 51*, 219–228. doi:10.1097/00006199-200207000-00002

Birks, J., & Craig, D. (2013). Galantamine for vascular cognitive impairment. *Cochrane Database Systematic Reviews*, CD004746. doi:10.1002/14651858.CD004746.pub2

Birks, J., & Harvey, R. J. (2006). Donepezil for dementia due to Alzheimer's disease. *Cochrane Database Systematic Reviews*, CD001190. doi:10.1002/14651858.CD001190.pub2

Birks, J., McGuinness, B., & Craig, D. (2013). Rivastigmine for vascular cognitive impairment. *Cochrane Database Systematic Reviews*, CD004744. doi:10.1002/14651858.CD004744.pub3

Birks, J. S., Chong, L. Y., & Grimley Evans, J. (2015). Rivastigmine for Alzheimer's disease. *Cochrane Database Systematic Reviews, 9*, CD001191. doi:10.1002/14651858.CD001191.pub4

Bombois, S., Derambure, P., Pasquier, F., & Monaca, C. (2010). Sleep disorders in aging and dementia. *Journal of Nutrition Health and Aging, 14*, 212–217. doi:10.1007/s12603-010-0052-7

Borroni, B., Agosti, C., & Padovani, A. (2008). Behavioral and psychological symptoms in dementia with Lewy-bodies (DLB): Frequency and relationship with disease severity and motor impairment. *Archives of Gerontology and Geriatrics, 46*, 101–106. doi:10.1016/j.archger.2007.03.003

Burns, A., Bernabei, R., Bullock, R., Jentoft, A. J. C., Frölich, L., Hock, C., . . . & Wimo, A. (2009). Safety and efficacy of galantamine (Reminyl) in severe Alzheimer's disease (the SERAD study): A randomised, placebo-controlled, double-blind trial. *Lancet Neurology, 8*, 39–47. doi:10.1016/S1474-4422(08)70261-8

Calati, R., Signorelli, M. S., Balestri, M., Marsano, A., De Ronchi, D., Aguglia, E., & Serretti, A. (2013). Antidepressants in elderly: Metaregression of double-blind, randomized clinical trials. *Journal of Affective Disorders, 147*, 1–8. doi:10.1016/j.jad.2012.11.053

Camberg, L., Woods, P., Ooi, W. L., Hurley, A., Volicer, L., Ashley, J., . . . & McIntyre, K. (1999). Evaluation of simulated presence: A personalized approach to enhance well-being in persons with Alzheimer's disease. *Journal of the American Geriatric Society, 47*, 446–452. doi:10.1111/j.1532-5415.1999.tb07237.x

Campbell, N., Ayub, A., Boustani, M. A., Fox, C., Farlow, M., Maidment, I., & Howard, R. (2008). Impact of cholinesterase inhibitors on behavioral and psychological symptoms of Alzheimer's disease: A meta-analysis. *Clinical Interventions in Aging, 3*, 719–728.

Carrasco, M. M., Agüera, L., Gil, P., Moríñigo, A., & Leon, T. (2011). Safety and effectiveness of donepezil on behavioral symptoms in patients with Alzheimer disease. *Alzheimer Disease and Associated Disorders, 25*, 333–340. doi:10.1097/WAD.0b013e318212ab7a

Chen, Y.-D., Zhang, J., Wang, Y., Yuan, J.-L., & Hu, W.-L. (2016). Efficacy of cholinesterase inhibitors in vascular dementia: An updated meta-analysis. *European Neurology, 75*, 132–141. doi:10.1159/000444253

Chung, J. C., Lai, C. K., Chung, P. M., & French, H. P. (2002). Snoezelen for dementia. *Cochrane Database Systematic Review,* CD003152. doi:10.1002/14651858.CD003152

Ciechanowski, P., Wagner, E., Schmaling, K., Schwartz, S., Williams, B., Diehr, P., . . . & LoGerfo, J. (2004). Community-integrated home-based depression treatment in older adults: A randomized controlled trial. *JAMA, 291*, 1569–1577. doi:10.1001/jama.291.13.1569

Cipriani, G., Lucetti, C., Nuti, A., & Danti, S. (2014). Wandering and dementia. *Psychogeriatrics, 14*, 135–142. doi:10.1111/psyg.12044

Cipriani, G., Vedovello, M., Ulivi, M., Nuti, A., & Lucetti, C. (2013). Repetitive and stereotypic phenomena and dementia. *American Journal of Alzheimer's Disease and Other Dementias, 28*, 223–227. doi:10.1177/1533317513481094

Clare, L., Linden, D. E. J., Woods, R. T., Whitaker, R., Evans, S. J., Parkinson, C. H., . . . &Yuen, K. S. L. (2010). Goal-oriented cognitive rehabilitation for people with early-stage Alzheimer disease: A single-blind randomized controlled trial of clinical efficacy. *American Journal of Geriatric Psychiatry, 18*, 928–939. doi:10.1097/JGP.0b013e3181d5792a

Cohen-Mansfield, J. (2001). Nonpharmacologic interventions for inappropriate behaviors in dementia: A review, summary, and critique. *American Journal of Geriatric Psychiatry, 9*, 361–381. doi:10.1097/00019442-200111000-00005

Cooper, C., Katona, C., Lyketsos, K., Blazer, D., Brodaty, H., Rabins, P., . . . & Livingston, G. (2011). A systematic review of treatments for refractory depression in older people. *American Journal of Psychiatry,* doi:10.1176/appi.ajp.2011.10081165

Courtney, C., Farrell, D., Gray, R., Hills, R., Lynch, L., Sellwood, E., . . . & AD2000, C. G. (2004). Long-term donepezil treatment in 565 patients with Alzheimer's disease (AD2000): Randomised double-blind trial. *Lancet, 363*, 2105–2115. doi:10.1016/S0140 6736(04)16499-4

Cuijpers, P., van Straten, A., & Smit, F. (2006). Psychological treatment of late-life depression: A meta-analysis of randomized controlled trials. *International Journal of Geriatric Psychiatry, 21*, 1139–1149. doi:10.1002/gps.1620/abstract

Culang, M. E., Sneed, J. R., Keilp, J. G., Rutherford, B. R., Pelton, G. H., Devanand, D. P., & Roose, S. P. (2009). Change in cognitive functioning following acute antidepressant treatment in late-life depression. *American Journal of Geriatric Psychiatry, 17*, 881–888. doi:10.1097/JGP.0b013e3181b4bf4a

Cummings, J., Lai, T.-J., Hemrungrojn, S., Mohandas, E., Yun Kim, S., Nair, G., & Dash, A. (2016). Role of donepezil in the management of neuropsychiatric symptoms in Alzheimer's disease and dementia with Lewy Bodies. *CNS Neuroscience Therapeutics, 22*, 159–166. doi:10.1111/cns.12484 de Vasconcelos Cunha, U. G., Lopes Rocha, F., Ávila de Melo, R., Alves Valle, E., de Souza Neto, J. J., Mendes Brega, R., . . . & da Costa Júnior, A. L. (2007). A placebo-controlled double-blind randomized study of venlafaxine in the treatment of depression in dementia. *Dementia and Geriatric Cognition Disorders, 24*, 36–41. doi:10.1159/000102570

Djernes, J. K. (2006). Prevalence and predictors of depression in populations of elderly: A review. *Acta Psychiatrica Scandinavica, 113*, 372–387. doi:10.1111/j.1600-0447.2006.00770.x

Doody, R. S., Geldmacher, D. S., Farlow, M. R., Sun, Y., Moline, M., & Mackell, J. (2012). Efficacy and safety of donepezil 23 mg versus donepezil 10 mg for moderate-to-severe Alzheimer's disease: A subgroup analysis in patients already taking or not taking concomitant memantine. *Dementia and Geriatric Cognitive Disorders, 33*, 164–173. doi:10.1159/000338236

Douglas, S., James, I., & Ballard, C. (2004). Non-pharmacological interventions in dementia. *Advances in Psychiatric Treatment, 10*, 171–177. doi:10.1192/apt.10.3.171

Farlow, M. R., Grossberg, G. T., Sadowsky, C. H., Meng, X., & Somogyi, M. (2013). A 24-week, randomized, controlled trial of rivastigmine patch 13.3 mg/24 h versus 4.6 mg/24 h in severe Alzheimer's dementia. *CNS Neuroscience Therapy, 19*, 745–752. doi:10.1111/cns.12158

Farlow, M. R., Salloway, S., Tariot, P. N., Yardley, J., Moline, M. L., Wang, Q., . . . & Satlin, A. (2010). Effectiveness and tolerability of high-dose (23 mg/d) versus standard-dose (10 mg/d) donepezil in moderate to severe Alzheimer's disease: A 24-week, randomized, double-blind study. *Clinical Therapy, 32*, 1234–1251. doi:10.1016/j.clinthera.2010.06.019

Fiske, A., Wetherell, J. L., & Gatz, M. (2009). Depression in older adults. *Annual Review of Clinical Psychology, 5*, 363–389. doi:10.1146/annurev.clinpsy.032408.153621

Folstein, M. F., Folstein, S. E., & McHugh, P. R. (1975). "Mini-mental state": A practical method for grading the cognitive state of patients for the clinician. *Journal of Psychiatric Research, 12*, 189–198.

Forrester, L. T., Maayan, N., Orrell, M., Spector, A. E., Buchan, L. D., & Soares-Weiser, K. (2014). Aromatherapy for dementia. *Cochrane Database Systematic Review*, CD003150 . doi:10.1002/14651858.CD003150.pub2

Francis, J. L., & Kumar, A. (2013). Psychological treatment of late-life depression. *Psychiatric Clinics of North America, 36*, 561–575. doi:10.1016/j.psc.2013.08.005

Gauthier, S., Wirth, Y., & Möbius, H. J. (2005). Effects of memantine on behavioural symptoms in Alzheimer's disease patients: An analysis of the Neuropsychiatric Inventory (NPI) data of two randomised, controlled studies. *International Journal of Geriatric Psychiatry, 20*, 459–464. doi:10.1002/gps.1341

Gerson, S., Belin, T. R., Kaufman, A., Mintz, J., & Jarvik, L. (1999). Pharmacological and psychological treatments for depressed older patients: A meta-analysis and overview of recent findings. *Harvard Review of Psychiatry, 7*, 1–28. doi:10.3109/hrp.7.1.1

Gerson, S. C., Plotkin, D. A., & Jarvik, L. F. (1988). Antidepressant drug studies, 1964 to 1986: Empirical evidence for aging patients. *Journal of Clinical Psychopharmacology, 8*, 311–322. doi:10.1097/00004714-198810000-00002

Gildengers, A. G., Houck, P. R., Mulsant, B. H., Pollock, B. G., Mazumdar, S., Miller, M. D., . . . & Reynolds, C. F. (2002). Course and rate of antidepressant response in the very old. *Journal of Affective Disorders, 69*, 177–184. doi:10.1016/S0165-0327(01)00334-2

Grossberg, G. T., Manes, F., Allegri, R. F., Gutiérrez-Robledo, L. M., Gloger, S., Xie, L., . . . & Perhach, J. L. (2013). The safety, tolerability, and efficacy of once-daily memantine (28 mg): A multinational, randomized, double-blind, placebo-controlled trial in patients with moderate-to-severe Alzheimer's disease taking cholinesterase inhibitors. *CNS Drugs, 27*, 469–478. doi:10.1007/s40263-013-0077-7

Hao, Z., Liu, M., Liu, Z., & Lu, D. (2009). Huperzine A for vascular dementia. *Cochrane Database Systematic Review*, CD007365. doi:10.1002/14651858.CD007365.pub2

Hebert, L. E., Weuve, J., Scherr, P. A., & Evans, D. A. (2013). Alzheimer disease in the United States (2010–2050) estimated using the 2010 census. *Neurology, 80*, 1778–1783. doi:10.1212/WNL.0b013e31828726f5

Hogan, D. B. (2014). Long-term efficacy and toxicity of cholinesterase inhibitors in the treatment of Alzheimer disease. *Canadian Journal of Psychiatry, 59*, 618–623.

Howard, R., McShane, R., Lindesay, J., Ritchie, C., Baldwin, A., Barber, R., . . . & Holmes, C. (2012). Donepezil and memantine for moderate-to-severe Alzheimer's disease. *New England Journal of Medicine, 366*, 893–903. doi:10.1056/NEJMoa1106668

Howard, R. J., Juszczak, E., Ballard, C. G., Bentham, P., Brown, R. G., Bullock, R., . . . & Johnson, T. (2007). Donepezil for the treatment of agitation in Alzheimer's disease. *New England Journal of Medicine, 357*, 1382–1392. doi:10.1056/NEJMoa066583

Huang, A. X., Delucchi, K., Dunn, L. B., & Nelson, J. C. (2015). A systematic review and meta-analysis of psychotherapy for late-life depression. *American Journal of Geriatric Psychiatry, 23*, 261–273. doi:10.1016/j.jagp.2014.04.003

Hugo, J., & Ganguli, M. (2014). Dementia and cognitive impairment: Epidemiology, diagnosis, and treatment. *Clinical Geriatric Medicine, 30*, 421–442. doi:10.1016/j.cger.2014.04.001

Hwang, T.-Y., Ahn, I.-S., Kim, S., & Kim, D. K. (2016). Efficacy of galantamine on cognition in mild-to-moderate Alzheimer's dementia after failure to respond to donepezil. *Psychiatry Investigation, 13*, 341–348. doi:10.4306/pi.2016.13.3.341

Ikeda, M., Mori, E., Matsuo, K., Nakagawa, M., & Kosaka, K. (2015). Donepezil for dementia with Lewy bodies: A randomized, placebo-controlled, confirmatory phase III trial. *Alzheimer's Research and Therapy, 7*, 4. doi:10.1186/s13195-014-0083-0

Institute of Medicine (2012). *The mental health and substance use workforce for older adults: In whose hands?* (Institute of Medicine ed.). Washington, DC: The National Academies Press. doi:10.17226/13400

Kales, H. C., Gitlin, L. N., & Lyketsos, C. G. (2015). Assessment and management of behavioral and psychological symptoms of dementia. *BMJ, 350*, h369. doi:10.1136/bmj.h369

Kaneriya, S. H., Robbins-Welty, G. A., Smagula, S. F., Karp, J. F., Butters, M. A., Lenze, E. J., . . . & Dew, M. A. (2016). Predictors and moderators of remission with aripiprazole augmentation in treatment-resistant late-life depression: An analysis of the IRL-GRey randomized clinical trial. *JAMA Psychiatry*, doi:10.1001/jamapsychiatry.2015.3447

Katona, C., & Livingston, G. (2002). How well do antidepressants work in older people? A systematic review of number needed to treat. *Journal of Affective Disorders, 69*, 47–52. doi:10.1016/S0165-0327(00)00332-3

Katona, C. L. E., Hunter, B. N., & Bray, J. (1998). A double-blind comparison of the efficacy and safety of paroxetine and imipramine in the treatment of depression with dementia. *International Journal of Geriatric Psychiatry, 13*, 100–108. doi:10.1002/(SICI)1099–1166(199802)13:2%3C100::AID-GPS738%3E3.0.CO;2-J/abstract

Katz, I., de Deyn, P.-P., Mintzer, J., Greenspan, A., Zhu, Y., & Brodaty, H. (2007). The efficacy and safety of risperidone in the treatment of psychosis of Alzheimer's disease and mixed dementia: A meta-analysis of 4 placebo-controlled clinical trials. *International Journal of Geriatric Psychiatry, 22*, 475–484. doi:10.1002/gps.1792

Katz, M. J., Lipton, R. B., Hall, C. B., Zimmerman, M. E., Sanders, A. E., Verghese, J., . . . & Derby, C. A. (2012). Age-specific and sex-specific prevalence and incidence of mild cognitive impairment, dementia, and Alzheimer dementia in blacks and whites: A report from the Einstein Aging Study. *Alzheimer Disease and Associated Disorders, 26*, 335–343. doi:10.1097/WAD.0b013e31823dbcfc

Kok, R. M. (2013). What is the role of medications in late life depression? *Psychiatric Clinics of North America, 36*, 597–605. doi:10.1016/j.psc.2013.08.006

Kok, R. M., Nolen, W. A., & Heeren, T. J. (2012). Efficacy of treatment in older depressed patients: a systematic review and meta-analysis of double-blind randomized controlled trials with antidepressants. *Journal of Affective Disorders, 141*, 103–115. doi:10.1016/j.jad.2012.02.036

Kolanowski, A. M., Litaker, M., & Buettner, L. (2005). Efficacy of theory-based activities for behavioral symptoms of dementia. *Nursing Research, 54*, 219–228. doi:10.1097/00006199-200507000-00003

Konovalov, S., Muralee, S., & Tampi, R. R. (2008). Anticonvulsants for the treatment of behavioral and psychological symptoms of dementia: A literature review. *International Psychogeriatrics, 20*, 293–308. doi:10.1017/S1041610207006540

Krishnan, K. R., Hays, J. C., & Blazer, D. G. (1997). MRI-defined vascular depression. *American Journal of Psychiatry, 154*, 497–501. doi:10.1176/ajp.154.4.497

Kverno, K. S., Black, B. S., Nolan, M. T., & Rabins, P. V. (2009). Research on treating neuropsychiatric symptoms of advanced dementia with non-pharmacological strategies, 1998–2008: A systematic literature review. *International Psychogeriatrics, 21*, 825–843. doi:10.1017/S1041610209990196

Lai, M. K. P., Tsang, S. W. Y., Francis, P. T., Esiri, M. M., Keene, J., Hope, T., & Chen, C. P. L.-H. (2003). Reduced serotonin 5-HT 1A receptor binding in the temporal cortex correlates with aggressive behavior in Alzheimer disease. *Brain Research, 974*, 82–87. doi:10.1016/S0006–8993(03)02554-X

Laidlaw, K., Davidson, K., Toner, H., Jackson, G., Clark, S., Law, J., . . . & Cross, S. (2008). A randomised controlled trial of cognitive behaviour therapy vs treatment as usual in the treatment of mild to moderate late life depression. *International Journal of Geriatric Psychiatry, 23*, 843–850. doi:10.1002/gps.1993

Lenze, E. J., Mulsant, B. H., Blumberger, D. M., Karp, J. F., Newcomer, J. W., Anderson, S. J., . . . & Reynolds, C. F. (2015). Efficacy, safety, and tolerability of augmentation pharmacotherapy with aripiprazole for treatment-resistant depression in late life: A randomised, double-blind, placebo-controlled trial. *Lancet, 386*, 2404–2412. doi:10.1016/S0140-6736(15)00308-6

Leonpacher, A. K., Peters, M. E., Drye, L. T., Makino, K. M., Newell, J. A., Devanand, D. P., . . . & Pollock, B. G. (2016). Effects of citalopram on neuropsychiatric symptoms in Alzheimer's dementia: Evidence from the CitAD study. *American Journal of Psychiatry, 173*, 473–480. doi:10.1176/appi.ajp.2016.15020248

Liu, X., Zhang, J., Sun, D., Fan, Y., Zhou, H., & Fu, B. (2014). Effects of fluoxetine on brain-derived neurotrophic factor serum concentration and cognition in patients with vascular dementia. *Clinical Interventions in Aging, 9*, 411–418. doi:10.2147/CIA.S58830

Livingston, G., Johnston, K., Katona, C., Paton, J., & Lyketsos, C. G. (2005). Systematic review of psychological approaches to the management of neuropsychiatric symptoms of dementia. *American Journal of Psychiatry, 162,* 1996–2021. doi:10.1176/appi.ajp.162.11.1996

Locher, C., Kossowsky, J., Gaab, J., Kirsch, I., Bain, P., & Krummenacher, P. (2015). Moderation of antidepressant and placebo outcomes by baseline severity in late-life depression: A systematic review and meta-analysis. *Journal of Affective Disorders, 181,* 50–60. doi:10.1016/j.jad.2015.03.062

Loewenstein, D. A., Acevedo, A., Czaja, S. J., & Duara, R. (2004). Cognitive rehabilitation of mildly impaired Alzheimer disease patients on cholinesterase inhibitors. *American Journal of Geriatric Psychiatry, 12,* 395–402. doi:10.1176/appi.ajgp.12.4.395

Lonergan, E., Luxenberg, J., Colford, J., & Birks, J. (2002). Haloperidol for agitation in dementia. *Cochrane Database Systematic Review,* CD002852. doi:10.1002/14651858.CD002852

Lopez, O. L., Becker, J. T., Chang, Y.-F., Sweet, R. A., Aizenstein, H., Snitz, B., . . . & DeKosky, S. T. (2013). The long-term effects of conventional and atypical antipsychotics in patients with probable Alzheimer's disease. *American Journal of Psychiatry, 170,* 1051–1058. doi:10.1176/appi.ajp.2013.12081046

Loy, C., & Schneider, L. (2006). Galantamine for Alzheimer's disease and mild cognitive impairment. *Cochrane Database Systematic Review,* CD001747. doi:10.1002/14651858.CD001747.pub3

Lyketsos, C. G., DelCampo, L., Steinberg, M., Miles, Q., Steele, C. D., Munro, C., . . . & Brandt, J. (2003). Treating depression in Alzheimer disease: Efficacy and safety of sertraline therapy, and the benefits of depression reduction: the DIADS. *Archives of General Psychiatry, 60,* 737–746. doi:10.1001/archpsyc.60.7.737

Lyketsos, C. G., Sheppard, J.-M. E., Steele, C. D., Kopunek, S., Steinberg, M., Baker, A. S., . . . & Rabins, P. V. (2000). Randomized, placebo-controlled, double-blind clinical trial of sertraline in the treatment of depression complicating Alzheimer's disease: Initial results from the Depression in Alzheimer's Disease study. *American Journal of Psychiatry, 157,* 1686–1689. doi:10.1176/appi.ajp.157.10.1686

Magai, C., Kennedy, G., Cohen, C. I., & Gomberg, D. (2001). A controlled clinical trial of sertraline in the treatment of depression in nursing home patients with late-stage Alzheimer's disease. *American Journal of Geriatric Psychiatry, 8,* 66–74. doi:10.1097/00019442-200002000-00009

Malouf, R., & Birks, J. (2004). Donepezil for vascular cognitive impairment. *Cochrane Database Systematic Review,* CD004395. doi:10.1002/14651858.CD004395.pub2

McKeith, I., Del Ser, T., Spano, P., Emre, M., Wesnes, K., Anand, R., . . . & Spiegel, R. (2000). Efficacy of rivastigmine in dementia with Lewy bodies: A randomised, double-blind, placebo-controlled international study. *Lancet, 356,* 2031–2036. doi:10.1016/S0140-6736(00)03399-7

McKeith, I. G., Dickson, D. W., Lowe, J., Emre, M., O'Brien, J. T., Feldman, H., . . . & Perry, E. K. (2005). Diagnosis and management of dementia with Lewy bodies third report of the DLB consortium. *Neurology, 65,* 1863–1872. doi:10.1212/01.wnl.0000187889.17253.b1

McShane, R., Areosa Sastre, A., & Minakaran, N. (2006). Memantine for dementia. *Cochrane Database Systematic Review,* CD003154. doi:10.1002/14651858.CD003154.pub5

Mittmann, N., Herrmann, N., Einarson, T. R., Busto, U. E., Lanctôt, K. L., Liu, B. A., . . . & Shear, N. H. (1997). The efficacy, safety and tolerability of antidepressants in late life depression: A meta-analysis. *Journal of Affective Disorders, 46*, 191–217. doi:10.1016/S0165-0327(97)00107-9

Mori, E., Ikeda, M., & Kosaka, K. (2012). Donepezil for dementia with Lewy bodies: A randomized, placebo-controlled trial. *Annals of Neurology, 72*, 41–52. doi:10.1002/ana.23557

Mori, E., Ikeda, M., Nagai, R., Matsuo, K., Nakagawa, M., & Kosaka, K. (2015). Long-term donepezil use for dementia with Lewy bodies: Results from an open-label extension of Phase III trial. *Alzheimer's Research and Therapy, 7*, 5. doi:10.1186/s13195-014-0081-2

Murgatroyd, C., & Prettyman, R. (2001). An investigation of visual hallucinosis and visual sensory status in dementia. *International Journal of Geriatric Psychiatry, 16*, 709–713. doi:10.1002/gps.426

Nelson, J. C., Delucchi, K., & Schneider, L. S. (2008). Efficacy of second generation antidepressants in late-life depression: A meta-analysis of the evidence. *American Journal of Geriatric Psychiatry, 16*, 558–567. doi:10.1097/01.JGP.0000308883.64832.ed

Nelson, J. C., Delucchi, K. L., & Schneider, L. S. (2013). Moderators of outcome in late-life depression: A patient-level meta-analysis. *American Journal of Psychiatry, 170*, 651–659. doi:10.1176/appi.ajp.2012.12070927

Nelson, J. C., & Devanand, D. P. (2011). A systematic review and meta-analysis of placebo-controlled antidepressant studies in people with depression and dementia. *Journal of the American Geriatric Society, 59*, 577–585. doi:10.1111/j.1532-5415.2011.03355.x

Nyth, A. L., & Gottfries, C. G. (1990). The clinical efficacy of citalopram in treatment of emotional disturbances in dementia disorders: A Nordic multicentre study. *British Journal of Psychiatry, 157*, 894–901. doi:10.1192/bjp.157.6.894

Nyth, A. L., Gottfries, C. G., Lyby, K., Smedegaard-Andersen, L., Gylding-Sabroe, J., Kristensen, M., . . . & Syversen, S. (1992). A controlled multicenter clinical study of citalopram and placebo in elderly depressed patients with and without concomitant dementia. *Acta Psychiatrica Scandinavica, 86*, 138–145. doi:10.1111/j.1600–0447.1992.tb03242.x/abstract

O'Connor, D. W., Ames, D., Gardner, B., & King, M. (2009). Psychosocial treatments of psychological symptoms in dementia: A systematic review of reports meeting quality standards. *International Psychogeriatrics, 21*, 241–251. doi:10.1017/S1041610208008223

O'Neil, M. E., Freeman, M., Christensen, V., Telerant, R., Addleman, A., & Kansagara, D. (2011). *A systematic evidence review of non-pharmacological interventions for behavioral symptoms of dementia* (VA-ESP Project #05–225). Department of Veterans Affairs Washington, DC. Retrieved from http://www.hsrd.research.va.gov/publications/esp/Dementia-Nonpharm.pdf

Olazarán, J., Muñiz, R., Reisberg, B., Peña-Casanova, J., del Ser, T., Cruz-Jentoft, A. J., . . . & Sevilla, C. (2004). Benefits of cognitive-motor intervention in MCI and mild to moderate Alzheimer disease. *Neurology, 63*, 2348–2353. doi:10.1212/01.WNL.0000147478.03911.28

Olazarán, J., Reisberg, B., Clare, L., Cruz, I., Peña-Casanova, J., Del Ser, T., . . . & Muñiz, R. (2010). Nonpharmacological therapies in Alzheimer's disease: A systematic review of efficacy. *Dementia and Geriatric Cognitive Disorders, 30*, 161–178. doi:10.1159/000316119

Olin, J. T., Schneider, L. S., Katz, I. R., Meyers, B. S., Alexopoulos, G. S., Breitner, J. C., . . . & Devanand, D. P. (2002). Provisional diagnostic criteria for depression of Alzheimer Disease. *American Journal of Geriatric Psychiatry, 10*, 125–128. doi:10.1097/00019442-200203000-00003

Orgeta, V., Qazi, A., Spector, A., & Orrell, M. (2015). Psychological treatments for depression and anxiety in dementia and mild cognitive impairment: Systematic review and meta-analysis. *British Journal of Psychiatry, 207*, 293–298. doi:10.1192/bjp.bp.114.148130

Paleacu, D., Mazeh, D., Mirecki, I., Even, M., & Barak, Y. (2002). Donepezil for the treatment of behavioral symptoms in patients with Alzheimer's disease. *Clinical Neuropharmacology, 25*, 313–317. doi:10.1097/00002826-200211000-00007

Paulsen, J. S., Salmon, D. P., Thal, L. J., Romero, R., Weisstein-Jenkins, C., Galasko, D., . . . & Jeste, D. V. (2000). Incidence of and risk factors for hallucinations and delusions in patients with probable AD. *Neurology, 54*, 1965–1971. doi:10.1212/WNL.54.10.1965

Petracca, G., Tesón, A., Chemerinski, E., Leiguarda, R., & Starkstein, S. E. (1995). A double-blind placebo-controlled study of clomipramine in depressed patients with Alzheimer's disease. *Journal of Neuropsychiatry and Clinical Neuroscience, 8*, 270–275.

Petracca, G. M., Chemerinski, E., & Starkstein, S. E. (2001). A double-blind, placebo-controlled study of fluoxetine in depressed patients with Alzheimer's disease. *International Psychogeriatrics, 13*, 233–240. doi:10.1017/S104161020100761X

Pimontel, M. A., Culang-Reinlieb, M. E., Morimoto, S. S., & Sneed, J. R. (2012). Executive dysfunction and treatment response in late-life depression. *International Journal of Geriatric Psychiatry, 27*, 893–899. doi:10.1002/gps.2808

Pinquart, M., Duberstein, P. R., & Lyness, J. M. (2007). Effects of psychotherapy and other behavioral interventions on clinically depressed older adults: A meta-analysis. *Aging and Mental Health, 11*, 645–657. doi:10.1080/13607860701529635

Plassman, B. L., Langa, K. M., Fisher, G. G., Heeringa, S. G., Weir, D. R., Ofstedal, M. B., . . . & Rodgers, W. L. (2007). Prevalence of dementia in the United States: The aging, demographics, and memory study. *Neuroepidemiology, 29*, 125–132. doi:10.1159/000109998

Porsteinsson, A. P., Drye, L. T., Pollock, B. G., Devanand, D. P., Frangakis, C., Ismail, Z., . . . & Munro, C. A. (2014). Effect of citalopram on agitation in Alzheimer disease: the CitAD randomized clinical trial. *JAMA, 311*, 682–691. doi:10.1001/jama.2014.93

Prince, M., Bryce, R., Albanese, E., Wimo, A., Ribeiro, W., & Ferri, C. P. (2013). The global prevalence of dementia: A systematic review and metaanalysis. *Alzheimer's and Dementia, 9*, 63–75. doi:10.1016/j.jalz.2012.11.007

Raivio, M. M., Laurila, J. V., Strandberg, T. E., Tilvis, R. S., & Pitkälä, K. H. (2007). Neither atypical nor conventional antipsychotics increase mortality or hospital admissions among elderly patients with dementia: A two-year prospective study. *American Journal of Geriatric Psychiatry, 15*, 416–424. doi:10.1097/JGP.0b013e31802d0b00

Rands, G., & Orrell, M. (2000). Aspirin for vascular dementia. *Cochrane Database Systematic Review*, CD001296. doi:10.1002/14651858.CD001296

Raskind, M. A., & Wang, L. Y. (2014). Antipsychotic drugs for psychosis and agitation in dementia: efficacy, safety, and a possible noradrenergic mechanism of action. *International Psychogeriatrics, 26*, 879–883. doi:10.1017/S1041610214000477

Ravona-Springer, R., & Davidson, M. (2014). Considerations in psychotropic treatments in dementia—can polypharmacy be avoided? *International Journal of Neuropsychopharmacology, 17*, 1107–1117. doi:10.1017/S1461145713000412

Reifler, B. V., Teri, L., Raskind, M., Veith, R., Barnes, R., White, E., & McLean, P. (1989). Double-blind trial of imipramine in Alzheimer's disease patients with and without depression. *American Journal of Psychiatry, 146*, 45–49. doi:10.1176/ajp.146.1.45

Requena, C., Maestú, F., Campo, P., Fernández, A., & Ortiz, T. (2006). Effects of cholinergic drugs and cognitive training on dementia: 2-year follow-up. *Dementia and Geriatric Cognition Disorders, 22*, 339–345. doi:10.1159/000095600

Reynolds III, C. F., Butters, M. A., Lopez, O., Pollock, B. G., Dew, M. A., Mulsant, B. H., . . . & Mazumdar, S. (2011). Maintenance treatment of depression in old age: A randomized, double-blind, placebo-controlled evaluation of the efficacy and safety of donepezil combined with antidepressant pharmacotherapy. *Archives of General Psychiatry, 68*, 51–60. doi:10.1001/archgenpsychiatry.2010.184

Reynolds III, C. F., Dew, M. A., Pollock, B. G., Mulsant, B. H., Frank, E., Miller, M. D., . . . & Stack, J. A. (2006). Maintenance treatment of major depression in old age. *New England Journal of Medicine, 354*, 1130–1138. doi:10.1056/NEJMoa052619

Rogers, S. L., Doody, R. S., Pratt, R. D., & Ieni, J. R. (2000). Long-term efficacy and safety of donepezil in the treatment of Alzheimer's disease: Final analysis of a US multicentre open-label study. *European Neuropsychopharmacology, 10*, 195–203. doi:10.1016/S0924-977X(00)00067-5

Rolinski, M., Fox, C., Maidment, I., & McShane, R. (2012). Cholinesterase inhibitors for dementia with Lewy bodies, Parkinson's disease dementia and cognitive impairment in Parkinson's disease. *Cochrane Database Systematic Review*, CD006504. doi:10.1002/14651858.CD006504.pub2

Roose, S. P., & Schatzberg, A. F. (2005). The efficacy of antidepressants in the treatment of late-life depression. *Journal of Clinical Psychopharmacology, 25*, S1–S7. doi:10.1097/01.jcp.0000162807.84570.6b

Ropacki, S. A., & Jeste, D. V. (2005). Epidemiology of and risk factors for psychosis of Alzheimer's disease: A review of 55 studies published from 1990 to 2003. *American Journal of Psychiatry, 162*, 2022–2030. doi:10.1176/appi.ajp.162.11.2022

Rosenberg, P. B., Drye, L. T., Martin, B. K., Frangakis, C., Mintzer, J. E., Weintraub, D., . . . & Lyketsos, C. G. (2010). Sertraline for the treatment of depression in Alzheimer disease. *American Journal of Geriatric Psychiatry, 18*, 136–145. doi:10.1097/JGP.0b013e3181c796eb

Rosenberg, P. B., Nowrangi, M. A., & Lyketsos, C. G. (2015). Neuropsychiatric symptoms in Alzheimer's disease: What might be associated brain circuits? *Molecular Aspects of Medicine, 43–44*, 25–37. doi:10.1016/j.mam.2015.05.005

Rosness, T. A., Barca, M. L., & Engedal, K. (2010). Occurrence of depression and its correlates in early onset dementia patients. *International Journal of Geriatric Psychiatry, 25*, 704–711. doi:10.1002/gps.2411

Roth, M., Mountjoy, C. Q., & Amrein, R. (1996). Moclobemide in elderly patients with cognitive decline and depression: An international double-blind, placebo-controlled trial. *British Journal of Psychiatry, 168*, 149–157. doi:10.1192/bjp.168.2.149

Salzman, C., Wong, E., & Wright, B. C. (2002). Drug and ECT treatment of depression in the elderly, 1996–2001: A literature review. *Biological Psychiatry, 52*, 265–284. doi:10.1016/S0006-3223(02)01337-9

Scarpini, E., Bruno, G., Zappalà, G., Adami, M., Richarz, U., Gaudig, M., . . . & Schäuble, B. (2011). Cessation versus continuation of galantamine treatment after 12 months of therapy in patients with Alzheimer's disease: A randomized, double blind, placebo controlled withdrawal trial. *Journal of Alzheimer's Disease, 26*, 211–220. doi:10.3233/JAD-2011-110134

Schneider, J. A., Arvanitakis, Z., Bang, W., & Bennett, D. A. (2007). Mixed brain pathologies account for most dementia cases in community-dwelling older persons. *Neurology, 69*, 2197–2204. doi:10.1212/01.wnl.0000271090.28148.24

Schneider, L. S., Dagerman, K., & Insel, P. S. (2006a). Efficacy and adverse effects of atypical antipsychotics for dementia: Meta-analysis of randomized, placebo-controlled trials. *American Journal of Geriatric Psychiatry, 14*, 191–210. doi:10.1097/01.JGP.0000200589.01396.6d

Schneider, L. S., Dagerman, K. S., & Insel, P. (2005). Risk of death with atypical antipsychotic drug treatment for dementia: meta-analysis of randomized placebo-controlled trials. *JAMA, 294*, 1934–1943. doi:10.1001/jama.294.15.1934

Schneider, L. S., Tariot, P. N., Dagerman, K. S., Davis, S. M., Hsiao, J. K., Ismail, M. S., . . . & Stroup, T. S. (2006b). Effectiveness of atypical antipsychotic drugs in patients with Alzheimer's disease. *New England Journal of Medicine, 355*, 1525–1538.

Scogin, F., Welsh, D., Hanson, A., Stump, J., & Coates, A. (2005). Evidence based psychotherapies for depression in older adults. *Clinical Psychology Science and Practice, 12*, 222–237. doi:10.1093/clipsy.bpi033

Seitz, D. P., Adunuri, N., Gill, S. S., Gruneir, A., Herrmann, N., & Rochon, P. (2011). Antidepressants for agitation and psychosis in dementia. *Cochrane Database Systematic Review*, CD008191. doi:10.1002/14651858.CD008191.pub2

Serfaty, M. A., Haworth, D., Blanchard, M., Buszewicz, M., Murad, S., & King, M. (2009). Clinical effectiveness of individual cognitive behavioral therapy for depressed older people in primary care: A randomized controlled trial. *Archives of General Psychiatry, 66*, 1332–1340. doi:10.1001/archgenpsychiatry.2009.165

Sink, K. M., Holden, K. F., & Yaffe, K. (2005). Pharmacological treatment of neuropsychiatric symptoms of dementia: A review of the evidence. *JAMA, 293*, 596–608. doi:10.1001/jama.293.5.596

Sitzer, D. I., Twamley, E. W., & Jeste, D. V. (2006). Cognitive training in Alzheimer's disease: A meta-analysis of the literature. *Acta Psychiatrica Scandinavica, 114*, 75–90. doi:10.1111/j.1600-0447.2006.00789.x

Sneed, J. R., Culang, M. E., Keilp, J. G., Rutherford, B. R., Devanand, D. P., & Roose, S. P. (2010). Antidepressant medication and executive dysfunction: A deleterious interaction in late-life depression. *American Journal of Geriatric Psychiatry, 18*, 128–135. doi:10.1097/JGP.0b013e3181c796d2

Sneed, J. R., Rutherford, B. R., Rindskopf, D., Lane, D. T., Sackeim, H. A., & Roose, S. P. (2008). Design makes a difference: A meta-analysis of antidepressant response rates in placebo-controlled versus comparator trials in late-life depression. *American Journal of Geriatric Psychiatry, 16*, 65–73. doi:10.1097/JGP.0b013e3181256b1d

Spector, A., Davies, S., Woods, B., & Orrell, M. (2000). Reality orientation for dementia: A systematic review of the evidence of effectiveness from randomized controlled trials. *Gerontologist, 40*, 206–212. doi:10.1093/geront/40.2.206

Spector, A., Thorgrimsen, L., Woods, B., Royan, L., Davies, S., Butterworth, M., & Orrell, M. (2003). Efficacy of an evidence-based cognitive stimulation therapy programme for people with dementia: Randomised controlled trial. *British Journal of Psychiatry, 183*, 248–254. doi:10.1192/bjp.183.3.248

Steinberg, M., Shao, H., Zandi, P., Lyketsos, C. G., Welsh-Bohmer, K. A., Norton, M. C., . . . & Investigators, C. C. (2008). Point and 5-year period prevalence of neuropsychiatric symptoms in dementia: The Cache County Study. *International Journal of Geriatric Psychiatry, 23*, 170–177. doi:10.1002/gps.1858

Strachowski, D., Khaylis, A., Conrad, A., Neri, E., Spiegel, D., & Taylor, C. B. (2008). The effects of cognitive behavior therapy on depression in older patients with cardiovascular risk. *Depression and Anxiety, 25*, E1–E10. doi:10.1002/da.20302/abstract

Sultzer, D. L., Davis, S. M., Tariot, P. N., Dagerman, K. S., Lebowitz, B. D., Lyketsos, C. G., . . . & Schneider, L. S. (2008). Clinical symptom responses to atypical antipsychotic medications in Alzheimer's disease: Phase 1 outcomes from the CATIE-AD effectiveness trial. *American Journal of Psychiatry, 165*, 844–854. doi:10.1176/appi.ajp.2008.07111779

Tan, L., Tan, L., Wang, H.-F., Wang, J., Tan, C.-C., Tan, M.-S., . . . & Yu, J.-T. (2015). Efficacy and safety of atypical antipsychotic drug treatment for dementia: A systematic review and meta-analysis. *Alzheimer's Research and Therapy, 7*, 20. doi:10.1186/s13195-015-0102-9

Taragano, F. E., Lyketsos, C. G., Mangone, C. A., Allegri, R. F., & Comesaña-Diaz, E. (1997). A double-blind, randomized, fixed-dose trial of fluoxetine vs. amitriptyline in the treatment of major depression complicating Alzheimer's disease. *Psychosomatics, 38*, 246–252. doi:10.1016/S0033-3182(97)71461-0

Tárraga, L., Boada, M., Modinos, G., Espinosa, A., Diego, S., Morera, A., . . . & Becker, J. T. (2006). A randomised pilot study to assess the efficacy of an interactive, multimedia tool of cognitive stimulation in Alzheimer's disease. *Journal of Neurology Neurosurgery Psychiatry, 77*, 1116–1121. doi:10.1136/jnnp.2005.086074

Taylor, W. D., & Doraiswamy, P. M. (2004). A systematic review of antidepressant placebo-controlled trials for geriatric depression: Limitations of current data and directions for the future. *Neuropsychopharmacology, 29*, 2285–2299. doi:10.1038/sj.npp.1300550

Tedeschini, E., Levkovitz, Y., Iovieno, N., Ameral, V. E., Nelson, J. C., & Papakostas, G. I. (2011). Efficacy of antidepressants for late-life depression: A meta-analysis and meta-regression of placebo-controlled randomized trials. *Journal of Clinical Psychiatry, 72*, 1660–1668. doi:10.4088/JCP.10r06531

Teri, L., Logsdon, R. G., Uomoto, J., & McCurry, S. M. (1997). Behavioral treatment of depression in dementia patients: A controlled clinical trial. *Journals of Gerontology Series B Psychological Sciences and Social Sciences, 52*, P159–P166. doi:10.1093/geronb/52B.4.P159

Teri, L., McKenzie, G., & LaFazia, D. (2005). Psychosocial treatment of depression in older adults with dementia. *Clinical Psychology Science and Practice, 12*, 303–316. doi:10.1093/clipsy.bpi032

Thompson, L. W., Coon, D. W., Gallagher-Thompson, D., Sommer, B. R., & Koin, D. (2001). Comparison of desipramine and cognitive/behavioral therapy in the treatment of elderly outpatients with mild-to-moderate depression. *American Journal of Geriatric Psychiatry, 9*, 225–240. doi:10.1097/00019442-200108000-00006

Thompson, L. W., Gallagher, D., & Breckenridge, J. S. (1987). Comparative effectiveness of psychotherapies for depressed elders. *Journal of Consulting and Clinical Psychology, 55*, 385–390. doi:10.1037/0022-006X.55.3.385

Thompson, S., Herrmann, N., Rapoport, M. J., & Lanctôt, K. L. (2007). Efficacy and safety of antidepressants for treatment of depression in Alzheimer's disease: A meta-analysis. *Canadian Journal of Psychiatry, 52,* 248–255.

Toseland, R. W., Diehl, M., Freeman, K., Manzanares, T., Naleppa, M., & McCallion, P. (1997). The impact of validation group therapy on nursing home residents with dementia. *Journal of Applied Gerontology, 16,* 31–50. doi:10.1177/073346489701600102

Trinh, N.-H., Hoblyn, J., Mohanty, S., & Yaffe, K. (2003). Efficacy of cholinesterase inhibitors in the treatment of neuropsychiatric symptoms and functional impairment in Alzheimer disease: A meta-analysis. *JAMA, 289,* 210–216. doi:10.1001/jama.289.2.210

van Schaik, A., van Marwijk, H., Adèr, H., van Dyck, R., de Haan, M., Penninx, B., . . . & Beekman, A. (2006). Interpersonal psychotherapy for elderly patients in primary care. *American Journal of Geriatric Psychiatry, 14,* 777–786. doi:10.1097/01.JGP.0000199341.25431.4b

Vann Jones, S. A., & O'Brien, J. T. (2014). The prevalence and incidence of dementia with Lewy bodies: A systematic review of population and clinical studies. *Psychological Medicine, 44,* 673–683. doi:10.1017/S0033291713000494

Vigen, C. L. P., Mack, W. J., Keefe, R. S. E., Sano, M., Sultzer, D. L., Stroup, T. S., . . . & Lyketsos, C. G. (2011). Cognitive effects of atypical antipsychotic medications in patients with Alzheimer's disease: Outcomes from CATIE-AD. *American Journal of Psychiatry, 168,* 831–839. doi:10.1176/appi.ajp.2011.08121844

Viggo Hansen, N., Jørgensen, T., & Ørtenblad, L. (2006). Massage and touch for dementia. *Cochrane Database Systematic Review,* CD004989. doi:10.1002/14651858.CD004989.pub2

Vink, A. C., Bruinsma, M. S., & Scholten, R. J. P. M. (2004). Music therapy for people with dementia. *Cochrane Database Systematic Review,* CD003477. doi:10.1002/14651858.CD003477.pub2

Wallace, A. E., Kofoed, L. L., & West, A. N. (1995). Double-blind, placebo-controlled trial of methylphenidate in older, depressed, medically ill patients. *American Journal of Psychiatry, 152,* 929–931. doi:10.1176/ajp.152.6.929

Wang, L. Y., Shofer, J. B., Rohde, K., Hart, K. L., Hoff, D. J., McFall, Y. H., . . . & Peskind, E. R. (2009). Prazosin for the treatment of behavioral symptoms in patients with Alzheimer disease with agitation and aggression. *American Journal of Geriatric Psychiatry, 17,* 744–751. doi:10.1097/JGP.0b013e3181ab8c61

Weintraub, D., Rosenberg, P. B., Martin, B. K., Frangakis, C., Mintzer, J. E., Porsteinsson, A. P., . . . & Lyketsos, C. G. (2010). Sertraline for the treatment of depression in Alzheimer disease: Week-24 outcomes. *American Journal of Geriatric Psychiatry, 18,* 332–340. doi:10.1097/JGP.0b013e3181cc0333

Williams, C. L., & Tappen, R. M. (2007). Effect of exercise on mood in nursing home residents with Alzheimer's disease. *American Journal of Alzheimer's Disease and Other Dementias, 22,* 389–397. doi:10.1177/1533317507305588

Williams, J. W., Barrett, J., Oxman, T. E., Frank, E., Katon, W., Sullivan, M., . . . & Sengupta, A. (2000). Treatment of dysthymia and minor depression in primary care: A randomized controlled trial in older adults. *JAMA, 284,* 1519–1526. doi:10.1001/jama.284.12.1519

Wilson, K. C., Mottram, P. G., Sivanranthan, A., & Nightingale, A. (2001). Antidepressant versus placebo for depressed elderly. *Cochrane Database Systematic Review, 2,* CD000561. doi:10.1002/14651858.CD000561

Wilson, K. C., Mottram, P. G., & Vassilas, C. A. (2008). Psychotherapeutic treatments for older depressed people. *Cochrane Database Systematic Review, 1*, CD004853. doi:10.1002/14651858.CD004853.pub2

Woods, B., Aguirre, E., Spector, A. E., & Orrell, M. (2012). Cognitive stimulation to improve cognitive functioning in people with dementia. *Cochrane Database Systematic Review*, CD005562. doi:10.1002/14651858.CD005562.pub2

Xu, Z.-Q., Liang, X.-M., Juan-Wu, Zhang, Y.-F., Zhu, C.-X., & Jiang, X.-J. (2012). Treatment with Huperzine A improves cognition in vascular dementia patients. *Cell Biochemistry and Biophysics, 62*, 55–58. doi:10.1007/s12013-011-9258-5

Zeiss, A. M. (2003). Depression in older adults: Evidence-based treatment and current gaps in the evidence base. *The Gerontologist, 43*, 279–283. doi:10.1093/geront/43.2.279

13

Behaviorally Prescribed Psychopharmacology: Beyond Combined Treatments to Coordinated Integrative Therapy

Mark D. Muse

> *It is becoming clear, moreover, that targeted alterations of neurotransmitter balances in specific brain regions can lead to the same kinds of synaptic changes as those associated with learning experiences. The effects of psychopharmacological interventions would be massively improved, however, if they were not applied as indiscriminately ...*
>
> Klaus Grawe, 2007, p. 4

Perhaps the most overlooked yet potent psychosocial component to medication dispensing is its reinforcing qualities: the way in which a drug is taken can reinforce therapeutic goals, or undermine them (Muse, 2008; Muse & McFarland, 1994).

Psychologists have long studied the reinforcing qualities of temporal parings in classical conditioning and of reward/punishment contingencies in operant conditioning paradigms.[1] These are not theoretical postulates, but verified laws of behavior (Salamone & Correa, 2002). Behavioral pharmacologists have recognized for decades that drugs affect animal and human behavior by acting as functional stimuli in the context of operant and respondent conditioning (Thompson & Pickens, 1971). The temporal assignment and reinforcing circumstances in which medication is used inevitably become significant components in the outcome of such interventions.

The agoraphobic patient who carries around a single dose of benzodiazepine in her purse, "just in case" she feels panic coming on, is an example of poor outcome to a treatment in which the use of medication reinforced a sense of vulnerability and the need to avoid anxiety/panic, as is the example of a patient with generalized anxiety disorder who has been on a selective serotonin reuptake inhibitor (SSRI) for more than a decade because he is apprehensive of an increase in anxiety if the medication were discontinued. Neither of these patients is anxiety-free, and both rely on medication not as a temporary coping strategy that at one point may have facilitated recovery but, rather, as a defense mechanism which engenders psychological dependency and, in some cases, physical addiction.

There are numerous examples of how medication can be scheduled behaviorally to further reinforce therapeutic gains (Muse, 2010; Muse & Moore, 2012; Sudak, 2011),

Cognitive Behavioral Psychopharmacology: The Clinical Practice of Evidence-Based Biopsychosocial Integration, First Edition. Edited by Mark Dana Muse.

but none more convincing than in the treatment of chronic pain. Wilbur Fordyce (1976, 1984) outlined the operant contingencies of therapeutic interventions (Sigal, 1967) for patients suffering from chronic benign pain syndromes, giving examples of how PRN pain medications, improperly prescribed, can lead to an increase in pain behavior (Berni & Fordyce, 1977). The question of whether malprescribed medications actually increase the phenomenological perception of pain does not need to be answered in order to appreciate an increase in dysfunctional pain behavior such as moaning, rocking, pacing, complaining, and movement restriction, all of which are associated with poor practices in prescribing. If the patient "needs to be in pain" in order to justify dispensing a reinforcing narcotic agent, then, quite predictably, for the behaviorist anyway, pain-related behavior will reappear at the instrumental time. On the other hand, properly dispensing relief by administering an analgesic after completing prescribed exercises is an example of using a pharmacologic agent to support therapeutic direction: pain relief is associated with greater activity. In one instance, narcotic agents extend dependency and other dysfunctional pain behaviors, acting as a detour to recovery, whereas in the second example the propitious administration of the same agent reinforces and rewards more functional behavior, and promotes progress toward the therapeutic goal of greater mobility and greater independence. Similarly, the agoraphobic patient who is given a benzodiazepine long enough to become physically dependent on the drug may find his or her phobia perpetuated as an instrumental behavior for obtaining further prescriptions of the drug. In contrast, the housebound patient who follows a behavioral program to manage agoraphobia, and who is prescribed a benzodiazepine to use only when making behavioral efforts to reverse the condition by venturing outside of the house, is likely to make greater progress as a result of the reinforcing nature of this contingency.

Juxtaposed to the medical model that views psychiatric illness and its remedy as stemming largely from biological processes, the cognitive-behavioral model of acquired dysfunctional syndromes, while acknowledging biological components to mental health and mental illness, spells out the link between learned behavior and psychopathology, and demonstrates how cognitive-behavioral strategies, properly applied, provide a powerful therapeutic tool in the recovery from emotional disorders. Within this biopsychosocial paradigm, the potential reinforcing characteristics of various psychotropics may be appreciated (Salamone & Corea, 2012; Salamone, Correa, Nunes, Randall, & Pardo, 2012), and their enhanced use, emphasizing their inherently reinforcing properties, may be elaborated within the cognitive-behavioral paradigm for the treatment of an array of mental health conditions. This approach I have called "cognitive-behavioral psychopharmacology" (CBP).

CBP accepts a biopsychosocial orientation in the diagnosing and treatment of mental illness and, as such, embraces the idea that psychopathology may include biological as well as psychosocial components; it is the interplay of these components that argues for a judicious balance of biopsychosocial interventions to properly address a variety of mental health conditions. In this respect, medications and psychotherapies represent the vast majority of the mental health field's therapeutic options at the present. While there are certainly times in which psychotherapy is indicated without the use of medications, our focus is on those cases where medication is prescribed for more efficacious management. Some form of psychosocial intervention is assumed to be involved whenever psychotropics are recommended (Tasman & Riba, 2000; Tasman, Riba, & Silk, 2000), and the specific cognitive-behavioral implication for the use of medication with those cases where pharmacotherapy is employed is our special concern.

An understanding of the specific cognitive-behavioral implications of the use of psychotropic medication provides the possibility of an added effect in the interplay of integrated interventions, and contributes to a growing awareness toward the "science of prescribing."

The connection between illness and learning mechanisms involved in symptom acquisition is apparent to students of psychology, who have observed that each of the major learning modalities (classical, operant, social modeling, and cognitive) is implicated in the acquisition of psychiatric syndromes such as anxieties, depressions, psychoses, and impulse control disorders, to name a few. The special role of "incentive learning," as promoted through biochemical reinforcement (Ikemoto & Panksepp, 1999; Salamone, Cousins, & Snyder, 1997) of dysfunctional behavioral responses, is highlighted in the cognitive-behavioral model of symptom acquisition, as is the importance of temporal pairings of injurious events with unconditioned aberrant responses and their subsequent solidification through habit formation.

Cognitive-Behavioral Learning Theory and Acquired Psychopathology

Classical conditioning is unquestionably involved in the acquisition of anxiety disorders, especially the phobias. A case in point is John Watson's documentation in the early part of the last century of Little Albert's induced rabbit phobia, and the subsequent treatment and recovery from the same through behavioral techniques (Watson & Rayner, 1920). The mere temporal pairing of an innocuous rabbit with a loud and frightening noise gave rise to the acquired symptom of fear in the infant Albert while in the presence of furry objects. Along these same lines, posttraumatic stress disorder (PTSD) acquisition, with associative flashbacks, shows a strong relationship between amount of temporal exposure to trauma and subsequent severity of symptoms (Rudd, 2003), while the emotional state created at the time of trauma may act as a conduit posttraumatically, as predicted by the state-dependent learning paradigm of respondent conditioning (Overton, 1978, 1983; Weingartner, 1978; Weingartner, Miller, & Murphy, 1977); that is, PTSD symptoms may not only be elicited by environmental stimuli similar to those present at the time of the traumatic event, but an emotional state reminiscent of the original state (anxiety) may also elicit traumatic material through association (Muse, 1984; Overton, 1964).

The role of learning in creating and maintaining psychopathology is also evidenced in instrumental conditioning's influence on the acquisition and maintenance of symptomatology: the acquisition of compulsions secondary to anxiety-related obsessions in obsessive-compulsive disorder (OCD) exemplifies the negative reinforcing properties of anxiety reduction in the maintenance of the compulsive symptom. In this case, compulsions allow the patient to mitigate or escape the heightened anxiety and obsessions, the unintended outcome of which is to negatively reinforce further compulsive behavior; seemingly meaningless behavior serves the purpose of avoiding unwanted anxiety-provoking obsession. Self-mutilation in the form of "cutting," and the use of alcohol as "self-medication," fall within this same category of reinforced escape behaviors from anxiety. Learned helplessness in depression, with its concomitant symptoms of anergia, anhedonia, and withdrawal, can be conceptualized as a lack of environmental reinforcement for problem-solving effort, resulting in reduced effort over time. In the same vein, the reduction in an aversive internal state of boredom or frustration through cathartic acting out serves as an obvious reinforcer in the maintenance of impulse/behavioral disorders; if such inappropriate acting out receives greater attention, it may additionally provide secondary gain for the adolescent in need of, albeit negative, affirmation.

The interplay of cognitive-behavioral-social learning in the acquisition and maintenance of psychopathology is assumed to be present in nearly all psychiatric diagnoses. Anxiety syndromes such as OCD and phobias, for example, not only have their behavioral components (compulsions in the case of OCD, and avoidance in the case of phobias), which presumably exist because they alleviate anxiety and perpetuate the behavior through negative reinforcement, but they most certainly have cognitive aspects as well (egodystonic ruminations in the case of OCD, and belief in one's imminent vulnerability in the case of phobias) that promote internal conditioned stimuli which elicit and sustain anxiety (Muse, 1996). Moreover, the likelihood that one might develop an anxiety disorder rather than, for example, depression is augmented by social modeling and exposure to covert learning at an earlier age; by observing salient or repetitive behaviors in childhood models, such as parents, the developing adolescent/young adult who has acquired a repertoire of latent behavioral patterns is predisposed, under environmental conditions akin to those previously observed in childhood, to manifest vicariously learned dysfunctional responses of the past. The reverse of this is the influence of functional social conditioning, which promotes beliefs of self-efficacy, which moderate anxiety and feelings of vulnerability (Bandura, 1997) and ultimately provide resiliency, as evidenced in studies of PTSD (Benight & Bandura, 2004). The child who has witnessed adult models successfully respond to adversity will be better equipped to bounce back from life's challenges, even extreme challenges as in the case of trauma.

Along these same lines, the experimental cognitivist Edward Tolman (1949) maintained that there are many ways of acquiring problematic behaviors, and that instrumental and respondent learning are but two forms. The acquisition of cognitive maps (Tolman, 1948), as well as the avoidance of cognitive dissonance (Festinger, 1957) as a special form of negative reinforcement, bring the cognitive—alongside the behavioral—within the realm of learning via conditioning. Even the radical behaviorist B. F. Skinner allowed that the "black box," or cognitive awareness of one's actions, is a force to be reckoned with in psychotherapy, when he acknowledged that it is essential that humans believe that they make choices in therapy, even when the choices are largely determined by the person's nature and circumstances (Skinner, personal correspondence, 1986). To believe in oneself is, arguably, the ultimate goal in mental health therapy; to trust in the therapist during psychotherapy (transference) or believe in medication in pharmacotherapy (expectancy) is but an intermediate stage to the patient gaining confidence in him or herself. The initial powerful belief in the outside agent (placebo), when it occurs, is short-lived, and it is incumbent upon the practitioner to make the most of this uniquely reinforcing dynamic.

To summarize, nothing in the cognitive-behavioral approach precludes biological predisposition and interplay in the formation and maintenance of psychopathology. Psychosocial learning principles of symptom acquisition, however, and the ultimate remediation of such symptoms through learning new ways of behaving and of thinking, hold true for anxiety syndromes, depression, schizophrenia, bipolar disorder, behavioral problems, psychosomatic syndromes, and drug dependency.

Carla, at the age of 7, was experiencing stress over her parents' temporary separation. She felt tense and fearful a good deal of the time as a result of family insecurity and parental arguments, and she had sensations of anxiety in the pit of her stomach. One day, at school, she observed a classmate who had stomach flu vomit in class, and Carla immediately felt an identification with the other girl, and vicariously experienced her predicament. She interpreted the queasiness of her own anxiety as imminent vomiting, and she was overcome with the conviction that she was about to vomit. She became increasingly anxious and finally felt a gag response that, indeed, precipitated reflux. She had never vomited, and the taste horrified her.

In the ensuing years, her fear of vomiting increased. She began to feel sick in the morning before going to school, and she begged to be allowed to stay home, which was intermittently consented to by her parents. By the age of 9, she now found herself highly sensitive to stomach queasiness or anything reminiscent of it, and she became convinced that riding on the school bus, sitting for quizzes, or participating in competitive sports would result in vomiting. She became increasingly avoidant as she was excused from these activities or accommodations were made to work around them. Her parents, who had since worked out their marital differences, now spent more time with their daughter because of her disability.

This case is not unlike many seen in clinical practice in which a multitude of reinforcers, largely social, tend to support and eventually contribute to the prolongation and augmentation of an original unconditioned response that was, in its day, elicited by stimuli which may have long since become irrelevant. The subsequent development of conditioned dysfunctional cognitive and behavioral components then forms the base of prolonged maladaptive syndromes.

Reinforcing and Aversive Properties of Pharmacological Agents

Awareness of the reinforcing potential of different psychotropics in the acquisition of new learning, both pathological and healthy learning, plays a significant role in the optimum management of pharmacotherapy. Quite apart from psychiatric medications' mechanism of action and intended pharmacological impact on the target symptoms of a given condition under treatment, the nature of collateral reinforcing effects of psycho tropics may be linked to their secondary role in the inadvertent maintenance of pathology or, conversely, in the furtherance of recovery. Aversive agents and undesirable side effects can also be linked to their impact on new learning within the context of therapy. Just as humans and other animals have evolved to seek healthy and pleasant stimuli, animated organisms are predisposed to avoid harmful and unpleasant stimulation. The pairing of reinforcing pharmacological agents that reduce unpleasant sensations, and enhance pleasant ones, to therapeutic thoughts, emotions, and behaviors furthers the acquisition of new functional learning. Along this same line, pairing aversive agents with undesirable behavior tends to reduce the unwanted behavior.

In classical or respondent conditioning, learning occurs when a contextual stimulus acquires informational value (by becoming a conditioned stimulus, or CS) through associational pairing with an original (desirable or undesirable) unconditioned stimulus (UCS). An example of this is the acquired value of pornography as a CS through pairings with sexual feelings of arousal (unconditioned response, or UCR) produced by masturbatory stimuli (UCS). Relearning or counterconditioning occurs with a new pairing of the CS with a different UCS that is linked to an antagonistic UCR, creating a competing stimulus–response association that attenuates or extinguishes the original pairing. Within the therapeutic context, an example of the process of acquiring desirable avoidant behavior through classical conditioning would be the viewing of pornography while sniffing smelling salts, thus creating an associational bond between the pornography (CS) and smelling salts (UCS) that now links pornography to physical distress (the new UCR) and results in avoidant behavior in the form of reduced accessing of pornographic material.

In operant or instrumental conditioning, learning occurs when approach or avoidant behavior is rewarded with obtaining or averting a desired or undesirable stimulus, such as in the case of reducing pain with an analgesic after the patient has exercised. Although the exercise may increase pain somewhat, the overall pain level is improved by administering an opioid postexercise that will not only suppress the exercise-related pain, but will also reduce the more chronic, pre-exercise pain. In operant conditioning, a response that reduces an undesired effect or increases a desired one is strengthened by the result produced. In strict behavioral terms, a reinforcer, by operational definition, is anything that increases the likelihood of a given behavior being repeated. A positive reinforcer increases instrumental behavior to obtain the reinforcer, whereas a negative reinforcer increases a particular behavior that results in escaping from an aversive situation. Reinforcers certainly play a role in psychotherapy, and social reinforcement within the counseling setting may account for much of the *common factor* (Grencavage & Norcross, 1990; Laska, Gurman, & Wampold, 2014) found in the effectiveness of psychotherapies across the various schools and approaches.

Reinforcers, ultimately, derive their potency from their ability to access and stimulate the motivational areas of the brain. Much research has lately centered on identifying the neurophysiology and neurochemistry behind motivation (Schultz, 2000); and, to understand the physiological reinforcement potential of drugs in general, it is opportune to revisit the neurophysiology of drugs of abuse (Cannon & Palmiter, 2003), which act as powerful rewards by exerting direct influence over dopaminergic neurons in the mesolimbic pathway (Adinoff, 2004; Beninger, Hoffman, & Mazurski, 1989; Ikemoto, Glazier, Murphy, & McBride, 1997;), which includes the medial forebrain bundle, the ventral tegmental area, and the nucleus accumbens. Alternatively, other drugs, such as the majority of prescribed psychiatric medications, alter the activity of adjacent receptors through gabanergic, opioidergic, oxytocinergic, endocannabinoidergic, serotonergic, cholinergic, and noradrenergic transmitters that indirectly exert modulatory influence over the mesolimbic dopaminergic pathway (Hernandez, et al., 2006; Salamone, 2006, 2010; Salamone & Corea, 2002; Salamone, Correa, Farrar, & Mingote, 2007; Tomlins & Sellers, 2001) and, thus, enhance learning and/or extinction (Lutz, 2007).[2] Of particular interest here is mounting evidence (de la Fuente-Fernandez & Stoessl, 2004) that the placebo effect also involves the ventral loop of the basal ganglia circuitry (de la Fuente-Fernandez, 2009), with the release of substantial amounts of endogenous dopamine in both the dorsal and ventral striatum (de la Fuente-Fernandez, Lidstone, & Stoessl, 2006), ultimately activating the nucleus accumbens (de la Fuente-Fernandez & Stoessl, 2002).

Once again, one is tempted to speculate about a "common factor" within the context of pharmacotherapy (Kirsch, 2011), just as within the psychosocial context. Such a common factor is derived from different means of evoking the same motivational/reinforcing centers of the brain, thereby ensuring a repetition of the behavior that resulted in mesolimbic stimulation of dopaminergic and other participating circuits. The common denominator might very well be activation of the motivational system, and the behaviors and cognitions that are instrumental in this activation are the ones that are reinforced.

Psychopharmacologically, it is interesting to consider placebo and nocebo responses as prototypes of reactions found to all psychotropics. The placebo can be thought of in a classical conditioning sense as an originally inert stimulus capable of eliciting a learned response, emanating, perhaps, from expectation of a forthcoming effect. That is, the placebo is a substitute stimulus that elicits a previously experienced response, and therefore is a form of second-order conditioning. The placebo effect may also be appreciated as "an evolutionarily adaptive trait and part of a healing mechanism operating across many levels-from genetic and cellular to social cultural" (Thompson, Ritenbaugh, & Nichter, 2009). That is, the placebo potential exists before it manifests itself, and reflects the switching on of an innate circuit (Colloca & Miller, 2011).[3] In this respect, placebo response is initially a UCR to social–cultural stimuli, presumably stimuli that increase expectation of a positive effect. Drug effects are significantly modulated by nonpharamcological factors (Siegel, 1989), and endogenous biological and psychological circuits may become activated by environmental stimuli, especially psychosocial stimuli, in a positive feedback loop that is further augmented by acquired conditioning bonds.

While the underlying biological structures for motivation exist innately and vary to some degree according to the sensitivity to reinforcement of any given individual (Smillie, 2008), it is important to acknowledge that sustained behavior derived from drug-induced motivation is not innate but acquired (Siegel & Ellsworth, 1986; Siegel, Marco, & Baptista, 2000). Indeed, innate biology is only a starting place, as biology itself is subject to modification through mechanisms of neuroplasticity and neurogenesis (Arden, 2010), and sustained behavioral modification is likely to be the result of internal gratification through the activation of the pleasure center, combined with supporting environmental stimuli and subject-initiated responses, reinforced by consequent-dependent effects (Geller & Seifter, 1960), all of which may result in biochemical and even structural changes in the nervous system. Drugs can enhance new associations by initially providing motivation through the reinforcement inherent to the dopaminergic activation of specific structures within the limbic system. In this respect, therapeutically reinforcing drugs, when administered behaviorally, tend to increase hitherto low frequency healthy behavior, but not high frequency pernicious behavior, which might be demonstrated as a rate dependency effect (Dews, 1958; Dews & Wenger, 1977; Sanger & Blackman, 1976).

Common factors inherent to drug administration notwithstanding, all drugs are not equally reinforcing. Drug preference varies according to the nature of the drug, and procedures for determining the comparative reinforcement potential of different drugs on humans have been developed along the lines of behavioral economics (Bickel, DeGrandpre, & Higgins, 1993; Bickel, Marsch, & Carroll, 2000; Heinz, Lilje, Kassel, & de Wit, 2012), which refers to methodology for experimentally quantifying relative pharmacological reinforcing efficacy. With the exception of hallucinogens, there is little difference between other mammals' and humans' preference for reinforcing psychoactive drugs (Griffiths, Bigelow, & Henningfield, 1980; Griffiths et al., 2016). Nonetheless, humans are complex subjects, and drugs do not necessarily have a homogeneous effect across all ages, genders, races, and socioeconomic/cultural groupings (Simoni-Wastila, 2000; Simoni-Wastila & Strickler, 2004). Hence, the need to be aware of patient variables—most notably novelty/sensation seeking tendencies (Stoops et al., 2007) and propensity for impulsivity (Bechara, 2005)—when determining the reinforcing potential for any given drug.

Some drugs have a strong reinforcing component and are prone to abuse, such as benzodiazepines and opioids, while others, such as the SSRIs, derive a subtler reinforcing property by, presumably, accessing the same dopaminergic pathway via indirect routing, either through a cascade effect of other neurotransmitters or through the placebo effect. In either case, the initial drug effect has a differential influence on learning, depending on the nature of the learning that is taking place. In classical conditioning associations, the pairing of respondent behaviors with environmental and proprioceptive stimuli enhances the bond between UCR and CRs within the stimulus context; for example, with cigarette consumption associated with listening to music, or beer drinking associated with social interaction within the context of a public bar (Perkins & Karelitz, 2013), environmental conditioned stimuli are capable of eliciting a biological response similar to that derived from smoking and drinking within psychosocial settings, even when the person has sworn off such substances. In the case of instrumental learning, behavior becomes an operant that allows access to the reward, and can be taken advantage of therapeutically by proper sequencing, such as in the case of making a cup of coffee contingent upon first completing an unwanted task, like studying (Battig, 2013).

Operant Reinforcers

Positive reinforcers are stimuli or responses that increase a specific behavior to obtain more of the same reinforcer; that is, the subject exhibits an increase in behavior that is instrumental in accessing the reinforcer. In our previous example, Fordyce demonstrated that groaning, which is rewarded with narcotics, may result, for some subjects, in further groaning.

The neuroanatomy of reinforcement was established by James Olds and Peter Milner (1954) in their proposal of a "pleasure center" within the septal region of the brain. Subsequent research has shown that drugs that act as positive reinforcers directly or indirectly activate the mesolimbic dopaminergic system and lead to increased activation of the nucleus accumbens (Wise, 1998). Certain drug-based reinforcers are fast-acting and present an immediate feeling of well-being or euphoria, such as barbiturates and benzodiazepines, which have different receptor sites on the gamma-aminobutyric acid (GABA) receptor–chloride ionophore complex; beyond their anxiolytic effect, they produce pleasure (Mintzer & Griffiths, 1998; O'Brien, 2005; O'Brien, Childress, McLellan, & Ehrman, 1992; Rosenbaum, 2005; Uhlenhuth, Balter, Ban, & Yang, 1999). Quetiapine, when administered intranasally, also has a rapid onset, and may demonstrate a pleasure-based reinforcing potential (Erdogan, 2010; Morin, 2007; Pinta, 2007; Reeves & Brister, 2007), whereas stimulants (analeptics/sympathomimetics) release dopamine directly within the nucleus accumbens of the mesolimbic system and act as powerful reinforcers (Boyd, McCabe, Cranford, & Young, 2006; Kalix, 1994). Of interest is that phasic (spike) release of amphetamine is more reinforcing than tonic (constant) release (Covey, Juliano, & Garris, 2013; Grace, 2000). Opioids are also powerful reinforcers, producing euphoria (Bieber et al., 2008) through mu, kappa, and delta receptors found within the nucleus accumbens or adjacent structures that communicate with the nucleus accumbens (Mansour et al., 1994).

Tobacco, alcohol, caffeine, and marijuana are all fast-acting drugs. Tobacco stimulates nicotinic cholinergic receptors that are found in cell bodies in the basal ganglia, ventral tegmental area, and nucleus acumens, where they in turn trigger the release of dopamine and norepinephrine when stimulated (Balfour, 1991; Levine, 1992). Alcohol activates receptors that lead to release of dopamine in the nucleus accumbens (Ma & Zhu, 2014; Yoshimoto et al., 2000), and caffeine, as an antagonist, activates adenosine receptor blockage, which in turn blocks GABA receptors and increases epinephrine through adrenal gland release, as well as impacting on dopamine receptors in much the same way as amphetamines (Garrett & Griffiths, 1997; McKim, 1980). Marijuana, on the other hand, stimulates cannabinoid receptors found in the nucleus accumbens, and may further act as a presynaptic signaler that potentiates the release of endogenous opioid peptides that, in turn, act as neuromodulators which increase dopamine levels in the mesolimbic reward system (Gardner, 1992; Tanda, Pontieri, & Chiara, 1997).

Not all drugs are reinforcers, or they are only partially reinforcing, and some drugs are quite the opposite and actually "dissuade" further drug-seeking behavior or compliance with therapeutically indicated consumption. Slow-acting psychotropics, for example, may eventually provide reinforcement in symptom relief, but they rarely provide a sense of euphoria or pleasure, and they oftentimes deliver unpleasant side effects. A case in point are antipsychotics, which do not produce pleasure; on the contrary, they work by blocking dopaminergic pathways, including the mesolimbic pleasure center, and are therefore not only inherently nonreinforcing but may be "amotivating" (McKim, 2007; Meltzer, 1990). What is more, neuroleptics tend to reduce aversion to noxious stimuli (Couvousier et al., 1953), thereby reducing negative reinforcing potential inherent in avoidant behaviors that lead the person away from dangerous or unpleasant situations. Equally as nonreinforcing, antidepressants and mood stabilizers do not directly motivate through providing enjoyment, but can actually act to mitigate pleasure/euphoria (Spiegle & Aebi, 1981). Some tricyclic antidepressants also reduce aversion avoidance (McMillan & Leander, 1976). The potential for both antipsychotics and antidepressants to serve as long-term reinforcers by acting over time as negative reinforcers that lessen distress and dyscontrol (Judd, Squire, Butters, Salmon, & Paller, 1987) can be offset by their interference with the normal mesolimbic pleasure/motivation centers, and noncompliance with these classes of medications due to their immediate negative effect on motivation can preclude the drug ever achieving the more distant reinforcing properties of symptom reduction.

And then there are a series of drugs that reinforce in a less direct fashion than agents that access the mesolimbic system directly. For example, hallucinogens, which act primarily as selective agonists of 5-HT_{2A} within the central nervous system, especially within the locus coeruleus and medial prefrontal cortex (Marek & Aghajanian, 1999), are reinforcing for sensation seekers. One might speculate that the reinforcing potential of the hallucinogens preys on curiosity and discovery, to eventually reward through secondary access to the nucleus accumbens. Socially reinforcing drugs, which provide reward in the form of assurance/social competence, include the cyclic guanosine monophosphate (cGMP)-specific phosphodiesterase type 5 inhibitors (sildenafil, etc.), which enhance sexual relating, and the entactogens (3, 4-methylenedioxy-methamphetamine (MDMA) as an oxytocinergic), which heighten empathic responding and act as social reinforcers. Along this same line, alcohol and marijuana may also potentiate secondary social reinforcement through lowering inhibition within a social context. The special case of conditioned compensatory responses to a drug within a familiar context (Siegel, Hinson, & Krank, 1982) illustrates how a drug can potentially reinforce social behavior through operant conditioning while the environmental context in which the drug is consumed acts to increase or decrease the effects of the drug through classical conditioning (Gerevich, Bácskai, Farkas,& Danics, 2005).[4]

Negative reinforcement increases the appearance of instrumental behaviors (e.g., drug-taking) that facilitate escape from an aversive situation. Fast-acting negative reinforcers include what might be called "distress-easers" such as the benzodiazepines, barbiturates, and alcohol, which allow escape from anxiety/fear (DeMartini & Carey, 2011). Marijuana use has been linked to facilitating escape from emotional memories (Mariscano & Lafenetre, 2009), and alcohol may be analogous to an emotional "anesthetic" in promoting escape from emotional pain through enhancement of GABA as well as enhanced inhibitory effect of glycine, and the additional attenuation of the N-methyl-D-aspartate (NMDA) receptor of the excitatory neurotransmitter glutamate (Balster, 1998; Kennedy & Longnecker, 1996). Along this same line, beta blockers can serve as negative reinforcers by providing a chemical escape from social anxiety and embarrassment, which is further reinforced by enhanced social competence and resulting social reward.

While the apparent negative reinforcing qualities of the slower-acting psychotropics is not as readily apparent, their ability to ease long-term emotional suffering places them in the category of "malaise-easers," and serves to motivate their continued use through compliance when there are few associated side effects and when the patient is not ambivalent about giving up targeted symptoms. In the long run, antipsychotics avoid emotional dyscontrol and thought disorder, antidepressants ease dysphoric mood and/or chronic anxiety, and mood stabilizers avert catastrophic consequences of hypomanic behavior. In this sense, all have the potential to act as negative reinforcers.

Respondent Conditioners

Apart from the recent use of "cognitive enhancers" for therapeutic learning, which we will take up momentarily, classical conditioners—not technically reinforcers, *per se*—are UCSs that provoke a reflexive response that can, subsequently, become conditioned to a set of neutral stimuli. This works in two directions: drugs, as UCSs, can produce UCRs that are subsequently associated with environmental stimuli; environmental stimuli, on the other hand, can modify a drug's impact by conditioning the response to it.

For example, a stimulant, at higher dosing, triggers the UCR of dopamine-related pleasure, which can be secondarily conditioned to surrounding stimuli present during the response. Hence, amphetamine taken while a student is studying has the potential to associate the feeling of well-being produced by the drug with the activity of studying. Studying, at a future date, would then elicit the now conditioned feeling of well-being without the presence of amphetamine. Paradoxically, a drug may interact with learning in a reciprocal manner. That is, the effect of the drug can be conditioned by the context in which it is taken: the same dose of amphetamine used for studying but now taken recreationally at a party where everyone is happy can provide double the effect, and result in feelings of euphoria. The chemical effect of the drug is mixed with endogenous reactions to pleasurable social context, and the drug-taker now experiences "twice the high." This reaction may account for a person becoming surprisingly "tipsy" at a party after consuming no more than his usual nightcap, which he normally consumes in the privacy of his home.

Just as there is no "reinforcer" *per se* in the classical conditioning paradigm, there is no "punishment" as such. Nonetheless, pairing aversive agents with unwanted CRs has been used therapeutically (Wolpe, 1973) to countercondition undesirable behavior by promoting a competitive escape behavior that displaces the original approach response. The use of disulfiram is a prime example of how pairing the UCR of flushing and vomiting to alcohol conditions drinking to a newly acquired feeling of nausea. The nausea is subsequently escaped by the CR of withdrawing from alcohol, setting up a segue for additional operant negative reinforcement. Smelling salts have been used in the same way (Muse & Frigola, 2003) through *in vitro* pairing of primitive olfactory repulsion with paraphilic ideation and impulse. One-trial learning has been demonstrated to be favored when pairings evoke primitive UCRs such as vomiting (Garcia, Kimeldorf, & Koelling, 1955), which are presumably innately wired to a survival mechanism.

Social/Cognitive Reinforcers/Conditioners

Social learning follows many of the tenets of operant and respondent conditioning inasmuch as social cues and reactions can be reinforced through reward or association; yet, social learning also has the unique component whereby conditioning can occur vicariously through observing a model receive reinforcement for his or her behaviors. Aggressive behavior such as that found in physical abuse can oftentimes be traced back to the initial learning of such behavior by observing a perpetrator rewarded for victimizing someone else (Bandura, 1973). Drug-taking and drug-experimenting is also inextricably related to early childhood exposure to drug behavior observed on the part of parental models and/or peer models during adolescence (Zucker, Donovan, Masten, Matson, & Moss, 2008). And social context can further play a prominent role in modulating the functional effects of the drug or medication used (Hughes, Gulliver, Amori, Mireanlt, & Fenwick, 1988): the social environment in which drugs are consumed has long been identified (Goode, 1972) as impacting on the subjective drug experience as well as on drug-induced behaviors (Bardo, Neisewander, & Kelly, 2013). Social learning, beyond mere vicariously acquired reinforcement, may also contribute a major cognitive component whereby social rules and regulations are applied to future/novel situations, and thus may condition the subject's future response by way of expectation of results generalized from previous learning. An example of this is the placebo response elicited from counterfeit cocaine, marijuana, or nicotine, when the substance is actually inert (Hughes et al., 1989; Poling & Byrne, 1992; Poling, Byrne, & Morgan, 2000). Finally, the effect of the interplay of drugs upon social behavior and, vice versa, the influence of social context upon the effect of the drug, is complex and worthy of further study. At least one study (Bershad, Seiden, & de Wit, 2015) has demonstrated how opioid receptors are involved in modulating social stimuli, by demonstrating that buprenorphine increases the rewarding effects of positive social interactions while reducing the punitive impact of negative social interaction.

Cognitive Enhancers in Classical, Instrumental and Social Therapeutic Learning

Cognitive enhancers have traditionally included neuromodulators such as acetylcholinesterase inhibitors (donepenzil, rivastimine) and NMDA receptor antagonists (memantine) for the treatment of neurodegenerative disorders such as Alzheimer's disease, Parkinson's disease with dementia, and dementia with Lewy bodies (Husain & Mehta, 2011). More recently, neuromodulators have been used to boost cognitive-behavioral rehabilitation through enhancing learning, and other cognitive enhancers have been added to the traditional neuromodulators to obtain these same effects; the list of agents used to this end now includes dopamine/noradrenaline reuptake inhibitors (methylphenidate and amphetamine), nonselective adenosine receptor antagonist (caffeine), nicotinic cholinergic receptor agonist (nicotine), orexin modulation (modafinil), noradrenaline reuptake inhibitors (atomoxetine, reboxetine), and a host of other agents (Gualtieri, 2004).

The use of cognitive enhancers in psychotherapy is being increasingly explored, and this is now considered a hopeful line of inquiry (Singewald, Schmuckermair, Whittle, Holmes, & Ressler, 2015), if actual clinical protocols are still experimental. The ability to separate pharmacologically induced neurocognitive enhancement of therapeutic learning from motivational reinforcement factors intertwined with the use of these drugs has proved difficult; nonetheless, that motivational factors have a role to play among cognitive enhancers is becoming explicit (Ilieva & Farah, 2013). The possibility of placebo as an active cognitive enhancer needs also to be recognized. The expectation that medication creates in many patients may carry over into the therapeutic learning situation and act as a powerful therapeutic enhancer. If this is true, nearly any psychoactive substance that provided proprioceptive cues of "something happening" could enhance the therapeutic material through classical conditioning association (Colloca & Miller, 2011; Siegel, 2002), as well as through operant-reward mechanisms. The neurobiological mechanisms of the placebo effect have been studied extensively (Benedetti, Mayberg, Wager, Stohler, & Zubieta, 2005), and in many ways these mechanisms parallel the pathways known to form part of the motivation-pleasure center; that is, dopaminergic mesolimbic projections to the nucleus accumbens, and parallel endogenous opioid activity (Finniss, Kaptchuk, Miller, & Benedetti, 2010).

Unintended Conditioning Outcomes of Medication Side Effects

Inadvertent adverse reactions to medications can lead to antitherapeutic effects if the prescriber is not aware of emotional/behavioral, and not just physical, side effects of psychotropics. The unwanted side effects of antipsychotics, antidepressants, anxiolytics, sympathomimetics, and mood stabilizers can outweigh therapeutic reinforcement: drug-induced problems with sexual arousal and performance, cognitive blunting, retrograde amnesia, akathisia, emotional deadening, and induced paranoia (Breggin, 2008; Veselinovic et al., 2013) can erase the long-term negative reinforcement in the form of symptom reduction that psychotropics pretend to provide. Paradoxically, however, unwanted medication side effects provide the astute clinician with a unique opportunity to capitalize on a new form of negative reinforcement, and harness it in benefit of accelerating progress toward therapeutic goals. Offering strategies for "getting off" medication can provide the patient with motivation to work toward this eventual escape. Once the patient has achieved reduction or discontinuation of the offending medication, previous efforts toward improved functioning are rewarded by negative reinforcement inherent in avoiding the original side effects of the discontinued drug.

Nocebo effects—that is, adverse effects following placebo administration—are well known, and confound many clinical trial interpretations (Mitsikostas, Mantonakis, & Charlarakis, 2010), and may contribute to lack of adherence to clinical treatment schedules (Colloca & Miller, 2011). Curiously, nocebo has also been correlated with greater therapeutic effect (Ciaramella, Paroli, & Poli, 2013), begging the question, again, of second-order conditioning in which side effects of past medications are associated with overall improvement (Häuser, Hansen, & Enck, 2011); subsequently, the associational expectation of improvement is transferred to the new therapeutic setting. Such an explanation might account for both the appearance of nocebo in the therapeutic setting, and its subsequent correlation with therapeutic improvement.

Mr. McLean was noncompliant with a large part of his treatment plan for bipolar disorder and attention deficit hyperactivity disorder (ADHD). He stopped his mood stabilizer because he felt it took away the fun in his life, and he smoked heavily to reduce the effectiveness of his neuroleptic for the same reason. He tended to rely on stimulant medication to pick him up, and did not take it as prescribed. The patient appeared to be in a constant search for feelings of pleasure, and found gambling to be his main source of excitement. He frequented casinos until early morning, and his sleep regulation was, at best, irregular. He self-medicated with alcohol and benzodiazepines to be able to sleep.

A behavioral contract was subsequently drawn up in which staying off the mood stabilizer (negative reinforcement) was made conditional upon completing other aspects of his therapy. His access to nicotine was made contingent upon getting up on time, and going to bed on time, and he was dispensed a daily allotment of cigarettes according to the night's previous "lights out–lights on" performance (positive reinforcement schedule). His neuroleptic was increased slightly to compensate for the initial cigarette consumption, and scheduled to be reduced if cigarette consumption were decreased. An immediate-release stimulant was dispensed during his most onerous moment of the day, which was bathing his invalid mother, and this activity was eventually associated with a degree of complacency if not gratification (classical conditioning). The excitement he derived from gambling was transferred to supervised stock market investing, and his ingestion of alcohol was limited to those Friday nights when he had completed his behavioral program (Premack principle[5]), which included staying on his neuroleptic medication and abstaining from benzodiazepines. His sustained effort was further reinforced by the gradual discontinuation of his mood stabilizer. The patient eventually voluntarily suggested reducing tobacco intake as a prelude to decreasing his neuroleptic medication.

Targeting Symptoms with Specific Cognitive-Behavioral Psychopharmacology Interventions

Managing the reinforcing nature of biopsychosocial approaches for the optimal integration of psychotherapy and medication is the thesis of CBP. With CBP, symptoms of each of the major conditions (anxiety, depression, psychosis, etc.) can be addressed individually, and the proper interface of pharmacotherapy with psychotherapeutic techniques may be used to treat the specific conditions with a synergy that surpasses the normal "combined treatment" approaches.

Anxiety

> Using benzodiazepines on an as-needed basis and providing CBT may be the worst method of combining treatment because the rapid relief from symptoms that ensues after taking benzodiazepines is a potent reinforcer of medication use and eliminates the chance of exposure and active coping.
>
> *(Sudak, 2011, p. 113)*

The possible interference of medication with cognitive-behavioral therapeutic goals in the treatment of anxiety has long been recognized, and is perhaps better understood than the potential for increasing new learning of functional behavior by intertwining medication within a behavioral treatment strategy. With anxiety disorders, such new behavior would stem largely from counterconditioning dysfunctional respondent behaviors to more functional responses (Jones, 1924), and, in this vein, CBP has the potential for accelerating clinical improvement by judiciously and punctually applying pharmacology at critical junctures, thus increasing the reinforcing value of subsequent pharmacological and psychotherapeutic effects. Such an approach, for example, might be kept in reserve for the patient who is otherwise unable to face the fear needed to undergo exposure therapy. In the specific case of systematic desensitization, the response of paralyzing anxiety is changed to one of competence and self-assurance through the use of anxiolytics combined with exposure therapy, conditioning a new relaxed response and a sense of self-mastery to the original fearful stimulus (e.g., social interaction, large crowds, noisy subways, etc.). Benzodiazepines (Hollister, 1986), beta blockers (Khalil, 2013), or even marijuana derivatives (Rabinaka et al., 2013) could be administered during *in vivo* exposure. Rather than desensitizing along a hierarchy of graded anxiety-provoking stimuli (situations), the hierarchy is composed of inverse graded amounts of an anxiolytic, prescribed during *in vivo* exposures to the full stimulus. For example, a public speaking phobia might be treated by prescribing 2 mg of alprazolam 1 h prior to the delivery of a speech before a group, followed on a separate occasion with 1 mg, a third exposure with 0.5 mg, and a fourth exposure with 0.25 mg; finally, several further exposures without the benzodiazepine would firm up the now established new conditioned response of confidence.[6] Such a contingency allows for rapid exposure to the highest item on the hierarchy of Subjective Units of Distress (SUD), by adding the reinforcing qualities of benzodiazepine just prior to and during the initial exposures, and then withdrawing the drug when the experience of competently delivering a speech becomes self-reinforcing.

On the other hand, implosion therapy for anxiety and phobia would appear to improve in certain cases with the use of antidepressant medication, in particular imipramine

(Mattick, Andrews, Hadzi-Pavlovic, & Christensen, 1990; Mavissakalian, 1990). Imipramine is dosed on a continuous basis rather than only during the exposure trial. The exact mechanism of the learning-enhancing effect of imipramine has not been adequately explicated, but it is tempting to place it in the category of other "cognitive enhancers," which span many classes of medications with diverse mechanisms of action, adding to the impression of a "common factor" component to medication administration with behavioral therapy (Muse & Moore, 2012). In contrast, an example of single trial implosion therapy paired with administration of amobarbital in the treatment of PTSD demonstrates how discrete administration of a pharmacologic agent to coincide with specific behavioral interventions can increase the effectiveness of exposure techniques (Muse, 1984; Overton, 1964). A novel twist in counterconditioning through implosion techniques is the possibility of "extinction-enhancing" compounds like cannabis resin in the treatment of traumatic memory. Endocannabinoids exert amnesic effect and may facilitate extinction (forgetting) of aversive memories (Marsicano et al., 2002; Passie, Emrich, Karst, Brandt, & Halpern, 2012).

The potential use of pharmacological agents to *enhance in vitro* anxiety during implosion exposure has not been previously explored, leaving one to mere speculation. In the *in vitro* treatment of panic disorder, for example, feelings of hyperarousal—one component of anxiety/panic—could theoretically be elicited through the use of epinephrine, either injected or sublingual administration, while training for cognitive acceptance of the subjective experience, and while practicing relaxation technique to mitigate tension and fear. However, what little research that has been done with epinephrine's effect on conditioning tends to argue against this use since epinephrine itself acts as a powerful UCS for eliciting fear and for stamping the fear in through enhanced memory retrieval (Flint, Bunsey, & Riccio, 2007; Toth, Ziegler, Sun, Gresack, & Risbrough, 2013; Weinberger, Gold, & Sternberg, 1984); the point of implosion therapy is not, of course, to leave the patient with more fear than before.[7] Nonetheless, therapeutic counterconditioning occurs only once the initial fear response diminishes in the face of continued exposure, and so the possibility of prolonged sessions in which the patient rides out the initial burst of anxiety from epinephrine administration and learns the all-so-important lesson of panic attack management, "what (anxiety) goes up must come down," is not completely beyond possibility. A different approach to pharmacologically recreating the anxiety response while undergoing covert exposure might, for example, use elevated dosing of amphetamine during *in vitro* deconditioning of, say, test anxiety. In such a case, the accelerated "racing mind" and physiological correlates of hyperarousal caused in great part by norepinephrine may be approximated with this inherently reinforcing (dopaminergic-based) agent, while avoiding introducing the unconditioned fear aspect associated with induced epinephrine arousal. To the contrary, one might speculate that in the case of test anxiety, for example, contextual conditioning[8] (Childs & de Wit, 2013) would render the experience of arousal under the influence of amphetamine, while exposed to increasingly competent test taking, more rewarding with repetitive exposure.

While clomipramine and the SSRIs as standalones have proved less effective than desired with OCD symptom regulation, behavioral therapy with response prevention has become first-line treatment (Muse, Moore, & Stahl, 2013). Traditional combining of these two modalities does not appear to have much advantage (Franklin, Abramowitz, Bux, Zoellner, & Feeny, 2002). Nonetheless, exposure with response prevention in the treatment of OCD could theoretically be enhanced by pairing a fast-acting anxiolytic such as benzodiazepine, delivered intra-muscularly after successful response prevention.

Here, conditioning defies intuition: the anxiolytic, to be a reinforcer of anxiety tolerance, is best applied *after* exposure to increased anxiety, and not in anticipation of it. No such studies have been done to date, and so one is left to yearn for randomized controlled trials (RCTs) with novel pairings of cognitive-behavioral therapy (CBT) and anxiolytics (Pull, 2007).[9] Still, rewarding prolonged response prevention in severe OCD would be most helpful with those patients who find it exceedingly hard not to succumb to the compulsion (Pence, Sulkowski, & Jordan, 2010), and there is likely to be no reinforcer more potent in such circumstances than the promise of a rapidly acting anxiolytic after response prevention. This contingency is quite different from prescribing an anxiolytic *pro re nata* to avoid anxiety. Such sequencing rewards drug-taking, while dispensing an anxiolytic after self-exposure rewards, and reinforces, anxiety tolerance.

Barbara routinely spent 2 h getting to and from work by taking several buses, rather than brave the subway escalator that she had avoided for the past 5 years. She was able to work through a hierarchy of related fears with imagined exposure, and she was eventually able to ride small escalators of one-story height in vivo, but she could not get herself to take the four-story-high escalator down the Bethesda underground station to the boarding platform. She was prescribed 2 mg of alprazolam,[10] taken 60 min before arriving at the station escalator, which proved to be sufficient for her to—with difficulty—ride the escalator down. At the end of the day's work, she took the same dose of anxiolytic and was able to ride the escalator back up to the entrance of the same Metro station. The dose was successively reduced by 0.5 mg per week, until she was able to ride the escalator daily without pharmacological support.

Depression

Anergia is a common symptom associated with depression, especially major depression. Therapeutic approaches to reduce anergia are largely based on the observation that increasing the patient's level of activity breaks a self-reinforcing cycle of inactivity and, subsequently, mitigates sedentary-induced feelings of fatigue and boredom. Activation techniques such as increased behavioral investment in social and physical activities could potentially be reinforced by the use of psychostimulants, administered just prior to the prescribed effort. Vegetative signs of depression have been effectively moderated with adjunctive stimulants in a variety of populations, including the elderly (Emptage & Semla, 1996) and patients with medical conditions (Huffman & Stern, 2004; Frierson, Wey, & Tabler, 1991; Kaufmann, Cassem, Murray, & Jenike, 1984; Rosenberg, Ahmed, & Hurwitz, 1991; Woods, Tesar, Murray, & Cassem, 1986). The use of amphetamine and methylphenidate to momentarily overcome depression and, for example, allow medical patients to follow rehabilitation exercises is one potential immediate benefit. Apart from providing the depressive patient a sense of relief from anergia, stimulant medications affect the nucleus accumbens directly and tend to momentarily mitigate dysphoria, thus providing an incentive to work for this reward when stimulant medication dispensing is made contingent upon completing a prescribed therapeutic activity. A parallel use of caffeine to overcome inertia and lack of motivation associated with anhedonia is based upon the well-established "Premack principle" (Premack, 1959), in which access to desired behavior normally engaged in by the subject (drinking coffee) is made contingent upon first completing an undesired behavior such as taking a shower (Robinson & Lewinsohn, 1973; Williams, 1984); in such a contingency, the response, rather than a stimulus, provides reinforcement.

Procrastination, another ubiquitous symptom associated with depression, may be addressed behaviorally with antidepressants when such medications are made to serve as "reinforcement enhancers" (O'Donnella, Marekb, & Seidenc, 2005; Seiden, Dahms, & Shaughness, 1985), especially when applied to a differential-reinforcement-of-low-rate (DRL) operant schedule. Imipramine has been shown to have a reward-enhancing effect for depressed patients, who more positively appraise the activity engaged in while on the drug (Wichers et al., 2008), and imipramine and citalopram treatment in socially stressed rats appears to restore anhedonia and motivational deficits (Rygula et al., 2006; Von Frijtag, Van den Bos, & Spruijt, 2002). Antidepressants, then, would appear to have the potential to facilitate the learning of new behavior by enhancing the reinforcing quality of an obtained reward once an operant behavior has been exhibited. Applying DRL, which is an operant contingency that requires behavioral suppression in order to gain a reward, reductions in targeted unhealthy behavior such as procrastination may be more effectively reinforced with concomitant administration of an antidepressant. By the patient withholding a response for a brief period of 1 min ("DRL60s") such as avoiding sitting on the couch, the subject is rewarded with a desired activity such as watching TV, whose reinforcing value is now augmented by concomitant use of an antidepressant. Administration of antidepressant medication, especially the tricyclic imipramine, with a DRL regimen has the potential of facilitating a decrease in response rate of behavioral symptoms associated with depression.

In the treatment of depression, CBP emphasizes time-limited, well-targeted use of medication to further the attainment of defined therapeutic goals by reinforcing cognitive-behavioral treatment strategies. While there are exceptions, notably with bipolar disorder and major depression with psychotic features where long-term pharmacotherapy may be indicated (Blier, Keller, Pollack, & Dunner, 2007), the great majority of depression, be that major depression, dysthymia, or adjustment disorder, is guided, where possible, toward a drug-free goal within the CBP paradigm.

Joseph, a 70-year-old retiree, became depressed to the point that he failed to maintain his personal hygiene, and would spend all day in bed. He had been on SSRIs for years, but no attempt had been made during that period to integrate medication with behavioral therapy. A new regime was instituted that left the SSRI in place for its adjunctive reinforcing potential while he was rewarded for getting out of bed and showering with a psychostimulant that he felt returned some degree of energy. In his case, the stimulant was dispensed 30 min before the activities of daily living (ADLs) were attempted. Finally, he was rewarded with his much-sought-after morning espresso upon completion of the ADLs.

Psychosis

Neuroleptic medications are inherently antireinforcing (Ettenberg, 1989) in the sense that they reduce the availability of dopamine and other catecholamines in the mesolimbic system (Anscombe, 1987; Cornblatt, Lenzenweger, Dworkin, & Erlenmeyer-Kimling, 1983; Fibiger, 1978; Salamone, 1987; Salamone, Correa, Nunes, Randall, & Pardo, 2012), thereby producing an antagonistic effect on the motivation centers of the brain, potentially resulting in a degree of drug-induced anhedonia.[11] The cognitive-behavioral psychopharmacologist is aware of this, and attempts to either offset the drug's undesirable effect by increasing reinforcement to compensate for the higher stimulus threshold needed to experience pleasure, or by reducing or discontinuing the neuroleptic when feasible to reestablish greater access to the reinforcing nature of unimpeded dopaminergic pathways. In other words, the key to overcoming the demotivating influence of neuroleptics is to make up for the desensitizing of pleasure by turning up reinforcing input, or by getting the patient off this class of medication as soon as possible.

Prescribing minimal doses of neuroleptics (McGorry, Alvarez-Jimenez, & Killackey, 2013), reducing dosing (Wunderink, Nieboer, Wiersma, Sytema, & Nienhuis, 2013), and phasing out antipsychotics (Harrow, Jobe, & Faull, 2012) or interrupting continuous use (Harrow & Jobe, 2013) have been found in some cases to be as or more effective than the more established practice of continuous, indefinite prescribing (Torrey, 2014) in the long-term management of psychosis. What is more, reducing antipsychotic medication potentially mitigates negative symptoms of psychosis by allowing for greater access to reinforcement derived from social contact, vocational competence, and personal development (Isel, 2013), all of which are therapeutic goals in themselves, but which are also experienced as rewarding and gratifying (Gumley & Schwannauer, 2006). The CBP approach emphasizes blending medications in a reinforcing manner with cognitive-behavioral goals of treatment, and the reduction in antipsychotic medication, where appropriate, can itself be presented as a therapeutic goal that motivates the patient to exert effort to avoid the need for medication. It also further reinforces recovery by potentially reducing negative symptoms associated with schizophrenia and by increasing the patient's availability to do therapeutic work, for even the most recalcitrant symptoms of schizophrenia are amenable to therapeutic change through behavioral modification strategies that increase access to greater reinforcement (Mitchell & Stoffelmayr, 1973).

William, a 50-year-old diagnosed with schizophrenia, had been on neuroleptics since he was in his late adolescence. He had not had any active positive signs of psychosis for more than a decade, but he was plagued with multiple negative symptoms, including flat affect, cognitive blunting, a seeming lack of interest in other people, and an inability to feel pleasure or act spontaneously. He was motivated to discontinue antipsychotic medications for years, but when he attempted to do so he usually met with skepticism from his treating prescriber, and so he would drop out of therapy and stop taking his medication against medical advice, only to find that his decision was followed by rough periods in which his blunted affect turned into anxiety as he was unable to change his social isolation on his own.

After consulting a CBP-minded practitioner, William agreed to work toward reducing his neuroleptic medication to the degree that he was able to keep up an effort to become more socially engaged. His belief, and the belief of his provider, that he could remain off psychiatric medications under proper conditions allowed him to feel more optimistic, and he found the energy and commitment to attend group therapy, and to venture into new social venues. His medication was reduced slowly, and several of the negative symptoms improved, allowing for more expressiveness and greater social success. Parenthetically, he had no recurrence of positive symptoms of schizophrenia at a 1-year follow up.[12]

Other syndromes

ADHD is remarkably responsive to stimulant medication, which not only increases the ability to attend through activating the dopaminergic pathways along the cortico-striato-thalamo-cortical loop that runs from the dorsolateral prefrontal cortex to the striatal complex and back (Stahl, 2013), but also enhances reward appreciation by potentiating the orbitofrontal reward/motivational pathway (Rubia et al., 2009), as well as the mesolimbic reward system. The possibility that ADHD is derived in part from a reward deficiency syndrome (Blum et al., 2008) that reduces motivation for compliance and may even contribute to oppositional defiant disorder (ODD) is corroborated by neuroimaging research showing that activity in the nucleus accumbens of the ventro-striatal dopamine reward system is reduced in children and adults with ADHD (Carmona et al., 2009; Volkow, 2009).

The behavioral management of ADHD relies largely on the patient's motivation to make an "extra effort" to overcome the interference of inattention and impulsivity, and certain contingencies that activate the dopaminergic-related reward system may better reinforce such an effort. Phasic dopamine firing patterns, composed of bursts and pauses, are generally found to be more rewarding than equivalent tonic firing. Nonetheless, receptor occupancy, ultimately, is dependent on the balance between tonic and phasic firing modes (Dreyer, Herrik, Berg, & Hounsgaard, 2010), and amphetamine, while eliciting both phasic and tonic release like methylphenidate (Covey et al., 2013), tends to favors phasic release over methylphenidate preparations (Devilbiss & Berridge, 2007), as methylphenidate may be more disposed to suppress phasic firing at clinical doses by augmenting inhibitory autoreceptors (Offermanns & Rosenthal, 2008). In this regard, phasic dopamine release creates greater immediate reward-seeking behavior (Aboitiz, 2007; Redgrave & Gurney, 2006), while the ultimate long-term effect of motivation on instrumental rates of responding is mediated through dopamine's influence on the net reward rate, which predicts sustained motivational states are better enhanced by tonic dopamine release (Niv, 2008). In addition, the reward component to psychostimulants is greatly enhanced at doses greater than the low clinical doses standardly used in ADHD treatment. Implications for therapy of these different firing patterns have not been clarified, but it may be worth keeping in mind that the use of low-dose tonic release methylphenidate may be more conducive to sustained learning over time, which is, after all, the goal of ADHD management, while higher-dosed phasic release preparations such as amphetamine may provide more of a reward for discrete, extra efforts such as preparing for major exams. Also, the greater immediate effect of phasic dopamine release over tonic release is likely to have implications for Pavlovian conditioning, where greater appreciable effect is more readily bonded in associational pairings. An area for future study may be the effect of psychostimulants in Pavlovian-to-instrumental-transfer (PIT) (Talmi, Seymour, Dayan, & Dolan, 2008). In this sense, one might speculate that a phasic release medication initially paired with studying, to countercondition previous opposition to studying, might best be followed by a tonic release preparation for greater sustained motivation and effort.

Jordan was prescribed detroamphetamine salt for ADHD without much improvement in his school performance. Although he was compliant to the extent that he took the medication, when he took it it was more on his terms, and more often than not he took the drug on the weekend rather than during hours of instruction or study. He routinely missed his CBT appointments with his psychologist but kept his psychiatry appointments to renew the amphetamine prescription. Subsequently, with coordinated informed consent involving the patient and his parents, the formulary and protocol for dispensing his medication was changed in order to capitalize on drug-seeking behavior: sequenced in accordance with the Premack principle to reinforce behavioral therapy and school attendance, Jordan's stimulant medication was made available only after perfect attendance in behavioral therapy. The medication was changed to methylphenidate during the school week, and was then only dispensed by the school nurse at the beginning of the school day; his parents subsequently dispensed amphetamine on the weekends but only during study periods at home. His therapy and school absenteeism fell sharply when he was not given stimulant medication on the days he missed school or his behavioral therapy appointment, and his homework improved with the aid of extra medication dispensed during times of home study.

Chronic Pain is replete with examples of how classical conditioning (Waschulewski-Floruss, Miltner, Brody, & Braun, 1994) and instrumental learning (Fordyce et al., 1973) are involved in the acquisition and maintenance of chronic pain syndromes. Most therapeutic recommendations for behaviorally dispensing pain medications are meant to avoid or reduce any connection between perceived pain and subsequent drug-seeking behavior. Scheduling opioids on a set temporal contingency, rather than dispensing pain medicine on demand, is one way to disassociate pain from drug use. Providing CBT to reinforce low-abusing drug-seeking behavior (Jamison et al., 2010) by making future access to narcotic contingent upon demonstrated moderate use is another way of managing opioid use in chronic pain. Increasing the rate of administration according to the activity level of the patient through "activity-contingent" dispensing is still another way of using pain medication to increase activity level. In activity-contingent dispensing, the pain-augmenting activity is initially anticipated and pain medication is given prior to the activity in order to reduce discomfort during it (Ries, Miller, & Fiellin, 2009). Such a regimen has the potential for increasing activity not only because the pain's interference is temporarily reduced by analgesics but also because the pleasant nature of moderately high doses of opioids acts as a UCR that is later associated with activity. Respondent conditioning notwithstanding, from an operant conditioning vantage, however, it may be argued that dispensing the opioid *after* activity is completed better propels the therapeutic goal of increased exercise and activity. In this sense, increase in activity level is one of the central behavioral goals in the treatment of chronic benign pain, and pain medication can acts as the horse that pulls the cart if it is made contingent upon first participating in physical exercise and social interaction. In such a case, it is wise to keep, at least initially, the reinforcer–response–cost low in order to motivate effort (Bennett, Stoops, & Rush, 2013; Stoops Lile, Glaer, Hays, & Rush, 2011); for, if too much effort is required, or the reinforcer is insufficiently strong, patients might very well forego the reward, and avoid the activity.

Joanne's consumption of pro re nata narcotic analgesics doubled and then tripled over a period of 1 month as she continued to complain of severe neuralgia. She was counseled that her level of consumption was unsustainable, and she agreed to a gradual reduction to initial dose levels, which were dispensed on an invariant time-determined schedule. She further agreed to the plan that additional medication would be administered following increases in activity, and the level of activity would be increased gradually. In 1 month, she was consuming half as much medication and performing 500% more activity.

Addictions provide an opportunity to appreciate the interface between biology—especially pharmacology—and biopsychosocial learning. Incentive sensitization theory of addictions (Robinson and Berridge, 2008) suggests that Pavlovian association between the abused substance and UCR of pleasure derived in the mesolimbic system can, with repeated exposure, potentiate a heightened response to the substance through additional learned CRs; what is more, co-occurring instrumental behavior can become resistant to change through operant conditioning that increases reward value, and reinforces learned drug-seeking behavior through a circular stimulus–response–reward loop.

Treatment based on the classical condition paradigm is perhaps best exemplified by cue exposure techniques in which *in vivo* or *in vitro* exposure techniques are used to reduce craving for drugs/alcohol through extinction strategies for counterconditioning CSs that were associated with cravings (Eliany & Rush, 1992). Such cues include the smell of alcohol, the sound of music present in clubs where drugs were purchased or consumed, etc. Studies have found that patients can maintain cue-reassigned avoidant activity after substance abuse treatment (Chiauzzi & Liljegren, 1993), and cue exposure has demonstrated improved abstinence (Blakely & Baker, 1980; Hodgson & Rankin, 1982), while *in vivo* exposure has proven more effective than covert exposure (Rankin, Hodgson, & Stockwell, 1983).

An example of operant conditioning turned, inadvertently, classical conditioning is that of alcohol deterrent therapy with disulfiram, which has been shown to be effective in a meta-analysis that included 35,000 patients (Elkins, 1991). Deterrent therapy works by negatively reinforcing efforts to avoid the punishing effects of alcohol consumption while on disulfiram. Krampe, Stawicki, and Wagner (2007) also showed in a 7-year follow up that supervised administration of disulfiram as an adjunctive to substance abuse treatment increased abstinence. Nonetheless, "deterrent therapy" often becomes aversion therapy when the patient consumes alcohol while on disulfiram. To this author's knowledge, there are no controlled studies on programmed aversion therapy in this area, where the patient would consume alcohol while on disulfiram in the presence of a behavioral therapist. It begs the question of whether the patient is best served by allowing such adverse effects to occur randomly outside of the therapeutic milieu, when deterrent therapy inadvertently, and perhaps inevitably, becomes unsupervised aversion therapy.

Operant conditioning approaches in substance abuse treatment emphasize the use of reward to increase motivation to avoid substances. Increasing compliance with drug management goals (Viswanathan et al., 2012) is a therapeutic challenge that has found some success in contingency contracting in substance abuse treatment (Higgins, Silverman, & Heil, 2010). Stitzer, Bigelow, and Liebson (1980), for example, showed that using cash to pay for drug-free urine samples was successful, and in separate studies voucher exchange for retail items has been successfully used as reinforcers (Silverman et al., 1996a, 1996b). Liebson, Tommasello, and Bigelow (1978) found that dispensing methadone contingent upon taking disulfiram among dual addiction patients with dependency on alcohol and narcotics resulted in a significant reduction in drinking. On the other hand, Soyka and Rösner (2008) found in a metanalysis that the opiate antagonist naltrexone reduced pleasure associated with alcohol and may be helpful in abstinence management of problematic drinking. Nonetheless, if naltrexone were to inadvertently raise the threshold for derived pleasure from other activities, it could, in the long run, set the patient up for increased pleasure-seeking behavior that could, ultimately, lead him or her back to substance abuse. Other pharmacological agents that show promise for being woven into a behaviorally driven treatment approach for substance abuse include nalmefene and Suboxone® (buphrenorphine and naloxone).

Janet had a drinking problem before she became addicted to oxycodone following a low back injury. After detox from both substances, she was placed on naltrexone and disulfiram, concurrent with behavioral therapy. One phase of her treatment consisted of a single trial of cue exposure therapy in the prescriber/therapist's office in which the smell and taste of alcohol were counterconditioned by provoking a reaction to disulfiram through ingesting a small amount of alcohol; her bottle of oxycodone, as well as the sight of displayed pills, were also paired with the nausea generated in the same session.

Sexual disorders can be divided, for the sake of convenience, into performance disorders (dysfunctions) and impulse disorders (paraphilias). Most psychosexual performance disorders are anxiety-based and respond to the same desensitization approaches used in treating phobias, and are therefore best treated with CBT alone. Nonetheless, there is limited use for SSRIs for initially retarding ejaculation in the very anxious male with premature ejaculation, just as the initial use of sildenafil may be indicated for the otherwise-nonresponsive male with erectile disorder (Muse, 2012). In both cases the drug is used in conjunction with cognitive-behavioral approaches, and gradually discontinued as therapeutic progress is made. Diazepam has been used in much the same way with vaginismus, providing initial anxiolytic and muscle relaxant effects at the beginning of an otherwise unresponsive case. For trauma-derived vaginismus, abreaction therapy (Poole, Wuez, & Agrawal, 2010) with the use of amobarbital has been used successfully (Mikhail, 1976). While the use of SSRIs and benzodiazepines are incorporated into a systematic desensitization paradigm, abreaction therapy may be conceived of, from a behaviorist's perspective, as a variety of implosion therapy.

The classical conditioning explanation of paraphilia is based on the assumption that whatever stimuli were present during an early sexual experience may become paired with the UCR of sexual arousal and orgasm (Atkins, 2004; Marshall, 2007; O'Donohue & Plaud, 1994). In the example of fetishism, masturbation (UCS) to orgasm (UCR) while wearing lingerie (CS) may later leads to arousal (CR) in the presence of lingerie. Paraphilic interest may develop from both a biological predisposition toward risk taking and sensation seeking (Kafka, 1997; Kafka & Hennen, 1999), plus early exposure to aberrant stimuli involved in fetishism, voyeurism, etc. (Wiederman, 2003). Social learning theory further suggests that the paraphilic behavior is learned from watching someone else model in a similar fashion (Bradford, Bowlet, & Pawlak, 1992).

Aversion therapy for the treatment of paraphilia makes use of induced anxiety, paired with CS associated with paraphilic interest, to generate a competing conditioned behavior. Pairings of smelling salts with CS such as pornographic material provides for a new conditioned avoidant response. Along these lines, operant conditioning can be added to Pavlovian pairing by holding one's breath for an extended time while viewing pornographic material; such an approach creates the conditions for learning a conditioned escape behavior of therapeutic value (looking away from pornography is reinforced with escaping the anguish associated with relative oxygen deprivation as the patient is subsequently instructed to breathe in).

John attempted treatment of premature ejaculation only to experience precipitous orgasm with his partner before the behavioral "start–stop" technique could begin. He was placed on fluoxetine and experienced a greater latency period to ejaculation, which allowed him to subsequently practice the stop–start technique and to gain confidence as well as competence with the technique before fluoxetine was gradually discontinued.

Anthony had a long history of exhibitionism, and he had just lost his security clearance for exposing himself to women as he drove next to them on the beltway. He was placed on paroxetine,[13] *which reduced his libido and gave him a sense of control over his impulse that he had never experienced before. He was then asked to imagine exposing himself to women while he held his breath in session with his therapist. He soon found that he lost his arousal after 20 s of holding his breath, and that his interest in the exhibitionist fantasy vanished at the same time. Still, he was encouraged to hold his breath another 30 s while forcing the fantasy forward. Ultimately he found great relief when instructed to breathe again after he was told he could drop the fantasy from his mind.*

Conclusion

CBP is based on the biopsychosocial paradigm in which health and disease/dysfunction are conceptualized as balance vs. disequilibrium within and among the major systems (biological, psychological, social) comprising the individual. Integrated mental health treatment reaps benefits from looking at the whole individual diagnostically, weighing the relative importance of the various systems involved in a given presenting problem, and from attending to multimodal intervention options, sized to the need of the particular case. Beyond this integrated approach, however, is the possibility of harvesting an even greater therapeutic effect by cultivating the provider's awareness of not only how different therapeutic modalities can complement each other, but also by discovering what such diverse modalities have in common: how do they reinforce therapeutic progress and improvement through conditioned learning?

Beyond the occasional use of psychotherapy to reinforce medication compliance (Wright, & Thase, 2010),[14] and beyond the combination of medication with psychosocial approaches to bolster treatment through a combined, dualistic approach, CBP offers the possibility of a dialectical synthesis, a new outcome that is greater than the mere combination of treatments, by fusing psychopharmacology with psychosocial treatment through their common basis in conditioning.

Unfortunately, the role of medication as a potential reinforcer for attaining psychotherapeutic goals has not received its due attention. In stark contrast to the evidence-based treatment recommendations of the previous chapters in this book, much of what has been presented in the present chapter is extrapolated from serendipitous observations and deduced from theoretical extensions, rather than derived from inductive conclusions based on multiple controlled studies. Herein lies the challenge: how can the clinician apply principles of learning to the integration of psychopharmacology with psychosocial approaches when the evidence supporting such an approach is scant to nonexistent?

Perhaps it is the promise that allures, the promise of something beyond the current combinations and permutations of treatment approaches; something that may guide research along established principles of learning, to look for effect where one might predict it, rather than pairing approaches randomly to see if a discernable difference is determined through *a posteriori* statistical analyses.

For the clinician, awareness of potential conditioning effects, even in the paucity of published studies, cannot be a disadvantage. While it is too early for CBP to be guided by established best practices, the sagacious clinician, mindful of the potential effects of conditioned learning, may be his or her own guide to more effective therapeutic results.

Notes

1 Conditioning paradigms (classical, operant, and social learning) are the foundation upon which psychology rests; analogous, arguably, to the theory of evolution for biology, or quantum mechanics for physics.

2 There is some evidence that other neural pathways within the brain, independent of the mesolimbic system, may also have a reinforcing/motivating component to their activation (Ikemoto, 2010; Robertson, 1989). These pathways include the prefrontal cortex, among other structures.

3 If placebo is the CS that elicits a conditioned response (feeling better), then the innate UCR of feeling enhanced well-being is elicited from the UCS of benevolent human contact, directly through talk therapy or indirectly through prescribing, and this, I contend, is the "common factor" that has eluded our understanding. That is, the initial basis of the common response to therapeutic intervention, including the placebo, is a respondent behavior, which may be further potentiated, and directed toward specific therapeutic goals, by operant contingencies that subsequently reinforce the healthy direction through maximizing rewards that activate the motivational centers of the brain.

4 Siegel, Hinson, and Krank, 1982, showed that situation-specific tolerance is capable of preventing the fatal consequence of a lethal-sized opiate overdose. When rats were given a large dose of morphine following morphine dosing in an environment substantially differing from the one in which they experienced the effects related to morphine, signs of overdose rapidly appeared, and in a few cases led to death. In contrast, rats given lethal-sized morphine doses in the same circumstances where morphine was previous

consumed had a substantially smaller effect; presumably, because the substance was given in the accustomed environment, the associated environmental cues elicited a modulating physical response to the substance. Gerevich et al. (2005) later found evidence of the same mechanism within a fatal overdose of a young man.

5 See page 340–341 for further discussion of the Premack principle.

6 Chronic use of benzodiazepines without behavioral therapy in treating social anxiety favors the reinforcement–loss hypothesis (Corfield-Sumner & Stolerman, 1978; Schuster, Dockens, & Woods, 1966; Wolgin, 1989), which in this case predicts increased drug tolerance when the drug interferes with social skills (Smith, 1990). Contingent tolerance will emerge in situations where the initial effect of the drug is to produce a loss of reinforcement (e.g., sedation causes further social withdrawal), but, when used in conjunction with cognitive-behavioral approaches, the drug's sedating effects can be woven into the therapeutic task of increased social interaction, thereby obviating any tolerance due to loss of reinforcement through failed social interaction. In fact, one might hope that success with social interaction increases reinforcement and, if not enhancing the drug effect, makes subsequent reduction in drug dosage less noticeable.

7 Stanley Schachter and Jerome Singer (1962) demonstrated the cognitive component to emotional response to epinephrine in which subjects forewarned that the drug was arousing were less frightened of the biological correlates of injection. Hence, the need to pay attention to the cognitive repercussions of the verbal delivery of any recommended therapeutic approach.

8 That is, experiencing D-amphetamine in a consistent environment produces context-dependent enhancement of its rewarding efficacy.

9 Until experimental evidence is available on such a novel pairing, I do not advocate applying a similar procedure in clinical practice.

10 Alprazolam presents, of the benzodiazepines, the most attractive profile for counterconditioning purposes as it is fast acting, early peaking, and short lasting in its anxiolytic effects.

11 Hence, the prevalence of nicotine intake by patients on antipsychotic medication in an attempt to mitigate the effects of neuroleptics (Šagud et al., 2009): Smoking stimulates dopaminergic activity in the brain by inducing its release and inhibiting its degradation, and may reduce deficits relative to dopamine hypofunction in prefrontal cortex. Cigarette smoke also increases the activity of CYP 1A2 enzymes, thus decreasing the concentration of many drugs and, in turn, alleviating cognitive deficit, reducing extrapyramidal side effects induced by antipsychotic medication, and rekindling a degree of pleasure associated with increased levels of dopamine.
Paradoxically, there is evidence that some D_2-specific neuroleptics administered at a lower dose may demonstrate a "prohedonic" property that potentiates reinforcement (Guyon, Assouly-Besse, Biala, Puech, & Thiébot, 1993).

12 In discontinuing antipsychotic medication, it is essential that a good deal of patient education occur previously, in which the patient is instructed on prodromal signs of impeding relapse that argue for reinitiating the medication.

13 Paroxetine, in a meta-analysis, has been shown to be the most sexually deadening among the SSRIs (Reichenpfader et al., 2014.)

14 Festinger (1957) might argue compliance is increased if the patient feels he has made the choice to start medication, rather than being persuaded or "convinced" by the clinician; ergo, informed consent for every medication change is a potent reinforcer of that medication's effectiveness. Moreover, informed consent is not only ethically essential but, as Skinner (1986) states, it is good conditioning practice. While a subject does not need to be aware of reinforcement contingencies for them to be effective, the patient is not only a subject, but a person, and voluntary participation in any learning task is a distinct advantage.

References

Aboitiz, F. (2007). Dynamics of a neuromodulator—I. The role of dopaminergic signaling in goal-directed behavior. In F. Aboitiz, & D. Cosmelli (Eds.), *From attention to goal-directed behavior: Neurodynamical, methological and clinical trends*. New York: Springer.

Adinoff, B. (2004). Neurobiologic processes in drug reward and addiction. *Harvard Review of Psychiatry, 12*, 305–320.

Arden, J. (2010). *Rewire your brain: Think your way to a better life.* Oxford: John Wiley and Sons.

Atkins, C. K. (2004). The role of Pavlovian conditioning in sexual behaviour: A comparative analysis of human and nonhuman animals. *International Journal of Comparative Psychology, 17*, 241–262.

Anscombe, F. (1987). The disorder of consciousness in schizophrenia. *Schizophrenia Bulletin, 13*, 241–260.

Balster, R. (1998). The neural basis of inhalant abuse. *Drug and Alcohol Dependence, 51*, 207–214.

Bandura, A. (1973). *Aggression: A social learning analysis*. Oxford: Prentice-Hall.

Bandura, A. (1997). *Self-efficacy: The exercise of control*. New York: Freeman.

Battig, K. (2013). Nicotinic and non-nicotinic aspects of smoking: Motivation and behavioral effects, In J. Snel, & M. Lorist (Eds.), *Nicotine, caffeine and social drinking: Behavior and brain function.* New York: Routledge.

Balfour, D. (1991). The influence of stress on psychopharmacological response to nicotine. *British Journal of Addictions, 86*, 489–493.

Bardo, M., Neisewander, J., & Kelly, T. (2013). Individual differences and social influences on the neurobehavioral pharmacology of abused drugs. *Pharmacological Reviews, 65*, 255–290.

Bechara, A. (2005). Decision making, impulse control and loss of willpower to resist drugs: A neurocognitive perspective. *Nature Neuroscience, 8*, 1458–1463.

Benedetti, F., Mayberg, H., Wager, T., Stohler, C. S., & Zubieta, J.-K. (2005). Neurobiological mechanisms of the placebo effect. *Journal of Neuroscience, 25*, 10390–10402.

Benight, C. & Bandura, A. (2004). Social cognitive theory of posttraumatic recovery: The role of perceived self-efficacy. *Behaviour Research and Therapy, 42*, 1129–1148.

Beninger, R., Hoffman, D., & Mazurski, E. (1989). Receptor subtype-specific dopaminergic agents and conditioned behavior. *Neuroscience and Biobehavioral Reviews, 13*, 113–122.

Bennett, J., Stoops, W., & Rush, C. (2013). Alternative reinforcer response cost impacts methamphetamine choice in humans. *Pharmacology Biochemistry and Behavior, 103*, 481–506.

Bershad, A., Seiden, J., & de Wit, H. (2015). Effects of buprenorphine on responses to social stimuli in healthy adults. *Psychoneuroendocrinology, 63*, 43–49.

Berni, R., & Fordyce, W. (1977). *Behavior modification and the nursing process.* Maryland Heights, MO: Mosby.

Bickel, W., DeGrandpre, R., & Higgins, S. (1993). Behavioral economics: A novel experimental approach to the study of drug dependence. *Drug and Alcohol Dependence, 33*, 173–192.

Bickel, W., Marsch, L., & Carroll, M. (2000). Deconstructing relative reinforcing efficacy and situating the measures of pharmacological reinforcement with behavioral economics: A theoretical proposal. *Psychopharmacology, 153*, 44–56.

Bieber, C., Fernandez, K., Borsook, D., Brennan, M. J., Butler, S. F., Jamison, R. N., . . . & Katz, N. P. (2008). Retrospective accounts of initial subjective effect of opioids in patients treated with pain who do and do not develop opioid addiction: A pilot case-control study. *Experimental Clinical Psychopharmacology, 16*, 429–434.

Blakely, R., & Baker, R. (1980). An exposure approach to alcohol abuse, *Behaviour Research and Therapy, 18*, 319–325.

Blum, K., Chen, A., Braverman, E., Comings, D. E., Chen, T. J. H., Arcuri, V., . . . & Oscar-Berman, M. (2008). Attention-deficit-hyperactivity disorder and reward deficiency syndrome. *Neuropsychiatric Disease and treatment, 4*, 893–917.

Boyd, C., McCabe, S., Cranford, J., & Young, A. (2006). Adolescents' motivation to abuse prescriptive medications. *Pediatrics, 118*, 2472–2480.

Bradford, J. M., Boulet, J., & Pawlak, A. (1992). The paraphilias: A multiplicity of deviant behaviours. *Canadian Journal of Psychiatry, 37*, 104–108.

Breggin, P. (2008). *Brain disabling treatments in psychiatry.* New York: Springer.

Cannon, C., & Palmiter, R. (2003). Reward without dopamine. *Journal of Neuroscience, 23*, 10827–10831.

Carmona, S., Proal, E., Hoekzema, E., Gispert, J. D., Picado, M., Moreno I, . . . & Vilarroya, O. (2009). Ventro-striatal reductions underpin symptoms of hyperactivity and impulsivity in attention deficit/hyperactivity disorder. *Biological Psychiatry, 66*, 972–977.

Chiauzzi, E. J., & Liljegren, S. (1993). Taboo topics in addiction treatment: An empirical review of clinical folklore, *Journal of Substance Abuse Treatment, 10*, 303–316.

Childs, E, & de Wit, H. (2013). Contextual conditioning enhances the psychostimulant and incentive properties of d-amphetamine in humans. *Addict Biology, 18*, 985–992.

Ciaramella, A., Paroli, M., & Poli, P. (2013). An emerging dimension in psychosomatic medicine: The nocebo phenomenon in the management of chronic pain. *International Scholarly research Notices: Neuroscience*, Article ID 574526.

Colloca, L., & Benedetti, F. (2005). Placebos and painkillers: Is mind as real as matter? *Nature Reviews/Neuroscience, 6*, 545–552.

Colloca, L. & Miller, F. (2011). How placebo responses are formed: A learning perspective. *Philosophical Transactions of the Royal Society B, 366*, 1859–1869.

Corfield-Sumner, P. & Stolerman, I. (1978). Behavioral tolerance. In D. Blackman, & D. Sanger (Eds.), *Contemporary research in behavioral pharmacology.* New York: Plenum.

Cornblatt, B., Lenzenweger, M. K., Dworkin, P., & Erlenmeyer-Kimling, L. (1983). Positive and negative schizophrenic symptoms, attention, and information processing. *Schizophrenia Bulletin, 11*, 397–408.

Covey, D., Juliano, S., & Garris, P (2013). Amphetamine elicits opposing actions on readily releasable and reserve pools for dopamine. *PLoS One, 3*, 8.
Couvousier, S., Fournel, J., Ducrot, R., Kolsky, M., & Koetschet, P. (1953). Propriété pharmacodynamiques du chlor-hydrate de chloro-3-10-phenorthiazine. *Archives Internationales de Pharmacodynamie et de Thérapie, 92*, 305–361.
De la Fuente-Fernandez, R. (2009). The placebo-reward hypothesis: Dopamine and the placebo effect. *Parkinsonism Related Disorders, Supplement 3*, 72–74.
De la Fuente-Fernandez, R., Lidstone, S., & Stoessl, A. (2006). Placebo effect and dopamine release. *Journal of Neural Transmission, 70*, 415–418.
De la Fuente-Fernandez, R., & Stoess, A. (2002). The biochemical bases for reward: Implications for the placebo effect. *Evaluation and the Health Professions, 25*, 387–398.
De la Fuente-Fernandez, R., & Stoessl, A. (2004). The biochemical bases of the placebo effect. *Science and Engineering Ethics, 10*, 143–150.
DeMartini, K., & Carey, K. (2011). The role of anxiety sensitivity and drinking motives in predicting alcohol use: A critical review. *Clinical Psychology Review, 31*, 169–177.
Devilbiss, D., & Berridge, C. (2006). Low-dose methylphenidate actions on tonic and phasic locus coeruleus discharge. *Journal of Pharmacology and Experimental Therapeutics, 319*, 1327–1335.
Dews, P. (1958). Studies on behavior: Stimulant actions of methamphetamine. *Journal of Pharmacology and Experimental Therapeutics, 122*, 137–147.
Dews, P., & Wenger, G. (1977). Rate dependency of the behavioral effects of amphetamine. In Thompson & Dews (Eds.), *Advances in behavioral pharmacology*. New York: Academic Press.
Dreyer, J., Herrik, K., Berg, R., & Hounsgaard, J. D. (2010). Influence of phasic and tonic dopamine release on receptor activation. *Journal of Neuroscience, 30*, 14273–14283.
Blier, P., Keller, M., Pollack, M. & Dunner, D. (2007). Preventing recurrent depression: Long-term treatment of major depressive disorder. *Journal of Clinical Psychiatry, 9*, 214–223.
Eliany, M., & Rush, B. (1992). *The effectiveness of prevention and treatment programs for alcohol and other drug problems: A review of evaluation studies*. (Unpublished report). Ottawa: Health and Welfare Canada.
Elkins, R. (1991). An appraisal of chemical aversion (emetic therapy) approaches to alcoholism treatment. *Behaviour Research and Therapy, 29*, 387–413.
Emptage, R., & Semla, T. (1996). Depression in the medically ill elderly: a focus on methylphenidate. *Annals of Pharmacotherapy, 30*, 151–157.
Erdogan, S. (2010). Quetiapine in substance abuse disorders, abuse and dependence possibility: A review. *Turkish Journal of Psychiatry, 21*, 167–175.
Ettenberg, A. (1989). Dopamine, neuroleptics and reinforced behavior. *Neuroscience and Biobehavioral Reviews, 13*, 105–111.
Festinger, L. (1957). *A theory of cognitive dissonance*. Stanford, CA: Stanford University Press.
Fibiger, H. (1978). Drugs and reinforcement mechanisms: A critical review of the catecholamine theory. *Annual Review of Pharmacology and Toxicology, 18*, 370–56.
Finniss, D., Kaptchuk, T., Miller, F., & Benedetti, F. (2010). Placebo effect: Biological, clinical and ethical advances. *Lancet, 20*, 686–695.
Flint, R., Bunsey, M., & Riccio, D. (2007). Epinephrine-induced enhancement of memory retrieval for inhibitory avoidance conditioning in preweanling Sprague-Dawley rats. *Developmental Psychobiology, 49*, 303–311.

Fordyce, W. (1976). *Behavioural methods for chronic pain and illness.* Maryland Heights, MO: Mosby.
Fordyce, W. (1984). Behavioural science and chronic pain. *Postgraduate Medical Journal, 60,* 865–868.
Fordyce, W., Fowler, R., Lehmann, J., Delateur, B. J., Sand, P. L., & Trieschmann, R. B. (1973). Operant conditioning in the treatment of chronic pain. *Archives of Physical Medicine and Rehabilitation, 54,* 399–408.
Franklin, M., Abramowitz, J., Bux Jr., D., Zoellner, L. A., & Feeny, N. C. (2002). Cognitive–behavioral therapy with and without medication in the treatment of obsessive–compulsive disorder. *Professional Psychology: Research and Practice, 33,* 162–168.
Frierson, R., Wey, J., & Tabler, J. (1991). Psychostimulants for depression in the medically ill. *American Family Physician, 43,* 163–170.
Garcia J., Kimeldorf, D., & Koelling, R. (1955). Conditioned aversion to saccharin resulting from exposure to gamma radiation. *Science, 122,* 157–158.
Gardner, E. (1992). Cannabinoid interactions with brain reward systems: The neurobiological basis of cannabinoid abuse. In L. Murphy, & A. Bartke (Eds.), *Marijuana/cannabinoids neurology and neurophysiology.* Boca Raton, FL: CRC Press.
Garrett, B., & Griffiths, R. (1997). The role of dopamine in the behavioral effects of caffeine in animas and man. *Pharmacology Biochemistry and Behavior, 57,* 533–541.
Geller, I., & Seifter, J. (1960). The effects of meprobamate, barbiturates, d-amphetamine and promazine on experimentally-induced conflict in the rat. *Psychopharmacologia, 1,* 482–492.
Gerevich, J., Bácskai, E., Farkas, L., & Danics, Z. (2005). Case report: A case report: Pavlovian conditioning as a risk factor of heroin "overdose" death. *Harm Reduction Journal, 2,* 11.
Goode, E. (1972). A sociological perspective on drugs and drug use. In E. Goode, *Drugs in american society.* New York: Alfred A. Knopf, Inc.
Grace, A. (2002). The tonic/phasic model of dopamine system regulation and its implications for understanding alcohol and psychostimulant craving. *Addiction, 95,* S119–S128.
Grawe, K. (2007). *Neuropsychotherapy.* London: Lawrence Erlbaum Associates.
Grencavage, L. M., & Norcross, J. C. (1990). Where are the commonalities among the therapeutic common factors? *Professional Psychology: Research and Practice, 21,* 372–378.
Griffiths, R., Bigelow, G., & Henningfield, J. (1980). Similarities in animal and human drug taking behavior. In N. K. Mello (Ed.), *Advances in substance abuse,* Vol. I, 1–90. Greenwich, CT: JAI Press.
Griffiths, R. Johnson, M., Carducci, M., Umbricht, A., Richards, W. A., Richards, B. D., . . . & Klinedinst, M. A. (2016). Psilocybin produces substantial and sustained decreases in depression and anxiety in patients with life-threatening cancer: A randomized double-blind trial. *Journal of Psychopharmacology, 30,* 1181–1197.
Gualtieri, T. (2004). *Brain injury and mental retardation: Cognitive enhancers and neuroprotectors.* London: Lippincott, Williams & Wilkins.
Gumley, A., & Schwannauer, M. (2006). *Staying well after psychosis: A cognitive interpersonal approach to recovery and relapse prevention.* Chichester: Wiley.
Guyon, A., Assouly-Besse, F., Biala, G., Puech, A. J., & Thiébot, M. H. (1993). Potentiation by low dose of selected neuroleptics of food-induced conditioned place preference in rats. *Psychopharmacology, 110,* 460–466.

Heinz, A., Lilje, T., Kassel, D., & de Wit, H. (2012). Quantifying reinforcement value and demand for psychoactive substances in humans. *Current Drug Abuse Review, 5,* 257–272.

Hernandez, G., Hamdani, S., Rajabi, H., Conover, K., Stewart, J., Arvanitogiannis, A., & Shizgal, P. (2006). Prolonged rewarding stimulation of the rat medial forebrain bundle: Neurochemical and behavioral consequences. *Behavioral Neuroscience, 120,* 888–904.

Hollister, L. (1986). Pharmacotherapeutic considerations in anxiety disorders. *Journal of Clinical Psychiatry, 47,* 33–36.

Harrow, M., & Jobe, T. (2013). Does long-term treatment of schizophrenia with antipsychotic medications facilitate recovery? *Schizophrenia Bulletin, 39,* 962–965.

Harrow, M., Jobe, T., & Faull, R. (2012). Do all schizophrenia patients need antipsychotic treatment continuously throughout their lives? A 20-year longitudinal study. *Psychological Medicine, 42,* 2145–2155.

Häuser, W., Hansen, E., & Enck, P. (2012) Nocebo phenomena in medicine: Their relevance in everyday clinical practice. *Deutsches Ärzteblatt International, 109,* 459–465.

Higgins, S., Silverman, K., & Heil, S. (2010). *Contingency management in substance abuse treatment.* New York: Guilford Press.

Hodgson, R. J., & Rankin, H. J. (1982), Cue exposure and relapse prevention. In W. M. Hay, & P. E. Nathan (Eds.), *Clinical case studies in the behavioral treatment of alcoholism.* New York: Plenum.

Hughes, J., Gulliver, S., Amori, G., Mireanlt, G. C., & Fenwick, J. F. (1989). Effects of instructions and nicotine on smoking cessation, withdraw symptoms and self-administration of nicotine gum. *Psychopharmacology, 99,* 486–491.

Huffman, J., & Stern, T. (2004). Using psychostimulants to treat depression in the medically ill. *Care Companion to Journal of Clinical Psychiatry, 6,* 44–46.

Husain, M., & Mehta, M. (2011). Cognitive enhancement by drugs in health and disease. *Trends in Cognitive Science, 15,* 28–36.

Ikemoto, S. (2010). Brain reward circuitry beyond the mesolimbic dopamine system: A neurobiological theory. *Neuroscience and Biobehavioral Reviews, 35,* 129–150.

Ikemoto, S., Glazier, B., Murphy, J., & McBride, W. J. (1997). Role of dopamine D_1 and D_2 receptors in the nucleus accumbens in mediating reward. *Journal of Neuroscience, 17,* 8580–8588.

Ikemoto, S., & Pankseppb, F. (1999). The role of nucleus accumbens dopamine in motivated behavior: a unifying interpretation with special reference to reward-seeking. *Brain Research, 31,* 6–41.

Isel, T. (2013). Antipsychotics: Taking the long view. *Director's Blog,* NIMH.

Jamison, R. N., Ross, E. L., Michna, E., Chen, L. Q., Holcomb, C. & Wasan, A. D. (2010). Substance misuse treatment for high-risk chronic pain patients on opioid therapy: A randomized trial. *Pain, 150,* 390–400.

Jones, M. C. (1924). A laboratory study of fear: The case of Peter. *Pedagogical Seminary, 31,* 308–315.

Judd, L., Squire, L., Butters, N., Salmon, D. P., & Paller, K. A, (1987). Effects of psychotropic drugs on cognition and memory in normal humans and animals. In H. Y. Meltzer (Ed.), *Psychopharmacology: A third generation of progress.* New York: Raven.

Kafka, M. (1997). Hypersexual desire in males: An operational definition and implications for males with paraphilias and paraphilia-related disorders. *Archives of Sexual Behaviour, 26,* 505–526.

Kafka, M., & Hennen, J. (1999). The paraphilia-related disorders: An empirical investigation of nonparaphilic hypersexuality disorders in outpatient males. *Journal of Sex Marital Therapy, 25*, 305–319.

Kalix, P. (1994). Khat, an amphetamine-like stimulant. *Journal of Psychoactive Drugs, 26*, 69–74.

Kaufmann, M., Cassem, N., Murray, G., & Jenike, M. (1984). Use of psychostimulants in medically ill patients with neurological disease and major depression. *Canadian Journal of Psychiatry, 29*, 46–49.

Khalil, R. (2013). Non-antidepressant psychopharmacologic treatment of specific phobias. *Current Clinical Pharmacology, 10*, 133–138.

Kennedy, S., & Longnecker, D. (1996). History and principle of anesthesiology. In A. Hardman, & L. S. Limbird (Eds.), *Pharmacological basis of therapeutics*. New York: McGraw-Hill.

Kirsch, I. (2011). *The emperor's new drugs: Exploding the antidepressant myth*. New York: Basic Books.

Krampe, H., Stawicki, S., & Wagner, T. (2006). Follow-up of 180 alcoholic patients for up to 7 years after outpatient treatment: Impact of alcohol deterrents on outcome. *Alcoholism: Clinical and Experimental Research, 30*, 86–95.

Laska, K. M., Gurman, A. S., & Wampold, B. E. (2014). Expanding the lens of evidence-based practice in psychotherapy: A common factors perspective. *Psychotherapy: Theory, Research, Practice, Training, 51*, 467–481.

Levine, E. (1992). Nicotinic systems and cognitive function. *Psychopharmacology, 108*, 417–431.

Liebson, I., Tommasello, A., & Bigelow, G. A behavioral treatment of alcoholic methadone patients. *Annals of Internal Medicine, 89*, 342–344.

Ilieva, I., & Farah, M. (2013). Enhancement stimulants: Perceived motivational and cognitive advantages. *Frontiers in Neuroscience, 7*, 1–6.

Lutz, B. (2007). The endocannabinoid system and extinction learning. *Molecular Neurobiology, 36*, 92–101.

Ma, H., & Zhu, G. (2014). The dopamine system and alcohol dependence. *Shanghai Archives of Psychiatry, 26*, 61–68.

Mansour, A., Fox, C., Burke, S., Meng, F., Thompson, R. C., Akil, H., & Watson, S. J. (1994). Mu, delta and kappa opioid receptor mRNA expression in rats: An in situ hybridization study. *Journal of Comparative Neurology, 350*, 412–438.

Marek, G., & Aghajanian, G. (1999). 5-HT2A receptor or alpha 1-adrenoreceptor activation induces excitatory postsynaptic currents in layer V pyramidal cells of the medial prefrontal cortex. *European Journal of Pharmacology, 367*, 197–206.

Marshall, W. (2007). Diagnostic issues, multiple paraphilias, and comorbid disorders in sexual offenders: Their incidence and treatment. *Aggression and Violent Behaviour, 12*, 16–35.

Mariscano, G., & Lafenetre, P. (2009). Roles of the endocannabinoid system in learning and memory. *Current Topics in Behavioral Neuroscience, 1*, 201–230.

Marsicano, G., Wotjak, C., Azad, S., Bizogno, T., Rammes, G., Grazia Cascio, M., . . . & Lutz, B. (2002). The endogenous cannabinoid system controls extinction of aversive memories. *Nature, 418*, 530.

Mattick, R., Andrews, G., Hadzi-Pavlovic, D., & Christensen, H. (1990). Treatment of panic and agoraphobia: An integrated review. *Journal of Nervous Mental Disorders, 178*, 567–576.

Mavissakalian, K. (1990). Sequential combination of imipramine and self-directed exposure in the treatment of panic disorder with agoraphobia. *Journal of Clinical Psychiatry, 51,* 184–188.

McGorry, P., Alvarez-Jimenez, M., & Killackey, E. (2013). Antipsychotic medication during the critical period following remission from first-episode psychosis: Less is more. *JAMA Psychiatry, 70,* 898–900.

McKim, W. (1980). The effects of caffeine, theophylline, and amphetamine on the operant responding of the mouse. *Psychopharmacology, 68,* 135–138.

McKim, W. (2007). *Drugs and behavioral: An introduction to behavioral pharmacology* (6th ed.). Princeton, NJ: Pearson Hall.

McMillan, D. & Leander, J. (1976). Effects of drugs on schedule-controlled behavior. In Glick & Goldfarb (Eds.), *Behavioral Pharmacology.* St. Louis, MO: Mosby.

Meltzer, H. (1990). Clozapine: Pattern of efficacy in treatment resistant schizophrenia. In H. Y. Meltzer (Ed.), *Novel antipsychotic drugs.* New York: Raven.

Mikhail, A. (1976). Treatment of vaginismus by I.V. diazepam abreaction interviews. *Acta Psychiatrica Scandinavica, 53,* 328–332.

Mintzer, M., & Griffiths, R. (1998). Flurazepam and triazolam: A comparison of behavioral effects and abuse liability. *Drug and Alcohol Dependence, 56,* 49–66.

Mitchell, W., & Stoffelmayr, B (1973). Application of the Premack Principle to the behavioral control of extremely inactive schizophrenics. *Journal of Applied Behavior Analysis, 6,* 419–423.

Mitsikostas, D., Mantonakis, L., & Charlarakis, N. (2010). Nocebo is the enemy, not placebo. A meta-analysis of reported side effects after placebo treatment in headache. *Cephalagia, 31,* 550–561.

Morin, A. (2007). Possible intranasal quetiapine misuse. *American Journal of Health System Pharmacy, 64,* 723–725.

Muse, M. (1984). Narcosynthesis in the treatment of posttraumatic chronic pain. *Rehabilitation Psychology, 29,* 113–118.

Muse, M. (1996). *Introducció a la teràpia conductual-cognitiva: Pautes teòriques.* Girona: Mensana Publications.

Muse, M. (2008). Convergencia de psicoterapia y psicofamacología: El uso de regímenes conductistas en el manejo de medicamentos psicoactivos. *Revista de Psicoterapia, 69,* 5–10.

Muse, M. (2010). Combining therapies in medical psychology: When to medicate and when not. *Archives of Medical Psychology, 1,* 19–27.

Muse, M. (2012). *Tratamiento de disfunciones sexuales.* Madrid: TEA.

Muse, M., & Frigola, G. (2003). La evaluación y tratamiento de las parafilias. *Revista de Medicina Psicosomática, 65,* 55–72.

Muse, M., & McFarland, D. (1994). The convergence of psychology and psychiatry: The use of behaviorally prescribed medications. *Second International Congress of Eclectic Psychotherapy*, Lyon, France.

Muse, M., & Moore, B. (2012). Integrating clinical psychopharmacology within the practice of medical psychology. In M. Muse, & B. Moore (Eds.), *Handbook of clinical psychopharmacology for psychologists.* Hoboken, NJ: Wiley.

Muse, M., Moore, B., & Stahl, S. (2013). Benefits and challenges of integrated treatment. In S. Stahl, & B. Moore (Eds.), *Clinical handbook of anxiety disorders: Psychopharmacology and psychotherapy practice.* Abingdon: Routledge Press.

Niv, Y. (2008). *Cost, benefit, tonic, phasic: What do response rates tell us about dopamine and motivation*? Princeton, NJ: Princeton University.
O'Brien, C. (2005). Benzodiazepines use, abuse, and dependence. *Journal of Clinical Psychiatry, 66*, 28–33.
O'Brien, C., Childress, A., McLellan, A., & Ehrman, R. (1992). Classical conditioning in drug-dependent humans. *Annuals of the New York Academy of Science, 28*, 400–415.
O'Donnella, J., Marekb, G., & Seidenc, L. (2005). Antidepressant effects assessed using behavior maintained under a differential-reinforcement-of-low-rate (DRL) operant schedule. *Neuroscience and Biobehavioral Reviews, 29*, 785–798.
O'Donohue, W., & Plaud, J. (1994). The conditioning of human sexual arousal. *Archives of Sexual Behaviour, 23*, 321–344.
Offermanns, S., & Rosenthal, D. (2008). *Encyclopedia of molecular pharmacy*. New York: Springer.
Olds, J., & Milner, P. (1952). Positive reinforcement produced by electrical stimulation of the septal area and other regions of the rat brain. *Journal of Comparative and Physiological Psychology, 47*, 419–427.
Overton, D. A. (1964). State-dependent or "dissociated" learning produced with pentobarbital. *Journal of Comparative and Physiological Psychology, 57*, 3–12.
Overton, D. A. (1978). Theories of state-dependent learning. In B. T. Ho D. Richardson, & D. Chute (Eds.), *Drug discrimination and state dependent learning*. New York: Academic Press.
Overton, D. A. (1983). State dependent learning and drug discrimination. In L. Iverson, S. Iverson, & S. Snyder, S. et al. (Eds.), *Handbook of psychopharmacology*. New York: Plenum.
Passie, T., Emrich, H., Karst, M., Brandt, S. D., & Halpern, J. H. (2012). Mitigation of post-traumatic stress symptoms by cannabis rein: A review of the clinical and neurobiological evidence. *Drug Testing and Analysis, 4*, 649–659.
Pence, S., Sulkowski, M., & Jordan, C. (2010). When exposures go wrong: Trouble-shooting guidelines for managing difficult scenarios that arise in exposure-based treatment for obsessive-compulsive disorder. *American Journal of Psychotherapy, 64*, 39–53.
Pinta, E. (2007). Quetiapine (Seroquel) addiction? *American Journal of Psychiatry, 164*, 174.
Perkins, K., & Karelitz, J. (2013) Reinforcement enhancing effects of nicotine via smoking. *Psychopharmacology, 228*, 479–486.
Poling, A., & Byrne, T. (1992). Rule-governed behavior and human behavioral pharmacology: A brief commentary on an important topic *Analysis of Verbal Behavior, 10*, 37–41.
Poling, A., Byrne, T., & Morgan, T. (2000). Stimulus properties of drugs. In A. Poling, & T. Byrne (Eds.), *Behavioral pharmacology*. Oakland, CA: New Harbinger.
Poole, N., Wuez, A., & Agrawal, N. (2010). Abreaction for conversion disorder: Systematic review with meta-analysis. *British Journal of Psychology, 197*, 91–95.
Premack, D. (1959). Toward empirical behavioral laws: Instrumental positive reinforcement. *Psychological Review, 66*, 219–233.
Pull, C. (2007). Combined pharmacotherapy and cognitive-behavioural therapy for anxiety disorders. *Current Opinion in Psychiatry, 20*, 30–35.
Rabinaka, C., Angstadta, M., Sripadaa, C., Abelson, J. L. Liberzon, I., Milad, M. R., & Luan Phan, K. (2013). Cannabinoid facilitation of fear extinction memory recall in humans. *Neuropharmacology, 64*, 396–402.

Rankin, H., Hodgson, R., & Stockwell, T. (1983), Cue exposure and response prevention with alcoholics: A controlled trial. *Behaviour Research and Therapy, 17,* 389–396.
Redgrave, P., & Gurney, K. (2006). Opinion: The short-latency dopamine signal: A role in discovering novel actions? *Nature Reviews Neuroscience, 7,* 967–975.
Reeves, R., & Brister, J. (2007). Additional evidence of the abuse potential of quetiapine. *Southern Medical Journal, 100,* 834–836.
Reichenpfader, U., Gartlehner, G., Morgan, L., Greenblatt, A., Nussbaumer, B., Hansen, R. A., . . . & Gaynes, B. N. (2014). Sexual dysfunction associated with second-generation antidepressants in patients with major depressive disorder: Results from a systematic review with network meta-analysis. *Drug Safety, 37,* 19–31.
Ries, R., Miller, S., & Fiellin, D. (2009). *Principles of addiction medicine.* Philadelphia, PA: Lippincott, Williams & Wilkins.
Robertson, A. (1989). Multiple reward systems and the prefrontal cortex. *Neuroscience and Biobehavioral Reviews, 13,* 163–170.
Robinson, J., & Lewinsohn, P. (1973). Experimental analysis of a technique based on the Premack Principle changing verbal behavior of depressed individuals. *Psychological Reports, 32,* 199–210.
Robinson, T. & Berridge, K. (2008). The incentive sensitization theory of addiction: Some current issues. *Philosophical Transactions of the Royal Society B, 363,* 3137–3146.
Rosenbaum, J. (2005). Benzodiazepines: Revisiting clinical issues in treating anxiety disorders. *Primary Care Companion to the Journal of Clinical Psychiatry, 7,* 23–24.
Rosenberg, P., Ahmed, I., & Hurwitz, S. (1991). Methylphenidate in depressed medically ill patients. *Journal of Clinical Psychiatry, 52,* 263–267.
Rubia, K., Halari, R., Cubillo, Mohammad, A. M., Brammer, M., & Taylor, E. (2009). Methylphenidate normalizes activation and functional connectivity deficits in attention and motivation networks in medication-naïve children with ADHD during a rewarded continuous performance task. *Neuropharmacology, 57,* 640–652.
Rudd, M. (2003). Severity of combat exposure, psychological symptoms, social support and suicide risk in OEF/OIF veterans. *Archives of Medical Psychology, 4,* 1–11.
Rygula, R., Abumaria, N., Flugge, G., Hiemke, C., Fuchs, E., Rüther, E., Havemann-Reinecke, U. (2006). Citalopram counteracts depressive-like symptoms evoked by chronic social stress in rats. *Behavioral Pharmacology, 17,* 19–29.
Salamone, J. (1987). The actions of neuroleptic drugs on appetitive instrumental behaviors. In L. L. Iversen, & S. Snyder (Eds.), *Handbook of psychopharmacology: New directions in behavioral pharmacology.* New York: Springer.
Salamone, J. (2006).Will the last person who uses the term "reward" please turn out the lights? Comments on processes related to reinforcement, learning, motivation and effort. *Addiction Biology, 11,* 43–44.
Salamone, J. (2010). Motor function and motivation. In G. F. Koob, M. Le Moel, & R. F. Thompson, et al. (Eds.), *Encyclopedia of behavioral neuroscience,* Volume 3. Oxford: Academic Press.
Salamone, J., & Correa, M. (2002). Motivational views of reinforcement: Implications for understanding the behavioral functions of nucleus accumbens dopamine. *Behavioural Brain Research, 137,* 3–25.
Salamone, J., & Correa, M. (2012). The mysterious motivational functions of mesolimbic dopamine. *Neuron, 76,* 470–485.

Salamone, J., Correa, M., Farrar, A., & Mingote, S. M. (2007). Effort-related functions of nucleus accumbens dopamine and associated forebrain circuits. *Psychopharmacology, 191*, 461–482.
Salamone, J., Correa, M., Nunes, E., Randall, P. A., & Pardo, M. (2012). The behavioral pharmacology of effort-related choice behavior: Dopamine, adenosine and beyond. *Journal of the Experimental Analysis of Behavior, 97*, 125–146.
Salamone, J., Cousins, M., & Snyder, B. (1997). Behavioral functions of nucleus accumbens dopamine: Empirical and conceptual problems with the anhedonia hypothesis. *Neuroscience and Biobehavioral Reviews, 21*, 341–359.
Sanger, D., & Blackman, D. (1976). Rate-dependent effects of drugs: A review of the literature. *Pharmacology Biochemistry and Behavior, 4*, 73–83.
Šagud, M., Mihaljević-Peles, A., Mück-Seler, D., Pivac, N., Vuksan-Ćusa, B., Brataljenović, T., & Jakovljević, S. (2009). Smoking and schizophrenia. *Psychiatria Danubina, 21*, 371–375.
Schachtner, S., & Singer, J. (1962). Cognitive, social, and physiological determinants of emotional state. *Psychological Review, 69*, 379–399.
Schultz, W. (2000). Multiple reward signals in the brain. *Nature Reviews Neuroscience, 1*, 199–207.
Schuster, C., Dockens, W., & Woods, J. (1966). Behavioral variables affecting the development of amphetamine tolerance. *Psychopharmacologia, 9*, 170–182.
Siegel, S. (1989). Pharmacological conditioning and drug effects. In A. Goudie and M. Emmett-Oglesby (Eds.), *Psychoactive drugs: Tolerance and sensitization*. New York: Springer.
Siegel, S. (2002). Explanatory mechanisms for placebo effect: Pavlovian conditioning. In H. A. Guess, A. Kleinman, J. W. Kusek, & L. W. Engel (Eds.), *The science of the placebo: Towards an interdisciplinary research agenda*. London: BMJ Books.
Siegel, S., & Ellsworth, D. (1986). Pavlovian conditioning and death from apparent overdose of medically prescribed morphine: A case study. *Bulletin of the Psychonomic Society, 24*, 278–280.
Siegel S., Hinson, R., & Krank, M. (1982). Heroin "overdose" death: Contribution of drug-associated environmental cue. *Science, 216*, 436–443.
Siegel, S., Marco, A., & Baptista, J. (2000). Pavlovian psychopharmacology: The associative basis of tolerance. *Experimental and Clinical Psychopharmacology, 8*, 276–293.
Seiden, L., Dahms J., & Shaughness, R. (1985). Behavioral screen for antidepressants: The effects of drugs and electroconvulsive shock on performance under a differential-reinforcement-of-low-rate schedule. *Psychopharmacology, 86*, 55–60.
Sigal, J. (1967). Operant conditioning and some aspects of the psychotherapeutic process. *Journal of the Canadian Psychiatry Association, 12*, 3–8.
Silverman, K., Higgins, S., Brooner, R., Montoya, I., Cone, E., Schuster, C., & Preston, K. (1996a). Sustained cocaine abstinence in methadone maintenance patients through voucher-based reinforcement therapy. *Archives of General Psychiatry, 53*, 409–415.
Silverman, K., Wong, C., Higgins, S., Brooner, R., Montoya, I., Contoreggi, C., . . . & Preston, K. (1996b). Increasing opiate abstinence through voucher-based reinforcement therapy. *Drug and Alcohol Dependence, 41*, 157–165.
Simoni-Wastila, L. (2000). The use of abusable prescription drugs: The role of gender. *Journal of Women's Health and Gender-Based Medicine, 9*, 289–297.

Simoni-Wastila, L., & Stickler, G. (2004). Risk factors associated with problem use of prescription drugs. *American Journal of Public Health, 94*, 266–268.

Singewald, N., Schmuckermair, C., Whittle, N., Holmes, A., & Ressler, K.J. (2015). Pharmacology of cognitive enhancers for exposure-based therapy of fear, anxiety and trauma-related disorders. *Pharmacology and Therapeutics 149* 150–190.

Skinner, B. F. (1986). Correspondence with Mark Muse. *November 5*, 1986.

Smillie, L. (2008). What is reinforcement sensitivity? Neuroscience paradigms for approach-avoidance process theories of personality. *European Journal of Personality, 22*, 359–384.

Soyka, M., & Rösner, S. (2008). Opioid antagonists for pharmacological treatment of alcohol dependence: A critical review. *Current Drug Abuse Review, 1*, 280–291.

Spiegle, R., & Aebi, H. (1981). *Psychopharmacology: An introduction*. Chichester: Wiley.

Stahl, S. (2013). *Stahl's essential psychopharmacology* (4th ed.). Cambridge: Cambridge University Press.

Stitzer, M., Bigelow, G., & Liebson, I. (1980). Reducing drug use among methadone maintenance clients: Contingent reinforcement for morphine-free urines. *Addictive Behavior, 5*, 333–340.

Stoops, W., Lile, J., Glaer, P., Hays, L. R., & Rush, C. R. (2011). Alternative reinforcer response cost impacts cocaine choice in humans. *Progress in Neuropsychopharmacology and Biological Psychiatry, 10*, 189–193.

Stoops, W., Lile, J., Robbins, C., Martin, C. A. Rush, C. & Kelly, T. H. (2007). The reinforcing, subject-related, performance, and cardiovascular effects of D-amphetamine: Influence of sensation-seeking status. *Addictive Behavior, 32*, 1177–1188.

Sudak, D. (2011). *Combining CBT and medication: An evidence-based approach*. Hoboken, NJ: John Wiley & Sons.

Talmi, D., Seymour, B., Dayan, P., & Dolan, R. J. (2008). Human Pavlovian–instrumental transfer. *The Journal of Neuroscience, 9*, 28, 360–368

Tanda, G, Pontieri, F., & Chiara, G. (1997). Cannabinoid and heroin activation of mesolimbic dopamine transmission by common 1 opioid receptor mechanism *Science, 276*, 2048–2050.

Tasman, A., & Riba, M. (2000). Psychological management in psychopharmacologic treatment. In J. Lieberman & A. Tasman (Eds.), *Handbook of psychiatric drugs*. Philadelphia, PA: WB Saunders.

Tasman, A., Riba, M., & Silk, K. (2000). *The doctor–patient relationship in pharmacotherapy*. New York: Guilford

Thomas, T., & Pickens, R. (1971). *Stimulus properties of drugs*. New York: Appleton-Century-Croft.

Thompson, T., & Pickens, R (1971). *Stimulus properties of drugs*. New York: Appleton-Century-Crofts.

Tolman, E. (1948). Cognitive maps in rats and men. *Psychological Review, 55*, 189–208.

Tolman, E. (1949). There is more than one kind of learning. *Psychological Review, 56*, 144–155.

Tomlins, D., & Sellers, E. (2001). Addiction and the brain: The role of neurotransmitters in the cause and treatment of drug dependence. *Canadian Medical Association Journal, 164*, 817–821.

Thompson, J., Ritenbaugh, C., & Nichter, M. (2009). Reconsidering the placebo response from a broad anthropological perspective. *Cultural Medicine and Psychiatry, 33*, 112–152.

Torrey, E. (2014). Better off without antipsychotic drugs? *Psychiatric Times*, June 18.

Toth, M., Ziegler, M., Sun, P., Gresack, J., & Risbrough, V. (2013). Impaired conditioned fear response and startle reactivity in epinephrine-deficient mice. *Behavioral Pharmacology, 24*, 1–9.

Uhlenhuth, E. H., Balter, M. B., Ban, T. A., & Yang, K. (1999). International study of expert judgment on therapeutic use of benzodiazepines and other psychotherapeutic medications: VI. Trends in recommendations for the pharmacotherapy of anxiety disorders, 1992–1997. *Depression and Anxiety, 9*, 107–116.

Veselinovic, T., Schorn, H., Vernaleken, I., Hiemke, C., Zernig, G., Gur, R., & Gründer, G. (2013). Effects of antipsychotic treatment on cognition in healthy subjects. *Journal of Psychopharmacology, 27*, 374–385.

Viswanathan, M., Golin, C., Jones, C., Ashok, M., Blalock, S. J., Wines, R. C., . . . & Lohr, K. N. (2012). Interventions to improve adherence to self-administered medications for chronic disease in the United States. *Annals of Internal Medicine, September 11*, 1–11.

Volkow, N., Wang, J., Kollins, S., Wigal, T. L., Newcorn, J. H., Telang, F., . . . & Swanson, J. M. (2009). Evaluating dopamine reward pathway in ADHD: Clinical implications. *JAMA, 302*, 1084–1091.

Von Frijtag, J., Van den Bos, R., & Spruijt, B. (2002). Imipramine restores the long-term impairment of appetitive behavior in socially stressed rats. *Psychopharmacology, 162*, 232–238.

Waschulewski-Floruss, H., Miltner, W., Brody, S., & Braun, C. (1994). Classical conditioning of pain response. *International Journal of Neuroscience, 78*, 21–32.

Watson, J. B., & Rayner, R. (1920). Conditioned emotional reactions. *Journal of Experimental Psychology, 3*, 1–14.

Weinberger, N., Gold, P., & Sternberg, D. (1984). Epinephrine enables Pavlovian fear conditioning under anesthesia, *Science, 10*, 605–607.

Weingartner, H., Miller, H., & Murphy, D. (1977). Mood-state-dependent retrieval of verbal associations. *Journal of Abnormal Psychology, 86*, 276–284.

Weingartner, H. (1978). Human state-dependent learning, in B. T. Ho, D. Richardson, & D. Chute (Eds.), *Drug discrimination and state-dependent learning.* New York: Academic Press.

Wichers, M., Barge-Schaapveld, D., Nicolson, N., Peeters, F., de Vries, M., Mengelers, R., & van Os, J. (2009). Reduced stress-sensitivity or increased reward experience: The psychological mechanism of response to antidepressant medication. *Neuropsychopharmacology, 34*, 923–931.

Wiederman, M. W. (2003). Paraphilia and fetishism. *The Family Journal: Counseling and Therapy for Couples and Families, 11*, 315–321.

Williams, M. (1984). *The psychological treatment of depression: A guide to the theory and practice of cognitive behavioral therapy.* New York: Routledge.

Wise, R. (1998). Drug-activation of brain reward pathways. *Drug and Alcohol Dependence, 51*, 13–22.

Wolgin, D. (1989). The role of instrumental learning in behavioral tolerance to drugs. In A. Goudie, & M. W. Emmett-Oglesby (Eds.), *Psychoactive drugs: Tolerance and sensitization*. New York: Springer.

Wolpe, J. (1973). *The practice of behavioral therapy* (2nd ed.). Oxford: Pergamon.

Woods, S., Tesar, G., Murray, G., & Cassem, N. H. (1986). Psychostimulant treatment of depressive disorders secondary to medical illness. *Journal of Clinical Psychiatry, 47*, 12–15.

Wright, J., & Thase, M. (2010). Combining high-yield CBT methods and pharmacotherapy in brief sessions. *Psychiatric Times*, November 2.
Wunderink, L., Nieboer, R., Wiersma, D., Sytema, S., & Nienhuis, F. J. (2013). Recovery in remitted first-episode psychosis at 7 years of follow-up of an early dose reduction/discontinuation or maintenance treatment strategy: Long-term follow-up of a 2-year randomized clinical trial. *JAMA Psychiatry, 70*, 913–920.
Yoshimoto, K., Ueda, S., Kato, B., Takeuchi, Y., Kawai, Y., Noritake, K., & Yasuhara, M. (2000). Alcohol enhances characteristic release of dopamine and serotonin in the central nucleus of the amygdala. *Neurochemistry International, 37*, 369–376.
Zucker, R., Donovan, J., Masten, A., Matson, M. E., & Moss, H. B. (2008). Early developmental processes and the continuity of risk for underage drinking and problem drinking. *Pediatrics, 121*, S252–S272).

Index

Cognitive Behavioral Psychopharmacology: The Clinical Practice of Evidence-Based Biopsychosocial Integration, First Edition. Edited by Mark Dana Muse.

d

www.ingramcontent.com/pod-product-compliance
Ingram Content Group UK Ltd.
Pitfield, Milton Keynes, MK11 3LW, UK
UKHW050943290926
15470UKWH00005B/1609